HEALTH INFORMATION TECHNOLOGY

Nadinia Davis
Melissa LaCour

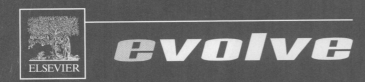

To access your Student Resources, visit:

http://evolve.elsevier.com/Davis/HIT/

Evolve® Student Resources for *Davis and LaCour: Health Information Technology*, **2nd Edition** offer the following features:

Student Resources

- **WebLinks**
  A resource that links the Evolve site to carefully chosen online resources to supplement and reinforce the content of the textbook.

- **Content Updates**
  The latest content updates from the author of the textbook to keep you current with recent developments in the area of health information management.

- **Sample Forms**
  Sample blank forms common in the field of health information management.

- **Links to Related Resources**
  See what other health information management related resources Elsevier has to offer.

HEALTH INFORMATION TECHNOLOGY

Second Edition

Nadinia Davis, MBA, CIA, CPA, RHIA, FAHIMA
Assistant Professor
Health Information Management
Kean University
Union, New Jersey

Melissa LaCour, RHIA
Program Director
Health Information Technology
Delgado Community College
New Orleans, Louisiana

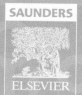
SAUNDERS
ELSEVIER

SAUNDERS
ELSEVIER

11830 Westline Industrial Drive
St. Louis, Missouri 63146

HEALTH INFORMATION TECHNOLOGY, Second Edition

ISBN-13: 978-1-4160-2316-6
ISBN-10: 1-4160-2316-X

Notice

Neither the Publisher nor the Authors assume any responsibility for any loss or injury and/or damage to persons or property arising out of or related to any use of the material contained in this book. It is the responsibility of the treating practitioner, relying on independent expertise and knowledge of the patient, to determine the best treatment and method of application for the patient.

The Publisher

ISBN-13: 978-1-4160-2316-6
ISBN-10: 1-4160-2316-X

Executive Editor: Susan Cole
Developmental Editors: Josh Rapplean, Colin Odell
Publishing Services Manager: Julie Eddy
Project Manager: Gail Michaels
Senior Designer: Jyotika Shroff

Working together to grow
libraries in developing countries

www.elsevier.com | www.bookaid.org | www.sabre.org

ELSEVIER   BOOK AID International   Sabre Foundation

Printed in the United States of America

Last digit is the print number: 9   8   7   6   5   4   3

This book is dedicated to all of those individuals who have inspired us to enter the Health Information Management profession, to participate in the educational process, and to volunteer with the associations and to all of our friends and colleagues who supported our efforts post-Katrina.

FOREWORD

he purpose of this text is to introduce the reader to health information technology both as a work-based, task-oriented function and as a part of a larger profession of health information management.

Ever since physicians and other caregivers have been documenting their care of patients, they have had individuals working with them to help, at a minimum, store and retrieve that documentation. In the late nineteenth century and early twentieth century, the individuals who performed that function, most notably in hospitals, were the medical record librarians. (We like to imagine these people in the basement with cobwebs and dust mites, scurrying around trying to file and retrieve charts.)

The health information management profession has grown over the last 75+ years as a result of health information management professionals, both individually and collectively, assuming increasing responsibilities as health care delivery has become a more complex industry. The field of health information management embraces a variety of individual functions and professional capacities, and a number of national and international professional organizations reflect the diversity of the profession in general. Notably, the American Health Information Management Association (AHIMA), based in Chicago, provides the national leadership for the broad-based management and technical aspects of health information management. AHIMA is an association of over 50,000 professionals, students, and associate members, all of whom have the common goal of ensuring "quality health care through quality data."

The field of health information management today is so broad that its elements and the knowledge that individuals must acquire in order to successfully practice cannot be contained in one volume. This book is designed to meet the needs of students at the beginning of their course of study in health information. It can easily fit into a one-quarter or one-semester course as an introduction to health information technology or introduction to medical records science, both in degree programs and in certificate courses such as coding and tumor registry. It can also be used by individuals who wish to acquire some basic knowledge of health information technology and how it fits into the health care arena.

On the basis of feedback from instructors and students who have used the first edition, we have made the following changes in the second edition:

- The workbook exercises have been incorporated into the text.
- We have broken out the statistics discussion from Chapter 1 and moved it to its own chapter. This is necessarily brief, as the topic of health statistics is the subject of entire books; however, it will give the new student a foundation for learning.
- Special health records have been given their own chapter—again, just an overview, but we have added accreditation and major health information management issues.
- Because health information management is moving to an increasingly electronic environment, we have added a chapter on computer-based health systems to help students understand the changes as they occur.
- The legal chapter incorporates Health Insurance Portability and Accountability Act privacy regulations.

One thing in particular that has not changed is the tone of the narrative. Our students have told us repeatedly that this is a very easy book to read and understand. As that was our original goal, we are pleased to maintain that aspect of the text.

For whatever reason you are reading this book, remember that it is the beginning of the journey. The understanding of health information technology is not achieved by the end of Chapter 14. Additional skills must be obtained. One must acquire additional knowledge from other sources in order to be a successful practicing professional in this field. Also, the industry and the profession are changing constantly. We have no doubt that elements in this book will be outdated the moment it goes to press. However, that is the challenge of life-long learning.

We believe that health information technology is an exciting and rewarding career choice for students, and we have tried our best to infuse the narrative with that enthusiasm. We hope you enjoy using this text and would welcome any comments that you may have to improve it for our next edition.

ACKNOWLEDGMENTS

I would particularly like to thank Marion Gentul, RHIA, CCS, for her constant support and guidance. You were right—this is a very exciting profession!

Thanks to my colleague at Kean University, Barbara Manger, MPA, RHIA, CCS, FAHIMA, for her support and encouragement.

To Susan Cole, our Elsevier Acquisitions Editor, and all of the editorial and production staff who worked with us, thank you for your faith in us, and apologies for the missed deadlines!

To the reviewers, thank you for your encouragement and thoughtful comments.

Thanks to our contributors for helping to make this a more useful text.

A special thanks to my Development & Retention class for allowing me to adapt your homework assignments for use in the second edition.

Thank you to JFK Medical Center / Solaris Health System for the tour of your electronic health record systems.

Thanks to Kathleen Frawley, JD, MBA, RHIA, Chairperson, HIT Program, DeVry University, North Brunswick, New Jersey, for your excellent technical advice (at a moment's notice) and continued support.

Many thanks to my coauthor, Missy LaCour. You are an inspiration!

Finally, thank you to all of our students, past and present. We didn't write this book for ourselves, we wrote it for you. Thank you for actually reading it!

Nadinia Davis

I hope that a deep heartfelt thank you expresses my true sentiment to Nadinia Davis for a second edition and especially for all of your help and support post-Katrina. I could not have finished this otherwise.

With much thanks to Ricky, Brett and Beth, here's another book to add to our library. A special thanks to my sister, Christy Billiot, for support, reviews, and manuscript prep; you came through in a pinch. To my parents, your love and encouragement is motivating.

Special thanks to Josh Rapplean, the most detail-oriented man I have ever worked with. To Susan Cole, thanks for believing in us, and continuing to support our project. And thanks also to the Elsevier team for all of the behind the scenes work that made this 2nd edition a reality.

Finally, I have to thank the students I have known and those yet to come; it is a privilege to be your instructor/advisor and be motivated by your goals, expectations, and dreams.

Missy LaCour

NADINIA DAVIS, MBA, CIA, CPA, RHIA, FAHIMA

Nadinia Davis is an Assistant Professor of Health Information Management at Kean University in Union, New Jersey. She holds a bachelor's degree in political science from Villanova University in Pennsylvania and an MBA with a concentration in accounting from Fairleigh Dickinson University in New Jersey. Nadinia worked for twelve years in the financial services industry before returning to school to obtain her postbaccalaureate certificate in health information management from Kean University. Nadinia has worked in a variety of capacities in acute care facilities and has been a coding consultant and a director of medical records in a rehabilitation facility. She began teaching full-time in 1996 and has been with Kean since 1999.

Nadinia is a past president of the New Jersey Health Information Management Association and received the NJHIMA Distinguished Member Award in 1999. She served for 3 years on the Board of Directors of the American Health Information Management Association. In 2004 she was granted Fellowship in the AHIMA. Nadinia has recently been inducted into the Honor Society of Phi Kappa Phi, Kean University Chapter.

MELISSA LaCOUR, RHIA

Melissa LaCour, most often known as Missy, is Assistant Professor and Program Director of the Health Information Technology Department at Delgado Community College in New Orleans. Melissa joined Delgado in August of 1996 after holding a variety of positions in health information management, including manager of health information management at a rehabilitation center, release of information/clerical supervisor, assistant director, and director of health information in acute care. Melissa earned a BS in Medical Record Administration from Louisiana Tech University in 1990 and is currently enrolled in the Masters program in Health Information Management.

She also volunteers her time with the Greater New Orleans Health Information Management Association, of which she is past president, and the Louisiana Health Information Management Association and was awarded the LHIMA Career Achievement Award in 2004.

*In 2002, Nadinia and Melissa won the AHIMA Legacy award for the first edition of this book.

ABOUT THE CONTRIBUTORS

MARION GENTUL, RHIA, CCS

Marion is a self-employed consultant, using her 30 years of health information management experience to provide coding and auditing services to clients in New Jersey and surrounding states. Marion holds a bachelor's degree in psychology from the University of Rhode Island and completed her health information management education at SUNY Downstate Medical Center. She is currently an adjunct coding instructor in the HIM Program at Kean University and a member of their advisory board. Marion is a past president of the New Jersey Health Information Management Association and has served in several chair positions on the Society for Clinical Coding Board. She is coauthor of two chapters in AHIMA's publication *Effective Management of Coding Services*. Marion received AHIMA's Triumph Mentor Award, was named a Distinguished Alumna by SUNY Downstate Medical Center, and is also a recipient of the NJHIMA Distinguished Member Award.

JACKIE JONES, MS, RHIA

Jackie is an instructor in the Health Information Technology Program at Delgado Community College. She has a bachelor's degree in Medical Record Administration from University of Louisiana at Lafayette. She also earned her MS degree from the University of St. Francis. Jackie has 27 years of experience as a Director of Health Information Management, Quality Management, Risk Management, Utilization Review, and Joint Commission on Accreditation of Healthcare Organizations planning at an acute care facility. She worked with an electronic medical record as an Health Information Management Supervisor in the New Orleans area. She has been teaching health information technology for 2 years. She is a past president of the Greater New Orleans Medical Record Association and has volunteered on several committees as a member of the Louisiana Health Information Management Association.

MARIELA TWIGGS, MS, RHIA, CHP, CDIA, FAHIMA

Mariela holds a bachelor's degree in Medical Record Administration and a master's degree in Health Care Administration. She has worked as a Director of Medical Records in various hospitals and managed a release of health information outsourcing business for many years. She now owns her own companies, MTT Enterprises, LLC and VELFILE, LLC, providing document management solutions, temporary services, consulting services, and release of information services. In addition to her health information credentials, she is a Certified Document Imaging Architect (CDIA+), with expertise in electronic record management. She has been very active in professional associations, serving as president and treasurer of the Louisiana and the Greater New Orleans Health Information Management associations. She is a fellow of the American Health Information Management Association and is certified in health care privacy (CHP). In addition, she is an active member of the Health Information and Management Systems Society, the Association for Image & Information Management, and the American Records Management Association. She serves on the advisory boards of the University of Louisiana and Delgado Community College Health Information programs. Mariela also received the Louisiana Health Information Management Association's Distinguished Member Award in 1995.

EDITORIAL REVIEW BOARD

CONTENTS

UNIT I

ENVIRONMENT OF HEALTH INFORMATION

Chapter 1

Health Care Delivery Systems

CHAPTER OUTLINE

Health Care Professionals

Physicians

Nurses
Licensed Practical Nurse
Registered Nurse
Advanced Practice Nursing Specialties

Allied Health Professionals
Occupational Therapist
Physical Therapist
Registered Dietitian
Phlebotomist
Health Unit Coordinator
Social Workers

Health Information Management

Credentials

Patient Care Plan

Comparison of Facilities

Types of Facilities
Acute Care Facilities
Ambulatory Care
Long-Term Care Facilities
Behavioral Health Facilities
Rehabilitation Facilities
Hospice
Home Health Care

Facility Size
Number of Beds
Discharges

Ownership

Financial Status

Patient Population

Services

Continuum of Care
Childhood
Adult Care
Special Health Issues
Elder Care
Impact of Mergers and Acquisitions

Legal and Regulatory Environment

Federal

State
Licensure
Reporting

Local

Accreditation
Joint Commission on Accreditation of Healthcare
    Organizations
Commission on Accreditation of Rehabilitation
    Facilities
Commission on Accreditation for Health
    Informatics and Information Management
    Education

Professional Standards

Chapter Activities

Chapter Summary

Review Questions

Professional Profile

Application

2

By the end of this chapter, the student should be able to

- Identify and describe the major medical specialties.
- Distinguish among nursing occupations.
- Identify and describe the major allied health professions and their principal occupational settings.
- Distinguish between inpatients and outpatients.
- Describe the differences among health care facilities.
- Describe government involvement in health care.
- Define accreditation.
- Define licensure.
- List two major accrediting organizations and the facilities they accredit.

VOCABULARY

accreditation

activities of daily living

acute care facility

admission

allied health professionals

assisted living

bed count

behavioral health facility

children's hospital

Conditions of Participation

continuum of care

deemed status

diagnosis

discharge

ethics

health information management (HIM)

health information technology (HIT)

home health care

hospice

hospital

inpatients

integrated delivery systems

licensed beds

licensure

long-term care facility

medical specialty

mental health facility

nurse

outpatient

palliative care

patient care plan

physician

primary care physician

procedure

psychiatrist

referral

rehabilitation facility

resident

he purpose of this chapter is to acquaint you with the basic structure and terminology of the health care industry. Most of us have experienced the need for health care at one time, whether it was at the time of our birth or for treatment for a particular illness. In fact, you may know a lot about certain types of health care because of your own illness or the illness of a family member or friend. Try to recall your experiences. Link what you are learning as you read this chapter to your previous experiences and understanding of the health care industry.

HEALTH CARE PROFESSIONALS

Increasing demand for health care workers and the special emphasis on particular groups of patients has led to a proliferation of professional associations and credentials. One of the primary roles of a professional association is to improve the practice of the profession. Therefore professional associations play a critical role in the development of professional standards and improvement in health care delivery. One of the most obvious ways that professional practice can be improved is through the mandatory education of practitioners. The outcome of this formal education process is the qualification to sit for an examination. That examination is designed to measure the competence of the individual. The specific level of competence varies from entry-level (basic) competence to advanced or specialty practice.

The health care industry comprises professionals in many disciplines. These professionals vary from physicians and nurses to therapists and technicians to administrative and financial personnel. Each of these professionals plays a vital role in the delivery of health care. Physicians generally direct the delivery of care. They make decisions about the patient's condition and advise treatment. Nurses and therapists often work on teams with physicians, helping to make those decisions and carrying out the recommended treatments. Technical and administrative personnel support the teams by administering and evaluating tests, organizing data, and evaluating processes and procedures. Here are examples of some of the specific professions you will encounter in the health care industry.

PHYSICIANS

A **physician** is a person who is licensed to practice medicine. The practice of medicine is regulated by each individual state, which administers the examination and issues the license. To become licensed, a physician attends college and medical school, then serves a residency in his or her specialty. A **resident** performs professional duties under the supervision of a fully qualified physician. Residency can last from 4 to 8 years, depending on the specialty. The medical licensing examination can be taken after the first year of residency. The United States Medical Licensing Examination results are provided to the individual state medical boards for licensing purposes.

A physician earns a degree as a Doctor of Medicine (MD) or a Doctor of Osteopathy (DO). The schools that train MDs and DOs focus on different philosophies of medical treatment and diagnosis. Historically, DOs relied on physical manipulation of the patient, particularly the spine, to alleviate symptoms of disease. MDs, on the other hand, used drugs and surgery, also called *conventional* medicine, to treat patients. You may see the term *allopathic* in reference to the conventional approach. In the United States, DOs take a whole-body approach and are likely to use both manipulation (osteopathic manipulative treatment) and conventional methods. However, in other countries, the historical differences remain. All states in the United States license both MDs and DOs. As a general rule, both are eligible to practice medicine in hospitals; however, that is a decision of individual hospitals (*About Osteopathic Medicine* 2005).

Physicians are generally classified by **medical specialty**. They can specialize in a particular disease or condition, a body or organ system, or a task. For example, an oncologist is a physician who diagnoses and treats cancers. An obstetrician specializes in fertility and pregnancy. A gastroenterologist specializes in diseases of the digestive system. A urologist specializes in diseases of the urinary system. Several of the tasks that physicians perform are considered specialties even though many physicians may perform them to a certain extent. For example, a radiologist interprets x-rays and other types of examinations that generate film records of internal organs. A gastroenterologist may know how to read an x-ray, but it is not his or her specialty. Some specialties may focus more narrowly on the patient's age group. A pediatric oncologist deals with children's cancers. Table 1-1 lists some common medical specialties.

Medicine typically requires a minimum 10 years of study after high school. For example, a physician who intends to specialize in family practice attends college for 4 years and medical school for another 3 years. He or she then applies for a residency of 3 years in family practice,

TABLE 1-1	Common Medical Specialties
PHYSICIAN SPECIALTY	**DESCRIPTION**
Allergist	Diagnoses and treats patients who have strong reactions to pollen, insect bites, food, medication, and other irritants
Anesthesiologist	Administers substances that cause loss of sensation, particularly during surgery
Cardiologist	Diagnoses and treats patients with diseases of the heart and blood vessels
Dermatologist	Diagnoses and treats patients with diseases of the skin
Family practitioner	Delivers primary health care for patients of all ages
Gastroenterologist	Diagnoses and treats patients with diseases of the digestive system
Gynecologist	Diagnoses and treats disorders of, and provides well care related to, the female reproductive system
Neonatologist	Diagnoses and treats diseases and abnormal conditions of newborns
Obstetrician	Cares for women before, during, and after delivery
Oncologist	Diagnoses and treats patients with cancer
Ophthalmologist	Diagnoses and treats patients with diseases of the eye
Orthopedist	Diagnoses and treats patients with diseases of the muscles and bones
Pathologist	Studies changes in cells, tissue, and organs in order to diagnose diseases and/or to determine possible treatments
Pediatrician	Delivers primary health care to children
Psychiatrist	Diagnoses and treats patients with disorders of the mind
Radiologist	Uses x-rays and other tools to diagnose and treat a variety of diseases

Hit-Bit

Medical Terminology

If you have not yet studied medical terminology, here is a brief lesson. Medical terms consist of combining forms, prefixes, and suffixes. These parts are assembled to form words, which can easily be deciphered when you know the definitions of the parts. For example, we just used the word *oncologist*. This word is assembled from the following parts:

onc/o = cancer
-logy = process of study
-ist = one who specializes

Therefore an oncologist is one who specializes in the study of cancer. The following are the word parts of some of the other specialties we mentioned:

gastr/o = stomach
enter/o = intestine
ped/i = children
iatr/o = treatment
-ic = pertaining to
oste/o = bone
pathy = process of disease

Can you decipher the words in Table 1-1 now that you know their parts?

Hit-Bit

Alphabet Soup

The decoding of professional credentials is simplified by familiarity with a few guidelines:

R   generally stands for *Registered*. Individuals who are registered have complied with the standards of the registering organization. Standards may include passing an examination, completing academic requirements, and demonstrating experience in the field.

C   means the individual is *Certified*. This term is synonymous with *Registered*.

F   is a *Fellow*. A Fellow has generally demonstrated long-term, significant contribution to his or her discipline or a specific high level of competence. Fellowship is granted in a professional organization. For physicians, board certification is expressed as a fellowship.

L   refers to a *License*. Separate from other designations, licensure denotes compliance with state regulations. Individuals may be licensed. Facilities may also be licensed. In some disciplines, licensure is a prerequisite to practice.

These guidelines refer to the acronyms of the credential. Some credentials imply dual meanings. For example, registered nurses (RNs) are so designated when they are licensed to practice.

studying internal medicine, pediatrics, obstetrics and gynecology, psychiatry, and geriatrics. An additional year of residency is required if the physician wants to further specialize in geriatrics, adolescent, or sports medicine ("Family Practice" 2005; *Diplomate Statistics* 2005).

Beyond licensing and completing the residency, physicians may pursue additional training and take an examination to become board certified. Board certification is developed and administered by the specialty board that sets standards of education for the physician's specialty. The American Board of Medical Specialties is an umbrella group representing the 24 medical specialty boards (http://www.abms.org/member.asp). Among the 24 medical specialties, there are additional subspecialties. As noted previously, geriatrics is a subspecialty of family medicine. A board-certified family practitioner is also referred to as a *Diplomate of the American Board of Family Medicine*. See Figure 1-1 for a list of medical specialty boards.

Most individuals have a relationship with a family practitioner. This physician is trained to identify and treat a wide variety of conditions. However, the family practitioner will also seek guidance from other specialists as needed. For example, the family practitioner may identify a suspicious skin problem and send the patient to a dermatologist for evaluation and treatment. The process of sending a patient to another physician in this manner is called a **referral.** The family practitioner refers the patient to a dermatologist to be diagnosed or treated. Alternatively, the family practitioner may ask the dermatologist to evaluate the patient's condition and confirm the family practitioner's ideas or give recommendations for treating the patient. This process is called a consultation. A physician who coordinates the care of a patient, through referrals and consultations, is called a **primary care physician** (PCP). A family practitioner is most often the PCP for his or her patients. However, not all PCPs are family practitioners. For example, some women choose to use their gynecologists as their PCPs. A pediatrician is frequently the PCP for a child.

NURSES

A **nurse** is a clinical professional who has received post–secondary school training in caring for patients in a variety of health care settings. There are several levels of nursing education, each qualifying the nurse for different positions. Historically, most nurses graduated from a hospital-based certificate program. Another large percentage received their training through associate degree programs. A growing number of nurses have a bachelor's or master's of science degree in nursing, and today, almost all nurses are college educated at some level. Nurses, like doctors, take licensing examinations. Table 1-2 lists the various levels of nursing and their educational requirements.

AMERICAN BOARD OF MEDICAL SPECIALTIES

Member Boards

The American Board of Allergy & Immunology
The American Board of Dermatology
The American Board of Internal Medicine
The American Board of Nuclear Medicine
The American Board of Orthopaedic Surgery
The American Board of Pediatrics
The American Board of Preventive Medicine
The American Board of Surgery
The American Board of Anesthesiology
The American Board of Emergency Medicine
The American Board of Medical Genetics
The American Board of Obstetrics & Gynecology
The American Board of Otolaryngology
The American Board of Physical Medicine & Rehabilitation
The American Board of Psychiatry & Neurology
The American Board of Thoracic Surgery
The American Board of Colon & Rectal Surgery
The American Board of Family Medicine
The American Board of Neurological Surgery
The American Board of Ophthalmology
The American Board of Pathology
The American Board of Plastic Surgery
The American Board of Radiology
The American Board of Urology

◆ **Figure 1-1**
Medical specialty boards.

TABLE 1-2	Levels of Nursing Practice
TITLE	**GENERAL DESCRIPTION AND REQUIREMENTS**
Licensed Vocational Nurse; Licensed Practical Nurse	High school graduate or equivalent; graduation from a 1- to 2-year state-approved Health Occupations Education practical/vocational nurse program; pass NCLEX-PN examination. Licensed by state of employment or by the National Federation of Licensed Practical Nurses.
Registered Nurse	Minimum high school graduation or equivalent; programs leading to registration are offered at the associate, bachelor's, and master's degree levels. Examination and licensure in state of practice.
Nurse Practitioner	Registered nurse; completion of an accredited course in nurse practitioner training.
Advanced Practice Nursing examples: Acute Care Nurse Practitioner Adult Nurse Practitioner Family Nurse Practitioner Gerontological Nurse Practitioner Pediatric Nurse Practitioner	Complete practice requirements and examinations offered by the American Nurses Credentialing Center, a subsidiary of the American Nursing Association.

From American Nurses Association: http://www.nursingworld.org/ancc/certification/certs.html; and All Nursing Schools: http://www.allnursingschools.com/faqs/lpn.php

Licensed Practical Nurse

A licensed practical nurse (LPN), sometimes referred to as a *vocational nurse,* receives training at a hospital-based, technical, or vocational school. The training consists of learning to care for patients' personal needs and other types of routine care. LPNs work under the direction of physicians or registered nurses or both. The extent of their practice depends on the rules of the state in which they are licensed.

Registered Nurse

In addition to caring for patients' personal needs, a registered nurse (RN) administers medication and renders other care at the order of a physician. RNs particularly focus on assessing and meeting the patients' need for education regarding their illness. RNs may specialize in caring for different types of patients. For example, a nurse may assist in the operating room or care for children or the elderly, each of which requires special skills and training. RNs who want to move into management-level or teaching positions generally pursue a master's degree, a doctoral degree, a specialty certification, or some combination thereof.

Advanced Practice Nursing Specialties

In response to physician shortages and nurses' desire for greater independence, several advanced specialties in nursing practice have developed under the general title of nurse practitioner. Examples of these specialties are nurse midwives and nurse anesthetists. A nurse midwife focuses on the care of women during the period surrounding childbirth: pregnancy, labor, delivery, and after delivery. A nurse anesthetist is trained to administer anesthesia and to care for the patient during the delivery of anesthesia and recovery from the process. Nurse practitioners have a minimum of a master's degree and additional training and certification beyond the RN certification.

The American Nurses Credentialing Center, a subsidiary of the American Nursing Association, offers a variety of advanced practice certifications in subspecialties such as diabetes management and pediatrics (American Nurses Credentialing Center 2006).

ALLIED HEALTH PROFESSIONALS

Allied health (or health-related) **professionals** can be both clinical and nonclinical professionals who provide a variety of services to patients, generally at the request of or under the direction of a physician or RN. A clinical professional is one who provides health care services to a patient. Nonclinical professionals support the clinical staff and provide other types of services to a patient. Allied health professions include x-ray technicians, a variety of therapists, and health information management professionals. Table 1-3 provides examples of allied health professions, their principal work environments, and their basic educational requirements.

Occupational Therapist

Occupational therapists (OTs) are clinical professionals who focus on returning the patient to his or her maximal functioning in **activities of daily living** (ADLs). The American Occupational Therapy Association refers to ADLs as "skills for the job of living," which include but are not limited to self-care, driving, and shopping. OTs are primarily employed in rehabilitation facilities but may work in virtually any health care environment. OTs serve a wide variety of clients, including those suffering from traumatic injuries, the after-effects of stroke, and the loss of limbs. OTs may specialize in the treatment of specific conditions or specific age groups. The increasing life span and greater activity of today's elderly are important factors in the demand for OTs.

Many practitioners have a bachelor's degree; however, the profession has moved to an entry-level master's requirement, with all new practitioners required to hold a master's degree in Occupational Therapy as of 2007. Certification (registration) can be obtained from the American Occupational Therapy Association. Licensure is also required in most states as a prerequisite for practicing occupational therapy.

Occupational therapy professionals also include occupational therapy assistants (OTA) and aides. OTAs have completed training in accredited programs and passed a national certification exam. Occupational therapy aides receive on-the-job training and are not eligible for certification or licensing (*What Is Occupational Therapy?* 2006).

Physical Therapist

Physical therapists (PTs) focus on strength, gait, and range of motion training to return patients to maximum functioning in ADLs. They are primarily employed in rehabilitation facilities but may work in virtually any health care environment. A master's degree is required, and many schools now offer doctoral preparation. In order to practice, PTs must take a national licensing exam. Practice requirements vary from state to state (*About APTA* 2005).

Registered Dietitian

A registered dietitian (RD) manages food services and evaluates patients' nutritional needs, including planning menus and special diets and educating patients and families. RDs are primarily employed in health care facilities. A bachelor's degree in dietetics and at least 900 hours of clinical practice are required. A national registration exam is offered by the American Dietetic Association upon completion of the minimum requirements. Similar to other professions described in this chapter, there is another level of practice, a dietetic technician, registered (DTR), which requires a minimum of an associate degree, a passing grade on an examination, and 450 hours of clinical practice (*Registered Dietician Information Sheet* 2006).

Phlebotomist

A phlebotomist draws blood for donation and testing, which may be analyzed, for example, by a medical technologist (biology and chemistry-based, college and clinical training) or a clinical pathologist (a physician). Phlebotomists are primarily employed in health care facilities, testing labs, and community blood banks and must have graduated from high school (or the equivalent) and completed a certification program in a hospital, physician's office, or laboratory. College courses are not required, but completion of a vocational education program as a phlebotomist is desirable. The National Phlebotomy Association accredits phlebotomy educational programs and promotes public awareness of the profession (*About Phlebotomy and Our Goals* 2006).

Health Unit Coordinator

A health unit coordinator transcribes the physician's orders and prepares and compiles records during patient hospitalization. Practitioners are primarily employed in acute care, long-term care, and clinics. Practitioners are high school graduates (or the equivalent), have community college or hospital training, or have completed a vocational education program in the area of ward clerk, unit secretary, or health unit coordinator.

In June of 1982, the first National Association of Health Unit Coordinators (NAHUC) annual national convention was held in San Antonio, Texas. At this convention, the Code of Ethics and Standards of Practice for unit coordinating were adopted. Education and recognition as a health profession were two of the main concerns of the founders of NAHUC. Accordingly, a subsidiary Certification Board was established and the first National Certification Examination was given in May 1983. By the end of 1991, approximately 15,000 health unit coordinators had become certified. Two other subsidiary boards, the Education Board and the Accreditation Board, were formed to work toward accreditation of programs and to establish an official listing of unit coordinator competencies (The History of Health Unit Coordinating).

Social Workers

Social workers are among the behavioral health specialists who work with individuals with special needs. For example, a patient who leaves the hospital after surgery may need to rest. This is a problem if the patient lives alone and has no caregiver at home. A social worker helps the patient to identify and obtain the needed assistance. Social workers also provide education and assistance to individuals with chronic illnesses, including human immunodeficiency virus (HIV) and substance abuse problems. The National Association of Social Workers promotes high professional standards and public awareness and administers the credentialing process (*About NASW* 2006). Some states offer licensure of trained social workers with master's degrees under a variety of different designations. The LMSW (*Licensed Master Social Worker*) and the LCSW (*Licensed Clinical Social Worker*), for example, are designations offered by the state of New York (*LMSW License Requirements* 2005).

TABLE 1-3	Examples of Health-Related Professions

TITLE	DESCRIPTION	REQUIREMENTS
Certified Coding Specialist or Certified Coding Specialist/ Physician-office based or Certified Coding Associate Health Unit Coordinator	Assigns, collects, and reports codes representing clinical data. Primarily employed in health care facilities. Transcribes physician's orders, prepares and compiles records during patient hospitalization. Primarily employed in acute care, long-term care, and clinics.	Certification by examination from the American Health Information Management Association. High school graduate or equivalent; community college; hospital training program; completion of a vocational education program in the area of ward clerk, unit secretary, or health unit coordinator. Certification available from the National Association of Health Unit Coordinators.
Occupational Therapist	Focuses on returning patient to maximal functioning in activities of daily living. Primarily employed in rehabilitation facilities, but may work in virtually any health care environment.	Bachelor's degree; licensure required in most states; certification (registration) can be obtained from the American Occupational Therapy Association.
Phlebotomist	Draws blood for donation and testing. Primarily employed in health care facilities and community blood banks.	High school graduate or equivalent. Completion of 10- to 20-hour certification program in a hospital, physician's office, or laboratory. Completion of a vocational education program as a phlebotomist.
Physical Therapist	Focuses on strength, gait, and range of motion training to return patients to maximal functioning in activities of daily living. Primarily employed in rehabilitation facilities but may work in virtually any health care environment.	Bachelor's or master's degree; licensure by state of practice.
Registered Dietitian	Manages food services; evaluates nutritional needs, including planning menus and special diets and educating patients and family. Primarily employed in health care facilities.	Bachelor's degree; registration can be obtained from American Dietetic Association; licensure, certification, or registration required in many states.
Registered Health Information Technician	Provides administrative support targeting the collection, retention, and reporting of health information. Employed primarily in health care facilities but may work in a variety of different settings, including insurance and pharmaceutical companies.	Associate degree from accredited Health Information Technology program; registration by examination from the American Health Information Management Association.

TABLE 1-3	*(cont'd)*	
TITLE	**DESCRIPTION**	**REQUIREMENTS**
Registered Health Information Administrator	Provides administrative support targeting the collection, retention, and reporting of health information, including strategic planning, research, and systems analysis and acquisition. Employed primarily in health care facilities but may work in a variety of different settings, including insurance and pharmaceutical companies.	Bachelor's degree from accredited Health Information Administration program; registration by examination from the American Health Information Management Association.
Respiratory Therapist	Delivers therapies related to breathing. Employed primarily in health care facilities.	Associate or bachelor's degree; licensure or certification required in most states; registration can be obtained from the National Board for Respiratory Care.

HEALTH INFORMATION MANAGEMENT

Health information management (HIM) encompasses all the tasks, jobs, titles, and organizations involved in the administration of health information, including collecting, storage, retrieval, and reporting of that information. HIM professionals perform or oversee the functions that support these activities.

One area in the broad field of health information management is **health information technology (HIT)**. HIT focuses on the day-to-day activities of HIM. Because this is an introductory text, it is primarily concerned with the HIT activities and daily functions that support the collecting, storing, retrieving, and reporting of health information.

Literally hundreds of different jobs with many different titles are performed by HIM professionals throughout the world. This text presents specific job descriptions and job titles that will assist you in planning your career in HIT.

CREDENTIALS

The American Health Information Management Association (AHIMA) offers certification at progressively higher levels of education and experience. According to the AHIMA Web site (*Certification*), the organization offers the following:

■ Coding credentials (see Chapter 6 for a detailed discussion of coding issues):
■ Certified Coding Associate (CCA), the entry-level credential for coding. The credential is available by examination. No specific formal training is required; however, coding courses or on-the-job training are recommended. A high school education (or equivalent) is required.
■ Certified Coding Specialist (CCS), the mastery credential for coding. The credential is available by examination. No specific formal training is required; however, coding courses or on-the-job training are recommended. A high school education (or equivalent) is required.
■ Certified Coding Specialist/Physician-office based (CCS-P), the mastery credential for physician office coding. The credential is available by examination. No specific formal training is required; however, the examination is designed to measure proficiency. Therefore significant study of coding or several years of experience (or both) are recommended. A high school education (or equivalency) is required.

General HIM credentials include the following:

- Registered Health Information Technician (RHIT), the credential that demonstrates entry-level competency at the associate degree level. Graduation from an accredited HIT program is required to sit for the national examination.
- Registered Health Information Administrator (RHIA), the credential that demonstrates entry-level competency at the baccalaureate or master's level. Graduation from an accredited Health Information Administration program or an approved master's program is required to sit for the national examination.

Advanced and specialty practice credentials include the following:

- Certified in Health Care Privacy (CHP), a specialty credential that demonstrates advanced competency in privacy aspect of HIM practice. The CHP is an AHIMA credential.
- Certified in Health Care Security (CHS), a specialty credential that demonstrates advanced competency in privacy aspect of HIM practice. The CHS is a Healthcare Information Management and Systems Society (HIMSS) credential and is administered by AHIMA.

Eligibility for the CHP and CHS is the same: a bachelor's degree with 4 years of HIM experience, a master's degree (or higher) with 2 years of HIM experience, or an RHIT, RHIA, or Certified Professional in Healthcare Information and Management Systems (CPHIMS) with a bachelor's degree and 2 years of management experience. (CPHIMS is an HIMSS credential.)

- Certified in Healthcare Privacy and Security (CHPS) is a specialty credential that demonstrates advanced competency in privacy and security aspects of HIM practice. Originally, individuals who were eligible for and who passed both the CHP and CHS examinations were designated CHPS. At the time of this writing, AHIMA has recently announced that the CHP and CHS credentials will no longer be offered separately and that a single CHB exam will be available in early 2007. Individuals holding existing CHP or CHS designations may retain them. Eligibility criteria and testing requirements are posted on the AHIMA Web site.

The examinations for all of the previously mentioned credentials are offered through computer-based testing 6 days per week, year round, at locations nationwide. Additional information, including examination fees and continuing education requirements, may be found at http://www.ahima.org/certification.

The AHIMA supports the health care industry by promoting high-quality information standards through a variety of activities, including but not limited to accreditation of schools, continuing education, professional development and educational publications, and legislative and regulatory advocacy.

HIM professionals work in virtually every area of the health care delivery system, from physician offices and hospitals to insurance companies and government agencies. They are also employed by suppliers, such as computer software vendors, and educational institutions as well as consulting firms. Throughout this text, you will find discussions of historical roles, emerging roles, and the future of the HIM profession. As you discover the many opportunities available to HIM professionals, check industry publications and Web sites for information about specific jobs in your geographical area and around the world.

Patient Care Plan

All the previously discussed professionals work together to care for the patient. Developing a diagnosis is generally the responsibility of the physician. However, the treatment of the patient involves many different individuals, including the patient. The **patient care plan** may be as simple as instructions to "take two aspirin and drink plenty of fluids," or it may be a multiple-page document with delegation of responsibilities. For example, suppose a patient has been diagnosed with insulin-dependent diabetes mellitus (IDDM), a disease characterized by chronic high blood glucose that can be controlled only with medication (i.e., insulin).

- A nurse may be responsible for educating the patient about medication regimens.
- A psychologist can help the patient deal with the stress of chronic illness.
- An HIM professional can provide the patient with documentation of the diagnosis and treatment for continuing patient care.
- A social worker may help the patient's family learn about IDDM and what to do in a crisis.
- If the patient is elderly and lives alone:
    - A home health care worker may be brought in to check the patient's blood sugar at home.

Hit-Bit

Diagnosis and Procedure

Physicians identify and treat illnesses. They can also help prevent illnesses through patient education and various types of inoculations. Nurses and professionals in other health-related disciplines help physicians prevent, identify, and treat illnesses. Identification of the illness is the **diagnosis**. A **procedure** is performed to help in the identification and treatment processes.

Diagnosis	Procedure	
	Diagnostic	*Therapeutic*
A disease or abnormal condition	The evaluation or investigative steps taken to develop the diagnosis or monitor a disease or condition	The steps taken to alleviate or eliminate the cause or symptoms of a disease
Examples		
Appendicitis	Physical examination Blood test	Appendectomy
Cerebrovascular accident (stroke)	Physical examination Neurological examination Computed tomography scan	Medication Physical therapy Occupational therapy Speech therapy Psychological counseling
Myocardial infarction (heart attack)	Physical examination Blood test Electrocardiogram	Medication Coronary artery bypass graft

■ A registered dietitian may provide the patient with education about proper diet.

■ A physical therapist may provide the patient with training for safe conditioning exercises. The patient, of course, must be involved every step of the way. A well-documented patient care plan helps all members of the interdisciplinary care team work together to deliver the best possible care to the patient.

Exercise 1-1

Health Care Professionals

1. List as many medical specialties as you can remember, and describe what they do. Refer to Table 1-1 in the text to see how well you did.
2. What is the difference between an RN and an LPN?
3. What is the purpose of advanced practice nursing credentials?
4. Physicians diagnose diseases and perform certain procedures, both diagnostic and therapeutic. Distinguish between *diagnosis* and *procedure*. Give examples of both.
5. Much of the care for patients is performed by various allied health professionals. List as many allied health professionals as you can remember, and describe what they do. Refer to Table 1-2 in the text to see how well you did.
6. List the health information management professional credentials and what they represent.
7. What is a patient care plan?

COMPARISON OF FACILITIES

There are many different types of facilities, which are discussed in detail in Chapters 4 and 7. However, this section gives some general examples of how to identify different types of facilities.

This chapter also discusses how facilities of the same type, such as two acute care facilities, can be compared. Because no single characteristic separates one hospital from another, the comparison of hospitals requires consideration of their many different characteristics to obtain a real understanding of the differences between the facilities.

TYPES OF FACILITIES

Many facilities are expanding to offer a variety of different services. In the following discussion, the distinctions are based primarily on the length of time during which the patient is treated and the services provided.

Acute Care Facilities

Now that you have an idea of "who's who" in health care, let's turn our attention to the facilities in which health care professionals work. The first type of facility is the **acute care** (or short stay) **facility**, a type of hospital. The word *acute* means sudden or severe. Applied to illnesses, it refers to a problem that generally arises swiftly or severely. An acute care facility treats patients who require an acute level of care that can be provided only in the acute care setting. The typical patient in an acute care facility either is acutely ill or has some problem that requires the types of evaluation and treatment procedures that are available in the facility. In recent literature, the term *short stay facility* is being used synonymously with acute care. However, because the term *short stay* can also refer to the length of time a patient is in a facility and is occasionally used to describe facilities that are not also acute care facilities, this text will continue to use the term *acute care.*

The acute care facility is a type of hospital. When we say that a patient is going to the hospital, we frequently mean that he or she is going to an acute care facility. However, the term *hospital* has a broader definition. Fundamentally, a **hospital** provides room and board and services for patients to stay overnight. Diagnostic and therapeutic care is provided to patients as directed by physicians. Round-the-clock nursing care is also offered. Hospitals are licensed by the state in which they operate, and each state defines hospitals for that purpose, usually in their licensure regulations. Some states include the requirement for an "organized medical staff" in their definition of a hospital.

Hospitals have a characteristic shared or dual authority in their governance. There is a board of directors or a board of trustees, which is ultimately responsible for the facility and its activities. From the board run two separate lines of authority: administration and medical staff. The administration, headed by the chief executive officer, is responsible for the day-to-day operations of the facility. The medical staff is responsible for the clinical care rendered in the hospital. Figure 1-2 shows an example of the organization of the upper management of a hospital and some of the departments that might report to those administrators.

Therefore an acute care facility is a type of hospital. Typically, an acute care facility is distinguished by the presence of an emergency department and surgical (operating) facilities. In other words, the facility is able to treat patients who need immediate medical care for serious injuries or illnesses. The facility is also able to provide services for surgical procedures, such as appendectomies and hip replacements.

In an acute care facility, patients are cared for as **inpatients**. Inpatients typically remain in the facility at least overnight and are, therefore, patients whose evaluation and treatment result in admission to and discharge from the facility on different days. Exceptions can occur, such as if a patient dies or is transferred on the day of admission. However, these patients are still considered inpatients because the physician's order to admit the patient reveals the intention of the physician to keep the patient at least overnight.

Admission is the process that occurs when the patient is registered for evaluation or treatment in a facility upon the order of a physician. In most facilities, the admission process involves a variety of data collection activities (see Chapter 4). The *admission date* is defined as the actual calendar day that the patient is registered. Therefore whether the patient arrives at 1:05 a.m. or 11:59 p.m. on January 5, the admission date is the same: January 5.

Discharge is the process that occurs when the patient leaves the facility. Discharge implies that the patient has already been admitted to the facility. The *day of discharge* is defined as the actual calendar day that the patient leaves the facility. Note that a physician's order for a patient to leave the facility is required for a normal discharge. However, as mentioned earlier, certain events might also cause a discharge. A patient may die, may leave against medical advice, or may be transferred to another facility. All of these events are discharges as of the calendar day on which they occur.

By definition, in state licensure standards, the average time that patients stay in an acute care facility is less than 30 days. Exceptions can and do occur; patients with greater lengths of stay are not uncommon and do not have an impact on the facility's acute care designation. Actually, the average number of days that a patient spends in a given acute care facility depends on what types of patients are treated in the facility. Many acute care facilities have an average patient stay between 3 and 6 days, significantly less than 30 days. For a detailed explanation of average (patient) length of stay (ALOS), see Chapter 9.

Historically, acute care facilities have been *stand-alone* hospitals. Although they may have provided a variety of different services to the community, they did not have a formal business affiliation with other hospitals. In recent years, as a result of economic pressures, hospitals are consolidating. Sometimes they merge, which means that two or more hospitals combine their

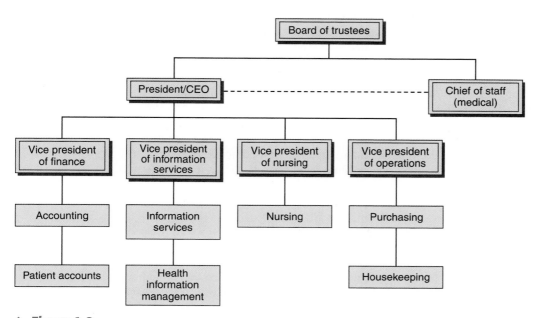

◆ **Figure 1-2**

Hospital organization chart. This is a very simple example of the possible organization of a hospital. There are many more possible departments than those depicted here and many different organizational structures. For example, an HIM department may report to any of the vice presidents—even Nursing.

Hit-Bit

Abbreviations and Acronyms

You may have noticed that many of the terms and phrases used in health care frequently are shortened to a few recognizable letters. An abbreviation made from the initial letters or parts of a term is called an *acronym*. Acronyms and other abbreviations shorten writing time and save space. However, acronyms can also cause confusion. AMA, for example, means "against medical advice." It is also the abbreviation for the American Medical Association and the American Management Association. There are also interdisciplinary issues with abbreviations. *Dr.* means doctor to a health care professional. To an accountant, it means debit. Therefore abbreviations should be used carefully. Health care facilities must define acceptable abbreviations and should restrict the use of abbreviations only to those that have been approved.

resources. Other times, one hospital acquires (purchases) the other. The differences between a merger and an acquisition are primarily organizational and financial.

In recent years, partly as a cost-cutting measure and partly for increased customer service, acute care facilities have expanded into ambulatory care and other services. They have done this in three ways: ambulatory surgery, clinics, and ancillary services (see Chapter 7: Alternative Settings).

Ambulatory Care

In an ambulatory care facility, patients are admitted and discharged on the same day. A patient whose evaluation or treatment is intended to occur within 1 calendar day is an ambulatory care patient, also known as an **outpatient.** The concepts of admission and discharge have little relevance in an ambulatory care facility because both processes typically are intended to take place on the same day. An ambulatory care admission, then, is referred to as a *visit* or an *encounter.*

Physician's Offices

A physician's office is one type of ambulatory care facility. Most of us have been to a physician's office. Most physicians maintain an office where patients can visit. There are many different types of physicians, as discussed earlier. Some physicians have offices attached to their homes; others have space in office buildings; still others are associated with specific facilities.

Ancillary Services

Some facilities offer a broad range of evaluation services, such as radiology and laboratory services. The radiology department performs and reviews x-rays. The laboratory analyzes body fluids, such as blood. These evaluation services are called *ancillary,* or *adjunct, services.* Many of these services are offered in freestanding facilities. Even when they are associated with acute care or other facilities, the services are often also offered on an outpatient basis. Some freestanding services lease space in other health care facilities, such as acute care hospitals, so that it is not always obvious that the service is not part of the hospital.

Long-Term Care Facilities

You may be more familiar with the term "nursing home." For many years, these were primarily facilities that took care of elderly patients who were ill or whose families could no longer care for them at home. Patients often moved into a nursing home and lived there until they died. Today, a **long-term care facility** treats a wide variety of patients who need more care than they would be able to get at home but who do not generally need the intensity of care provided by an acute care facility. In addition, the philosophy of these facilities has changed so that the focus is less on making a home for the patient and more on maintaining the patient's health and preparing him or her to go home, if possible.

In long-term care, we refer to those inpatients as *residents.* By definition, a long-term care facility has an ALOS in excess of 30 days. This is an important difference between acute care and long-term care. Because the ALOS is over 30 days, we know that a long-term care facility manages its residents on an inpatient basis.

Hit-Bit

Mergers and Acquisitions

Although this is not a strict rule, two hospitals that have combined often get a new name. If two hospitals combine and their group name is different from either of the original names, it usually indicates a merger. If the group name is the same as one of the original hospitals, it may indicate an acquisition. For example, if Community Hospital and Spencer Hospital combine to form Star Health System, the two hospitals probably merged. If they combine to form Spencer Health System, then Spencer Hospital probably acquired Community Hospital.

Behavioral Health Facilities

Behavioral health facilities are defined by their patient population. Patients in a **behavioral health facility** either have or are being evaluated for psychiatric illnesses. Such a facility may also be referred to as a **mental health facility** or psychiatric facility. These facilities can be inpatient, outpatient, or both. Large behavioral health facilities may be administered by the state or county government. In addition, there are many small, private facilities. There is no standard in terms of ALOS. Outpatient services may be provided in stand-alone clinics or as part of an inpatient facility.

Rehabilitation Facilities

The focus of *rehabilitation* is to return the patient to the maximal possible level of function in terms of ADLs. ADLs include self-care functions such as bathing and toileting as well as practical concerns such as ironing and cooking. This type of rehabilitation is referred to as *physical medicine and rehabilitation.* These facilities may be inpatient, outpatient, or both.

A **rehabilitation facility** treats patients who have suffered a debilitating illness or trauma or who are recovering from certain types of surgery, such as a patient who survived a car accident but has suffered a head trauma and other injuries that require extensive therapy or a patient who has had knee replacement surgery and needs therapy to learn to function with the prosthetic joint.

Hospice

A **hospice** provides palliative care for the terminally ill. **Palliative care** involves making the patient comfortable by easing his or her pain and other discomforts. Hospice care can be delivered to the patient in an inpatient, residential setting or in the home. A hospice also provides support groups and counseling for both the patient and his or her family and friends. Hospice services may continue for the survivors after the patient's death.

Home Health Care

As the name implies, **home health care** involves a variety of services provided to patients in the home. Services range from assistance with ADLs to physical therapy and intravenous drug therapy. Personnel providing these services also vary, from aides to therapists, nurses, and doctors.

FACILITY SIZE

One way of distinguishing one facility from another is by the facility's size. Frequently, not only is a facility described as being *acute care* or *long-term care* or *ambulatory care* or *rehabilitation*, but it also is differentiated by number of beds or number of discharges. The size of an ambulatory care facility is defined by the number of encounters or the number of visits. These concepts are detailed in the following sections. Figure 1-3 summarizes some comparisons of different types of facilities.

Number of Beds

In an inpatient facility, beds are set up for patients to occupy. There are two basic ways to view beds: licensed beds and bed count. **Licensed beds** are the number of beds that the state has approved the hospital to have. For now, think of licensed beds as the maximum number of beds allowed to the facility.

Facilities do not always need all of their licensed beds. For example, a facility may not have enough patients to fill all of its beds. It is very expensive to maintain the equipment and staff members for an empty room. Facility administrators look at beds in terms of whether they are occupied. If the percentage of occupied beds is low over a period of time, then administrators may decide to close some of the beds. Therefore a facility may equip and staff only as many beds as it needs for the foreseeable future. This number of beds, which can be less than the number of licensed beds but not more, is called the *bed count*. **Bed count** is the number of beds that the facility actually has set up, equipped, and staffed—in other words, the beds that are ready to treat patients.

In comparing facilities, the size of the facility is often referred to in terms of its licensed beds. It is also useful to analyze a facility's licensed beds versus bed count over time. A seasonal or otherwise short-term closing of beds is not automatically a matter of concern and may, in fact, indicate sound administration. Long-term low bed count (as compared to licensed beds), on the other hand, may indicate serious problems. Over the last 10 years, many hospitals have been forced to

---

HEALTH CARE FACILITIES

Some facilities are defined by length of stay:

Ambulatory care facility:	Patients are admitted and discharged on the same day
Acute care facility:	Patients remain at least overnight and, on average, stay less than 30 days
Long-term care facility:	Patients remain at least overnight (inpatient) and, on average, stay longer than 30 days

Other facilities are defined by the medical specialty or by the types of patients they treat:

Rehabilitation facility:	Physical medicine, physical therapy, and occupational therapy; may be inpatient or outpatient
Behavioral health facility:	Psychiatric diagnosis; may be inpatient or outpatient
Children's hospital:	Treats only children, usually 16 years old and younger; may be inpatient or outpatient

◆ **Figure 1-3**
Comparison of health care facilities by characteristics and patients.

close beds as a result of the health care industry shift from acute care to ambulatory care. Because licensed beds are granted on the basis of the needs of the community, long-term reduction of bed count may signal that the facility is no longer needed in its community.

Discharges

Another measure of the size of a facility is the number of discharges in a period, usually expressed monthly or annually. Number of discharges is a measure of activity, as opposed to a measure of physical size. Although two acute care facilities may each have 250 beds, one of them may discharge 15,000 patients per year while the other discharges 25,000 patients per year. Higher numbers of discharges require larger numbers of administrative and other support staff.

Occupancy, the percentage of available beds that have been used over a period of time, is one explanation for the difference in the number of discharges. To calculate occupancy, divide the number of days that patients used hospital beds by the number of beds available. If the number of days that patients used hospital beds is 7000, and the number of beds available is 8000, then the occupancy rate is 87.5%. The number of beds available can be based on either bed count or licensed beds. A facility may use bed count internally to monitor the rate at which available beds are being used, but it may use licensed beds to compare use over time because licensed beds are less likely to change.

Length of stay is another explanation for different discharge numbers. The longer a patient stays in the hospital, the fewer individual patients can be treated in that particular bed. Therefore if a hospital has an ALOS of 6 days, it can treat half as many patients as a hospital of the same size with an ALOS of 3 days. For example, to calculate the ALOS of a 200-bed hospital in the month of June, multiply 200 beds by 30 days in June to equal 6000 "beds" or "days" available to treat patients. If the ALOS is 6 days, then the hospital is able to treat an estimated 1000 patients for 6 days (6000 divided by 6 equals 1000). If the ALOS is 3 days, then the hospital is able to treat an estimated 2000 patients—twice as many as the hospital with an ALOS of 6 days. That means twice as many admissions, twice as many discharges, and twice as much work for many of the administrative support staff who process these activities (see Chapter 4).

OWNERSHIP

Health care facilities may exist under many different types of ownership. Some facilities, such as physician group practices and radiology centers, are owned by individuals or groups of individuals. Facilities may be owned by corporations, government entities, or religious groups. Frequently, the ownership of the organization has an impact on both the operations and the services provided by the facility. For example, a facility owned by a religious organization may not allow abortions to be performed by their physicians. A government-owned facility may require supplies to be purchased from government-approved vendors.

FINANCIAL STATUS

Another way to distinguish institutions from one another is by their tax status: for-profit or not-for-profit. A for-profit, or proprietary, organization has owners. It can have few or many owners or shareholders. Ford Motor Company is an example of a for-profit organization with many shareholders. A not-for-profit institution operates solely for the good of the community and is considered to be owned by the community. It has no shareholders who have a vested interest in the economic viability of the organization.

The tax status of an organization has little or no impact on the day-to-day operations of the organization. The fundamental impact is on the distribution of net income. In a not-for-profit organization, net income must be reinvested in the organization or the community. In a for-profit organization, net income may, at the discretion of the board of directors, be distributed in whole or in part to the shareholders of the organization.

PATIENT POPULATION

As previously discussed, facilities may differ in terms of the types of patients that they treat. Rehabilitation facilities and mental health facilities treat patients with different types of problems. Many facilities specialize in treating only certain types of diseases. For example, Deborah Heart and Lung Center in New Jersey specializes in treating cardiac and respiratory problems. It would not accept a patient whose only problem is a broken leg. Another common type of specialty hospital is a **children's hospital.** The medical treatment of children requires smaller equipment as well as specialized equipment and clinical skills. A children's hospital would not normally accept a 35-year-old patient.

SERVICES

Depending on the type of patients that they treat, facilities offer a variety of different services. These services are often organized into departments. For example, an acute care facility has an emergency department and a surgery department. It also offers radiology, laboratory, and pathology services. If an acute care facility offers physical therapy, it may be a small department. Often, therapy is provided at the patient's bedside. A rehabilitation facility does not have an emergency department, but it may have a room set aside for the performance of minor surgical procedures. It may have radiology and laboratory services, but it probably does not have a pathology department. Because physical therapy is a major component of rehabilitation, physical therapy is a large department. A large amount of space is available for treatment, including a variety of specialized equipment.

CONTINUUM OF CARE

With so many different caregivers working in such a variety of facilities, communication among them is essential. The coordination among caregivers to treat a patient is called the **continuum of care.** Continuum of care is a concept with two separate but related elements. First, it refers to communication among all the patient's care providers in a facility from his or her admission to discharge. As a patient moves from place to place in a facility, communication among all his or her caregivers ideally should be as smooth and coordinated as possible. Second, continuum of care refers to all the patient's experiences from one facility to another, either throughout a particular illness or throughout the life of the patient. We illustrate the continuum of care from birth to death for a female patient in the subsequent text and in Figure 1-4.

Childhood

The patient, Emily, is born in an acute care facility. As a child, Emily is treated by a pediatrician. The pediatrician is her PCP. She receives extensive well-child care: preventive vaccinations, check-ups, and developmental assessments.

Adult Care

As Emily ages and grows into adulthood, she visits a family practitioner as her new PCP. The family practitioner would benefit from having information about all of the patient's childhood diseases, immunizations, and problems that she has experienced previously. Emily sees her PCP on a regular basis. As she becomes an adult, she also visits a gynecologist for regular examinations.

Special Health Issues

When Emily becomes pregnant, she is examined and followed by her obstetrician throughout the pregnancy and cesarean delivery. Later in life, as she becomes older, other illnesses arise. For example, in her late 30s, Emily develops diabetes. Her PCP refers her to an endocrinologist for treatment of the diabetes. After Emily discovers a lump in her breast, she undergoes a mammography and is referred to a surgeon for a diagnosis. Then she enters an acute care facility to have a lumpectomy. Note that at this point, Emily has had at least three admissions to an acute care facility and has visited at least three specialists in addition to her PCP. How confusing would it be if none of these physicians was aware of the treatment that she had received from the others?

Practitioners	Pediatrician	Primary care physician	Obstetrician Endocrinologist Surgeon	Orthopedic surgeon Physiatrist	Gerontologist Neurologist Psychiatrist
Facilities	Children's specialized		Women's health center	Rehabilitation	Long-term care
	Ambulatory care — Physician's office or clinic				
	Acute care				
Patient					
Baby	Birth				
Child	Preventive vaccinations, checkups, and developmental assessments				
Young adult		Checkups			
Adult			Childbirth Lumpectomy Diabetes		
Older adult				Hip fracture	Alzheimer's

◆ **Figure 1-4**
Continuum of care example.

Elder Care

As an elderly woman, Emily falls and breaks her hip. She needs to have a hip replacement and is treated by an orthopedic surgeon in an acute care facility for hip replacement surgery, after which she is transferred to a rehabilitation facility for a couple of weeks of rehabilitation to enable her to resume her ADLs. Eventually, Emily becomes incapacitated and is unable to take care of herself. She develops Alzheimer's disease and is seen by a neurologist and a **psychiatrist**. Ultimately, she is admitted into a nursing home for round-the-clock nursing care.

Throughout these encounters with various facilities and specialists, the previous history of Emily's encounters should follow her smoothly. The orthopedic surgeon will want to know her experiences under anesthesia when she had breast surgery and her reaction to anesthesia when her baby was born. This information should be available to subsequent surgeons.

Table 1-4 compares some of the onsite services provided by various types of facilities. Note that many services are provided across the continuum of care.

Impact of Mergers and Acquisitions

As noted previously, hospital mergers have increased in recent years. Many health care organizations are consolidating along the continuum of care. In other words, they are not just buying multiple acute care facilities; they are buying physician's office practices, rehabilitation facilities, and long-term care facilities as well as acute care facilities. Thus they are able to provide patients with seamless coordination of care along this continuum. Such enterprises are referred to as

TABLE 1-4	Comparison of Onsite Services Provided in Health Care Facilities			
SERVICE OR DEPARTMENT	**PHYSICIAN'S OFFICE**	**ACUTE CARE**	**LONG-TERM CARE**	**REHABILITATION**
Nursing	Maybe	Yes	Yes	Yes
Medical staff	One, two, or many	Many; visit many patients daily	Many; visit patients as needed or defined	Many; visit many patients daily
Patient registration	Yes	Yes	Yes	Yes
Dietary	Not usually	Yes	Yes	Yes
Health information management	Not a separate department in small facilities	Yes	Not always a separate department	Usually
Patient accounts	Yes	Yes	Yes	Yes
Volunteers	Only in large facilities	Yes	Yes	Yes
Radiology	Maybe	Yes	Limited, if any	Usually
Laboratory	Maybe	Yes	Limited	Limited
Physical therapy	May be associated within group practice	Small department	Varies; may have small department	Large department
Occupational therapy	May be associated within group practice	Small department	Varies; may have small department	Large department
Emergency Services	Urgent care	Yes	No	No
Surgery	Minor procedures	Yes	Minor procedures	Minor procedures
Pathology	No: Physician usually uses a freestanding or hospital-based service	Yes	Limited	Limited

integrated delivery systems (IDSs). Many see this as an efficient delivery of health care throughout the lifetime of a patient.

Exercise 1-2

Comparison of Facilities

1. Patients whose care requires them to remain in the hospital overnight are called _____.
2. What are the characteristics of a hospital?
3. Define *admission* and *discharge.*
4. If a patient is admitted as an inpatient on Monday at 10 a.m. but dies on Monday at 3 p.m., is that patient still considered an inpatient?
5. A hospital with an average length of stay of less than 30 days, an emergency department, operating suite, and clinical departments to handle a broad range of diagnoses and treatments is most likely a(n) _____.
6. A specialty inpatient facility that focuses on the treatment of individuals with psychiatric disorders is a(n) _____.
7. Care for the terminally ill is the focus of _____ care.
8. _____ focuses on treating patients where they reside.
9. Chapone Health Care is an organization that owns a number of different health care facilities: three acute care hospitals, two long-term care facilities, and a number of physician offices. Chapone also owns a rehabilitation hospital and an assisted living facility, which also delivers home care. They deliver care to patients at every point along the continuum of care. Chapone Health Care can be described as a(n) _____.
10. The broad range of services that may be required by a patient in his/her lifetime is referred to as the _____.
11. A(n) _____ provides care to patients at all or most points along the continuum of care.
12. The Community Care Center has 200 beds. It has an average length of stay of 2 years. Most of the patients are elderly, but there are some younger patients with serious chronic illnesses. Community Care Center is most likely a(n) _____.

▌ LEGAL AND REGULATORY ENVIRONMENT

In addition to the issues previously discussed, various facilities have different ways of operating or functioning. More often, the guidance or mandate under which activities are performed arises from legislation, regulation, and accreditation issues. In this section, the legal environment of health care is explained. Because this is frequently a topic of another entire text or course, the discussion is limited to the issues that bear directly on the activities of the HIT professional. Federal, state, and local government all have an impact in varying degrees on health care institutions and delivery. Table 1-5 summarizes the impact of the government on health care.

FEDERAL

The federal government has a major impact on health care through regulatory activity. The federal legislature (Congress and the Senate) enacts laws, which the executive branch (the President) must then enforce. Enforcement arises from the delegation of executive responsibilities to various agencies. In terms of health care, the critical regulatory agency is the Department of Health and Human Services (DHHS), which houses the Centers for Medicare and Medicaid Services (CMS), which administers Medicare and part of Medicaid.

Medicare is an entitlement to health care benefits for persons of advanced age (over 65) or those with certain chronic illnesses (e.g., end-stage renal disease). Health care facilities are not

TABLE 1-5	**Federal Agencies Involved in Health Care**	
DEPARTMENT	**AGENCY**	**HEALTH-RELATED FUNCTIONS**
Department of Health and Human Services	Food and Drug Administration	Ensures safety of foods, cosmetics, pharmaceuticals, biological products, and medical devices
	Centers for Medicare and Medicaid Services	Oversees Medicare and the federal portion of Medicaid
	National Institutes of Health	Supports biomedical research
	Centers for Disease Control and Prevention	Provides a system of health surveillance to monitor and prevent outbreak of diseases
	Health Resources and Services Administration	Helps provide health resources for medically underserved populations
	Indian Health Service	Supports a network of health care facilities and providers to Native Americans, including Alaskans
Department of Defense	Military Health Services System	Maintains a network of health care providers and facilities for service personnel and their dependents
Department of Veterans Affairs	Veterans Affairs facilities	Maintains a network of facilities and services for armed services veterans and sometimes their dependents
Department of Labor	Occupational Safety and Health Administration	Regulates workplace health and safety

automatically eligible for reimbursement from Medicare simply on the basis of treating a Medicare patient. To be eligible for reimbursement from Medicare, a health care facility must comply with Medicare's **Conditions of Participation** (COP). COP addresses the quality of providers, certain policies and procedures, and financial issues and is updated in the *Federal Register.* Another important area of federal regulation concerns the release of information pertaining to patients with drug and alcohol diagnoses (discussed in Chapter 11).

STATE

The impact of state government on health care organizations varies from state to state. Here we discuss some of the more common involvements, licensure and reporting.

Licensure

For operation of any health care facility, a license must be obtained from the state in which the facility will operate. The process of **licensure** varies among states. Often, the state's legislature passes a hospital licensing act or a similar law that requires hospitals to be licensed and delegates the authority to regulate that process to a state agency, possibly the state's Department of Health. The delegated agency then develops and administers the detailed regulations, which are part of the state's administrative code. The licensure regulations contain a great deal of useful information pertaining to the operations of a health care facility, including the minimum requirements for maintaining patient records. Some states' regulations are very detailed and specific as to the organization and structure of a facility, including such items as services to be provided, medical staff requirements, nursing requirements, committees, and sanitation. Licensure is specific to the type of health care facility being operated. The regulations governing acute care facilities differ somewhat from the regulations governing long-term care facilities, which are in turn different from regulations governing rehabilitation facilities.

It is fundamentally the responsibility of the board of directors or board of trustees of a facility to ensure compliance with each of the requirements of the license. The board delegates the day-to-day operations of the facility to management, through the chief executive officer or administrator of the hospital.

Many state agencies visit hospitals regularly and review the hospital operations and the documentation for compliance with the license of the facility. Of particular note are long-term facilities, which tend to be scrutinized very closely. Many states defer their acute care facility reviews to alternative methods, such as relying on the reviews of accrediting bodies, which is discussed next.

Reporting

There is a tremendous amount of reporting that occurs among health care facilities and state agencies. Typically, reporting includes information about general patient data, cancer, trauma, birth defects, and infectious disease. Additional reporting may result from health care workers' observation of inappropriate activities, such as child abuse; health care workers have an obligation to report to the authorities certain types of suspected abuses. The relationship between state government and health care facilities is often extensive.

LOCAL

Local government may also become involved in health care organizations, particularly in the aspect of zoning regulations. Because the facility is an important member of the local community, its activities may become deeply intertwined with those of the community.

ACCREDITATION

Up to this point, federal statutes and regulations and the impact of licensure have been discussed. Another issue that has a visible impact on the operation of a health care facility is voluntary accreditation. Whereas licensure is mandatory to operate a health care facility within a given state, accreditation is voluntary.

Accreditation begins with voluntary compliance with a set of standards that are developed by an independent organization. That organization then audits the facility to ensure compliance. Numerous accrediting bodies exist for different industries. Table 1-6 lists some health care accrediting bodies and the subjects of their activities.

Joint Commission on Accreditation of Healthcare Organizations

Within the health care profession, the most important accrediting body is the Joint Commission on Accreditation of Healthcare Organizations (JCAHO). The JCAHO is an organization, located in Chicago, that sets standards for acute care facilities, ambulatory care networks, long-term care facilities, and rehabilitation facilities, as well as certain specialty facilities, such as hospice and home care.

The standards set by the JCAHO reflect optimal industry practice and in many ways define how the health care facility should operate in terms of patient care, the clinical flow of data, and documentation standards. Much of the activity of the JCAHO stems from the original 1913 American College of Surgeons (ACS) medical documentation standardization project. For many years after that project, ACS not only maintained the development of the standards of documentation for hospitals but also conducted the approval proceedings. In 1951, the ACS, along with the American Hospital Association, the American Medical Association, and the Canadian Medical Association, formed the Joint Commission on Accreditation of Hospitals, which took over that accrediting function. In 1987, the Joint Commission changed its name to reflect the variety of different organizations that were seeking accreditation.

The JCAHO has a tremendous impact on health care facilities for a number of reasons. First, on-site accrediting surveys take place on a scheduled 3-year (maximum) cycle. Therefore at least every 3 years, the facility is subject to an intensive onsite review. The accreditation standards change to

TABLE 1-6	Accrediting Organizations in Health Care

ACCREDITING ORGANIZATION	FACILITIES/ORGANIZATIONS ACCREDITED
Health Care Facilities	
Accreditation Association for Ambulatory Health Care (AAAHC)	Ambulatory care facilities, including
American Osteopathic Association (AOA)	Osteopathic hospitals
Joint Commission on Accreditation of Healthcare Organizations (JCAHO)	Acute care, ambulatory care, behavioral health, long-term care, and rehabilitation facilities
Commission on Accreditation of Rehabilitation Facilities (CARF)	Rehabilitation facilities
National Committee for Quality Assurance (NCQA)	Managed care organizations
Community Health Accreditation Program (CHAP) (National League for Nursing)	Home- and community-based health care organizations
Educational Programs	
Accreditation Council for Occupational Therapy Education	Occupational therapist and occupational therapy assistant programs
American Physical Therapy Association	Physical therapist and physical therapist assistant programs
Committee on the Accreditation of Allied Health Education Programs	Education programs for multiple allied health specialties, including anesthesiologist assistant, cardiovascular technologist, blood bank technologist, medical assistant, exercise science, and respiratory therapist
Commission on Accreditation of Health Informatics and Information Management Education	Health information and informatics programs
Commission on Accreditation/Approval for Dietetics Education of the American Dietetic Association Chapter 1	Dietitian/nutritionist and dietetic technician programs
Liaison Committee of the Association of American Medical Colleges and the American Medical Association	Medical schools
National League for Nursing Accrediting Commission	Nursing schools

differing degrees annually, with interim changes as needed. Therefore within the 3-year cycle of review, facilities are required to stay abreast of the changes and implement procedures to comply.

Second, whether a facility attains favorable accreditation status has an impact on its relationship with government entities. As was previously discussed, the CMS, through Medicare, allows reimbursement from Medicare to those facilities that comply with Medicare's COP. This ordinarily entails a survey to ensure that the facility complies with COP. However, a facility that is accredited by the JCAHO is not normally required to be subject to the COP review. This is called **deemed status** because the facility is deemed to have complied with the COP. In addition, in some states JCAHO accreditation reduces or eliminates the need for state licensure surveys. So, in some cases, the voluntary accreditation by the JCAHO can alleviate two additional surveys: the state department of health and Medicare COP.

Finally, accreditation is also desirable for marketing purposes. As the public becomes more aware of quality issues in a facility, JCAHO accreditation becomes a symbol of quality to a certain extent.

Commission on Accreditation of Rehabilitation Facilities

Another important accrediting body is the Commission on Accreditation of Rehabilitation Facilities (CARF), also known as the Rehabilitation Accreditation Commission, which focuses on facilities that provide physical, mental, and occupational rehabilitation services. Accreditation of adult day

CODE OF ETHICS

Ethical Principles: The following ethical principles are based on the core values of the American Health Information Management Association and apply to all health information management professionals.

Health information management professionals:

I. Advocate, uphold and defend the individual's right to privacy and the doctrine of confidentiality in the use and disclosure of information.
II. Put service and the health and welfare of persons before self-interest and conduct themselves in the practice of the profession so as to bring honor to themselves, their peers, and to the health information management profession.
III. Preserve, protect, and secure personal health information in any form or medium and hold in the highest regard the contents of the records and other information of a confidential nature, taking into account the applicable statutes and regulations.
IV. Refuse to participate in or conceal unethical practices or procedures.
V. Advance health information management knowledge and practice through continuing education, research, publications, and presentations.
VI. Recruit and mentor students, peers and colleagues to develop and strengthen professional workforce.
VII. Represent the profession accurately to the public.
VIII. Perform honorably health information management association responsibilities, either appointed or elected, and preserve the confidentiality of any privileged information made known in any official capacity.
IX. State truthfully and accurately their credentials, professional education, and experiences.
X. Facilitate interdisciplinary collaboration in situations supporting health information practice.
XI. Respect the inherent dignity and worth of every person.

Revised & adopted by AHIMA House of Delegates–July 1, 2004

◆ **Figure 1-5**
AHIMA Code of Ethics. Revised and approved by the AHIMA House of Delegates July 2004. (Used with permission from the American Health Information Management Association, Chicago, Illinois.)

care, **assisted living,** and employment and community services are also available. The JCAHO also accredits rehabilitation facilities, but it has slightly different requirements and standards, adapting acute care and ambulatory care requirements. In fact, many rehabilitation facilities may be accredited by both the JCAHO and CARF. The focus of the two reviews is slightly different, and rehabilitation facilities that are accredited by the JCAHO find themselves in something of a dilemma in complying with both sets of requirements. CARF requirements tend to be more prescriptive, and surveyors focus beyond physician/nurse documentation to emphasize documentation of occupational, physical, and other therapies. In recent years, JCAHO and CARF have collaborated to offer joint survey options to facilities. In this way, the surveys can be simultaneous and partially coordinated to reduce duplication of effort.

Many organizations accredit health care facilities and health care professional education programs. A partial list of these organizations and the facilities and institutions that they accredit is provided in Table 1-6.

Commission on Accreditation for Health Informatics and Information Management Education

If you are studying health information management in a college that has an accredited health information management program, your program is accredited by the Commission on Accreditation for Health Informatics and Information Management Education (CAHIIM).

CAHIIM serves the public interest by establishing quality standards for the educational preparation of future health information management (HIM) professionals. When a program is accredited by

CAHIIM, it means that it has voluntarily undergone a rigorous review process and has been determined to meet or exceed the standards set by the sponsoring professional organization—the American Health Information Management Association (AHIMA)—in cooperation with the Commission. CAHIIM accreditation is a way to recognize and publicize best practices for HIM Education Programs. (*Welcome to CAHIIM on the Web!* 2006)

PROFESSIONAL STANDARDS

In addition to licensure and accreditation requirements, there is yet another level of requirements that must be followed in a health care organization. This last set of requirements is professional standards. On the one hand, licensure and accrediting bodies take a general overview of the facility and tend not to specifically address the day-to-day activities of individual practitioners. Professional standards, on the other hand, are developed by the professional organizations that grant the credentials to the individuals who are performing health-related tasks.

In addition to professional standards that govern the behavior of a variety of health care professionals, many of those professionals are also licensed by the state in which they practice and come under those licensing regulations as well. Specifically, physicians are licensed to practice medicine in the same way that health care facilities are licensed to operate, and the requirements for licensure may vary from state to state.

Professional standards play an important role in determining the activities of health care professionals. Often, it is the professional standards of the individual practitioner that dictate the type and extent of documentation that is required in the performance of any type of therapy or evaluation of patients.

In the field of HIM, professional standards tend to revolve around issues of **ethics** and best practices. They also tend to target data quality, confidentiality, and access to health information. It is important in the practice of HIT that practitioners know and adhere to these professional standards. Professional standards in HIM are developed by AHIMA and take the form of an ethics statement as well as practice briefs and position papers, which are routinely published in the *Journal of the American Health Information Management Association*. Figure 1-5 shows the AHIMA Code of Ethics ("*AHIMA Code of Ethics*" 2004).

Exercise 1-3

Legal and Regulatory Environment

1. List and describe the purposes of the agencies within the Department of Health and Human Services.
2. Medicare is administered by_____.
3. Medicare waives compliance audits for appropriately accredited facilities by granting them _____.
4. Voluntary compliance with a set of standards developed by an independent agency is part of the _____ process.
5. Health care professionals must adhere to their discipline's _____.

■ WORKS CITED

"About APTA." 2005. American Physical Therapy Association. 29 November 2005 <http://www.apta.org/AM/Template. cfm?Section=About_APTA&Template=/TaggedPage/TaggedPageDisplay.cfm&TPLID=41&ContentID=23725>.

"About NASW." 2006. National Association of Social Workers. 6 June 2006 <https://www.socialworkers.org/nasw/ default.asp>.

"About Osteopathic Medicine." 2005. American Osteopathic Association (AOA). 29 November 2005 <http://www.DO-Online.org>.

"About Phlebotomy and Our Goals." 2006. National Phlebotomy Association. 6 June 2006 <http://www.nationalphlebotomy.org/ 230374.html>.

"AHIMA Code of Ethics." 2004. American Health Information Management Association. 29 November 2005 <http://library.ahima.org/xpedio/groups/public/documents/ahima/bok1_024277.hcsp?dDoc Name=bok1_024277>.

American Nurses Credentialing Center. (2006). *Certified nursing excellence.* Retrieved June 6, 2006, from the American Nursing Association Web site: <http://www.nursingworld.org/ancc/inside.html>.

"Certification." 2005. American Health Information Management Association. 29 November 2005 <http://www.ahima.org/certification/>.

"Certified Nursing Excellence." 2006. American Nurses Credentialing Center. 6 June 2006 <http://nursaingworld.org/ancc/inside.html>.

"Diplomate Statistics." 2005. American Board of Family Medicine. 29 November 2005 <https://www.theabfm.org/about/stats.aspx>.

"Family Practice. Careers in Medicine: Specialty Information – Family Practice." 2005. American Association of Medical Colleges. November 29 2005 Web site: <http://www.aamc.org/students/cim/pub_fp.htm>.

"LMSW License Requirements." 2005. New York State Education Department, Office of the Professions <http://www.op.nysed.gov/lmsw.htm>.

"Registered Dietician Information Sheet." 2006. American Dietetic Association. 6 June 2006 <http://www.eatright.org/cps/rde/xchg/ada/hs.xsl/home_6658_ENU_HTML.htm>.

"The History of Health Unit Coordinating and NAHUC." 2006. National Association of Health Unity Coordinators. 6 June 2006 <http://www.nahuc.org/nahuc_hi.htm>.

"Welcome to CAHIIM on the Web!" 2006. Commission on Accreditation for Health Informatics and Information Management Education. 6 June 2006 <http://www.cahiim.org/>.

"What is Occupational Therapy?" 2006. American Occupational Therapy Association. 6 June 2006 <http://www.aota.org/featured/area6/index.asp>.

■ SUGGESTED READING

Peden, Ann H. *Comparative Health Information Management.* 2nd ed. Clifton Park, NY: Delmar, 2005.

Sultz, Harry and Kristina Young. *Health Care USA: Understanding Its Organization and Delivery.* 2nd ed. Gaithersburg, MD: Aspen, 1999.

WEB SITES

The Evolve companion site has links to various government agencies, health care facilities, and professional associations at http://evolve.elsevier.com/productPages/s_0721683533.html

American Dietetic Association: http://www.eatright.org

American Health Information Management Association: http://www.ahima.org

American Hospital Association: http://www.aha.org.

American Occupational Therapy Association: http://www.aota.org/

American Osteopathic Association: http://www.DO-Online.org

American Physical Therapy Association: http://www.apta.org/

Department of Health and Human Services: http://www.os.dhhs.gov

Department of Labor: http://www.dol.gov

National Library of Medicine: http://www.nlm.nih.gov

National Association of Health Unit Coordinators: http://www.nahuc.org/

National Association of Social Workers: http://www.naswdc.org/

National Phlebotomy Association: http://www.nationalphlebotomy.org/index.html

United States Medical Licensing Examination: http://www.usmle.org/

Veterans Administration: http://www.va.gov

CHAPTER ACTIVITIES

CHAPTER SUMMARY

Health care is provided by a variety of different practitioners, including physicians, nurses, and therapists. Practitioners in multiple disciplines work together to care for the patient. Physicians may maintain their own offices as solo practitioners or work with other physicians in group practices. Physicians' offices are a type of ambulatory care facility. Other types of facilities are acute care, long-term care, and a variety of specialty facilities, including rehabilitation facilities, mental health facilities, and children's hospitals. Facilities can be classified by length of stay, inpatient versus outpatient services, and financial status (i.e., for-profit or not-for-profit).

Government plays a role in the health care industry. Federal and state governments enact laws and enforce them through regulations. Health care facilities are licensed through the state, and there are a number of very specific reporting requirements. Another aspect of facility organization is accreditation status. Accreditation is very important to ensure quality and efficient reimbursement. Lastly, professional standards play a role in determining the activities of a facility because each profession has its own standards of both care and documentation.

Review Questions

1. List six medical specialties, and describe what those professionals do. Research five medical specialties that were not listed in the text, and discover what those professionals do.

2. Identify and describe five allied health professions and their principal occupational settings. Research four health-related professions that were not listed in the text, and discover what those professionals do.

3. Describe government involvement in health care.

4. The fundamental difference between ambulatory care and acute care is the patient's length of stay. Ambulatory patients are called *outpatients,* and acute care patients are called *inpatients.* In your own words, describe the differences between the two. What problems arise in an acute care facility in distinguishing between an outpatient and an inpatient? What are some other differences between ambulatory care and acute care?

5. Health care facilities can be compared in many ways other than length of stay. Organizational structure and ownership are two of those ways. List and describe in your own words how facilities can be different from one another.

6. Several types of health care settings were mentioned in this chapter. List as many different settings as you can remember. Identify and distinguish the various health care settings.

7. Health care facilities must be licensed to conduct business. However, they often choose to be accredited as well. What is licensure? What is accreditation? What is the difference between licensure and accreditation?

8. Many different organizations accredit health care facilities and educational programs. List as many accrediting bodies that you can remember and which facilities or programs they accredit.

9. If you were just diagnosed with diabetes, how would you go about finding a physician to care for you?

10. Identify a facility in your area by looking in the telephone book or on the Internet. Find out as much as you can about the facility, including the types of services that it offers. Describe the facility in terms of size, organization, patients, and average length of stay. What type of facility is it?

11. Log on to the AHIMA Web site (http://www.ahima.org). Explore the site. What does AHIMA say about careers in health information management? How many schools offer degrees in health information management? What courses are included in these programs?

12. What is the difference between occupational therapy and physical therapy? If you have trouble explaining the difference, try logging on to the Internet and find the Web sites for their national professional associations. What do those sites have to offer the public in terms of information about the profession?

13. The lines between inpatients and outpatients may become blurred under certain circumstances. An emergency department patient who is treated and released is clearly an outpatient. However, if the patient enters the emergency department at 11 p.m. and leaves at 4 a.m., the patient clearly arrived on one day and left on the next. Is this patient an inpatient or an outpatient? Why?

14. Some patients are kept in the hospital for observation. This is a special category of patients, neither outpatients nor inpatients, who may stay in the hospital for up to 24 hours without being admitted as inpatients. Can you think of a reason that this category of patients was created?

15. Match the diagnosis, activity, or patient group on the left with the name of the specialty on the right.

_____ 1. Administers substances that cause loss of sensation	A. Allergist
_____ 2. Cares for cancer patients	B. Anesthesiologist
_____ 3. Provides care related to the female reproductive system	C. Cardiologist
_____ 4. Cares for women before, during, and after delivery	D. Dermatologist
_____ 5. Delivers primary health care for children	E. Family practitioner
_____ 6. Delivers primary health care for patients of all ages	F. Gastroenterologist
_____ 7. Treats diseases and abnormal conditions of newborns	G. Gynecologist
_____ 8. Treats diseases of the digestive system	H. Neonatologist
_____ 9. Treats diseases of the heart and blood vessels	I. Obstetrician
_____ 10. Treats diseases of the muscles and bones	J. Oncologist
_____ 11. Treats diseases of the skin	K. Ophthalmologist
_____ 12. Deals with disorders of the mind	L. Orthopedist
_____ 13. Provides care related to eye diseases	M. Pathologist
_____ 14. Treats patients who have strong reactions to pollen and insect bites	N. Pediatrician
_____ 15. Studies changes in cells, tissue, and organs	O. Psychiatrist

16. Match accrediting bodies on the left with the type of organization on the right. Some accrediting bodies accredit more than one type of organization.

_____ 1. AAAHC	A. Acute care
_____ 2. AOA	B. Ambulatory care facilities
_____ 3. CARF	C. Home health care
_____ 4. CHAP	D. Managed care organizations
_____ 5. JCAHO	E. Osteopathic hospitals
_____ 6. NCQA	F. Rehabilitation facilities

Physician Office Liaison

My name is Melanie, and I have a very interesting position at a community hospital. I am a physician office liaison. I am responsible for helping the hospital maintain good relationships with the physicians on our staff. We are a small community hospital with 250 licensed beds. Our physicians are not employees of the hospital; they have privileges. This means that the hospital allows the physicians to admit their patients for treatment at the hospital. These physicians have private practices with their own offices and staff. It's my job to know them, to help with any problems they may have communicating with the hospital, and to coordinate the filing of their professional documentation.

I like my job because I get to meet many really interesting people, and I learn about their jobs as well. Even though I'm learning something new every day, I had to know a lot to get this job in the first place.

To be able to help a physician's office staff member, I have to know the various professionals who might work in an office and what they might do. It really helps that I know the difference between a medical assistant and a nurse practitioner. It's important that I know how a group practice works so that I can help the hospital keep track of which physicians can cover for each other.

The hospital collects statistics on physicians: how many patients they admit, what diagnoses they are treating, what procedures they are performing, and other information. I collaborate with other hospital departments to collect these reports and help present them at medical staff meetings. To do this, I have to know all the departments in the hospital and how they are related. I also need to understand the reports.

One of my most important tasks is credentialing. When a physician applies for privileges, I do a background check, collect the licensing documentation, and prepare a presentation for the credentialing committee. Because privileges aren't permanent, I remind the physicians when they need to reapply and help gather the updated documentation. I need to understand the differences among the medical specialties and what board certification means.

Finally, I coordinate continuing education sessions for physicians and their office staff. My next project is to develop a newsletter of hospital and physician activities that I can e-mail to the physicians' offices.

How did I get this job? I'm a registered health information technician. I have an associate degree in health information technology (HIT) from my local community college. In the HIT program, I learned a lot about physicians, hospitals, and other health-related professions. The hospital administrators were very happy to find a candidate for the job who already understood the system.

APPLICATION

An Ethical Dilemma

Vanessa is the supervisor of health information management at Community Hospital. She is a member of AHIMA and is studying to become a registered health information technician. Community Hospital has a new chief operating officer, Brad, who is new to the hospital and comes from another state. Brad is concerned that too many physicians are not completing their paperwork when patients are discharged. He would like Vanessa and her staff to send the paperwork out of the hospital to the physicians' offices for completion because he thinks that the physicians would be more likely to do the work if it were on their desks. Vanessa knows that the state licensure regulations prohibit the removal of the paperwork from the hospital under normal circumstances.

Should Vanessa comply with Brad's request? Is compliance with Brad's request a violation of the AHIMA Code of Ethics?

Chapter 2

PAYING FOR HEALTH CARE

CHAPTER OUTLINE

CHAPTER OBJECTIVES

By the end of this chapter, the student should be able to

- Identify and explain major reimbursement methods.
- Identify and describe the players in third party reimbursement.
- Explain the impact of a reimbursement method on the care provider.
- Explain the role of government in paying for health care.

VOCABULARY

admission denial

capitation

clinical pathway

continued stay denial

deductible

discharge planning

discounted fee for service

fee for service

fiscal intermediaries

flexible benefit account

group practice model HMO

health maintenance organization

(HMO)

indemnity insurance

independent practice association (IPA) model HMO

insurer

managed care

Medicare

Medicaid

per diem

preferred provider organization (PPO)

premiums

prospective payment

reciprocal services

risk

staff model HMO

Tax Equity and Fiscal Responsibility Act of 1982 (TEFRA)

third party payer

Title XVIII

Title XIX

usual and customary fees

utilization review

wraparound policies

REIMBURSEMENT

This section provides a general discussion of how reimbursement is accomplished in the health care industry, who is involved in the reimbursement process, what methodologies are used to calculate reimbursement, and how health information management (HIM) professionals are involved in the process. One of the most visible roles that HIM professionals play in health care today involves the reimbursement process (e.g., as a coding professional or clinical data manager).

The term *reimbursement* is something of a misnomer. It is generally used today to refer to the payment provided to a physician or other health care provider in exchange for services rendered. Actually, however, *reimbursement* means to be repaid. For example, a business traveler may pay for his or her hotel room with a personal credit card. After the traveler returns, his or her company repays, or reimburses, the traveler the amount of the hotel charges. With respect to reimbursement in health care, the same sequence of events occurs when a patient pays a physician directly for services rendered and then that patient requests reimbursement from the insurance company (the **insurer**). However, in general, the health care industry has come to call the direct payment from a payer for services provided by a physician or facility *reimbursement*, regardless of who is actually remitting the funds and when. In a hospital setting, for example, a hospital will provide services and supplies to a patient, thus incurring costs or charges, under the assumption that it will be reimbursed for these expenses after the patient has been discharged. Insurance plans today do not typically require a patient to reimburse a hospital and then submit a claim to the insurance company for reimbursement. Given the high costs of treatment today, many patients would not be able to pay a bill for hospitalization even if they were going to be reimbursed by their insurer later.

TYPES OF REIMBURSEMENT

Reimbursement takes many different forms. Historically, it was not uncommon for a physician to be "paid in kind." For example, a physician might have made a house call to treat a patient and then received chickens as payment, or compensation. These types of bartering arrangements were mutually acceptable to both physician and patient. Reimbursement today is generally monetary, especially for hospitalization services, but in many parts of the world and in the United States, bartering for services is common and acceptable.

Historically, a physician did not necessarily receive the payment that he or she charged but rather the payment that the patient thought the physician's services were worth. In the early twentieth century, this practice changed to paying what the physician charged. More recently, the amount of compensation given to the physician or health care provider is decided not by the patient or physician but by the insurance company. Insurance introduces a third party into the physician/patient relationship. **Third party payers** are usually insurance companies or government entities that have assumed the risk that a particular group of patients will require health care services and therefore incur the cost of paying for the services. In the following discussion, reimbursement is categorized according to the control that the health care provider exerts over the fees that are charged.

Fee for Service

As previously mentioned, a physician or other health care provider does not necessarily need to receive money as compensation. Perhaps chickens, bread, or other food is acceptable under certain circumstances. In other circumstances, services might be bartered (e.g., "You treat my pneumonia, and I will take care of your plumbing."). This is known as an exchange of services, or **reciprocal services**. The parties involved will decide the value of each service (e.g., how many hours of plumbing would be equal in value to how many hours of physician treatment). Again, however, monetary compensation is still the generally accepted reimbursement method in the United States.

Fee for service is the term assigned to the payment for services rendered by a physician, health care provider, or facility. It is sometimes referred to as "pay as you go" because this is how many patients without any insurance pay for treatments. The patient is essentially "buying" services or supplies. For example, a patient goes to, or "visits," the physician's office because of a runny nose. The physician examines the patient and determines that the patient is allergic to a house pet. This

Hit-Bit

Risk: The Big Picture

Risk is the danger that an activity will lead to an undesired outcome. In health care, risk applies to the patient, the physician, and the insurance company. The physician risks making an error in either the diagnosis or the treatment of the patient (obviously, this also presents a risk to the patient). There is also the risk that the physician will not be paid for the services rendered. The patient faces the risk that the cost of health care will be greater than the patient can bear, which would lead to excessive debt. For the payer, the risk is that claims for payment and administrative costs will exceed the premiums received. The payer may raise premiums to compensate; however, in so doing, the payer may lose subscribers. Overall, the financial risks and rewards in the health care industry are a delicate balancing act.

service, which comprises an office visit and examination, costs $100.00. This $100.00 is the "fee." Suppose this same patient also needs an allergy shot, and this shot costs $20.00. In this case, the total cost of (or fee for) the visit is $120.00. As this example shows, there are fees that correspond to the services rendered—hence, "fee for service."

If you compare the fees charged by physicians in a particular state or geographic area, you will find that the fees for services are similar. Ignoring the very high and very low fees in your comparison, you would be able to determine the **usual and customary fees** charged by physicians in that area. To determine usual and customary fees, it is necessary to compare not only the services but also the specialties of the physicians providing the services. The term *usual and customary fees* commonly appears in the language of insurance contracts because this is the fee that third party payers are willing to reimburse for services. For example, a physician may decide to charge $100.00 for an office visit, but the insurer will reimburse only $80.00, if $80.00 is the usual and customary fee for that specialty in that area.

Discounted Fee for Service

Within this category of reimbursement are other negotiated fees. For a typical discounted fee, the third party payer (in this case, the insurer) negotiates a payment that is less than the provider's normal rate. For example, the provider may charge $100 for a service. The insurer assumes that the volume of patients added to the provider's business would warrant a 10% discount from the normal rate. Therefore the payment for the service would be $90.

Some insurers reimburse at flat rates, known as **per diem** (daily) rates, for service. A per diem rate is basically a flat fee, negotiated in advance, that an insurer will pay for each day of hospitalization. For inpatient health care providers or facilities, per diem rates may represent a significant discount from the actual accumulated fees for each individual service performed, but again the provider or facility benefits by gaining that payer's business. Per diem rates are most commonly negotiated with providers who serve a limited patient population, such as providers of rehabilitation services.

Prospective Payment

Prospective payment is a method of determining the payment to a health care provider on the basis of predetermined factors, not on individual costs for services. Numerous insurers and government agencies use prospective payment systems for reimbursement, most notably the Medicare Prospective Payment System (PPS), which is discussed in detail in Chapter 6. PPSs are based on the statistical analysis of large quantities of historical health care data for the purpose of evaluating the resources used to treat specific diagnoses and effect certain treatments. On the basis of this evaluation, it has been determined that certain diagnoses and procedures consume sufficiently similar resources, such that reimbursement to the facility for these patients should be the same. For this purpose, resources are measured in both costs and days. Essentially, the provider receives a payment that represents the historical average cost of treating patients with that particular combination of diagnoses and procedures.

For example, suppose a review of 10,000 uncomplicated appendectomies reveals that patients are hospitalized for an average of 2 days. The statistical average charges for these hospitalizations, based on the 10,000 uncomplicated appendectomy cases, is $5,000.00. An insurer who uses a prospective payment system to reimburse a facility will pay that facility $5,000.00, regardless of how long a given patient who received an uncomplicated appendectomy was actually hospitalized or what the actual charges were. If the charges for that hospitalization were actually $4,500.00, the facility would still receive $5,000.00. If the charges for that hospitalization were actually $5,500.00, the facility would still receive $5,000.00. The use of the term *prospective* in this type of reimbursement system means that both the facility and the insurer know, *in advance*, how much each type of case will be reimbursed.

From the payer's perspective, prospective payment can be an extremely effective budgeting tool. Utilization trends can be followed, types of cases can be analyzed in groups, and reimbursement costs can be better controlled through rate setting for each type of case. From the perspective of the provider or facility, there is greater motivation to keep costs under tight control. If there are inefficiencies within the facilities or among physicians, facilities may lose income. However, critics of PPSs, including some physicians, maintain that prospective payment focuses only on the financial aspects of treating a patient and does not take into consideration individual, case-by-case clinical management.

Capitation

Another type of payment is **capitation.** Capitation requires payment to a health care provider regardless of whether the patient is seen or how frequently the patient is seen during a given period of time. For example, a physician might receive $5.00 a month for each patient under an insurance plan whose patients choose him or her as their primary care physician. If there are 100 patients who choose this physician as their primary care physician, the physician receives $500.00 a month for those patients—even if none comes in for a visit. If all 100 patients are seen in one month, the physician still receives $500.00. Generally, however, the more patients who choose this physician under a capitation plan, the greater the odds that that physician will receive adequate overall payment for his or her services, especially if that group of patients is relatively healthy and does not make many office visits. The insurer will still benefit if it is less costly to pay a known monthly capitation fee rather than reimburse an unpredictable amount of money to the physician each month.

COMPARISON OF REIMBURSEMENT METHODS

Table 2-1 summarizes the four methods of reimbursement previously discussed: fee for service, discounted fee for service, prospective payment, and capitation. To distinguish among these methods, remember the previous example of the patient's visit to the doctor's office for an allergy shot. That visit, under fee for service, cost $100. Under **discounted fee for service**, perhaps a

TABLE 2-1	Comparison of Reimbursement Methods
METHOD*	**DESCRIPTION**
Fee for service	Pay for services rendered
Discounted fee for service	Pay for services rendered but at a rate lower than the usual fee for a service
Prospective payment	Pay a flat rate based on diagnoses, procedures, or a combination of the two
Capitation	Pay a regular, flat rate to the provider regardless of whether services are rendered

*There are numerous variations on these methods, and exceptions to a normal method of payment are made under certain circumstances. For example, under prospective payment, additional compensation can sometimes be obtained if it is medically necessary for the patient to be hospitalized far in excess of the average length of stay for the diagnosis or procedure.

contract was negotiated for payment based on a discount of 10% of the fee for service. Therefore under discount fee for service, the same visit would cost $90. Under a PPS, based on a statistical analysis of costs associated with office visits for allergy shots, the insurance company may reimburse the physician $85. Under capitation, the insurance company would not pay the physician anything for a particular visit, paying instead $5.00 each month for that patient, which would amount to $60 annually but may involve additional visits.

These methods vary widely, and exceptions to a normal method of payment are made under certain circumstances. For example, under PPS, additional compensation sometimes can be obtained if it is medically necessary for the patient to be hospitalized far in excess of the average length of stay for the case.

Exercise 2-1

Reimbursement

1. The payer had an agreement with the physician to pay the usual and customary fee, less 10%. This is an example of _____.
2. What incentive do physicians have to operate under each of the four methods of reimbursement discussed?
   Use the following scenario to answer Questions 3 and 4:
   The 82-year-old patient came to the physician's office for a routine physical examination. He gave the receptionist two cards proving his primary, government-funded insurance plan, which pays for most of the bill, and an additional private plan that covers the remaining charges.
3. The patient's primary insurance is most likely _____.
4. The patient's secondary insurance is called _____.
5. The physician charged the patient $75 for the office visit. The patient paid the physician $5, and the patient's insurance company paid the physician $70. This method of reimbursement is called _____.
6. The physician charged the patient $75 for the office visit. The patient paid the physician $5, and the patient's insurance company paid the physician $70. The patient's portion of the payment is called _____.
7. Match the definition on the left with the health insurance terminology on the right.
   1. Amount of cost that the beneficiary must incur before the insurance will assume liability for the remaining cost
   2. Contractor that manages the health care claims
   3. One who is eligible to receive or is receiving benefits from an insurance policy or a managed care program
   4. Party who is financially responsible for reimbursement of health care cost
   5. Payer's payment for specific health care services or, in managed care, the health care services that will be provided or for which the provider will be paid
   6. Payment by a third party to a provider of health care
   7. Request for payment by the insured or the provider for services covered

   A. Beneficiary
   B. Benefit
   C. Claim
   D. Deductible
   E. Fiscal intermediary
   F. Payer
   G. Reimbursement

INSURANCE

HISTORY

Insurance companies have existed for centuries. Notably, Lloyds of London insured cargoes on merchant ships, which were frequently subject to loss from piracy, inclement weather, and other catastrophes. The beginnings of insurance in health care date only to the mid-nineteenth century, when companies insured railroad and paddleboat employees in the event of catastrophic injury or death. A lump sum was paid to the employee or employee's family after these events.

The origins of modern health care insurance, as we know it today in the United States, began after the Great Depression of 1929. The decline in health care industry income prompted the development of hospital-based insurance plans. For example, for a payment of a small sum, a hospital guaranteed a specific number of days of hospital care at no additional charge. The most successful of these plans was developed at Baylor University (Sultz and Young 28), which eventually became the model for what we know today as Blue Cross Hospital Insurance. Table 2-2 contains definitions of several terms that are useful during any discussion of health insurance.

In the early days of the industry, health care insurance was paid for by the recipient, sometimes through the employer, union, or other organization. In the original Baylor University scheme, teachers paid $0.50 a month, which entitled them to 21 days of hospital care should they need it (Sultz and Young 2006). The insurance company became a third party payer in the relationship between the provider and patient.

After World War II, employers began offering their employees certain benefits, including health insurance. Benefits packages became useful in enabling employers to hire and retain employees.

TABLE 2-2	Terminology Common to Health Insurance Policies
TERM	**DESCRIPTION**
Benefit	Amount of money paid for specific health care services or, in managed care, the health care services that will be provided from an insurance policy or a managed care program
Beneficiary	One who is eligible to receive or is receiving benefits from an insurance policy or a managed care program
Benefit period	Time frame in which the insurance benefits are covered; varies from insurance policy to policy
Claim	Request for payment by the insured or the provider for services covered
Co-payment	Type of cost-sharing in which the insured (subscriber) pays out-of-pocket a fixed amount for health care service
Coverage	Types of diseases, conditions, and diagnostic and therapeutic procedures for which the insurance policy will pay
Deductible	Amount of cost that the beneficiary must incur before the insurance company will assume liability for the remaining cost
Exclusion	Specific conditions or hazards for which a health care policy will not grant benefit payments; often includes preexisting conditions and experimental therapy
Fiscal intermediary	Contractor that manages health care claims
Insurance	Purchased contract (policy) in which the purchaser (insured) is protected from loss by the insurer's agreement to reimburse for such loss
Out-of-pocket costs	Money that the patient pays directly to the health care provider
Payer	Party who is financially responsible for reimbursement of health care cost
Premium	Payment required to maintain policy coverage; usually paid periodically
Preexisting condition	Disease, injury, or condition identified as having occurred before a specific date
Reimbursement	Payment by a third party to a provider of health care
Rider	Policy amendment that either increases or decreases benefits
Policy	Written contract between insurance company and subscriber (insured) that specifies the coverage, benefits, exclusions, co-payments, deductibles, benefit period, and so on
Subscriber	Person who elects to enroll or participate in managed care or purchase health care insurance
Third party payer	Party (insurance company, state or federal entity, other) that is responsible for paying the provider on behalf of the insured (subscriber, patient, member) for health care services rendered

From Mervat Abedlhak, Sara Grostick, Mary Alice Hanken, and Ellen Jacobs. *Health Information Management of a Strategic Resource*, Philadelphia, Saunders, 1996, p 37.

Employees benefited because they did not need to spend the money on **premiums** anymore, and employers benefited because health insurance benefits were a relatively low cost in the course of doing business. Insurance companies benefited from an increased client base. However, this thrust a fourth party into the provider/patient relationship: the employer.

Originally, the focus of insurance was on the coverage of services at the health care provider's fee. If the provider raised the fee, the insurance company raised its premiums to cover these costs. As health care costs increased, the premiums began to increase dramatically. Currently, many employers pay only a part of the premiums, with employees bearing the rest of the cost.

ASSUMPTION OF RISK

The previous example of the patient's office visit for an allergy shot and the comparison of possible financial outcomes based on type of reimbursement serve to illustrate and emphasize the concept of risk. There is a risk involved to each party under each reimbursement scenario; each party would like to minimize the risk of a financial loss for treating patients or for reimbursing providers. Each party negotiates contracts and attempts to minimize its risks by taking all potential treatment costs and circumstances into consideration. For example, a physician may agree to a capitation fee of $5.00 per patient monthly but only if the insurer's patient group has an average age of 45. The insurer also may insist that all patients covered under a discounted fee for service group plan be nonsmokers. Health care providers render services for which they expect to be fairly compensated. Patients need these services, but they would like someone else to pay for them because these services might otherwise be unaffordable. Insurance companies are willing to assume the risk of having to pay for expensive services, but they would like to balance their risk by insuring a large number of patients, many of whom will likely not need health care services at all. The assumption of risk is the foundation of the concept of insurance.

Insurance companies serve the public by assuming the risk of financial loss. If you own an automobile, you probably have auto insurance. You pay periodic premiums to the auto insurance company, which in turn covers all or part of the costs incurred in an accident. The auto insurance company, although assuming the risk of financial loss in the event of an accident, is gambling that you won't have one. In fact, it goes to great lengths to predict the likelihood of accidents in certain populations, geographic areas, and types of vehicles. If you pay $1,000.00 per year in auto insurance premiums for 40 years and never have an accident, then the insurance company keeps the $40,000.00 (plus interest) accumulated over the course of your policy. If the auto insurance company insures a very large number of drivers, in theory and under normal circumstances, only a small percentage of them will ever have a costly accident. In some states, auto insurance companies are permitted to choose which drivers they wish to insure. Obviously, they would prefer to choose drivers with good driving records and no history of accidents. In other states, insurers may not pick and choose and must offer insurance to anyone who applies for it. This requirement raises the risk that the insurer will be required to pay for the costs of accidents and resultant settlements, which in turn raises the cost of auto insurance for all unless the premiums of the high-risk drivers are raised significantly to compensate.

Health insurance works in a similar way. The insurer wants to cover large numbers of individuals so that the risk that someone will require expensive medical care is offset by large numbers of individuals who require less expensive care (Figure 2-1). In an environment of rising health care costs, increases in reimbursements trigger increases in premiums. The insertion of the employer into the patient/provider relationship has at least two effects: loss of control over the choice of individuals to cover and loss of total freedom to raise premiums. The insurer is pressured to accept all employees, reducing the insurer's ability to control risk by eliminating the choice as to which individuals to cover. If one individual cancels a policy, the impact is far less financially dramatic than if an employer cancels a group policy. Therefore the insurer is pressured to keep premiums low so as not to lose the employer's account.

TYPES OF INSURANCE

There are many different insurance plans, with an almost endless variety of benefits and reimbursement rules. Plans may set dollar-amount limits or visit limits on the benefits in given time

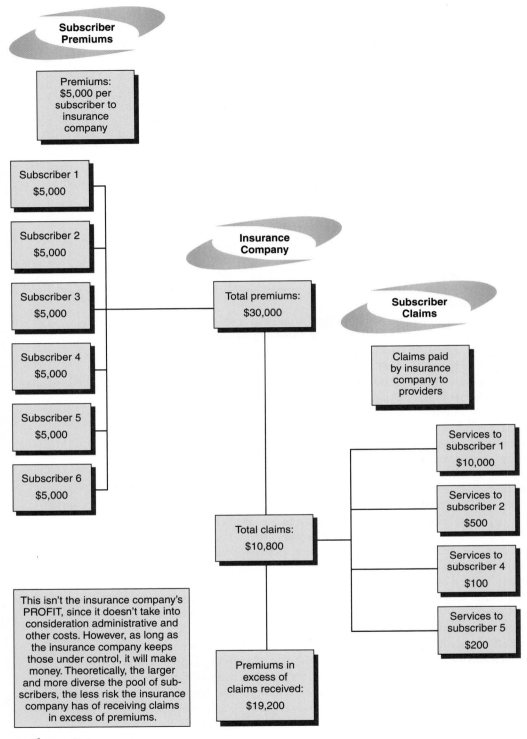

◆ **Figure 2-1**

How insurance companies reduce risk.

periods. Nevertheless, plans fall into one of two basic categories: indemnity and managed care. Managed care plans are further divided into two major types: preferred provider organizations and health maintenance organizations. The major features of these plans are discussed later in this chapter. The plans differ in the relationships among the physician, patient, and insurer. In addition, some plans are more likely than others to use certain reimbursement methods.

Indemnity

A typical insurance arrangement requires the patient to pay the physician or other health care provider and then submit the bills to the insurance company for reimbursement. Under the terms of the insurance contract is a list of services for which the insurance company agrees to pay: the covered services. If the patient receives a covered service, then the insurance company reimburses the patient. Some insurance companies pay 100% of the cost of certain covered services and a lower percentage of the cost of other covered services. This type of insurance, called **indemnity insurance**, was the predominant type of health insurance for many years. Indemnity insurance plans still exist, but managed care insurance plans have become more prevalent.

An important feature of indemnity insurance is the **deductible**. A deductible is the amount of for which the patient is personally responsible. It must be spent or paid before any insurance benefits are paid. For example, a patient with medical expenses of $5,000 and a deductible of $300 pays the first $300 out-of-pocket. Then the insurer pays whatever portion of the remaining $4,700 is covered by the policy. The patient is responsible for any noncovered expenses.

Depending on the insurance company plan, a deductible could apply for every encounter, every visit, or every hospitalization, or it could be applied on an annual basis. If your insurance plan covers your whole family, your deductible could be per person or per family. One effect of the deductible is that routine heath care costs often do not exceed the deductible amount. In these instances, the insurance company ultimately covers and pays for only unusual or extraordinary expenses. Conversely, indemnity contracts often specify limits for reimbursement of certain covered services. Thus if the benefit limit is $3000 for physician office visits and the patient's care (after the deductible) is $4000, then the patient is responsible for the additional $1000.

One of the ways in which indemnity insurance plans affected the health care industry was to contribute to the increase in dollars being spent on health care. In the physician/patient relationship, the patient bears the cost of the care and therefore has some influence on the fees. Individuals may choose not to go to the physician in the first place because they feel the fee is too high and they can't afford it, or they might be able to afford only some services. Because indemnity insurance plans, even with the deductible, reduce the out-of-pocket expense to the patient, they increase the likelihood that the services of the provider will be used regardless of the fees. Consequently, the number of people actually using health care services under indemnity plans may increase. In addition, if the insurance company reimburses for services without reviewing the need for those services, then physicians have no incentive to be conservative in diagnosis and treatment. The costs have risen still further with advances in diagnostic and therapeutic technologies, many of which are extremely costly in their initial phases. As these technologies become available and are more widely used, the cost of health care increases.

In addition to the technology-driven expenses, health care costs increased because a small portion of the health care community provided an excessive number of services to their patients. Two x-rays may have been taken when one would have sufficed, or a computed tomography scan or magnetic resonance imaging was used when a simple x-ray would have been sufficient to achieve the same diagnostic goal. Often, it is not entirely the provider's fault when these excesses occur. Some patients may feel entitled to the newest technologies even if they aren't necessary, and so they pressure their physicians into ordering these expensive treatments. The physician may not want to lose this patient's business or, worse, be subjected to a lawsuit later.

To meet the rising costs of health care, insurance companies raised health care premiums. Eventually, some employers could no longer afford to offer health insurance as a benefit. Many employers began shifting the cost of insurance to the employees. Other employers solved the problem by hiring more part-time employees, who were not eligible for benefits. Still other employers hired outside contractors to perform noncritical functions.

Some of the consequences of rising health care costs have been attempts by the insurance companies to control the amount of dollars actually being spent on health care. Insurance companies attempt to control costs in various ways. First, as previously discussed, they can impose deductibles. They can strictly limit the number and types of covered services. However, insurance becomes less attractive under these circumstances, and insurance companies want to remain in business. The insurance industry responded to these circumstances and factors, opening the door to the concept of managed care plans.

Managed Care

The term **managed care** is very broad. In general, it refers to the control that an insurance company or other payer exerts over the reimbursement process and the patient's choices in selecting a health care provider.

In the pure physician/patient relationship, the patient uses the physician of his or her choice. The patient arrives at the office with a medical concern, and the physician determines a diagnosis and develops a treatment plan. The patient agrees (or declines) to undergo the treatment plan, the physician bills the patient, and the patient pays the physician.

Under managed care, the insurer (payer) and the physician (provider) have a contractual arrangement with each other. These physicians participate in a particular managed care plan, which means that they are under contract with the managed care plan insurer to provide services to the insurer's patients. Managed care patients are referred to, depending on the insurer, as members, enrollees or covered lives. The primary insured member is the subscriber, with those covered under the subscriber's policy referred to as dependents or additional insured. The insurer's patients must choose their physicians from those participating in the managed care plan. The scope of services paid for is determined by the insurer's contract with the subscriber (or the subscriber's employer or group manager). Decisions about the appropriateness of specific services are made by the managed care organization, not necessarily by the patient's physician.

In a managed care scenario, the patient goes to the primary care physician (PCP) whom the patient has chosen from the list of participating physicians. The physician diagnoses and treats the patient according to guidelines from the managed care plan. The patient may pay the physician a small co-pay. The physician bills the managed care insurer directly for the visit. The managed care insurer may refuse to pay the physician if the physician does not obtain preapproval—or authorization for some treatments, such as hospitalization. The managed care insurer may also bill the patient if preapproval is not obtained. If the patient sees a physician outside of the plan, the patient may not be covered at all and may have to pay the physician himself or herself. In

Hit-Bit

The Insurance Contract

An insurance contract is essentially the promise to pay for certain health care costs incurred by the subscriber in return for the payment of a premium to the insurer by either the subscriber or another party. When the subscriber contracts directly with the insurer, the premium is not usually negotiable. However, when the subscriber is a member of a larger group, such as that provided by an employer, both the premium and the services for which the insurer will pay may be subject to negotiation.

Insurance companies (particularly managed care organizations) also negotiate with providers to determine the services that apply to that provider, how much the insurer is willing to pay for those services, and under what circumstances the provider may render those services. Providers apply to be included in insurer's lists of in-plan providers. Because subscribers are encouraged to choose providers from those lists, being on multiple lists is theoretically a good business decision for providers. However, if insurers reduce payments and restrict services, providers may decide to avoid these payer relationships entirely. In fact, physicians may elect not to accept insurance at all, requiring patients to file cumbersome claims for reimbursement with their insurers.

many instances, the patient cannot go to a specialist directly but must visit the PCP first. After examination and discussion with the patient, the PCP must justify the necessity for the involvement of a specialist and refer the patient to a specialist participating in the plan. The managed care organization scenario can vary in myriad ways, which are discussed later in this chapter.

Managed care organizations seek to reduce costs by controlling as much of the health care delivery system as possible. The underlying rationale for managed care is to reduce overall costs by eliminating unnecessary tests, procedures, visits, and hospitalizations through financial incentives if the plan is followed and financial punishment if the plan is not followed. A major controversy in this strategy lies in the definition of what constitutes unnecessary health care and who makes this determination. Traditionally, physicians have determined the care that they provide to patients, whereas managed care has shifted that determination to the insurer. It should be noted that managed care plans employ physicians who assist in making determinations, although critics of these plans claim that these physicians have an incentive to save the managed care insurer money rather than provide all treatments to patients. For example, many managed care insurers did not consider preventive care to be necessary and would not pay for it. It was only through years of study, investigation, and trial and error that they discovered that preventive care was one of the best ways to reduce health care costs. This fact is particularly salient with regard to pregnancy care. The costs of treating a pregnant woman through prenatal testing, education, and regular examinations, with the goal of delivering a healthy newborn, is significantly less than treating a newborn or new mother with complications that could have been prevented or treated earlier at less cost. The same holds true for dental care. Theoretically, if you have your teeth examined and cleaned routinely, you will not need expensive fillings and root canal treatments later because your dentist will help you detect and treat those problems early.

Beyond preventive care, the extent to which managed care organizations control the services provided continues to spark controversy. For example, by requiring preapproval and second opinions for some procedures, managed care organizations assert that they are delivering cost-effective, high-quality care. Low patient out-of-pocket costs and, in some instances, reduced paperwork are further enticements. However, patients are often frustrated by the preapproval process, the seeming incentive of physicians *not* to treat, and the sometimes limited choice of physicians.

Individuals who change jobs are often forced to find new health care providers if their previous physicians are not included in the new insurer's plan. The same may be true if the employer changes insurers. Patients who live at the outskirts of a plan's primary service area may be required to travel unacceptably long distances to receive covered health care services.

Physicians often feel a loss of control in the treatment process. They are sometimes frustrated by the emphasis on medical practice standards, what some call "cookbook medicine," and resistance to what they may see as individualized alternative approaches of care. Managed care organizations focus heavily on statistical analysis of treatment outcomes and scrutinize physicians whose practices appear to vary significantly from the norm. Managed care has forced physicians to become more aware of and active in managing their own resources by employing reimbursement methods other than fee for service that shift some financial risk to the physician.

Despite controversy and criticism, managed care has become an important presence in the health care arena. Managed care takes a number of different forms, and there are many variations in the relationship among managed care organizations and physicians and other health care providers who deliver their services. At the heart of managed care is the idea that the insurer can gain better control over cost of health care by delivering the services directly. The U.S. Congress supported this concept with the Health Maintenance Organization Act of 1973, which encouraged the development of **health maintenance organizations (HMOs)** and mandated certain employers to offer employees an HMO option for health care delivery.

Health Maintenance Organizations

An HMO is a managed care organization that has ownership or employer control over the health care provider. Essentially, the HMO is the insurer (payer) and the provider. Members must use the HMO for all services, and the HMO will not pay for out-of-plan services without prior approval. In some plans, approval to obtain health care services outside of the plan is granted only in emergency situations.

In the **staff model HMO**, the organization owns the facilities, employs the physicians, and provides essentially all health care services. In a **group practice model HMO**, the organization contracts with a group or a network of physicians and facilities to provide health care services. Finally, in an **independent practice association (IPA) model HMO**, the HMO contracts with individual physicians, a portion of whose practices is devoted to the HMO. Regardless of the HMO model, an HMO seeks to limit services to approved providers. Payment for out-of-plan care is extremely limited and usually requires preapproval.

Preferred Provider Organizations

A **preferred provider organization (PPO)** is another managed care approach in which the organization contracts with a network of health care providers who agree to certain reimbursement rates. It is from this network that patients are encouraged to choose their primary care physician and any specialists. If a patient chooses a provider who is not in the network, the PPO reimburses in the same manner as an indemnity insurer: for specified services, with specific dollar amounts or percentage limits, and after any deductible is paid by the insured.

A PPO is a hybrid plan that gives patients the option of choosing physicians outside the plan without totally forfeiting benefits. In addition, PPOs may offer patients a certain degree of freedom to self-refer to specialists. For example, some plans allow patients to visit gynecologists and vision specialists directly, without referral from the PCP.

Self-Insurance

Although not specifically a type of insurance, self-insurance (or self-funded insurance) is an alternative to purchasing an insurance policy. The term *self-insurance* should not be confused with patients who "self-pay," or those without any insurance or coverage plan at all. Self-insurance is really a savings plan in which an individual or employer puts aside funds to cover health care costs. In this way, the individual or company assumes the financial risk associated with health care. Because the assumption of risk rests with the company or the individual, this is not so much a type of insurance as it is an alternative to shifting the risk to an insurer.

An employer may choose to self-insure for all health care benefits, or it may self-insure to provide specific benefits that its primary insurance plan does not cover. For example, an insurance plan may cover preventive care, hospital and physician services, and diagnostic tests. However, it may not cover vision or dental care. The employer may designate to each employee a certain dollar amount with which the employee may then be reimbursed for these other services. Ordinarily, if the annual dollar amount is not spent, it is lost to the employee. Because the issue of confidentiality is so important, employers may choose to contract with an insurer to process health care claims, even if the employer self-insures.

Individuals may self-insure by saving money on a regular basis through their employer. These savings are designated for health care expenses. One formal plan that enables individuals to save in this manner is a **flexible benefit account** (or medical savings account). A flexible benefit account provides the individual with a savings account, usually through payroll deduction, into which a set amount determined by the employee can be deposited routinely. These funds can then be drawn on to pay out-of-pocket health care and some childcare expenses. The advantage to a flexible benefit account is that the funds are withdrawn from the individual's salary on a pre-tax basis, thereby reducing the individual's income tax liability. The disadvantage is that non-disbursed funds are forfeited at the end of the year. Table 2-3 summarizes the four types of insurance that have been discussed.

CLINICAL OVERSIGHT

In Chapter 1, the patient care plan was described as a collaborative process involving the physicians, nurses, and other allied health professionals. The patient care plan is more than just a series of instructions or recommendations for an individual patient. Clinicians typically follow established patterns of care that are based on experience, successful outcomes, and research. The formal description of these patterns of care is the **clinical pathway**. Each discipline has a specific clinical pathway that describes the appropriate steps to take, given a specific diagnosis or a specific set of signs and symptoms and based on the answers to critical questions. For example, a

TABLE 2-3	**Summary of Health Insurance Relationships**

INSURANCE	MAJOR FEATURES
Self-insurance	Employer may reserve funds to cover projected medical expenses. Covered employees may contribute to fund. Insured sets aside pretax dollars to cover specific medical expenses, such as vision care. Unused funds are lost.
Indemnity	Employer maintains group policy with insurer, thereby spreading the risk among many. Employer may pay all or part of the premium. Employer sets policy as to classification of eligible employees and collects employee share of premium, if any.
HMO	Providers are limited to those in the plan. Patient pays small co-payment. Covered services must be medically necessary. Providers tend to be employees of the HMO or to have exclusive contracts with HMO.
PPO	Combination of HMO and indemnity features. Providers are independent contractors.

patient with high blood glucose (hyperglycemia) must be tested to determine whether the patient is diabetic. If the patient is diabetic, further studies will identify whether the condition is insulin dependent or not. The physician will prescribe the appropriate medications and other regimens on the basis of that determination. Nursing staff will assess the patient's level of understanding of his or her condition and take the appropriate steps to educate the patient and possibly the family. Figure 2-2 illustrates a clinical pathway.

Case Management

Although the responsibility for patient care rests with the provider, there are often multiple providers, and possibly multiple facilities, involved in a patient's care. From the payer's perspective, case managers are necessary to coordinate the approval of and adherence to the care plan. From the provider's perspective, case managers are necessary to facilitate the continuum of care. Thus a given patient may have multiple case managers working from different perspectives, all helping to ensure that the patient is cared for appropriately and efficiently.

Utilization Review

Understanding clinical pathways and payer issues enables facilities to evaluate patient care, control the use of facility resources, and measure the performance of individual clinical staff. Staff members in a hospital's utilization review (UR) department work closely with all health care disciplines involved in caring for a patient who has been admitted. UR staff members are responsible, with physician oversight, for performing an admission review that covers the appropriateness of the admission itself, certifying the level of care for an admission (e.g., acute, skilled nursing), monitoring the intensity of services provided, and ensuring that a patient's length of stay is appropriate for that level of care. UR staff members may have daily contact with a patient's insurance company during the patient's admission to verify that the correct level of care payment will be received for the anticipated length of stay. UR staff also may make provisions for aftercare once the patient is discharged. This is called **discharge planning**.

For example, suppose a patient with insulin-dependent diabetes mellitus (IDDM) is admitted because the patient did a self-check at home and could not control his blood sugar even while taking the prescribed amounts of daily insulin. UR staff members will be notified that the patient has been admitted, and they will perform an admission review. This admission review entails an evaluation of the patient's medical record, including physician orders and any test results. In some cases, the admission will be deemed unnecessary. The admission might be unnecessary if the patient's blood glucose levels were all normal on admission. At that point, UR staff members would not certify the admission for reimbursement; this is called an **admission denial**.

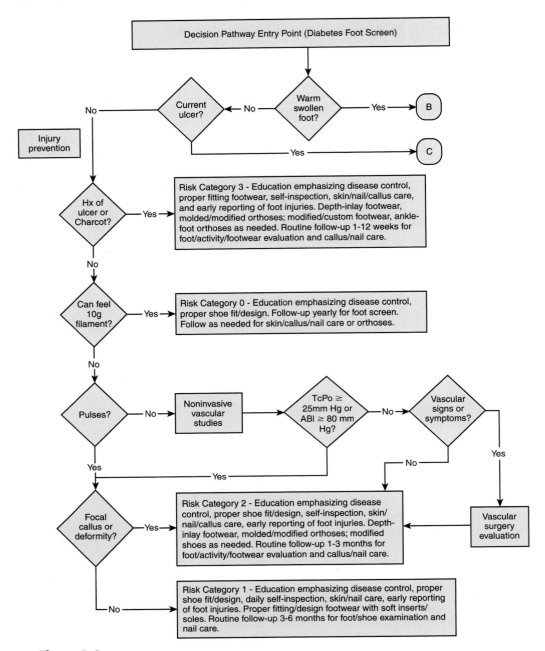

◆ **Figure 2-2**
Clinical pathways. (From Charles A. Patout Jr, James A. Birke, Wayne A. Wilbright, William C. Coleman, and Ronnie E. Mathews *Arch Phys Med Rehabil* 82 [2001]: 1724–8.)

If UR staff members deem the admission necessary, it will certify the admission. UR staff may contact the patient's insurer, verify the diagnosis of uncontrolled IDDM, and determine that the anticipated length of stay for that diagnosis is 2 to 3 days. The insurer agrees to reimburse the hospital for 3 days of acute care as certified by UR staff. During the hospitalization, UR staff members will discuss the aftercare, or discharge plan, with the attending physician. In this case, perhaps more home care services are warranted. On the third day, the patient is expected to be discharged. If the patient is not discharged on Day 3, members of the UR staff must review documentation and discuss the case further with the physician to justify additional hospitalization. If the additional days are not justified by the documentation in the medical record, the additional days may not be reimbursed by the insurer. This is called a **continued stay denial**. In these instances, the patient will be notified that he or she no longer needs to be in the hospital, that the insurer will not reimburse the hospital for any additional costs, and that the patient is responsible for all further costs. When this happens, the physician is also notified. The physician will either concur with the continued stay denial and discharge the patient or provide documentation justifying the additional care.

Exercise 2-2

Insurance

1. Each type of reimbursement has unique characteristics and a different approach to risk. Compare and contrast the four types of reimbursement, identifying the financial risk to the parties involved.
2. Health care insurance involves the assumption of the risk of financial loss by a party other than the patient. Describe how insurance companies can afford to assume such risk.
3. The text discussed three different types of health insurance. List them, and describe how they are different.

GOVERNMENT INFLUENCE ON REIMBURSEMENT

Although the United States does not have universal health care (i.e., government-subsidized health care for all citizens), the various levels of government do serve as the largest payer for health care services.

FEDERAL COVERAGE FOR SPECIFIC POPULATIONS

The U.S. federal government has historically allocated funds for the benefits of specific populations. In the case of health care, target populations of chronically ill or indigent patients have received low-cost or free health care. Until the 1960s, funding was not entirely predictable and health care providers were often required to provide a certain amount of charity care. In addition, there were large groups of individuals with limited incomes who were not eligible for federal assistance. The federal government took the plunge in the mid-1960s with the enactment of legislation that made it the largest single payer in the health care industry: Title XVIII and Title XIX of the Social Security Act, which established the Medicare and Medicaid programs.

In addition to Medicare and Medicaid, Congress also created the Civilian Health and Medical Program of the Uniformed Services (CHAMPUS), which provides health benefits for military personnel, their families, and military retirees. CHAMPUS is now called TRICARE. The federal government provides health services to veterans through the Veterans Health Administration (VHA). The Civilian Health and Medical Program of the Veterans Administration (CHAMPVA) was created in 1973 to provide health services for spouses and children of certain deceased or disabled veterans. TRICARE, VHA, and CHAMPVA are service benefits, not insurance, and are included here to illustrate the extent of the federal government's financial involvement in health care. (See the TRICARE and CHAMPVA Web sites for additional information.) Table 2-4 provides a summary of this involvement.

The Indian Health Services (IHS) provides care for American Indians and Alaska Natives. According to the IHS, the agency provides the following services:

- Assisting Indian tribes to develop their health programs
- Facilitating and assisting Indian tribes in coordinating health planning
- Obtaining and using health resources available
- Operating comprehensive health care services and health programs

- Providing comprehensive health care services
- Advocating in the health field to ensure comprehensive health services for American Indian and Alaska Native people. (http://www.ihs.gov)

MEDICARE

Title XVIII of the Social Security Act established the Medicare program in 1965. Originally enacted to provide funding for health care for the elderly, Medicare has grown to include patients with disabilities, those who require renal dialysis, and those who have undergone organ transplants. For some health care providers, Medicare represents more than 50% of their income. Medicare is an extremely important driving force in the insurance industry because many insurance companies follow Medicare's lead in adopting reimbursement strategies.

The Medicare program, although funded by the federal government and administered by the Centers for Medicare and Medicaid Services (CMS), does not process its own claims reimbursements. Reimbursements are processed by **fiscal intermediaries** located in different regions throughout the country. The Blue Cross and Blue Shield companies are the most common fiscal intermediaries. These companies are not-for-profit insurance companies.

Medicare coverage applies in four categories: Parts A, B, C, and D. Part A covers inpatient hospital services. Part B covers physician claims and outpatient services. Part C is a voluntary managed care option. Part D, implemented in 2006, is a prescription drug program.

Because there are limits to Medicare coverage, many beneficiaries choose to purchase additional insurance; such plans are called **wraparound policies** (supplemental policies) and are aimed at absorbing costs not reimbursed by Medicare. Many end-of-life hospital stays generate costs in the hundreds of thousands of dollars. Therefore wraparound policies can help to preserve estates and save surviving spouses from financial ruin.

Medicare beneficiaries also may enroll in a Medicare HMO program, called Medicare+Choice. Different HMOs have contracted with the federal government under the Medicare+Choice program to provide health services to these beneficiaries.

TABLE 2-4	Summary of Federal Involvement in Health Care Reimbursement	
ACRONYM	**DESCRIPTION**	**COVERED LIVES**
Medicare	Title XVIII of the Social Security Act (1965)	Elderly, disabled, renal dialysis, and transplant patients Part A: inpatient services Part B: outpatient services and physician claims Part C: managed care option Part D: prescription drug benefit
Medicaid	Title XIX of the Social Security Act (1965)	Low income patients
TRICARE	Medical services for members of the armed services, their spouses and families	Administered by the Department of Defense and applying to members of the: Army, Air Force, Navy, Marine Corps, Coast Guard, Public Health Service, or the National Oceanic and Atmospheric Administration
VHA	Veterans Health Administration	Health services for veterans
CHAMPVA	Civilian Health and Medical Program of the Department of Veterans Affairs (CHAMPVA)	U.S. Department of Veterans Affairs (Health Administration Center) administered programs for veterans and their families
IHS	Indian Health Service	Provides, or assists in providing and organizing, health care services to American Indians and Alaskan Natives

Ancillary and Physician Billing

Not all diagnostic testing and other services are billable by the health care facility. For example, a facility may not have a magnetic resonance imaging (MRI) machine. If this is the case, the patient is transported to the MRI provider, who bills either the payer or the original facility separately for both the diagnostic test and its interpretation, depending on the reimbursement method and payer. Additionally, unless the physician is an employee of the hospital, physicians bill separately for their services.

MEDICAID

In 1965, Congress enacted **Title XIX**, which created a formal system of providing funding for health care for low-income populations. Also administered by CMS, **Medicaid,** which is sometimes also called "Medical Assistance," is a shared federal and state program designed to shift resources from higher-income to lower-income individuals. Funds are allocated according to the average income of the residents of the state. Unlike Medicare, which reimburses through fiscal intermediaries, Medicaid reimbursement is handled directly by each individual state. The reimbursement guidelines vary from state to state. Some states have contracted with insurers to offer HMO plans to Medicaid beneficiaries.

Eligibility for Medicaid is determined by the individual states on the basis of the state's income criteria. The federal government mandates that the following services be included in each state's program: hospital and physician services, diagnostic services, home health, nursing home, preventive care, family planning, pregnancy care, and child care (see the CMS Web site for more information: http://www.cms.hhs.gov).

TAX EQUITY AND FISCAL RESPONSIBILITY ACT OF 1982

With the federal government's entry into the reimbursement arena, more citizens had access to health care services than ever before. The use of health care services rose accordingly, which in turn drove health care costs upward at an alarming rate. Improved access for the elderly meant better care and therefore longer life expectancy, which further increased costs. Thus cost containment became a critical issue. In the early 1970s, Professional Standards Review Organizations (PSROs) were established. PSROs conducted local peer reviews of Medicare and Medicaid cases for the purpose of ensuring that only medically necessary services were being rendered and appropriately reimbursed. Under the Peer Review Improvement Act of 1982, PSROs were replaced by Peer Review Organizations (PROs) through a federal law called the **Tax Equity and Fiscal Responsibility Act of 1982 (TEFRA).** TEFRA included a broad array of provisions, many of which had nothing to do with health care. For example, TEFRA raised taxes by eliminating previous tax cuts. In 2002, PROs were replaced by (or, more accurately, renamed) Quality Improvement Organizations (QIOs). More information about QIOs can be found on the CMS website, with links to local QIOs. Many HIM professionals are employed in QIOs because certain specialized skills, such as data analysis and coding expertise, are necessary to support various federal initiatives.

TEFRA's impact in health care included a modification of Medicare reimbursement for inpatient care to include a case mix adjustment based on diagnosis related groups. The following year, in 1983, Medicare adopted the prospective payment system (PPS), which uses the DRG classification system as the basis of its reimbursement methodology. The focus of treatment, patients' length of stay, and the individuals involved in the care plan differ from setting to setting. Because prospective reimbursement systems are based on just these types of factors, different systems must be developed for each health care setting. (See Chapter 6 for further discussion of prospective payment systems.)

Paying for health care is an ever-changing subject. HIM professionals must be aware of new developments that pertain to their practice and keep abreast of general reimbursement issues.

Exercise 2-3

Government Influence on Reimbursement

1. What is the difference between Medicare and Medicaid?
2. What is the difference between VHA and CHAMPVA?
3. Who benefits from the Indian Health Services?
4. Explain the impact of TEFRA on health care.

■ WORK CITED

Sultz, Harry and Kristina Young. *Health Care USA: Understanding its Organization and Delivery.* 5th ed. Sudbury, MA: Jones & Bartleu, 2006.

WEB SITES

BlueCross BlueShield Association: http://www.bcbs.com
CHAMPVA: http://www.va.gov/hac/hacmain.asp
Center for Medicare and Medicaid Services: http://www.cms.hhs.gov
Indian Health Services: http://www.ihs.gov/PublicInfo/PublicAffairs/Welcome_Info/ThisFacts.asp
Kaiser Permanente: http://www.kaiserpermanente.org/
Medical Group Management Association: http://www.mgms.com
Medicare: http://www.Medicare.gov
TRICARE: http://www.tricare.osd.mil

CHAPTER ACTIVITIES

CHAPTER SUMMARY

Health care providers may be reimbursed for their services by one or a combination of four ways: fee for service, discounted fee for service, prospective payment, and capitation. Providers traditionally are reimbursed on the basis of fee for service, but they may negotiate their fees depending on the provider's relationship with the payer. Insurance companies contract with employers and subscribers to offer coverage of health care costs under one or a combination of indemnity or managed care plans. Employers, and even employees, may choose to self-insure, accepting their exposure to the risk of high medical costs.

Government regulations greatly influence health care. The Social Security Act and the Tax Equity and Fiscal Responsibility Act had a serious impact on the way in which health care is provided and reimbursed. Federal entitlement programs include Medicare, Tri-Care, and the Indian Health Services. Medicaid is an additional program that is funded jointly by federal and state entities and administered at the state level.

Review Questions

1. List, compare, and contrast four reimbursement methodologies.
2. Compare and contrast indemnity health insurance plans with managed care plans.
3. Describe government involvement in health insurance.
4. What are the financial risks in health care delivery for providers, third party payers, and patients?

Practice Manager

My name is Sherri, and I am the Practice Manager for a group partnership of six physicians who specialize in internal medicine, Ridgewood Medical Associates. I use my expertise in physician billing and contract negotiations to ensure that Ridgewood Medical Associates receives the appropriate payments and reimbursement from our patients and insurers after services are rendered.

I began my career in health care by taking a coding certificate course at my local community college. Our course work included coding all types of patient records and outpatient encounters, and I realized that I preferred outpatient coding. After I completed the course, I sat for the American Health Information Management Association (AHIMA) Certified Coding Specialist—Physician-based (CCS-P) exam, passed it, and earned my credential as a CCS-P. I was fortunate to find a position working for a physician billing company. As a physician biller, I applied my knowledge of HCPCS/CPT-4 and ICD-9-CM coding, adding the correct codes to billing claims so that physicians could be reimbursed for services rendered. After a few years as a physician biller, I was ready for new challenges to further my career. I applied for the position of practice manager for Ridgewood Medical Associates and was hired.

To perform my job well, I must manage and oversee the many daily tasks and functions of a busy medical practice. First, I must make sure that every new and existing patient is registered in our patient billing system with the correct information according to insurance type. Because we accept all types of patient insurances and also accept self-pay patients, we need to know who must pay a deductible, who must pay a co-pay, and who will pay out-of-pocket fees. We store this information and patient demographic details electronically, and we anticipate adding clinical information as we move toward adopting an electronic health record (EHR). Our goal is to become a paperless office within 5 years. I keep abreast of the latest information concerning the EHR through my professional association, AHIMA. I am also a member of the Medical Group Management Association (see http://www.mgms.com).

Patients who are in managed care plans may require from one of our physicians a referral to see a specialist. It is my job to see that the referral process does not inconvenience either our patients or our physicians. To accomplish this goal, I need to know which managed care plans require a referral and for which specialties. I keep referral forms on-line and in paper format, if necessary, for the different insurers and managed care plans. These referral forms are made accessible to our physicians at all times; they can either retrieve the forms on-line or use one of the hard copies that are readily available in patient treatment areas. If our physician orders a referral to a different specialist outside of our group practice, I assist our patients by making appointments and ensuring that our referral form and any necessary medical records are forwarded to the different specialist in time for the appointment.

I supervise our billing staff and perform periodic audits of the codes submitted to insurers on claims submissions. We must submit accurate claims, including codes, to insurers to be properly reimbursed and also to avoid claims rejections. We submit most of our claims electronically. As a CCS-P, I stay abreast of any code changes or changes in claims submission requirements. I must also periodically remind our physicians to provide our billing staff with documentation that is complete and legible.

I also supervise our accounting staff. I receive detailed monthly reports that include an analysis of each insurer's payments to us. If I see that our expenses to treat a certain insurer's patients are not covered under the reimbursement we receive, I will negotiate with that insurer for a higher reimbursement to be applied for the next contract period. I must be able to review each insurer's contract and understand contract language so that I go into negotiations well prepared.

As a practice manager, I am involved in every nonclinical aspect of Ridgewood Medical Associates. I look forward to going to work each day because of the variety of functions that I oversee, and I also feel that I am helping our patients. The physicians value my work because I minimize the time that they must spend filling out paperwork and worrying about reimbursement. When I perform my job well, I enable our physicians to devote their time and clinical expertise to our patients.

Patient Registration

You are the manager of patient registration at a community hospital. When registering patients, your staff is required to obtain insurance information. The largest employer in your town has recently changed its employee benefit plan from an indemnity plan to a managed care plan. As manager of patient registration, you must educate your staff as to the differences in registering patients in a managed care plan versus an indemnity plan. For example, what will be your process for obtaining co-pays? How will your staff handle cash or checks? How will you ensure that cash or check co-pays are correctly credited to each patient's account? What will you instruct your staff to do if a patient with managed care insurance comes to the hospital for admission but their physician is not a participant in the patient's managed care plan?

Chapter 3

COLLECTING HEALTH CARE DATA

By the end of this chapter, the student should be able to

- Define data.
- Define health data.
- List and explain key data categories.
- Distinguish among characters, fields, records, and files.
- Describe how data are organized in a health record.

VOCABULARY

assessment	field	plan of treatment
character	file	problem-oriented record
clinical data	financial data	record
computerized patient record	guarantor	rule out
data	health data	SOAP format
data accuracy	health information	socioeconomic data
data collection devices	health record (medical record)	source-oriented record
data dictionary	indicative data	subjective
data validity	information	symptom
demographic data	integrated record	
epidemiology	objective	

hapter 1 contained a discussion of various health care professionals and the settings in which they work. While caring for patients, health care workers listen to the patients and make observations. They record those observations, along with their evaluations and plans for treatment. This chapter focuses on the ways that health care workers record what they observe and what they do.

It often surprises patients when health care workers record their observations on paper. Popular literature and cinema often present a futuristic view of health care delivery, one that will not be accurate for some years. Nevertheless, in some health care systems, computer-supported recording is the norm. Because this country is making the transition from paper- to computer-based standards, both will be addressed to the extent that is practical in this small volume.

BASIC CONCEPTS

Before proceeding, you should have an understanding of some basic terminology. Although these terms may be meaningful to you in other ways, it is important that you understand them in the context of health care.

HEALTH

Because this book is about health information, you should certainly have an understanding of what *health* is. Health begins with the absence of *disease*. For the purposes of this discussion, consider a disease to be an abnormality caused by organic, environmental, or congenital problems. Therefore a person with no diseases is considered "healthy." Suppose a person has no diseases but is very emotionally upset about events in his or her life: Is that person healthy? Not really. Long-term emotional upheaval can lead to a number of serious diseases. Consequently, emotional concerns detract from health. What about a child who does not get enough to eat but is currently free from disease? Won't that child eventually deteriorate and become unhealthy over time? Of course. Thus health is a broader concept than merely the absence of disease. A person who is healthy is free of disease and is also free of outside physical, social, and other problems that could lead to a disease condition.

DATA

Health information starts with **data.** Data are items, observations, or raw facts. We can collect data without understanding them. We can collect temperatures, blood pressures, or number of patients, but unless these items are structured or organized, they are only data, not meaningful in themselves.

INFORMATION

To interpret data—to make sense of the facts and use them—we organize the items of data. We use our knowledge of the data: once they are organized, data become **information.** The terms

---

Hit-Bit

Data: Plural or Singular?

Is *data* a plural word or a singular word? "Datum" is the singular form of the Latin word, and it represents a single item, observation, or fact. However, we rarely refer to one item of knowledge. Generally, we discuss a group of similar items, such as the temperatures listed in Figure 3-1, and we call the group *data*. In this book, the plural form is used to refer to items of related data ("the *data are* significant").

data and *information* are often used synonymously, but they are not the same. "Get me the data" usually really means "get me useful information." Data are the units of observation, and information is data that we have organized. On the left in Figure 3-1 is a list of data pertaining to Maria Gomez. We cannot tell what the data on the left mean until we determine that they are her oral temperature, taken at 1-hour intervals. Only then does the information become useful. The primary purpose of this book is to discuss data in the health care setting; how data are organized, stored, and retrieved; and how we can create information from data.

In Figure 3-1, the temperatures are listed in chronological order. On the basis of these few observations, it is easy to see that Maria's temperature is going down. If we took her temperature every hour for 5 days, we would have more than 100 items of data, but even listing them in order would not be helpful. Therefore the most useful information is often a picture, such as the graph shown in Figure 3-2. Here, we can see that Maria's temperature went up on day 2 but returned to normal and stayed there. The figure shows that the usefulness of data depends on their organization and presentation. (See Chapter 9 for further discussion of data presentation.)

HEALTH DATA

Health data are items in reference to an individual patient or a group of patients. We can list all of the diseases that a patient has or all of the patients who have a certain disease. In fact, our example of data in Figure 3-1 is really an example of health data: We collected a series of temperatures from one patient.

Similarly, we can obtain vast quantities of data on individual patients or groups of patients. Imagine a list of 10,000 patients and their diseases. Are these useful data? What could you do with these data? Unless you are prepared to organize it yourself, the list is not very informative. However, a list of the top 10 most common diseases of 10,000 residents would be quite useful. This type of information is published frequently. For example, Figure 3-3 shows the top 10 causes of death in the United States in 1900 and 2002. Certainly, a list of the top 500 causes of death would not have been as useful.

DATA VS. INFORMATION

DATA		INFORMATION	
Definition:	Individual units of knowledge	Definition:	Data with a frame of reference
Example:	Maria Gomez	Example:	Maria Gomez Temperature (oral) March 15, 2002
	104		1 p.m. 104°
	105		2 p.m. 105°
	104		3 p.m. 104°
	103		4 p.m. 103°
	102		5 p.m. 102°
	101		6 p.m. 101°
	100		7 p.m. 100°
	99		8 p.m. 99°

On the left, the data about Maria Gomez are not useful, because we do not have a frame of reference. Those same data, within the frame of reference of date and time, tell a story that is clinically significant.

◆ **Figure 3-1**
A list of data with a frame of reference becomes information.

HEALTH INFORMATION

Health information is health data that have been organized. Health data related to 10,000 residents become health information when the data are organized in a way that is meaningful to the reader. Listing the top 10 diseases of your city's residents is useful health information. In Figure 3-1, the temperatures gathered become health information when we understand that those temperatures are for one patient at certain times of the day. This is information that physicians can use to make decisions. In Figure 3-3, the charts present interesting information that helps us to ask questions that lead to more information, and so on. For example, tuberculosis, and diarrhea/ enteritis are no longer on the list. Upon study, we find that the development of antibiotics, vaccines, and improvement in sanitation have significantly reduced the number of deaths caused by these conditions. The study of these types of health trends or patterns is called **epidemiology.**

Health information is a broad category. It may refer to the organized data that have been collected about an individual patient, or it can be the summary of information about that patient's entire experience with his or her physician. Health information can also be summary (also called aggregate data) information about all of the patients that a physician has seen. Further, we can take all of the physicians in a certain area and organize information about all of their patients and make broad statements on the basis of this array of information.

Health information therefore encompasses the organization of a limitless array of possible data items and combinations of data items. It can range from data about the care of an individual patient to the health trends of an entire nation.

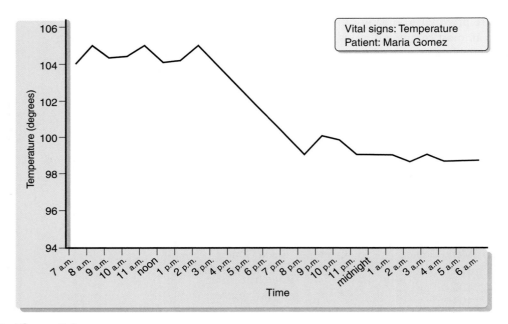

◆ **Figure 3-2**
The data presentation graph displays a large amount of data.

Exercise 3-1

Basic Concepts
1. Give two examples in your personal life of data and two examples of information. Think of two examples of ways that health data differ from health information.
2. How does data become information?
3. What is health information?

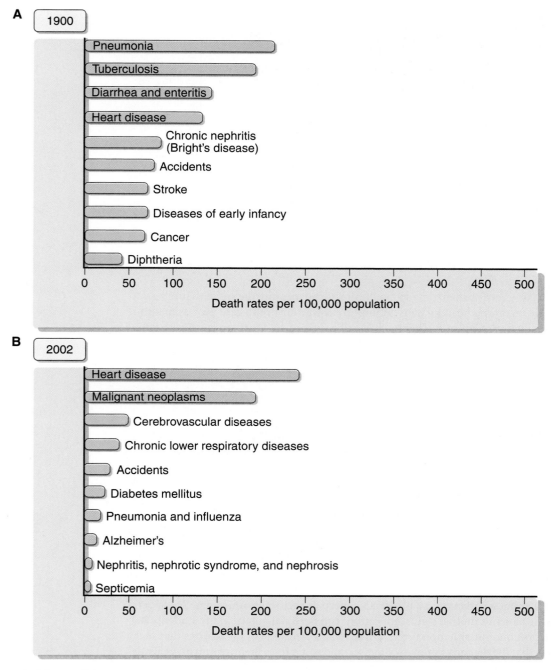

◆ Figure 3-3
A, The top ten causes of death in the United States: 1900. **B,** The top ten causes of death in the United States: 2002. (**A,** Modified from R. D. Grove and A. M. Hetzel. *Vital Statistics Rates of the United States, 1940-1960.* Washington DC: U.S. Government Printing Office, 1968; and D. L. Hoyert, K. D. Koehanek and S. I. Murphy. *Deaths: Final Data for 1997.* National Vital Stat Report 47, No.19, 30 June 1999. **B,** From R. N. Anderson and B. L. Smith. "Deaths: Leading Causes". *National Vital Statistics Reports,* Vol. 53, No. 17, 7 March 2006.)

▮ KEY DATA CATEGORIES

The primary purpose of recording data is communication, which is necessary for a variety of reasons. For example, the medical assistant may take a patient's vital signs for the physician's

> ## DEMOGRAPHIC DATA
>
> Definition: Data that help the user to contact the patient or to distinguish one patient from another
>
> Name
> Address
> Home telephone number
> Work telephone number
> Social Security number
> Birth date

◆ **Figure 3-4**
Sample indicative data.

reference. The physician records patient data so that he or she can measure the patient's progress at a later date. Therefore recording health data is an important way for health care professionals to communicate and facilitate patient care. Chapter 8 describes other uses for recording health data.

Most of us have visited a physician at one time or another. Consider what happens in a physician's office in the context of the data that are being collected about the patient. You may use your knowledge of this activity to organize the data into meaningful categories.

DEMOGRAPHIC DATA

The first thing the physician wants to know is the patient's name and address. The physician needs the patient's name and address to develop a relationship with the patient and, perhaps, to send him or her correspondence, follow-up notices, or a bill. Other necessary data include the home phone number, place of employment, work telephone number, and Social Security number. The physician needs these data both to contact the patient and to distinguish one patient from another. This type of data about a patient is called **demographic data.** In other industries, this type of data may be called **indicative data**. Figure 3-4 shows a list of demographic data. The demographic data are the foundation of the master patient index, which is discussed in Chapter 8.

SOCIOECONOMIC DATA

Another type of data about a patient that a physician collects is **socioeconomic data.** These personal data include the patient's marital status, education, and personal habits. Many students ask why the patient's socioeconomic situation is relevant to health care. One of the reasons that such data are important is that the diagnosis of many illnesses, and sometimes their treatment, depends on the doctor's understanding of the patient's personal situation. A list of socioeconomic data is presented in Figure 3-5.

Obviously, an asthma patient who smokes will be advised by his or her physician to quit smoking. This is an example of a personal habit that directly affects a disease condition. In addition, the socioeconomic situation or personal life of a patient sometimes dictates whether the patient will be compliant with a medication regimen or even whether he or she is able to obtain treatment. For example, if an elderly patient has just undergone a hip replacement, sending that patient home to a third-story walk-up apartment is going to be counterproductive to therapy. It will be very difficult for the patient to get in and out of the house and certainly very difficult for the patient to leave the home for therapy, particularly if there is no caregiver at home. Home health care may be the appropriate alternative. Longer-term inpatient therapy may also be an option. Therefore understanding a patient's personal life and living situation is important when planning how to care for the patient.

Sometimes the knowledge that a patient travels widely on business can lead a physician to suspect an illness that he or she would not consider if the patient never traveled. This patient's travels

SOCIOECONOMIC DATA

Definition: Personal data that give the user clues about potential problems and assistance in planning care

Marital status
Profession
Occupation
Employer
Religion
Sexual orientation
Personal habits
Race
Ethnicity

◆ **Figure 3-5**
Sample socioeconomic data.

in certain areas of the world could have caused exposure to parasites not prevalent in his or her native area. The patient's complaint of gastrointestinal disturbances would lead the physician to suspect a parasite, whereas ordinarily the physician would consider only bacterial or viral causes.

FINANCIAL DATA

When undergoing treatment in a health care facility, you should expect at some point that an invoice will be generated that either you or your insurance company must pay. The physician requests information about the party responsible for paying the bill. This information comprises the **financial data.** Financial data, obviously enough, relate to the payment of the bill for services rendered.

As discussed in Chapter 2, the person or organization responsible for paying the bill is the payer. The payer is frequently an insurance company. It may also be a government agency, such as Medicare or Medicaid. Many patients have more than one payer. The primary payer is approached first for payment. A secondary payer is approached for any amount that the primary payer did not remit. For example, many elderly patients who are covered by Medicare have supplemental or secondary insurance with a different payer. The physician first sends the bill to Medicare. Any amount that Medicare does not pay is then billed to the secondary payer.

Ultimately, the patient is responsible for payment of services that he or she has received. If the patient is a dependent, a person other than the patient may be ultimately responsible for the bill. This person is called the **guarantor.** For example, if a child goes to the physician's office for treatment, the child, as a dependent, cannot be held responsible for the invoice. Therefore the parent or legal guardian is responsible for payment and is the guarantor. Figure 3-6 lists financial data required by a health care facility.

CLINICAL DATA

Clinical data are probably the easiest to understand and relate to the health care field. **Clinical data** comprise all of the data that have been recorded about the patient's health, including diagnoses and procedures. The following example illustrates clinical data.

Imagine that you are a patient going to the physician's office for pain in the abdomen. The physician knows that pain in the abdomen can be caused by a variety of conditions. The pain is merely a **symptom,** a description of what the patient feels or is experiencing. Other symptoms may include nausea, dizziness, and headache. The physician orders tests and performs a physical examination to determine which of those conditions is responsible for the abdominal pain. Some of

FINANCIAL DATA

Definition:	The identities of the parties responsible for paying the invoice:
	Primary payer
	Secondary payer(s) (if any)
	Guarantor

Example:
Patient: Samantha Clooney

Primary
payer: Medicare
                    Account number

Secondary
payer: Pennsylvania Blue Cross
                    Group number
                    ID number

Guarantor: Samantha Clooney

◆ **Figure 3-6**
Sample financial data.

these tests include x-rays and blood tests. Ultimately, the physician may conclude that the abdominal pain is caused by an inflamed appendix, or appendicitis. Appendicitis is the diagnosis, and the blood test and physical examination are the procedures. The physician records both the findings of the examination and the results of the tests in the patient's record. Clinical data comprise the bulk of any patient's record. All of the previous data that we have discussed—demographic, socioeconomic, and financial—can usually be contained in one or two pages in the front of a patient's health record. The rest of the record is the clinical data. Figure 3-7 lists examples of clinical data.

Exercise 3-2

Key Data Categories
1. List and describe the four key data categories.
2. For each category of data, give four examples of data elements that would be contained in that category.

MEDICAL DECISION MAKING

A logical thought process supports the medical evaluation process, or development of a medical diagnosis. Data are collected in one of four specific categories: the patient's subjective view, the physician's objective view, the physician's opinion, and the care plan. In conducting the evaluation, the physician collects data sufficient to develop a medical diagnosis. Initially, the data may support several different diagnoses. The physician continues to collect data until a specific diagnosis can be determined. For example, chest pain and shortness of breath can be symptoms of many conditions, including myocardial infarction, congestive heart failure, and pneumonia. The physician examines the patient and orders sufficient tests to conclude which diagnosis (or diagnoses) applies in each individual case.

> ### CLINICAL DATA
>
> Definition: Data specific to the patient's diagnosis and treatment
>
> Diagnosis
> Temperature
> Blood pressure
> Laboratory reports
> X-ray reports
> Medications
> Surgical procedures

◆ **Figure 3-7**
Sample clinical data.

SUBJECTIVE

The physician begins the medical evaluation process by asking the patient about the medical problem and the symptoms that he or she is experiencing. The patient's description of the problem, in his or her own words, is the **subjective** portion of the evaluation process. For example, the patient may have stomach pain. The patient may describe this as "abdominal pain," "pain in the belly," or "pain in the stomach." The physician's task is to narrow the patient's description through questioning. For instance, the patient can be assisted to identify the pain as a sharp, stabbing pain in the lower right portion of the abdomen. The physician also asks when the pain began, whether it is continuous or intermittent, and whether there are any other symptoms.

OBJECTIVE

Once the physician has obtained and recorded the patient's subjective impressions about the medical problem, the physician must look at the patient objectively. In other words, the physician conducts a physical examination, exploring the places at which the stomach pain may be located. The patient says his or her stomach hurts, but the physician records that the patient has "tenderness on palpation in the right lower quadrant." Tenderness on palpation in the right lower quadrant is a classic indication of appendicitis. Other possible diagnoses include ovarian cyst and a variety of intestinal disorders, such as diverticulosis. The physician's **objective** notation is the specific anatomical location of the pain and the results of any laboratory tests that the physician ordered. The physician orders tests to confirm a likely diagnosis or to **rule out,** or eliminate, a possible diagnosis. In our examples, the physician is looking for an elevation of the white blood cell count, which indicates the presence of an infection. Additional tests, such as an abdominal ultrasound, might be ordered if the blood test results are negative or inconclusive.

ASSESSMENT

Once the physician has obtained the patient's subjective view and has conducted an objective medical evaluation, he or she develops an **assessment.** The assessment is a description of what the physician thinks is wrong with the patient: the diagnosis or possible (provisional) diagnoses. Using the previous example, assume that the physician has determined that the patient has appendicitis.

PLAN

Once the physician has assessed what is wrong with the patient, he or she writes a **plan of treatment.** The plan may be for treatment or for further evaluation, particularly if the assessment includes several possible diagnoses. Figure 3-8 illustrates the pattern of data collection.

Physician notes	Physician orders	Radiology	Surgeon notes
S – Pt complains of intermittent sharp pain in abdomen O – Tenderness on palpation in RLQ A – R/O appendicitis, ovarian cyst P – Abd U/S			
	Abd U/S to rule out appendicitis vs ovarian cyst		
		Abd U/S performed: Report positive for appendicitis	
S – Pt states pain increasing in frequency O – Abd U/S positive for appendicitis A – Acute appendicitis Ovarian cyst ruled out P – Appendectomy			
	Refer pt to surgeon for appendectomy		
			S – Pt complains of intermittent sharp pain in abdomen, increasing in frequency O – Sharp pain on palpation in RLQ, abd U/S positive for appendicitis A – Acute Appendicitis P – Appendectomy

◆ **Figure 3-8**
Link between physician notes and orders.

This method of recording observations or clinical evaluations is called the **SOAP format:** *S*ubjective, *O*bjective, *A*ssessment, and *P*lan. Although physicians may not always follow this format exactly, they record their thoughts in this general manner. Table 3-1 lists the elements of a medical evaluation. It should be noted that an increasingly important component of the medical decision-making process is the outcome: the result of the plan. As noted in Chapter 2, insurance

TABLE 3-1	Elements of Medical Evaluation (SOAP)
DATA ELEMENT	**EXPLANATION**
Subjective	The patient's report of symptoms or problems
Objective	The physician's observations, including evaluation of diagnostic test results
Assessment	The physician's opinion as to the diagnosis or possible diagnoses
Plan	Treatment or further diagnostic evaluation

Hit-Bit

Rule Out

In recording the assessment of possible diagnoses, the physician will often make the following statement: *Rule Out.* This phrase indicates that the listed diagnosis is still provisional—that it may prove to be the final diagnosis (or one of them). On the other hand, if the statement reads *Ruled Out*, the diagnosis is no longer being considered.

Rule Out: CHF (congestive heart failure), pneumonia. This means that the patient may or may not have CHF and/or pneumonia.

CHF, pneumonia ruled out. This means that the patient has CHF and does *not* have pneumonia.

companies may use the history and trending of outcomes to determine which health care providers will be included in their networks.

Other clinical personnel also record their observations but not necessarily in the SOAP format. Many nursing evaluations are recorded by use of graphs or on preprinted forms. Graphs or preprinted forms are also used for clinical evaluations in physical therapy, respiratory therapy, and anesthesia records; also, some operative records and many maternity and neonatal records use preprinted or graphical forms.

Exercise 3-3

Medical Decision-Making Process

Match the physician progress note entry on the left with the SOAP note component on the right.

1. 60 mg pseudoephedrine every 4 hours; 100 mg Tylenol as needed for pain
2. Acute sinusitis with pharyngitis
3. Patient complaints of headache
4. Patient's frontal sinuses sensitive to percussion; lungs clear; throat slightly inflamed

A. Subjective

B. Objective
C. Assessment
D. Plan

DESCRIBING DATA

We collect data for a reason and store the data for later use. It's a little like grocery shopping. We buy food that we need now and store it in the proper place for future use. Similarly, we collect the data that we think we need and store these data in the proper places for future use.

Whether we are collecting data to be stored on paper or in a computer, the data must be organized in such a way that we can find them and retrieve them later. The first step in collecting the data is determining what data are needed. Earlier in this chapter we started to explain the process of collecting data as it relates to health care by defining the types of data that we need.

To take the analogy of grocery shopping further: Just as food comes in appropriate containers, data also come in packages. Data are collected and stored in logical segments. Individual data items are collected and packaged into useful bundles, according to the category of data. Think about our appendicitis example. What data did the physician need? How were the data obtained? Data are collected piece by piece in logical segments. The logical segments are called *characters, fields, records,* and *files.*

CHARACTERS

This chapter focuses on data that are represented by written communication. Such data can be collected on paper or directly entered into a computer database. With regard to computers, the smallest segment of data is referred to as a *bit.* A bit is the computer's electronic differentiation between two choices: on and off. Strings of bits in specific combinations of on/off patterns make *bytes,* which are represented on the computer screen as *characters.*

A **character** is a letter, a single-digit number, or a symbol. "A" is a character, as well as "3" and "&." A character is the smallest unit of data that we can collect. Characters are the building blocks of data. When we put characters together, we make words and larger numbers and other types of written communication. The physician needs to know what characters to combine to make the words that are the patient's name, for example. Placing the characters in the correct order is important so that we collect the correct data.

FIELDS

A **field** is a series of related characters that have a specific relationship to one another. Usually, a field is a word, a group of related words, or a specific type of number. The number 07036 could be a field containing a zip code. Therefore the field "zip code" contains five characters: 0, 7, 0, 3, and 6. Other typical fields that create a logical data segment are first name, last name, Social Security number, and telephone number.

Fields are defined by the type of data that they contain. A field containing nothing but characters would be an *alphabetic* field. For example, a field for first name would be an alphabetic field (abbreviated as *alpha*). A field containing only numbers would be a *numeric* field. A field for dollars is an example of a numeric field. A fields can also be a combination of alphabetic and numeric characters; this is called an *alphanumeric* field. A field for street address is an alphanumeric field.

Fields are generally given logical names to identify them. Figure 3-9 illustrates data fields and definitions. The listing of fields is one component of creating a **data dictionary.**

Hit-Bit

Formatting Fields

When creating fields in a computer, you may find it useful to tell the computer that a number is really alphanumerical. For example, if a zip-code field is labeled "numerical," most computer systems will drop the leading zeros. Zip code 07036 then becomes 7036 both on the screen and when printed out. This is not desirable if you are printing labels for mailing envelopes. Mail addressed this way would most certainly be delayed. Social Security numbers are another tricky field to define. Again, a field containing a Social Security number should be defined as alphabetical or text to preserve the zeros.

RECORDS

In the same way that characters combine to make fields, fields combine to make records. So, if we take a number of fields that have some logical connection to one another and group them together, we have created a **record.** A very simple example of fields that combine to make a record is an entry in a telephone address book. You can accumulate characters and create fields that are very familiar, such as first name, last name, street address, state, and city. Similarly, a physician keeps track of patients using groups of fields that combine to make a record of the patient's demographic data. A simple example of how fields combine to make a record is shown in Figure 3-10. Whether the data are collected on paper or in a computer, the size of the field must be considered to ensure uniformity in recording and retrieving the data.

FILES

Obviously, creating a record of a patient's name and address is really just the beginning of the data that a physician collects for a given patient. The physician collects numerous records of different types of data, and this group of related records is called a **file.** In Figure 3-11, the entire telephone address book is a file made up of individual records. Files can be large or small, depending on the number of records that they contain. A patient's entire health history can be contained in one file depending on how it is organized. An electronic patient record is developed by linking the data records collected for each patient. The special terminology and skills to accomplish this task are beyond the scope of this text.

Exercise 3-4

Describing Data

1. Create a file of five records that contain name, address, and telephone number. Begin by defining the fields in data dictionary format, and then show how you would represent these fields if you were trying to explain them to someone else.
2. Which of the following is the best example of a single field?
   a. J
   b. NJ
   c. New Jersey
   d. All of the above

Use the sample data dictionary below to answer Questions 3 through 5.

NAME	DEFINITION	SIZE	TYPE	EXAMPLE
FNAME	Patient's first name	15 Characters	Alphabetical	Jane
LNAME	Patient's last name	15 Characters	Alphabetical	Jones
HTEL	Patient's home telephone number	12 Characters	Alphanumerical	973-555-3331
TEMP	Patient's temperature	5 Characters	Numerical	98.6

3. Using 12 alphanumerical characters is one way to capture the patient's home telephone number. List at least one other way to capture that data.
4. List and describe two additional fields that would be needed to capture a patient's entire name.
5. Using the format above, define the fields that would be needed to capture a patient's diagnosis and a procedure. Refer to Chapter 1 for examples that you can use.

ORGANIZATION OF DATA ELEMENTS IN A HEALTH RECORD

All of the data that have been collected about an individual patient are called a **health record** or **medical record.** *Medical record* is the term that has been used historically in the United States.

DATA FIELDS AND DEFINITIONS

Name	Definition	Size	Type	Example
FNAME	Patient's first name	15 Characters	Alphabetic	Jane
LNAME	Patient's last name	15 Characters	Alphabetic	Jones
HTEL	Patient's home telephone number	12 Characters	Alphanumeric	973-555-3331
TEMP	Patient's temperature	5 Characters	Numeric	98.6

Here is a simple example of part of a basic data dictionary. Can you see why the telephone number is not 10 numeric characters? Why is the temperature 5 characters?

◆ **Figure 3-9**
Common fields of data, including definitions.

FIELDS COMBINE TO MAKE A RECORD

Name	Definition	Size	Type	Example
FNAME	Patient's first name	15 Characters	Alphabetic	Marion
LNAME	Patient's last name	15 Characters	Alphabetic	Smith
ADDRESS	Patient's home street address	25 Characters	Alphanumeric	23 Pine Street
CITY	City associated with ADDRESS	15 Characters	Alphabetic	Anywhere
STATE	State associated with ADDRESS	15 Characters	Alphabetic	IOWA
ZIP	Postal zip code associated with ADDRESS	5 Characters	Alphanumeric	31898
Telephone	Patient's home telephone number	14 Characters	Alphanumeric	(319) 555-1234

This record has seven fields:

Marion   Smith

23 Pine Street

Anywhere   Iowa   31898

(319) 555-1234

Each field is underlined to illustrate the number of characters allowed in the field, compared with the number that this record required. Is there a more efficient way to capture STATE? The telephone number is captured differently than the example in Figure 3-9. Can you see why? Can you think of a third way to capture it?

◆ **Figure 3-10**
Address book example of how fields combine to make a record.

Elsewhere, the term *medical record* may refer to the patient's record of a specific visit or group of visits to a health care facility, but *health record* refers to the patient's lifelong medical history. In the United States it has become increasingly more common to call a patient's collective data a *health record.* For the sake of clarity, we refer to a patient's information as the health record, whether it refers to a single visit or the patient's collective experience.

RECORDS COMBINE TO MAKE A FILE

	Telephone Address Book	
Character:	**A**	A single letter, digit, or symbol.
Field:	Marion	A related string of characters. This field has six characters.
Record:	**Marion** Smith 23 Pine Street Anywhere, Iowa 31898 (319) 555-1234	A related group of fields. This record has seven fields (the street and number are considered one field).
File:	**Harry** Jones 76 Elm Street Anywhere, Iowa 31898 (319) 555-4321 **Samuel** Davis 98 Sycamore Terrace Anywhere, Iowa 31898 (319) 555-4567 **Jake** Schoner 65 Spruce Run Anywhere, Iowa 31898 (319) 555-2727 **Marion** Smith 23 Pine Street Anywhere, Iowa 31898 (319) 555-1234	A related group of records. This file has four records.

◆ **Figure 3-11**

Address book example of how records combine to make a file.

The previous example of a telephone address book involved defining data in a certain useful format. Data collected in a health care environment can be similarly defined. Although the previous sections defined a health record and discussed health data, the way in which data are compiled into a patient's health record was not discussed. When health care workers collect items of data, they record them so that they remember them and can retrieve them later. Data can be recorded on paper or in an electronic format, such as a computer. This chapter explores the ways in which health data are collected and recorded. Chapter 8 delves into the intricacies of storing health data in both formats.

Data are collected in an organized fashion. In a paper-based environment, the data collection device is a form. Forms are specific to their purpose, as discussed later in this chapter. As the forms are collected into the record, they must be put into some kind of order so that users will be able to locate and retrieve the data. Paper records are sorted in one or a combination of three ways: by date, source, or diagnosis.

INTEGRATED RECORD

Pages in the record can be organized by order of date. In a completely **integrated record**, the data itself are also collected by date order (i.e., chronologically), regardless of the source of the data. The first piece of data is recorded with its date, and each subsequent piece of data is organized sequentially after the preceding piece of data. This method of recording data is particularly useful when we need to know when events happen in relation to one another. For practical purposes, different types of data are recorded on separate forms, but those forms are also placed in data order. Figure 3-12 illustrates the chronological organization of data.

This method of recording data in date order can also be called *date-oriented* or *sequential*. The organization of the data in date order is a fairly useful and efficient way to collect data sequen-

A

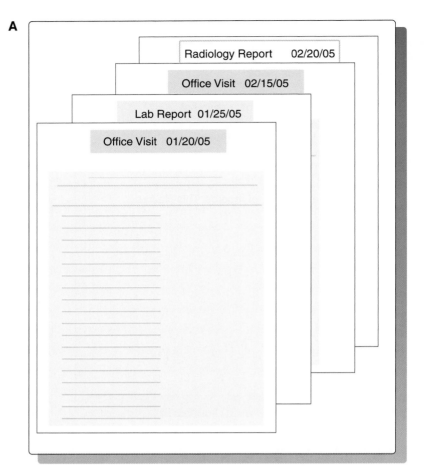

Radiology Report   02/20/05

Office Visit   02/15/05

Lab Report   01/25/05

Office Visit   01/20/05

◆ **Figure 3-12**
A, Integrated record.

tially during each episode of care and from one episode to the next. In a paper record, it is easier to place the most recent pages on top; therefore an integrated paper record may be organized in reverse chronological order, but this is still considered an integrated record.

Because of the ease of filing and the chronological picture such records provide, many physicians and other ambulatory care providers use an integrated record.

SOURCE-ORIENTED RECORD

In addition to being organized by date, data may be organized by source. In other words, all of the data obtained from the physician can be grouped together, all of the data obtained from the nurse can be grouped together, and all of the laboratory data can be grouped together. This method of organizing data produces a **source-oriented record.** Source-oriented records are complicated to file in paper format.

Organizing data by source is useful when there are many items of data coming from different sources. For example, a patient who is in the hospital for several days may require numerous laboratory and blood tests, and many pages of physician and nursing notes are compiled. If all of these pieces of data are organized in date order, you would have to know the exact date on which something occurred before you could find the desired data. Further, it would be very difficult to compare laboratory results from one date to the next. Consequently, in records that have numerous items from each type of source, the records tend to be organized in a source-oriented manner. Figure 3-13 illustrates a source-oriented record. Notice that within each source, the data are organized in chronological order so that specific items are more easily located.

B

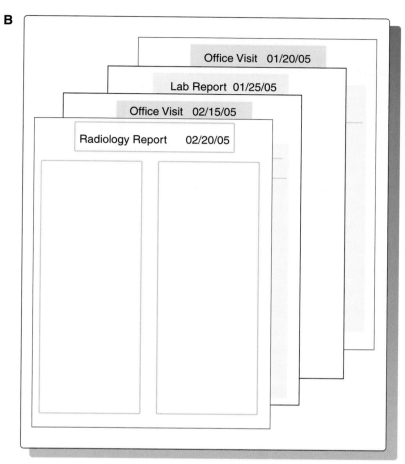

Office Visit   01/20/05

Lab Report 01/25/05

Office Visit   02/15/05

Radiology Report   02/20/05

◆ **Figure 3-12,** *cont'd*
B, Integrated record in reverse chronological order.

PROBLEM-ORIENTED RECORD

The data can also be organized by the patient's diagnosis, or problem. For instance, all of the data on a patient's appendicitis and appendectomy can be organized together. Similarly, all of the data that pertain to the patient's congestive heart failure can be organized together. Such a method greatly facilitates the monitoring of individual patient conditions. This method of organizing data produces a **problem-oriented record** and is useful when the patient has several major chronic conditions that may be addressed at different times. For example, if a patient has congestive heart failure, diabetes, and hypertension, the patient might not be treated for all three simultaneously. Therefore the records for each of the conditions may be kept separately. Problems that have been resolved are easily flagged, and current problems are more easily referenced. Figure 3-14 illustrates a simple problem-oriented record.

PROBLEM LIST

After several visits to an ambulatory care facility, a list of the patient's problems (diagnoses or complaints) is compiled. This problem list facilitates management of the patient's care and improves communication among caregivers. In a problem-oriented record, this list becomes an index to the record as well as a historical summary of patient care management. Therefore the problem list is an integral part of a problem-oriented record. A simple problem list is shown in Figure 3-15.

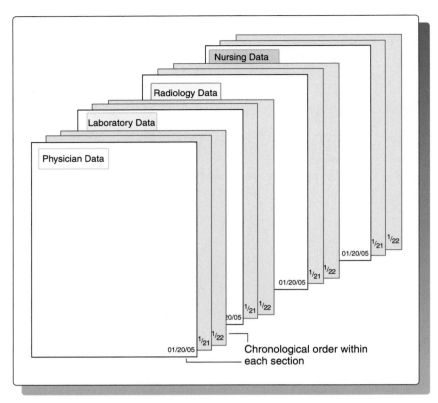

◆ **Figure 3-13**
Source-oriented record.

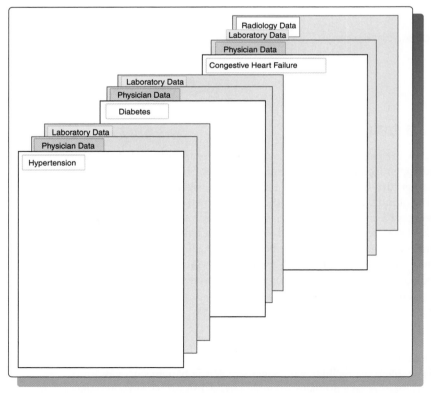

◆ **Figure 3-14**
Problem-oriented record.

PROBLEM LIST

Date	Problem #	Description	Date of Initial Diagnosis	Current Treatment	Comments
01/20/05	1	Hypertension	11/27/02	Diet	Follow-up 01/06
02/15/05	2	Sprain/right ankle	02/15/05	Wrap and rest Tylenol 1000 mg as needed	
03/15/05	2	Sprain/right ankle	02/15/05	None	Resolved

◆ **Figure 3-15**
Problem list.

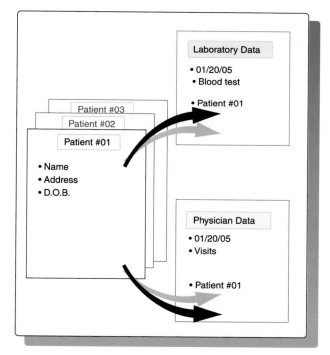

◆ **Figure 3-16**
Electronic patient record.

ELECTRONIC HEALTH RECORD

Computerization has had and will continue to have an impact on the health information management (HIM) profession. The terminology of computerization is often confusing. The terms *electronic, computerized, computer-assisted,* and *computer-based* are sometimes used interchangeably. At the time of this writing, the generally accepted term for a computerized patient record is *electronic health record (EHR)*.

In an EHR, data are collected in fields and records that are linked together in such a manner that the data can be referenced, displayed, or reported in any of the ways previously mentioned. This versatility is one of the major advantages of an EHR. The data are linked by reference numbers (e.g., medical record or billing number) so that all data about the patient are accessible. A complete discussion of a relational database is beyond the scope of this text, but Figure 3-16 shows one way in which computer records might be designed to link patient data together.

ADVANTAGES AND DISADVANTAGES

Each of these methods of organizing data elements has its own advantages and disadvantages. The integrated record is simple to file, but subsequent retrieval and comparison of data are more difficult. The source-oriented record is more complicated to file, but retrieval and comparison of source data are facilitated. The problem-oriented record lends itself best to the long-term management of chronic illnesses; however, filing is complicated, and duplication of data may be necessary so that laboratory reports related to different problems are included in all relevant sections. All of these methods are essentially paper-based organization systems. A well-designed computer-based system can solve filing and retrieval inefficiencies; however, cost and resistance to technology have prevented the universal implementation of computer systems.

It should be noted that the method of organizing a record is not patient specific. In other words, all patients' records are recorded in the same way. The method of organization is determined by its overall suitability to the particular environment and the needs that it satisfies.

Exercise 3-5

Organization of Data Elements in a Health Record

1. Think about a disease with which you are familiar, and create a list of all the data elements that you think a physician and allied health personnel in a physician's office would generate for this disease. You can make up the data, but make the list as complete as you can. This exercise will give you an idea of how complex health information is, even at the physician's office level.
2. The study of disease trends and occurrences is called _____.
3. Match the chart description on the left with the record order on the right:

   1. All of the information about the patient's congestive heart failure is together, the hypertension information is all together, and the appendicitis information is all together.   A. Integrated

   2. Data are collected and recorded by different health care workers and linked to other data about the patient by common data elements.   B. Source-oriented

   3. In the record, all of the physician's notes are together, the orders are together, the nursing notes are together, the medication sheets are together, and the laboratory reports are together.   C. Problem-oriented

   4. The record is organized in chronological order only.   D. Computer-based

■ DATA QUALITY

Have you ever heard the saying "garbage in, garbage out"? This expression is a humorous reflection on data quality in a computer environment. In other words, if the information you enter into the computer is wrong, all you will get out of the computer is wrong information. Therefore you must be extremely careful to ensure that your information is correct before you enter it. The same rule applies to data collected on paper. If your data on the paper record are incorrectly recorded, you will retrieve incorrect data when you review it. High-quality data collection starts with an understanding of the data needs of the user. Data collection devices (e.g., forms, computer screens) must be designed to capture the appropriate information efficiently.

DATA COLLECTION

Data collection is rarely the collection of a single data field but is more often a record of several data fields collected repeatedly over time. At this point, consider the way in which the data are collected.

While the patient is in the hospital, an entire team of clinical personnel is collecting and recording data about everything that happens to the patient. The primary difference between the data compiled in a physician's office record and the data collected in an inpatient facility lies in the volume of data collected about a patient and the way it is organized in a record. Even a patient with multiple complications who visits a physician's office will have a fairly brief record until he or she has visited many times. In a hospital, however, sometimes even the smallest procedures generate enormous volumes of data. Paper forms and computer screens are the primary **data collection devices** for health data.

Forms

In a paper-based record, most of the data are collected in a standard format that is devised by the individual facility. With some exceptions, notably neonates and patients with obstetrical issues, the forms in one hospital do not look the same as those in another hospital. The purposes of the forms are numerous:

1. A form reminds the user of which data have to be collected.
2. A form provides a structure for capturing that data so that the reader knows where to look for the desired data.
3. The forms ensure that complete data are collected according to the clinical guidelines of the facility and profession and according to regulation.

Paper forms are frequently created by committees of the people who use them. Some facilities have an oversight committee, simply called the *forms committee* or *documentation committee*. This committee may be charged with ensuring that forms are created only when necessary, that duplicate forms are not created, and that the forms conform to hospital guidelines.

The demographic, financial, and some of the socioeconomic data that are collected in the patient registration record usually fit on one paper form, called the *admission record* or *face sheet,* although several computer screens may be necessary to capture these data. Even facilities that collect the clinical data on paper tend to have computerized patient registration data.

Content

Many considerations go into the development of a health data form. For example, suppose you would like to create a form for a physician's order. You need to be creative because the form must satisfy every user's needs. First you must consider what data are necessary on a physician's order form. The purpose of this form is to record the physician's instructions to nurses, therapists, consultants, and radiologists and to record anything else the physician decides must be done to care for the patient. The form must be flexible enough to record the hundreds of different medications, therapies, and instructions that a physician might give. On a paper form, these data are recorded by the physician, who writes the orders in his or her own handwriting. The purpose of the form is the most important consideration in its creation. The form for a physician's order has the very important function of communicating the patient's care to all members of the health care team.

If a physician wants to tell a nurse to administer penicillin to a patient, the nurse needs to know the following:

■ To which patient to give the medication
■ The patient's medical record number (to ensure that the right patient receives the medication, given that two people can have the same name)
■ The exact medication
■ The exact dosage
■ The specific route of administration (e.g., oral or intravenous [via a needle into the bloodstream])
■ The ordered frequency of administration
■ When the order was given
■ Who gave the order

Given the purpose of the form and the specific information that must be conveyed, how would you create a form that is able to capture this information? Generally, the patient's name and medical record number are recorded in the top right-hand corner of every page. Patient identification data must be on every page so that the data can be matched to the correct patient. The patient data usually go in the right-hand corner of the page because most records, particularly when the patient is still in the hospital, are kept in three-ring binders. Having the patient's name and medical record number in the top right-hand corner makes the record easy to check and prevents misfiling.

In addition to identifying the patient on the form, you must also include some information identifying the particular form. Typically included are the name of the facility, the title of the form, and any special instructions about the form. The top left-hand corner of the page is a convenient place to put the name of the hospital and possibly its location (which is useful if the hospital has many facilities), along with the title of the form.

Format

How many physician's orders can be put on one page of a paper record? Should you create separate blocks for each order or design a form that has a lot of lines on which the physician may write as much as he or she desires for each order? This is a matter of personal preference. Forms with the orders in blocks, with each block containing only one set of orders, and forms that consist of a page of blank lines on which the physician may write free-form are both common.

A major consideration in constructing a form is the size of the fields that will be included. In the previous discussion about data dictionaries, the size of a field was illustrated. On a paper form, the size of the field in characters must be accommodated, as well as the space needed to handwrite the data.

You also must consider the size of the form on the page. How close to the edge of the page can the form be printed? Will holes be punched in the form? If so, where will they be and how much space should be allowed? Figure 3-17 shows a forms design template.

One problem with paper records is that clinicians may write an order but forget to sign it, which means that the order is not authenticated. In a computer system, authentication is captured by a key word, or code, that the physician enters when the order is complete. Authentication data may be captured in numerous ways. We call these methods *electronic signatures*. An electronic signature does not capture the person's actual signature into the computer. Rather, it is the

TABLE 3-2	**Data Collection Device Design Issues**
ISSUE	**CONSIDERATIONS**
Identification of user needs	Not limited to the collectors of the data; also necessary to consider subsequent users of both the device and the data it contains
Purpose of the data collection device	Necessary to ensure both data collection and controls for quality
Selection of the appropriate data items and sequencing of data collection activities	Should fulfill the purpose of the device, without unnecessary fields; important to consider the order in which data is collected
Understanding the technology used	Not just paper versus computer (e.g., how is the paper used, how is the computer used, what input devices are available and how will they be used?)
Use of standard terminology and abbreviations as well as development of a standard format	Communication among users improved by consistency in language and format
Appropriate instructions	Consistency improved by instructions on the form
Simplicity	The simpler the device, the easier to use

Modified from Mervat Abdelhak, Sara Grostick, Mary Alice Hanken, and Ellen Jacobs. *Health Information: Management of a Strategic Resource.* 2nd ed. Philadelphia: Saunders, 2001, p 164.

computer recognition of a unique code that only the author has in his or her possession. The computer can be programmed to reject orders that do not contain an appropriate authentication. The program would look for both the existence of the authentication (for data completeness) and the correct authentication (for data validity). Table 3-2 summarizes forms design issues.

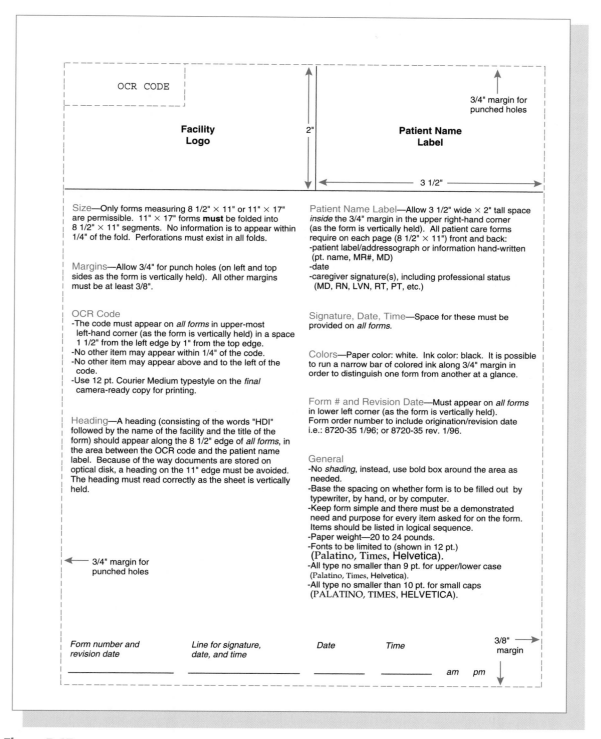

◆ **Figure 3-17**

Forms design template. (From Mervat Abdelhak, Sara Grostick, Mary Alice Hanken and Ellen Jacobs. *Health Information Management of a Strategic Resource*. 2nd ed. Philadelphia: Saunders, 2001, p 19.)

Compliance with licensure and accreditation standards is another consideration. If the Joint Commission on Accreditation of Healthcare Organizations (JCAHO) requires that physician's orders must be authenticated, then we should facilitate that process on the form. Two concepts are necessary to understand regarding authentication. The first concept is *authorship:* the author of an order is the person who wrote it. The second concept is *authentication*: the author's mark or signature. On a paper record, that mark or signature takes the form of the author's formal signature or his or her initials. Consequently, when you are designing the form, you must ensure that there is a place for the author's authentication and a note of the date and time of the orders. This detail is important from a clinical perspective because the time between the writing of the order and the execution of the order is often crucial.

Next, consider what other information will be necessary on the form. The physician's orders are written to communicate instructions to other health care providers. In a paper record, the physician's orders are maintained in the nursing unit near the patient. The orders are not directly accessible to the radiology department, laboratory department, pharmacy, and so on. Someone has to take the orders and communicate them to the correct party. Members of the nursing staff are usually charged with that responsibility. Therefore our form must contain an area for these staff members to indicate that they have read and executed the order. In the case of medication, the drug must be ordered from the pharmacy and then be administered to the patient. Figure 3-18 shows a completed physician's order on a form that leaves separate blanks for each order.

Other Considerations

Creation of a form involves many other considerations. So far, the focus has been on the data that must be recorded on the form. In a paper record, a number of other issues must be considered:

- How heavy should the paper be? Should it be heavy card stock or copy machine weight?
- Should the form be one part, two parts, or more?

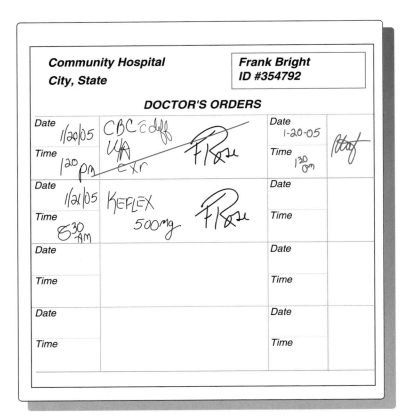

◆ **Figure 3-18**
Sample of a completed physician's order form.

- If it is a multipart form, should there be carbon paper between the pages or should it be NCR (no carbon required) paper?
- On what color paper should the form be printed? White is best for photocopying, but would another color help the users of the form?

These are considerations that the forms committee reviews to ensure that the form conforms to the institution's guidelines. Designing forms was once a difficult and time-consuming process because they had to be developed with a pencil and paper, given to a printer, printed, and then returned to the organization. Today, it is possible to create forms using word-processing software and reproduce them on a photocopy machine. Nevertheless, the great volume of forms required and the unique characteristics of some of the forms often require the assistance of professional printers to this day.

Forms Control

In a paper-based system, forms are used selectively depending on the type of patient record and the department using them. Someone in the hospital, frequently the director of the HIM department, must keep track of all approved forms. In reality, forms get passed around, photocopied, and shuffled from department to department. If a form is not used frequently, it often becomes lost. When the form is needed but not readily available, the health care provider creates a new form even though the old form still exists. Therefore a master forms file should be created and maintained. The master forms file contains every form used by the hospital and can be organized in any way that the hospital finds useful. One very efficient way to save a master forms file is to keep forms in the order of the departments that use them, for example, alphabetically by department name. Another way to maintain a master forms file is to give each form a numerical assignment and then save the forms in numerical order. In either case, the creation of an index and table of contents for the master forms file is necessary. The index is at the front of the file, and the title of each form and its individual number are listed in the table of contents. The responsibility for ensuring that forms are not duplicated and that each form conforms to the institution's needs usually lies with the forms committee, as previously mentioned.

The forms committee is an institution-wide committee that has the responsibility of reviewing all forms. Therefore representatives of all the major clinical services must be included. For example, the committee should include a representative from nursing, physician staff (probably several representatives if the facility offers numerous services), laboratory, and radiology. Because HIM personnel are frequently in charge of the master forms file, a representative from the HIM department should be included in the forms committee. In a computer-based environment, the forms are created and displayed on computer screens. The development of or addition to a computer system should be under the direction of a systems development team. However, only the clinicians and other health practitioners are truly aware of the data that must be collected and how the data should be organized. The data dictionary then becomes critical in the developmental process. The data fields that are collected; the staff members who have access to them; and whether those with access can print, change, or view the data become increasingly important considerations. Existing institutional committees become involved in this development according to institution policies. Often, groups are formed for these new roles. In any event, HIM personnel should be as directly involved in these new groups as they were in the old.

ELECTRONIC DATA COLLECTION

Paper-based forms are the traditional way to record health data, and the skills that you have learned creating paper-based forms can be transferred to the creation of computer-based forms. Even when you are recording data into a computer, you are still recording it on a form—the computer screen. It simply looks different. To create a computer-based form, you must have a name for the form, which should be input at the top of the computer screen. The patient's name and medical record number are carried forward onto every screen after the data have been entered. Computerized data capture facilitates the improvement of data quality. In a computer-based record, it is not necessary to "allow room" for variable handwriting; exactly enough room is allowed for the particular data field because the size of the field is already known. The computer may also be programmed to check the data for validity. In other respects, many of the data collection considerations for a paper-based record are applicable when developing a computer-based data record.

One consideration that is more important in computer data entry than in paper-record data collection is the sequence of data capture. On a paper-based form, the data can be entered in any order. Although the paper-based form may be designed to capture data in a logical sequence, as identified by the designers, recording items at the bottom of the form before recording items at the top does not pose a disadvantage if the data collector chooses to do it this way. With a computer-based data collection device, however, data collection may continue over several screens, or virtual pages. Flipping back and forth among the pages is confusing and time-consuming and may lead to errors and omissions. Although the computer may be programmed to check for incomplete data fields, this feature wastes time if the omission was caused by inefficient data capture. Consequently, computer-based data collection screens should collect data in the most efficient sequential order.

In the context of a computer program, forms actually improve the data collection. As previously discussed, on a paper-based form the patient's name and identification number go in the top right-hand corner, which is done manually: Someone has to write it in, stamp it in, or affix a label in the corner. On a computer screen, the patient's name and medical record number are collected in other ways. The person who enters the data may type it in the appropriate field. Alternatively, the patient's name and identification number may be in a directory from which the person who enters the data selects the patient's name and identification number and transfers it to the form. In both paper and electronic form design, the element of human error is still a hazard of form completion.

If the physician's order form is completed in the computer, the data can be obtained in additional ways. For example, instead of the physician's actually typing or writing out the name of the drug, the dosage, and the route of administration, this information may be included in pop-up windows from a menu-driven pharmacy directory. This method is particularly convenient because the only elements included in the list are items that are definitely on the facility's approved drug list. In this particular instance, the use of a menu-driven computer-based data collection system significantly reduces the error that might occur if a physician ordered a nonapproved drug. Such a mistake might very well happen if the physician has privileges at a variety of different hospitals because approved drug lists in various hospitals are not necessarily identical. Moreover, the order entry can be linked to the pharmacy, which might generate the medication request without nursing intermediation. In addition, the order entry system can be linked to health data that we have already collected about the patient, such as sex, height, weight, age, and diagnosis. Then, if a physician ordered a drug at a dosage that exceeds the maximal amount that is considered safe for a newborn, for instance, a computer system could automatically generate a warning statement that the drug dosage was inappropriate, thereby alerting the physician of his or her error before any harm was done.

DATA ACCURACY

To be useful, the data must be *accurate*. To understand the importance of **data accuracy,** think about how irritating it is to receive a telephone call from someone who has dialed the wrong number. Sometimes a person writes the wrong number in his or her telephone address book. In this case, the recorded data are inaccurate. However, receiving misdirected telephone calls is merely an annoyance, whereas receiving someone else's medication could be fatal. If data are not accurate, wrong information is conveyed to the user of the data.

DATA VALIDITY

Whether data are recorded on paper or electronically, their recording is subject to human error. **Data validity** ensures its usefulness. The term *validity* pertains to the data's conformity with an expected range of values. For example, "ABCDE" is not a valid U.S. Postal Service zip code. Currently, zip codes in the United States contain only numbers. Similarly, 287° Fahrenheit is not a valid temperature for living human beings. A computer can be instructed to check specific fields for validity and alert the user to a potential data collection error.

DATA SETS

In addition to a basic understanding of the concept of data—where it comes from, what types of things are collected, and why it is necessary—we must know how the data will be used. All of the health data available can be voluminous and confusing. Individual physicians use the data to improve the quality of their services and help treat individual patients. Health care consumers may use the data to select a physician or a treatment. Moreover, insurance companies and government agencies may also require health data to pay patients' bills or track health trends. The uses of health data are described in subsequent chapters. For most types of health care delivery, there is a minimum set of data that must be collected and reported for each patient. Those data sets are discussed in subsequent chapters in relation to the appropriate discussion of the health care setting.

Exercise 3-6

Data Quality

1. The nursing department in your facility has submitted a form to the forms committee for approval. The form is printed on dark gold paper so that it will stand out in the chart. You recommend a light yellow paper instead because it photocopies better than dark gold. This is an example of taking which of the following into consideration?
   a. The purpose of the data collection device
   b. The needs of all users of the device
   c. An understanding of the technology used
   d. Simplicity
2. Which of the following most closely describes the purpose of instructions on a data collection device?
   a. It ensures that the correct form is used.
   b. It helps users with complicated data collection.
   c. It helps ensure the consistency of data collection.
   d. It organizes the data in the correct sequence.

■ SUGGESTED READING

Johns, Merida. *Information Management.* Albany, NY: Delmar, 1996.

Koch, Gerda. *Basic Allied Health Statistics and Analysis.* 2nd ed. Albany, NY: Delmar, 1999.

Kuzma, Jan W. and Stephen E. Bohnenblust. *Basic Statistics for the Health Sciences.* 3rd ed. Mountain View, CA: McGraw-Hill, 1998.

Osborn, Carol. *Statistical Applications for Health Information Management.* Gaithersburg, MD: Aspen, 2000.

WEB SITES

Society for Medical Decision Making: http://www.smdm.org/

Foundation for Informed Medical Decision Making: http://www.fimdm.org/

CHAPTER ACTIVITIES

CHAPTER SUMMARY

This chapter contains a discussion of some basic concepts related to data. It explained the difference between data and information and defined the terms *health, health data,* and *health information.* A physician's office is one type of ambulatory care facility. It can be staffed by a variety of personnel, including receptionist, medical secretary, medical assistant, nurse, physician assistant, and nurse practitioner. In a physician's office, data are collected in these specific categories: demographic data, socioeconomic data, financial data, and clinical data. Health records are the patient's collective health information, and they include ambulatory visits as well as inpatient stays in a facility; health records cover all the health care services that the patient has received over a lifetime. Health information management professionals are concerned with the collection, storage, retrieval, and documentation of health information. Health information technology is one area of the health information management profession.

Data are collected in logical segments called *characters, fields, records,* and *files.* A patient's entire health history could be combined in one file depending on how it is organized. One of the useful aspects of collecting data is that it can be analyzed in a variety of ways, including by patient, physician, facility, or even country.

Review Questions

1. Explain the difference between data and information.
2. Distinguish among fields, records, and files.
3. For each of the elements of the Uniform Ambulatory Care Data Set, describe how you might define the field in a data dictionary.
4. Compare and contrast the considerations in developing paper-based versus computer-based data collection devices.

APPLICATION

Creating a Data Dictionary

You are a health information professional working for Dr. Heath in his private practice. Dr. Heath has a large practice with several ancillary services attached. He and his partner see 50 patients a day in the practice, many of whom receive on-site diagnostic procedures. The diagnostic areas that Dr. Heath has are x-ray, electrocardiography, and laboratory. He is concerned because a number of patients have complained that in each area of care, the health personnel seem to ask the same questions. The redundancy is annoying. He is considering computerizing his data collection to streamline the data collection process. Before he does, he wants to make sure that he understands the clinical flow of data in the facility. Dr. Heath seeks your advice and assistance in resolving his problem. What do you recommend? How would you go about implementing your recommendation?

UNIT II

CONTENT, STRUCTURE, AND PROCESSING OF HEALTH INFORMATION

Chapter 4

ACUTE CARE RECORDS

CHAPTER OBJECTIVES

By the end of this chapter, the student should be able to

- List and explain the elements of an admission record.

- Given a data element, identify the appropriate original source of the data.

- Given a specific clinical report, analyze the required data elements.

- List the elements of the Uniform Hospital Discharge Data Set.

VOCABULARY

admission record

admitting diagnosis

attending physician

authenticate

consultant

consultation

countersigned

discharge summary

etiologies

face sheet

history

laboratory tests

medications

nursing assessment

nursing progress notes

operation

operative report

physical examination

physician's orders

progress notes

radiology tests

standing orders

surgeon

treatment

Uniform Hospital Discharge Data Set (UHDDS)

his chapter introduces a number of concepts related to data and further explores concepts related to data quality. It also provides the details of how data are organized in a health record—both data components and the record as a whole. As you read through this chapter, refer to Appendixes A and B for examples of the specific data collection forms and screens being discussed.

Data collection begins with building the hospital's data set for a given patient. Each type of facility has its own particular data set that must be considered when planning data collection strategies. While you are reading this chapter, make a list of the items that you think would be appropriate to include in the minimum data set required in an acute care facility—the Uniform Hospital Discharge Data Set (UHDDS).

CLINICAL FLOW OF DATA

In any health care delivery encounter, there is a pattern of activity and data collection that is characteristic of the facility and the type of care being rendered. Although there are unique differences, as we will see in Chapter 7, most encounters have some basic points in common: patient registration, clinical data collection and evaluation, assessment, and treatment.

PATIENT REGISTRATION

All patients who seek treatment in any setting (e.g., emergency department, clinic, inpatient unit) within a hospital must be registered. Inpatient admissions usually correspond to one of four scenarios. When a patient goes to the hospital, sometimes it is unexpected, in which case the patient is taken to the emergency department and admitted as an *emergency admission*. At other times, the patient's visit is expected, in which case the patient has an appointment (i.e., the patient's physician or someone in the physician's office arranges for, or schedules, the admission). The patient may be admitted because of an exacerbation of a medical condition. A woman may be coming in to give birth by elective cesarean section. The physician or someone from the physician's office calls in advance in much the same way that a patient calls a physician's office and makes an appointment. This type of admission is referred to as a *direct admission*. Other patients may be admitted as *transfer patients* from other hospitals or skilled nursing facilities. *Newborns* are considered to be admitted at the time of birth and are registered soon thereafter. In all instances, with the exception of newborns, a physician must create an order to admit the patient.

Organization of the Department

Hospitals often have an entire department whose function is similar to the registration or reception area of a physician's office. The patient registration department (also called the *admissions department* or *patient access*) is responsible for ensuring the timely and accurate admission of patients. Employees who perform the clerical function of completing the paperwork may be called *admitting clerks, registrars,* or *patient registration specialists.* In a small hospital, the admissions department may consist of only one person; however, in a larger facility, a number of health care professionals are trained to register the patient.

If there is one place in the hospital where all registration activities are performed, the registration function is said to be centralized. In larger facilities, the registration function may be decentralized—that is, registrars are placed in locations throughout the facility. For example, registration areas may be located in the emergency department, clinics, and same-day surgery area, as well as in a general area. However registration is organized, it is a process and function that must be staffed around-the-clock, every day of the week.

Data Collection

After the patient arrives at the patient registration reception area, the registration clerk asks the patient for proof of identity and insurance, as well as demographic data, certain socioeconomic data, and financial data. These data are used to populate (or update) the master patient index. In a paper record, these data are printed together on a form known as a **face sheet** or an **admission record** (Table 4-1). It is important to file this form at the beginning of every record so that the patient is clearly identified to everyone who records or accesses data in it. In addition to printing out the admission record, employees in patient registration also provide the means by which clinical personnel can identify every page in the record, using either an identification plate for stamping pages or labels to affix to the individual pages. If the hospital uses a bar code system, labels with the patient's bar code are also provided.

The patient is also asked to sign an admission consent form, with the patient's signature witnessed by the registration clerk. If the patient is unable to sign this form, the registrar must make a note of this fact and follow up with an attempt to obtain a signature during the hospitalization. The admission consent form is important because it permits physicians and other hospital staff to provide general care.

In addition to beginning the data collection process for the health record and labeling the files, the staff member must also properly label the patients themselves. Many facilities use wristbands to identify each patient with relevant data. These data might include the patient's birth date, admission date, medical record number, account number, and the attending physician's name. Recent technology has enabled a picture of the patient to be included on the wristband as well. Once the wristband is donned, it is difficult to remove, which means that the patient can be clearly identified during the hospitalization or encounter at all times. Physicians and all hospital staff must check each patient's wristband before administering any treatments to confirm that they are performing the appropriate treatment for the right patient. Occasionally, the facility will require that patients be photographed for the purpose of identification. If photographs are taken, care must be taken to comply with all applicable rules to ensure patient privacy (see Chapter 11).

As mentioned earlier, some hospitals have an emergency department. Patients arriving in the emergency department are initially treated as ambulatory care patients because they are expected

TABLE 4-1	**Sample Data Included in an Admission Record**
DATA ELEMENT	**EXPLANATION**
Patient's identification number	Number assigned by the facility to this patient
Patient's billing number	Number assigned by the facility to this visit
Admission date	Calendar day: month, day, and year
Discharge date	Calendar day: month, day, and year
Patient's name	Full name, including any titles (MD, PhD)
Patient's address	Address of usual residence
Sex	Male or female
Marital status	Married, single, divorced, separated
Race and ethnicity	Must choose from choices given on the admissions form
Religion	Optional
Occupational	General occupation (e.g., teacher, lawyer)
Current employment	Specific job (e.g., professor, district attorney)
Employer	Company name
Insurance	Insurance company name and address
Insurance identification numbers	Insurance company group and individual identification numbers
Additional insurance	Some patients insured by multiple companies; all information to be collected
Guarantor	Individual or organization who is responsible for paying the bill if the insurance company declines payment
Attending physician	Name of the attending physician; may also include the physician's identification number
Admitting diagnosis	Reason the patient is being admitted

These are typical items that are included in an admission record. Remember that the admission record contains demographic, financial, and some socioeconomic data. What is missing from this list?

to be treated and released. Sometimes, however, the condition of the patient warrants admission to the hospital. In this case, a member of the emergency department staff contacts the patient registration department to arrange for admission. The registrar will arrange for the patient to be transported from the emergency department to a room or bed on a patient unit. Previously collected patient information is transferred to the patient registration department, and an inpatient stay is initiated. Clinical information accompanies the patient to the patient unit. Seriously ill pateients may not be able to walk to the patient registration area. Therefore, additional data collection often takes place at the patient's bedside or with the assistance of family members. A physician order is required to effect the admission. In these instances, the emergency department physician may order the admission; however, the emergency department physician will not be the patient's attending physician once the patient is admitted. The patient's attending physician may be the physician whom the patient regularly visits or a physician who has been assigned to them.

Precertification

As with a physician office visit, the patient registration staff must determine whether the patient has insurance and whether the insurance covers the care that the physician has requested. The physician must provide an **admitting diagnosis** to explain the reason for admission as part of the preapproval process. This preapproval, or precertification, process is extremely important to the hospital. Without the confirmation that the insurance company will pay for the patient's stay, the hospital is exposed to the risk of financial loss in the event that the patient is unable to pay for his or her treatment. Often, when the patient's hospitalization is planned, the patient will complete the initial registration process and some preadmission testing (e.g., laboratory and radiology tests) before the actual hospitalization. This slightly extended process gives members of the patient registration department a bit more time to obtain the necessary information.

The registration process can be somewhat complicated because the registrars must be able to handle any and all admission scenarios and understand various insurance rules. Because the registrar is often the first hospital staff member that patients and their families meet, providing excellent customer service is important. Many facilities require registrars to speak at least two languages, depending on the patient population. Many registration departments are staffed and managed by health information professionals. Registrars have their own professional association, the National Association of Healthcare Access Management (http://www.naham.org).

INITIAL ASSESSMENT

After being formally admitted, the patient is taken to the appropriate treatment area. Sometimes this area is the patient unit, and sometimes it is the preoperative area, where the patient is prepared immediately for surgery. In the treatment area, the patient is assessed by nursing staff in much the same way that a patient in a physician's office is assessed by a medical assistant or a nurse in the physician's office. After the nursing assessment has been completed, the physician performs an assessment of the patient. An important part of the initial assessment is the preliminary, or provisional, diagnosis.

Hit-Bit

Admission Consent Forms

Depending on the patient population that the hospital serves, admission consent forms may be printed in various languages, such as Spanish, Polish, Chinese, and Arabic as well as English. Great care must be taken when translating forms from English to other languages because this form becomes part of the legal patient record. Hospitals often send their forms to companies that specialize in such translations.

PLAN OF CARE

On the basis of the initial assessments, a plan of care is developed for the patient. Because the plan of care may involve many disciplines, often each patient is assigned to a patient care team that consists of various health care professionals, in addition to physicians. The initial plan may consist of tests and other diagnostic procedures. If the diagnosis has already been established, therapeutic procedures, such as surgery, may take place. All procedures, whether diagnostic or therapeutic, are undertaken only on the direct order of the physician. Orders may also specify whether the patient has bathroom privileges, requires a special diet, or can have visitors.

As you can see, an inpatient stay shares certain similarities with an ambulatory visit. The primary differences are length of stay and volume of patient data collected. Table 4-2 compares an ambulatory care visit with an acute care, inpatient stay. The physician always coordinates the care of the patient. The degree of collaboration with other disciplines in developing the plan of care depends on the patient's diagnosis and the health care setting. Rehabilitation facilities, for example, are characterized by highly interdisciplinary care plans because therapies play the largest role in patient care, and the physician relies on feedback from rehabilitation therapists to direct further treatment. Care plan meetings take place regularly and include patients and families. In acute care, the interdisciplinary activity often is not as formal or routine.

Physicians collaborate by asking one another for advice; this is called a **consultation.** The **attending physician,** who is responsible for the patient's overall care, requests a consultation, citing the specialty information needed and the specific reason for the consultation. The **consultant** evaluates the patient and responds to the request with specific diagnostic or therapeutic opinions and recommendations. For example, a patient admitted for treatment of a heart condition may develop severe diarrhea. The attending physician may request a consultation from a gastrointestinal specialist or an infectious disease specialist. Table 4-3 lists the data required for a consultation. In addition, the nursing staff advises physicians of changes in the patient's status or problems that may arise.

Although each patient is treated individually, the process of treating a patient is based on standards of medical practice. Nursing practice has evolved its own standards of practice, and nurses historically have been diligent in documenting and providing evidence for that practice.

TABLE 4-2	**Contrast Between Key Ambulatory and Acute Care Events**	
	AMBULATORY CARE (PHYSICIAN'S OFFICE)	**ACUTE CARE (HOSPITAL)**
How to choose	Referral, advertisement, or investigation Choices sometimes limited by insurance plan	Choices limited to facilities in which physician has privileges Choices sometimes limited by insurance plan
Initiate contact	Call for an appointment; walk-in, if permitted	Emergency department or attending physician orders admission
Collection of demographic and financial data	Receptionist, medical secretary	Patient registration, patient access, or admissions department personnel
Initial assessment	Vital signs and chief complaint recorded by physician, nurse or medical assistant	Nursing assessment Physician responsible for history and physical examination
Plan of care	Prescriptions, instructions, diagnostic tests, and therapeutic procedures performed on an ambulatory basis	Medication administration, instructions, and diagnostic tests performed on an inpatient basis

TABLE 4-3	Data Required for a Consultation
DATA ELEMENT	**EXPLANATION**
Patient's name	See Table 4-1
Patient's identification number	See Table 4-1
Physician's order	Required before the consultation is performed (see Table 4-6)
Date of request	Date that the attending physician requests the consultation
Specialty being consulted	Cardiology, podiatry, gastroenterology, etc.
Reason for consultation	Brief explanation of reason that the consultant's opinion is being sought
Authentication	Authentication of physician requesting consultation
Date of evaluation	When consultant saw patient
Consultant's opinion	Diagnosis or recommendations; may be an entire report, similar to an H&P (see Tables 4-4 and 4-5)
Report date	Date that consultant prepares report of the opinion
Authentication	Authentication of consultant

Exercise 4-1

Clinical Flow of Data

1. Upon admission, patient data is collected that helps to identify the patient and the payer for the services to be rendered. List as many data items (fields) as you can recall that would be included in an admission record.

CLINICAL DATA

An enormous volume and variety of clinical data can be collected in an inpatient setting. Physicians, nurses, therapists, and numerous ancillary and administrative departments contribute notes, reports, and documentation of events. This section covers the major data elements that each of these professionals contributes. Data elements are gathered in logical groups, or collections, according to the nature of the data being collected. Figure 4-1 shows the contributors of health data and the collections of data that they contribute.

PHYSICIANS

When the patient is admitted, the attending physician conducts a medical evaluation. This evaluation begins with the subjective history, the objective physical examination, the assessment of a preliminary diagnosis or diagnoses, and a plan of care, for which orders are recorded. Medical decision making is a complex activity that depends on the number of possible diagnoses, the volume and complexity of diagnostic data that must be reviewed, and the severity of the patient's condition. This complexity is reflected in the physician's documentation. Figure 4-2 illustrates the components of medical decision making.

History

A **history** is taken from the data that the patient reports to the physician regarding the patient's health. This information may be written by hand, but it is generally preserved in a dictated report that is later typed. In an ambulatory care setting, the history can be very short and focused. In an inpatient setting, however, the history is usually significantly more comprehensive. The history should consist of the chief complaint, the history of the present complaint, a description of relevant previous illnesses and procedures, and a review of the relevant organs or body systems. The

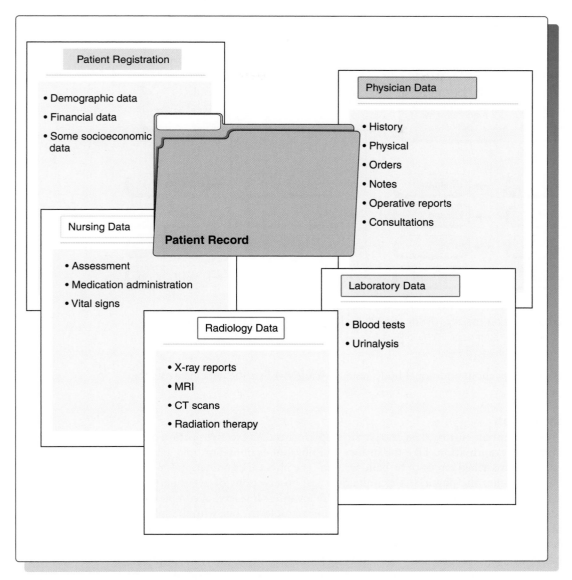

Patient Registration

- Demographic data
- Financial data
- Some socioeconomic data

Physician Data

- History
- Physical
- Orders
- Notes
- Operative reports
- Consultations

Nursing Data

- Assessment
- Medication administration
- Vital signs

Patient Record

Laboratory Data

- Blood tests
- Urinalysis

Radiology Data

- X-ray reports
- MRI
- CT scans
- Radiation therapy

◆ **Figure 4-1**

Sample data elements in a health record by source.

history is characterized by its complexity. The complexity of the history is directly related to the amount of data that the physician needs to evaluate the patient's problem.

For example, if a patient visits the physician's office because of a splinter in his or her finger, a simple, or problem-focused, history is directed toward the presenting problem, and very little else is discussed or observed. The history would probably contain nothing more than the events surrounding the occurrence of the splinter and possibly an inquiry as to whether the patient had received a tetanus vaccination in the past 10 years.

Sometimes, even in a fairly straightforward situation, the complexity of the issue may expand fairly rapidly. For example, the finger may appear to be infected, which might lead to a blood test. Perhaps the patient had fallen beforehand, which might cause the physician to suspect possible head trauma or fracture. The history becomes increasingly complex as the number of body systems are involved and the potential threat to the patient's life becomes more evident.

A patient admitted to an acute care facility requires more substantive evaluation, particularly when the underlying illness is still under investigation. In that case, the physician collects a comprehensive history. The physician makes more detailed inquiries about the patient's entire medical

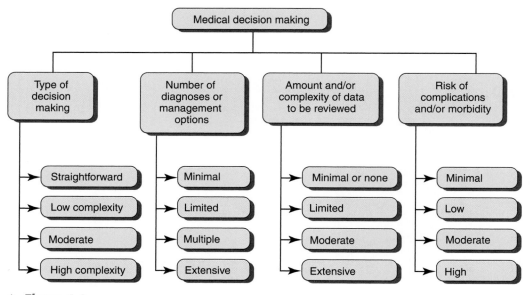

◆ **Figure 4-2**
Flowchart of medical decision making. (From Alice A. Andress. *Saunders' Manual of Medical Office Management.* Philadelphia: Saunders, 1996, p 96.)

history and asks questions about additional body systems. Table 4-4 lists the data elements that are collected in a history.

Physical Examination

After collecting the appropriate history data, the physician performs the objective portion of the evaluation: the **physical examination.** Like the history, the physical examination may take the form of a dictated and transcribed report or be hand written. The physical examination (or more briefly, the *physical*) includes the physician's examination and observations of every pertinent body system. We say *pertinent* because the physical generally follows the same level of complexity as the history. For example, the patient described in the previous example, the one with the splinter, may require only an examination of the affected finger. In the absence of infection or other trauma, a problem-focused physical examination is appropriate. Moreover, it is not appropriate for the physician to perform a comprehensive physical examination of the patient with a splinter in the absence of a history indicating its necessity. In many cases, gynecological and rectal examinations are frequently omitted, sometimes at the patient's request and also when no related abnormalities or disorders are suspected. The physical examination ends with the physician's assessment, also called the *impression,* and the initial plan of treatment. Table 4-5 lists data elements that are collected in a physical.

When the history and physical data are collected and reported together in a single, longer report, it is referred to as the *history and physical* (H&P). Note that the H&P follows the medical evaluation process previously described. The subjective data (the patient's history) are followed by the objective data (the physical), and then the assessment and the plan of care are recorded.

The data collected in these two reports are critical for patient management; therefore specific rules direct the completion of this data collection activity. For example, in an acute care facility, the Joint Commission on the Accreditation of Healthcare Organizations (JCAHO) requires that the history and physical be present in the record within 24 hours of admission or before any surgical procedure takes place. The physician collecting and recording the data must **authenticate** the data. Authentication can be, for example, a signature on a dictated and typed report, a signature at the bottom of a handwritten note, or a password entered into a computer. In some teaching hospitals, the H&P may be performed by a resident physician. The resident physician and the attending physician are both required to authenticate the data.

In an ambulatory care facility, the H&P may be the only data recorded at the time of the encounter, particularly if the patient's problem is minor. In an inpatient setting, the H&P is performed only on admission. In a residence setting, such as a long-term care facility, the H&P must

TABLE 4-4	**Data Elements in a History**

DATA ELEMENT	EXPLANATION
Chief complaint	The reason for the encounter, usually as expressed by the patient
History of present illness	The patient's report of the events, circumstances, and other details surrounding the chief complaint
Review of systems	The patient's responses to the physician's questions regarding pertinent body systems, including Constitutional symptoms Eyes Ears, nose, mouth, and throat Cardiovascular Respiratory Gastrointestinal Genitourinary Musculoskeletal Integumentary Neurological Psychiatric Endocrine Hematological/lymphatic Allergic/immunological
Past, family, and/or social history	Including the patient's prior illnesses and operations, socioeconomic concerns, and important family illnesses

All histories contain, at a minimum, the chief complaint and the history of present illness. The history can have four levels of complexity.

LEVEL OF HISTORY	HISTORY OF PRESENT ILLNESS	REVIEW OF SYSTEMS	PERSONAL, FAMILY, AND/OR SOCIAL HISTORY
Problem focused	Brief	N/A	N/A
Expanded problem focused	Brief	Problem pertinent	N/A
Detailed	Extended	Extended	Pertinent
Comprehensive	Extended	Complete	Complete

Data from the American Medical Association. Modified from Carol J. Buck. *Step-by-Step Medical Coding*. 3rd ed. Philadelphia: Saunders, 2000, pp 33-37.

be updated periodically so that it represents the patient's current status. Health information management professionals must know the regulatory and accreditation requirements of any data collection activity that occurs in facilities in which they are employed.

Orders

While the patient is in the facility, the physician makes decisions about the patient's **treatment,** including those pertaining to any further diagnostic testing. For example, a patient who is scheduled for an appendectomy may have entered the hospital with an admitting diagnosis of appendicitis. The plan of treatment includes the appendectomy. Other patients enter the hospital with vague or multiple symptoms, and the physician is not entirely sure which of several possible conditions the patient actually has. In the SOAP note example discussed in the previous chapter, you saw that right lower quadrant abdominal pain could have a number of different **etiologies,** or causes, which are investigated while the patient is in the hospital. In an acute care facility, the physician must specifically order the diagnostic procedures that will help reveal the patient's diagnosis.

The doctor's instructions for laboratory tests, radiological examinations, consultations, and medication are all contained in a separate data collection called **physician's orders.** Physician's orders may be recorded in a patient's record in numerous ways, from handwritten instructions on

TABLE 4-5	Data Elements in a Physical Examination
LEVEL OF EXAMINATION	**BODY AREA(S)/ORGAN SYSTEM(S)***
Problem focused	Affected body area (BA) and organ system (OS)
Expanded problem focuses	Affected BA and other BA/OS
Detailed	Extensive affected BA/OS
Comprehensive	Complete BA and complete OS

Organ Systems
- Eyes
- Ears, nose, mouth, and throat
- Respiratory
- Cardiovascular
- Genitourinary
- Hematological/lymphatic immunological
- Musculoskeletal
- Skin
- Neurological
- Psychiatric
- Gastrointestinal

Body Area
- Head
- Neck
- Chest
- Abdomen
- Genitalia, groin, buttocks
- Back
- Extremities

General
- Constitutional (vital signs, general appearance)

Data from the American Medical Association. Modified from Carol J. Buck. *Step-by-Step Medical Coding*. 3rd ed. Philadelphia: Saunders, 2000, pp 38-39.

a piece of paper to direct entry into a computer. No tests or treatment can take place without the physician's order. Orders must be dated and authenticated by the physician. Nursing staff execute the orders, or put them into effect, by notifying the appropriate department or outside agency of the order. For example, medications may be requested from the hospital pharmacy, radiological tests may be arranged, or a consultant may be contacted. The nurse who executes the order authenticates and dates the activity (see Figure 3-18).

Although each patient is treated individually, many conditions call for a predetermined plan of care. This predetermined plan may include a specific series of blood tests, x-rays, and urinalysis. It may also consist of a set of preoperative or pretherapeutic activities. Such predetermined plans are called **standing orders.** The direction to put a set of standing orders into effect comes from the physician, who is still required to authenticate and date the orders.

Orders may be directly entered by the physician or dictated to a registered nurse, who then enters the orders. Orders that are dictated to a registered nurse are called *verbal orders (VOs).* Verbal orders that are dictated over the telephone are called *telephone orders (TOs).* VOs and TOs are sometimes necessary in emergencies and in situations when the physician is unable to be present at the hospital at the time the orders are required. VOs and TOs must be authenticated by the physician, although they can be executed immediately. In an ambulatory care setting, orders may not be formally set apart from other data collections and may be incorporated in the end of the H&P or progress notes. Nevertheless, the data elements of the physician's orders as described previously are present. Table 4-6 lists the data contained in an order.

Progress Notes

While treating the patient, the physician continues to make observations and update the assessment and plan. These **progress notes** are important evidence of the care that the patient has received and serve to document the physician's activities and evaluation process. Notes are often documented in the SOAP format (see Chapter 3); some physicians even write the SOAP acronym on the note. In an ambulatory care setting, progress notes may immediately follow the H&P in the patient's medical record or may be omitted if all of the encounter data are included in the H&P. However, in an inpatient setting, progress notes become critical because days, weeks, or months may elapse from the time of the H&P taken at admission to the time of the patient's discharge. Notes must be authenticated and dated. In a facility in which physician residents are

TABLE 4-6	Data Contained in a Physician's Order

DATA REQUIRED FOR AN ORDER PERSONALLY ENTERED BY THE PHYSICIAN

DATA ELEMENT	EXPLANATION
Patient's name	See Table 4-1
Patient's identification number	See Table 4-1
Order date	Date the order is rendered
Time	Time the order is rendered
Order	Medication, test, therapy, consultation, or other action directed by the physician
Physician's authentication	Physician's signature or password
Executor's authentication	Signature or password of party effecting the order
Execution date	Date the order was effected
Execution time	Time the order was effected

An important element of a physician's order is the time that it is rendered. The interpretation of the requirement to authenticate verbal orders as soon as possible is often "within 24 hours." Implicitly, this requires a date and time attached to both the order and the authentication. If the physician personally makes the order, then the date and time of both are the same. If it is a verbal order, then the nurse taking the order must record the date and time, and the physician logs the appropriate date and time of the subsequent authentication. In a paper-based system, the time of the order is often omitted. However, in a computer-based order entry system, the time can be automatically affixed by the computer.

DATA REQUIRED FOR A VERBAL ORDER

DATA ELEMENT	EXPLANATION
Patient's name	See Table 4-1
Patient's identification number	See Table 4-1
Order date	Date the order is received
Time	Time the order is received
Nurse's authentication	Signature or password of party receiving the order
Order	Medication, test, therapy, consultation, or other action directed by the physician
Physician's authentication	Physician's signature or password
Physician's authentication date	Date the order is authenticated
Physician's authentication time	Time the physician authenticated the order
Executor's authentication	Signature or password of party effecting the order
Execution date	Date the order was effected
Execution time	Time the order was effected

training, the resident may collect and record the data for the note. In many situations, and always for unlicensed residents, the resident's note must also be authenticated, or **countersigned,** by the attending physician.

Consultations

Sometimes when a patient is in the hospital, the attending physician must call in an expert in a particular field. For example, if the patient undergoing an appendectomy in the previous example also has chronic obstructive pulmonary disease, emphysema, asthma, or other severe respiratory problem, the attending physician may elect to call in a pulmonary specialist to evaluate the patient's status before surgery. Some typical consultations that may be performed in an inpatient setting include an endocrinology consultation if the patient has diabetes mellitus; a podiatry consultation if the patient has overgrown toenails or onychomycosis; a cardiology consultation if the patient has some sort of heart condition; and, as mentioned previously, a pulmonary specialist if the patient has respiratory concerns. Another typical type of consultation is a psychiatric consultation, which would be appropriate if the patient suffers from depression or other behavioral health issues. Table 4-3 lists the data required in a consultation.

Discharge Summary

In an inpatient setting, a **discharge summary,** or case summary of the patient's care, is prepared by the attending physician or his or her designee. This summary should include a brief history of the problem, the discharge diagnosis and other significant findings, a list of treatments and procedures performed, the patient's condition on discharge, and any instructions given to the patient or patient's caregiver. As with other data, the discharge summary must be authenticated and dated. The recording of the discharge summary often takes the form of a dictated and transcribed report.

Some inpatient stays do not require a discharge summary, such as an admission of a normal newborn. Generally, stays of less than 48 hours' duration do not require a detailed discharge summary; a form called a *short stay form* may be completed instead. An exception to this occurs when a patient expires while in a hospital for less than 48 hours. In such cases, a full discharge summary is required.

NURSES

While the patient is in the hospital, the professionals who perform most of the patient's care, particularly in acute care and long-term care facilities, are the nurses and their ancillary staff. Nurses collect and record their own set of data for each patient. As with physician data, nursing data also requires authentication, dates, and times.

Nursing Assessment

Nurses perform an assessment of the patient when the patient first enters the facility. The purpose of the **nursing assessment** is not to diagnose the patient's illness—that is the responsibility of the physician—but to diagnose the patient's care needs. The assessment includes determining the patient's understanding of his or her condition and whether the patient has any particular concerns or needs that will affect nursing care. The nursing assessment includes an evaluation of the condition of the patient's skin, learning needs, and ability to perform self-care.

Notes

Nurses also must record **nursing progress notes.** During each shift, the nurse writes down particular events or interactions with the patient. Patient complaints and any activities of the nursing staff to address those complaints are noted. The elements of a nursing progress note are given in Table 4-7. In a paper-based record, these notes typically take the form of free text. In a computer-based record, the documentation may be guided and at least partially menu-driven.

TABLE 4-7	Data Required for a Nurse's Progress Note
DATA ELEMENT	**EXPLANATION**
Patient's name	See Table 4-1
Patient's identification number	See Table 4-1
Date	Date of the note
Time	Time of the note
Note	Nurse's comments, observations, and documentation of activities
Nurse's authentication	Nurse's signature or password

Notes should be written as soon as possible after the activity has occurred. Thus the date and time of the note coincide with the date and time of the occurrence. If a note is written after the fact, the date and time of the occurrence must be separately noted.

In a paper-based system, the note field is generally a large alphanumeric field in which the author can comment freely. In a computer-based system, this field may be replaced with a series of fields from which the nurse can compose comments from predetermined menus, in addition to a free field for more specific remarks. The actual content of the note is governed by nursing professional standards and facility requirements.

Vital Signs

Nurses are also responsible for observing and recording the patient's vital signs while the patient is in the health care facility. Vital signs include temperature, blood pressure, pulse, and respiration. Frequently, vital signs are recorded in a graphical format, which can be referenced easily while the patient is in the facility. Chapter 3 demonstrated how displaying a patient's temperature in a graph or picture facilitates review of the data (see Figure 3-2). In a computer-based record, the data are also entered into a field that can then be linked to previous data collections to produce a report that is a graphical representation of the cumulative data over time. Other data that nurses collect in graph format include fluid intake and output and mechanical ventilation readings.

Medication Administration

One of the most important nursing data collections involves the administration of **medications.** The name of the medication, dosage, date and time of administration, method of administration, and the nurse who administered it are important data elements.

LABORATORY DATA

In an inpatient setting, the physician frequently orders routine laboratory tests, such as a complete blood count (CBC) and a urinalysis (UA). The CBC and UA have many uses and may be ordered for specific diagnostic purposes. When these laboratory tests are performed at the time of the patient's admission, they help to identify preexisting infectious conditions. Infections identified after 72 hours of hospitalization are attributed to the facility: These are called *nosocomial infections.* **Laboratory tests** are performed only when ordered by the physician. The results of the tests are included in the health record. Laboratory results include both patient-specific data and data comparing the patient's test results against normative ranges of data. For example, the normal hemoglobin range is 12.0 to 15.0 for female adults. A female adult patient whose hemoglobin level is 14.3 is within normal limits.

In an ambulatory care setting, a single set of laboratory tests may be ordered. In an inpatient setting, the number of laboratory tests may increase dramatically. For some conditions, daily blood tests are appropriate. Therefore multiple data fields, in which the results of multiple tests can be recorded, are necessary. Once again, the usefulness of a computer-based record is evident. Once the test result data are collected, a computer can display them in whole or in part, as well as graphically.

RADIOLOGY DATA

Radiology tests generate two sets of data: the original diagnostic image and the interpretation. The original diagnostic image is usually retained separately from the patient's record, which includes only the interpretation of the images. For example, a chest x-ray produces a large film, which is retained in special envelopes or files, usually in the radiology department. The radiologist's interpretation of the image on the film, another type of data collection that often takes the form of a dictated and transcribed report, becomes part of the patient's record. Currently, facilities are increasingly relying on digital methods of radiographic imaging. These digital images may be downloaded to a disc with the reading software and given to the patient.

SPECIAL RECORDS

The previous discussion of clinical data includes only the basic data elements common to most patients. Depending on the diagnosis and the clinical setting, many other data elements are collected. The clinical flow of data is similar in every type of health care setting. Up to this point, the discussion has focused on ambulatory or physician's office settings and inpatient visits in an acute care hospital. Other types of health care facilities require special records, which are discussed in Chapter 7. However, even in an acute care facility, certain clinical situations require additional documentation or variations on the standard documentation described in the previous sections.

Operative Records

The previously discussed data elements are very common and occur in one form or another in almost all inpatient health records. However, physicians and nurses may collect and record other data in the health record, notably in the case of surgical procedures. The patient who undergoes a surgical procedure requires two sets of data: the operative data and the anesthesia data.

Operative Report

The **operative report** is recorded as a detailed, usually dictated and typed document. Transcribed operative reports are not immediately available to users; therefore a brief operative note in the progress notes is usually written. The operative report lists the preoperative and postoperative diagnosis, the **surgeon** and surgical assistants, the procedures performed, and a detailed description of the **operation,** including the patient's condition and any blood loss. The operative report should be completed immediately after the procedure. As with all physician activities, the operative report is authenticated and dated. Additional data, such as instrument counts, are collected and recorded by nursing staff and kept separate from the operative report.

Anesthesia Report

The anesthesiologist performs preoperative and postoperative evaluations of the patient's condition. These may be documented in the progress notes or on a specially designed data collection device. During the procedure, a graphical representation of the patient's status is recorded continuously.

Same-Day Surgery Records

A patient can enter a hospital, have surgery, and leave on the same day; this is called *same-day surgery.* In those cases, because of the simplicity of the procedure, the data collection is frequently compressed so that the H&P, some anesthesia information, and some procedural information (e.g., the operative report) are compressed into shorter documents. The short stay form may also be used for these types of cases.

Obstetrical Records

Obstetrical records differ from the ones that we have already discussed because of the type of data that are collected. When a woman is pregnant and regularly visits a physician's office or clinic for prenatal care, many data are collected on her progress and the progress of the fetus. Shortly before the woman is due to give birth, the data are transferred to the hospital in which she intends to deliver. The data are incorporated into the inpatient record. Upon admission for childbirth, pregnant patients are monitored for contractions, fetal activity, and stress during labor. Specific delivery data, such as the number of previous births, types of deliveries, and conditions of the newborns, are collected.

Neonatal Records

Neonatal records for healthy newborns are generally very short. Because these patients are in the hospital solely because of the mother's choice of delivery site, care is focused on promoting the infant's comfort and assisting the mother with learning care. The contents of a newborn record consist of an admission record, a brief physical that includes mention of any congenital anomalies, the birth record, nursing and pediatric progress notes, notes regarding medication administration, a note regarding the circumcision (if applicable), and a record of any testing done, such as a phenylketonuria (PKU) or hearing test. Newborns who exhibit signs of jaundice also will have notes in their records pertaining to therapeutic interventions taken, such as phototherapy.

Babies who are born ill require more intensive care. Neonatal intensive care units (NICUs) feature more technological options, a greater number of caregivers, and a correspondingly high volume of data collection.

Intensive Care Records

Sometimes, patients who are gravely ill when they enter the hospital are sent to special nursing care units called *intensive care units (ICUs).* A patient with a serious heart problem might be cared for in a coronary care unit (CCU). Because of the intensity of nursing care in CCUs, nurses prefer to use graphical forms, which provide a great deal of visual data at a glance. In a paper record, this may consist of heavy-stock foldout graphs, which can be as large as 8 × 14 inches or 8 × 17 inches. They represent 24 hours of care. Vital signs are plotted on graphs that illustrate the patient's progress and the way the patient is being treated. Some of these forms are difficult to photocopy; however, they greatly facilitate the recording of patient data.

The following are some examples of special care units for close monitoring and care:

- Intensive care unit: for medical treatment
- Surgical intensive care unit: for postsurgical treatment
- Cardiac care unit: for cardiac treatment
- Neonatal intensive care unit: for care of newborns

Exercise 4-2

Clinical Data

1. The first page in a paper record is usually the _____.
2. Describe the events that will occur when a patient is admitted to an acute care facility for an operation. What caregivers will be involved with the patient?
3. In this chapter, we discussed some of the actual data collection devices that are used in health care facilities, particularly acute care. Table 4-6 lists the key items in a physician order. List those items as fields and describe them in data dictionary format, as discussed in Chapter 3.
4. At the end of a hospital stay, a _____ is usually required to be completed, often as a dictated and transcribed report.
5. Routine documentation of the nurse's interaction with a patient is recorded in the _____.
6. Sometimes a physician needs to ask another physician for an opinion regarding the care of a patient. The physician whom he asks is referred to as the _____.
7. Match the definition on the left with the vocabulary word(s) on the right.

   1. Acronym that describes the medical decision-making process.
      Also refers to the way physicians organize their progress notes.
   2. Analysis of body fluids.
   3. Examination of a patient using x-rays.
   4. One or more surgical procedures performed at the same time.
   5. Record of all drugs given to a patient during the hospitalization.
   6. The diagnostic, therapeutic, or palliative measures that will be taken to investigate or treat the patient's condition or disease.
   7. The nurse's evaluation of the patient.
   8. The physician's directions regarding the patient's care. Also refers to the data collection device on which these elements are captured.
   9. The physician's documentation of a surgical procedure, usually dictated and transcribed.
   10. The physician's documentation of the examination of the patient, particularly at the initial visit.
   11. The physician's record of each visit with the patient.
   12. The predetermined, routine orders that have been designated to pertain to specific diagnoses or procedures. Must be ordered and authenticated by the appropriate physician.
   13. The process of systematically eliminating potential diagnoses. Also refers to the list of potential diagnoses.

   A. Laboratory tests
   B. Medication Sheet
   C. Nursing Assessment
   D. Operation
   E. Operative report
   F. Physical Exam
   G. Physician's orders
   H. Plan of treatment
   I. Progress notes
   J. Radiology tests
   K. Rule out
   L. SOAP format
   M. Standing orders

TABLE 4-8	Data Dictionary with Range of Valid Values				
NAME	**DEFINITION**	**SIZE**	**TYPE**	**EXAMPLE**	**VALID RANGE**
Day	Day of the month	Two characters	Numerical	15	1–31
Month	Month of the year	Two characters	Numerical	08	1–12
Temperature	Patient's temperature	Five characters	Numerical	98.6	85–110

These are simple data elements that may appear in a patient health record. Although validity checks may include the size of the field, the range of values is also an important evaluation tool to check to prevent data entry errors. Can you see a problem with the valid range of values for the Day column? How can you fix the problem?

When determining a valid range of values for clinical measures, you must be careful to include a sufficiently wide range so that extreme values can be entered; however, because some extreme values are not compatible with life, be careful to place reasonable limits on the values. Excessively wide ranges may jeopardize the accuracy of the data.

DATA QUALITY

In Chapter 3, data validity was discussed as a measure of data quality. Only valid data entered within a range of values that is legitimate for that type of data should be collected. For example, if you are collecting social security numbers, the computer is programmed to look for a nine-digit field. (Alternatively, you may choose to collect it as three fields of three, two, and four characters, respectively, or as 11 digits including the dashes.) If someone tries to enter a social security number with 11 digits, it is not recognized by the computer as a valid entry. The range of valid entries is an element of the data dictionary. Table 4-8 illustrates a data dictionary with this additional element.

Earlier in this chapter, you were asked to think of a list of data elements for an acute care facility that would correspond to the **Uniform Hospital Discharge Data Set (UHDDS).** Here are the major elements of the UHDDS. Some of the elements are self-explanatory. Where specific choices are permitted, they are noted in the following outline (Abdelhak et al 2001):

Person/Enrollment Data

1. Personal/unique identifier
   The patient's medical record number or other unique identifier. Although some advocate for the use of the Social Security number in this field, there are strong arguments against it.
2. Date of birth
   The year, month, and day of the patient's birth
3. Gender
   Male, female, or unknown/not stated
4. Race and ethnicity
   Race: American Indian/Eskimo/Aleut; Asian or Pacific Islander; Black; White; Other; Unknown/not stated
   Ethnicity: Hispanic Origin; Other; Unknown/not stated
5. Residence
   Full address and ZIP code of the patient's usual residence

Encounter Data

6. Health care facility identification number
   Identification number of the facility that treated the patient
7. Admission date
   The year, month, and day of admission for the current episode of care
8. Type of admission
   Was the admission expected or unexpected?
9. Discharge date
   The year, month, and day of discharge for the current episode of care

10. Attending physician's identification number

    The unique national identification number assigned to the clinician of record at discharge who is responsible for the discharge summary

11. Surgeon's identification number

    The unique national identification number assigned to the clinician who performed the principal procedure

12. Principal diagnosis

    The condition established after study to be chiefly responsible for occasioning the admission of the patient to the hospital (ICD-9-CM code: see Chapter 6)

13. Other diagnoses

    All conditions that coexist at the time of admission, or develop subsequently, which affect the treatment received, the length of stay, or both (also an ICD-9-CM code)

14. Qualifier for other diagnoses

    For each other diagnosis, was the onset prior to admission? (Yes or No)

15. External cause-of-injury code

    The cause of an injury, poisoning, or adverse effect that has been recorded as the principal or other diagnosis (also an ICD-9-CM code)

16. Birth weight of neonate

    If the patient is a newborn, the actual birth weight in grams is reported.

17. Principal procedure and date of procedure

    The procedure that was performed for definitive treatment, rather than one performed for diagnostic or exploratory purposes, or was necessary to take care of a complication. If more than one procedure qualifies, the one most closely related to the principal diagnosis should be selected.

18. Other procedure(s) and the date(s) of the procedure(s)

    All other procedures that qualify (see 17).

19. Disposition of the patient at discharge

    Discharged alive

        Discharged to home or self care (routine discharge)

        Discharged/transferred to another short-term general hospital for inpatient care

        Discharged/transferred to skilled nursing facility (SNF)

        Discharged/transferred to an intermediate care facility (ICF)

        Discharged/transferred to another type of institution for inpatient care or referred for outpatient services to another institution

        Home under care of organized home health service organization

        Home under care of a Home IV provider

        Left against medical advice or discontinued care

    Expired

    Status not stated

20. Expected source of payment

    A. Primary source of payment. The primary source is expected to be responsible for the largest percentage of the patient's current bill.

    B. Secondary sources of payment.

21. Categories of source of payment are as follows:

    1. Self-pay
    2. Worker's Compensation
    3. Medicare
    4. Medicaid
    5. Maternal and Child Health
    6. Other government payments
    7. Blue Cross
    8. Insurance companies
    9. No charge (free, charity, special research, or teaching)
    10. Other
    11. Unknown/not stated

22. Total charges

    All charges for procedures and services rendered to the patient during a hospitalization or encounter.

Exercise 4-3

Data Quality

1. When physician orders are entered in a computer-based system, the computer can check the authentication to ensure that the individual who entered the data is authorized to do so (that is, that the authentication is correct). This is an example of a computer being used to ensure what characteristic of data?

2. Medicare requires a specific list of data elements to be collected about each patient who is discharged from an acute care facility. This list is called the Uniform Hospital Discharge Data Set (UHDDS). List as many items as you can remember from the UHDDS.

ACCREDITATION

Accreditation refers to the voluntary compliance by a facility with standards set by an external organization that is independent of the facility. Virtually ever provider has accreditation standards. It is up to the provider to decide which organization's accreditation standards best reflect the goals of the facility.

JCAHO

The most common accreditation sought by acute care facilities is hospital accreditation by the JCAHO. The JCAHO was introduced in Chapter 1. JCAHO accreditation is evidence of compliance with a broad range of standards. Founded in 1952, the JCAHO accredits many types of

TABLE 4-9	**Joint Commission Standards**
COMPREHENSIVE ACCREDITATION MANUAL FOR HOSPITALS (CAMH)	
EXAMPLES OF CHAPTERS	**EXAMPLES OF TOPICS**
Ethics, rights and responsibilities	Patient rights
Provision of care, treatment and services	Assessments, testing, use of restraints
Medication management	Medication orders, formularies, medication storage
Leadership	Management issues
Management of environment of care	Disaster drills, emergency management, utilities maintenance
Management of human resources	Competency, criminal background checks
Management of information	Security, documentation
Medical staff	Credentialing, continuing education

These are examples of the types of issues covered in the JCAHO Standards for Hospitals. Practitioners must have a thorough knowledge of the detailed standards to ensure continuous compliance. The accreditation standards may be obtained through the JCAHO. All accredited facilities should have an updated copy of the current standards available for reference.

From "Standards Frequently Asked Questions." *Comprehensive Accreditation Manual for Hospitals.* 2006. Joint Commission on Accreditation of Healthcare Organizations. 13 June 2006 <http://www.jointcommission.org/AccreditationPrograms/Hospitals/Standards/FAQs/default.htm>.

health care facilities. The JCAHO updates the standards annually to reflect current practice and its experience in reviewing facilities throughout the United States. The JCAHO hospital standards are currently divided into 11 functional sections (Table 4-9). For health information management professionals, there is no single section of the standards to which we can easily refer for all of our guidance. Virtually all of the standards contain something of which we must be aware.

AMERICAN OSTEOPATHIC ASSOCIATION

Founded in 1897, the American Osteopathic Association (AOA) is the primary professional association for doctors of osteopathy. The AOA accredits medical schools of osteopathy as well as heath care facilities.

Exercise 4-4

Accreditation

1. Identify an acute care facility in your area by looking in the telephone book or on the Internet. Find out as much as you can about the facility, including the types of services it offers. Describe the facility in terms of size, organization, patients, and average length of stay.

■ WORKS CITED

Abdelhak, Mervat, Sara Grostick, Mary Alice Hanken, and Ellen Jacobs. *Health Information: Management of a Strategic Resource.* 2nd ed. Philadelphia: Saunders, 2001.

■ SUGGESTED READING

Andress, Alice A. *Manual of Medical Office Management.* Philadelphia: Saunders, 1996.
Clark, Jean. *Documentation of the Acute Care Record.* Chicago: AHIMA, 2004.
Moisio, Marie A., Moisio, E. *Understanding Laboratory and Diagnostic Tests.* Albany, NY: Delmar, 1998.
Skurka, Margaret. *Health Information Management: Principles and Organization for Health Record Services.* Rev ed. Chicago: American Hospital Publishing, 1998.

WEB SITES

New Jersey Department of Health and Senior Services—Hospital Licensure Standards: http://www.state.nj.us/health/hcsa/njac843g.pdf
Joint Commission on Accreditation of Healthcare Organizations: http://www.jcaho.org
Institute for Healthcare Improvement: http://www.ihi.org/ihi
American Hospital Association: http://www.aha.org

CHAPTER ACTIVITIES

CHAPTER SUMMARY

This chapter followed the clinical flow of data through an acute care visit. The clinical flow of a patient's data in an acute care facility was compared and contrasted with the flow of the patient's data in an ambulatory care setting. The chapter also described the various types of clinical data that are collected from physicians and nurses and laboratory and radiology personnel. You learned how to create a form and considered the differences in the way a paper form was designed as opposed to a computer-based input screen. The data quality concepts of data validity and data completeness were discussed in greater detail.

Review Questions

1. List and explain the elements of an admission record.
2. Identify the appropriate source of the following data:
   a. Patient's name and address
   b. Patient's latest blood test results
   c. Patient's ability to explain his or her condition
   d. Patient/family education activities
   e. Plan of treatment on a specific day
   f. Whether the patient had a consultation during the inpatient stay
3. List and describe the data elements of the medication administration sheet.
4. Develop a paper-based data capture device to record medication administration.
5. Compare and contrast the elements of the Uniform Hospital Discharge Data Set with the elements of the Uniform Ambulatory Care Data Set.

Transcriptionist

My name is Nicole, and I am a transcriptionist. I work for a large firm that performs transcription services for a lot of different facilities. I could work at home if I wanted to, but I like going into the office. I work in a nice cubicle, which is in a room full of similar cubicles. My responsibility is to listen to what the physician dictated and to type exactly what the physician says. I learned transcription and took classes such as medical terminology and anatomy and physiology in the health-related professions program at my high school. I worked in a physician's office for a while and took some additional courses at my local community college.

My job isn't just typing. In order to transcribe accurately, I have to understand what the physician is saying and what it means. That means I need to understand and use medical terminology correctly. I need to know the requirements of the various medical reports, such as the H&P and the discharge summary, so that I transcribe them in the right format. I also need to know the regulatory requirements pertaining to the reports. For example, I know that the H&P is more urgent than the discharge summary, so I always transcribe the H&P report first.

Some people think that my job will go away when computers can understand and transcribe human language quickly and accurately. I certainly won't need to type as much, but my skills will become more important in reviewing the clinical reports for completeness, accuracy, and other data quality issues. I'm looking forward to that. To better prepare myself for that function, I am studying to become a registered health information technician.

APPLICATION

Does Computerization Reduce the Use of Paper?

The term *paperless environment* is common when the computerization of functions is under discussion. The term is interesting and potentially misleading. *Paperless* implies that no paper is used at all. However, consider what happens when you computerize a patient's record. If you put the admissions data on a computer-based admissions form and the health record is still largely paper based, you still must print the admissions record on paper to include in the paper record. Many facilities that have a computer-based admissions record still print out the record for the benefit of those using the paper record.

The physician reports a history and physical that can be dictated into a computer; the transcriptionist listens to the dictation on the computer and transcribes it into the computer using a word processing program. What happens to the history and physical then? It is printed out as a paper record. In a computer-based environment, a transcription is not routinely printed out, but you will find that many individuals print it out anyway for more convenient review. Even though computer security and the confidentiality of health records have not yet been discussed (see Chapters 11 and 12), you should still think carefully about the appropriateness of this activity.

Think about the order entry system. The computer-based order entry system facilitates the entry of the order by the physician. However, when it is received in the pharmacy, the order is often printed out by the pharmacist while he or she is filling the order. More paper may be generated when a prescription is transferred to the nursing station for the patient. Still more paper is generated if the order is printed so that it can be filed in the health record. This excessive generation of paper often occurs when a facility is in transition from a paper-based record system to a computer-based system. This example alone demonstrates that computerization of a patient record does not necessarily reduce paper, at least not immediately. How would you stop the excessive printing of data that can be viewed on the computer?

Chapter 5

HEALTH INFORMATION MANAGEMENT PROCESSING

CHAPTER OUTLINE

CHAPTER OBJECTIVES

By the end of this chapter, the student should be able to

- List and explain the elements of data quality.
- List, explain, and give examples of the three types of controls.
- Explain the flow of postdischarge processing of health information.
- List and explain the major functions of a health information management department.
- Explain the principles and process flow of an incomplete record system.
- Compare and contrast paper-based versus computer-based processing.

VOCABULARY

abstracting

analysis

assembly

audit trail

batch control form

classification

coding

completeness

concurrent analysis

concurrent coding

corrective controls

countersignature

Current Procedural Terminology (CPT)

data entry

deficiencies

deficiency system (incomplete system)

delinquent

detective controls

discharge register (discharge list)

error report (exception report)

Healthcare Common Procedure Coding System (HCPCS)

loose sheets

nomenclature

postdischarge processing

preventive controls

quantitative analysis

retention

timeliness

universal chart order

he last two chapters focused on the elements of data, clinical data flow, and the organization of patient encounter data on paper- and computer-based forms in an ambulatory care facility and in an acute care inpatient facility. This chapter concludes the discussion of data elements and introduces you to the controls that ensure that data are accurate. To illustrate data control measures, the role of the health information management (HIM) professional is discussed in relation in postdischarge processing of patient data.

DATA QUALITY

Whether the data are recorded by hand or entered into a computer, the process of recording data into an information system is called **data entry.** In health care, a patient's life can depend on the correctness of the data entered. For example, if an incorrect blood type was recorded and a patient then received the wrong blood type during a blood transfusion, that patient may experience a life-threatening transfusion reaction. Consequently, the overall quality of the data that are recorded is critical. Chapters 1 and 2 introduced the concepts of data accuracy and validity. This chapter focuses on the additional concepts of data timeliness and completeness.

TIMELINESS

Timeliness refers to the recording of data in a reasonable amount of time, preferably concurrent with its collection. Numerous regulations, both on the licensure level from government and on the accrediting level from voluntary agencies, address the issue of when specific data must be recorded. The previous chapters discussed some of these regulations. For example, an operative report must be documented immediately after the operation. A history and physical (H&P) must be completed within 24 hours of admission or before a surgical procedure. Timeliness applies to many other activities, as subsequent chapters will demonstrate.

Timeliness is important, particularly from the health care facility's point of view, because the patient's health record is part of the normal business records of the facility (see the discussion of litigation in Chapter 11). Therefore data that are being entered into the health record must be recorded as soon as possible after the events that the data describe. For example, if a nurse is monitoring a patient at 3:00 p.m., then the note that he or she records in the medical record must be written very shortly thereafter. Writing that same note at 9:00 p.m., 6 hours after the actual observation, would impair the quality of the recorded note. Can the nurse really remember, 6 hours later, exactly what happened with the patient? Can a physician really remember, weeks later, exactly what happened on an operating table? Because this element is so important, a significant amount of time and energy is spent facilitating the timely completion of health records.

COMPLETENESS

Completeness refers to the collection or recording of data in their entirety. A recording of vital signs that is missing the time and date is incomplete. A comprehensive physical examination that omits any mention of the condition of the patient's skin is incomplete. A progress note that is not authenticated is incomplete. Table 5-1 summarizes the data quality concepts that have been discussed so far. Good data are complete; therefore to ensure that good data are collected, HIM professionals must develop and implement data controls.

CONTROLS

As you have learned from previous discussions about data collection in this book, there are many opportunities for errors to occur. Everyone knows that humans make mistakes. Errors may occur in the simple act of hand-writing the data. If an individual's handwriting cannot be read by another health professional, how can those data be considered valid or accurate? If only the author of the data can decipher the writing, the data are useless to others. If a nurse records a temperature of 98.6° F without the decimal point (986° F), the temperature recorded is not valid. Finally, if a

TABLE 5-1	Elements of Data Quality	
ELEMENT	**DESCRIPTION**	**EXAMPLE OF ERRORS**
Accuracy	Data are correct.	The patient's pulse is 76. The nurse recorded 67. That data entry was inaccurate.
Validity	Data fall within predetermined values or parameters.	99 degrees is a valid body temperature for humans; 990 degrees is not.
Timeliness	Data are recorded within a predetermined period.	Operative reports must be recorded immediately following surgery.
Completeness	Data exist in their entirety.	Date, time, or authentication missing from a record renders it incomplete.

This is a partial list of the elements of data quality. Data quality elements are discussed throughtout this book with regard to different aspects of health information management.

physician does not dictate an operative report until a month after the operation was performed, how can that operative report truly reflect what actually occurred on that specific day? The patient's record is incomplete until the report is added to the record, and the report fails the test of timeliness.

One way that data can be protected so that they are accurate, valid, timely, and complete is through the development and implementation of controls over the collection, recording, and reporting of the data. This chapter focuses on the collection and recording of data. Reporting of data is discussed in Chapter 9. There are three types of controls over the collection and recording of data: preventive, detective, and corrective (Table 5-2).

Preventive Controls

Preventive controls are designed to ensure that data errors do not occur in the first place. The best example of a preventive control is a computer validity check. For example, suppose you wanted to write a date into the computer and you indicated that the date was July 45, 2006 (i.e., 07/45/2006). If the computer is programmed to prevent you from entering invalid dates, it might send a message saying, "You have entered an invalid date—please re-enter." It might even make a loud sound or block the character 4 from being typed in the first position of the day field. This type of preventive control double checks data validity and proves that the computer is extremely useful for data collection.

The procedural checks required in a nursing unit to ensure that patients receive the appropriate medication are a non–computer-based example of preventive controls. For example, the nurse checks the patient's identification band before administering the medication to ensure that the medication is being given to the correct patient. The development of well-designed preprinted

TABLE 5-2	Processing Controls	
CONTROL	**DESCRIPTION**	**EXAMPLE**
Preventive	Helps to ensure that an error does not occur	Computer-based validity check during data entry; examination of patient identification before medication administration
Detective	Helps in the discovery of errors that have been made	Quantitative analysis (e.g., error report)
Corrective	Correction of errors that have been discovered, including investigation of the source of the error for future prevention	Incomplete record processing

DATA COLLECTION MENUS

Religion (choose one)	Sex (choose one)	Marital Status (choose one)
○ Protestant	○ Male	○ Single
○ Catholic	○ Female	○ Married
○ Jewish		○ Divorced
○ Muslim		○ Separated
○ Other		○ Widow/Widower

◆ Figure 5-1
Data collection menus improve data quality.

forms to collect data also helps to ensure that data collection is complete. Some facilities use a combination of paper and bar codes to collect data. However, as health care moves toward an electronic health record, health care providers in many facilities collect data using portable computer devices that are later downloaded into the facility's information system and linked with all entries for that patient during their visit or hospitalization. These are just a few examples of routine preventive controls in a health care facility.

Preventive controls can be expensive, especially in the transition to a paperless environment, and cumbersome to develop and implement. Health care providers might resist the implementation of preventive controls if they are burdensome and time-consuming. Therefore the cost of a preventive control must always be balanced against its expected benefits. It is relatively easy to justify checking medications, orders, and patient identification because the benefit to the patient is apparent. It is not quite as easy to justify developing a control to prevent the entry of an incorrect patient religion or ethnicity.

One simple way to prevent invalid data entries is with the use of multiple-choice questions on a printed form or computer screen. All of the valid choices are listed so that the recorder merely chooses the correct one for the particular patient (Figure 5-1). This method also prompts the user to complete the form. However, this method does not prevent inaccurate or untimely entries because it is still possible to hit the wrong key without realizing it. For example, the staff member may enter the wrong sex for a patient, and because the computer has no way of knowing if the patient is male or female, it does not prompt a correction. As you can see, comprehensive preventive controls may be quite complex.

Detective Controls

Detective controls are developed and implemented to ensure that errors in data are discovered. Whereas a preventive control is designed to help prevent the person recording the data from making the mistake in the first place, a detective control is in place to find the data error after it is entered. In the previous date example, a computer-based detective control might be programmed to print out a list of entries that the computer recognizes as problematic. Such a printout is called an **error report** or **exception report.** Error reports are also generated when the computer or other system encounters a problem with its normal processing. For example, a fax machine can be programmed to print an error report describing the reason a fax transmission was not completed. In the previous medication administration example, a detective control could verify the medication ordered against the medication received to ensure that the order was completed correctly. Errors of omission may also occur in an error report or exception report. For example, if the medication was ordered but not recorded as being received or given, this mistake could present serious implications regarding patient care.

Detective controls are critical in a paper-based environment. Because there is no practical way to completely prevent erroneous data entry in a paper-based environment, the process of looking for errors is necessary. For example, nursing medication records may be reviewed regularly to ensure that medication administration notes are properly entered. Also, if a physician fails to dictate an operative report in a timely manner, a control must be in place to detect the missing operative report. (The process of implementing detective controls is discussed later in this chapter.)

Detective controls are frequently the easiest and most cost-effective method to develop and implement, but as with preventive controls, they may be complex. The development of preventive and detective controls requires a thorough knowledge of the process being controlled as well as the potential negative impact of data errors in processing. For this reason and depending on the type and reason for the control, the process may be performed either facility-wide, under the auspices of an overall quality improvement plan, or by a specific department.

Corrective Controls

Corrective controls may be developed and implemented to fix an error once it has been detected. Corrective controls follow detective controls. In general, identifying an error wastes time and does no good if the facility does not correct the mistake. However, corrective controls, by their very nature, occur after the error has occurred. Thus if an error report identified an invalid date, such as July 45, the date would be corrected after the fact.

Nevertheless, some errors, such as the administration of incorrect medications, cannot be effectively corrected once they occur. In such cases, analysis of the error is necessary to determine whether sufficient controls are in place to prevent the error in the future. For example, if a patient received an injection of an incorrect medication, the medication cannot subsequently be withdrawn. However, the events leading up to the administration of the drug can be thoroughly examined to determine why the error occurred. Did the physician order the wrong medication? Was the order transmitted incorrectly to the pharmacy? Did the health care provider check the patient's wristband before administering the medication? Once the source of the error is determined, the appropriate correction to the process can take place. The process of determining the cause of an error is often referred to as a *root cause analysis*. Facilities in which serious errors take place, such as those resulting in death, may be required to report these errors with a root cause analysis and a corrective action plan to the appropriate regulatory agencies. Employee education and disciplinary action are two examples of typical corrective actions that may take place if procedures were in place but not followed. Health care professionals, such as nurses and physicians, may even lose their professional licenses if serious patient errors occur once or continue to occur even after the corrective action plan is in effect.

Earlier in the chapter, an unsigned progress note was used as an example of incomplete data. Authentication of the note was missing. In a paper-based environment, the HIM professional would have to obtain the record and read all of the progress notes in it to identify the incomplete note. In a computer-based environment, preventive controls, such as noises and verbal prompts, can be built into the program to encourage the authentication of the note at the time the note is originally recorded and also on subsequent access to the record. The computer may also be programmed to review the record and identify incomplete notes. In both paper-based and computer-based environments, the corrective control consists of alerting the physician to the omission and providing the physician with the opportunity to complete the note.

The health care profession is shifting from the use of paper-based to the use of computer-based and eventually electronic health records. Terminology used to describe the health record varies, and the terms *electronic patient record, computerized patient record,* and *computer-based patient record* all are currently used. You should be alert to the myriad terminology and pay particular attention to how the terminology is used as you are reading and learning about HIM.

Correction of Errors

The correction of errors is an important consideration in patient record keeping because nothing that is recorded should be deleted. Corrections must be made so that the error can be seen as easily as the corrected information. In a paper-based record, errors are corrected by drawing a line through the erroneous data and writing the correct data near it. It is important not to obscure the original entry because this may lead to the perception that someone attempted to cover up a mistake. The correction must be authenticated and dated. In addition, correction of errors cannot consist of destroying entire documents or pages of a record. All of the erroneous documents or pages must be clearly labeled as incorrect, authenticated and dated, and kept with the correct portions of the record.

In a computer-based record, errors can be corrected in several ways depending on the type of error and the data that are being changed. For example, suppose that a patient admitted to a facility had been treated there before. A record of the previous visit exists. The patient registration specialist looks at the previous record and discovers that the patient has moved. The address and telephone number are now incorrect. Therefore the patient registration clerk may delete the old data and re-enter them with the new data. In doing so, the computer may be programmed to create a historical file of the patient's previous addresses. Alternatively, the previous address could be wiped out completely and replaced by the new address. Because the patient's previous address may not be of future interest to the facility, either method is acceptable. However, in both cases, an **audit trail** should be created to indicate that the correction was made. An audit trail is a list of all activities performed in a computer. In addition to the date and time, the audit trail contains a list of the activities, the computer in which the activity took place, the user who performed the activity, and a description of the activity itself. In the case of changes, such as the one previously described, the audit trail also may be programmed to contain the predischarge and postdischarge data. Because the audit trail indicates the user, it can be used to determine whether errors are being made by certain staff members or in general.

Exercise 5-1

Data Quality

1. When creating a paper form for new patients to complete at registration in a hospital, you should implement what preventive control to ensure that the patient lists all significant childhood illnesses?
2. Maintaining high standards of data quality is essential for patient care and effective use of health data. Data quality has a number of characteristics, many of which were discussed in this chapter and the preceding chapters. List and define as many characteristics as you can remember.
3. The development and implementation of internal controls aid in the protection of data quality and integrity. List and define three fundamental types of internal controls.

POSTDISCHARGE PROCESSING

The understanding of data concepts and control issues is critical for the development and implementation of **postdischarge processing** procedures (Figure 5-2). Postdischarge processing is what happens to the patient data after the patient is discharged. In a paper-based environment, postdischarge processing is a series of procedures aimed at **retention,** mainly storage, of an accurate and completed record. In a computer-based environment, the goals are the same, but the procedures are different. Concepts to understand in the retention of records include storage, security, and access. Table 5-3 summarizes the components of record retention. Members of the HIM department and facility staff must adhere to requirements for record retention. These requirements vary from state to state.

TABLE 5-3	Components of Record Retention
COMPONENT	**DESCRIPTION**
Storage	Compiling, indexing or cataloging, and maintaining a physical or electronic location for data (see Chapter 8)
Security	Safety and confidentiality of data (see Chapter 11)
Access	Ability to retrieve data; release of data only to appropriate individuals or other entities (see Chapters 8 and 11)

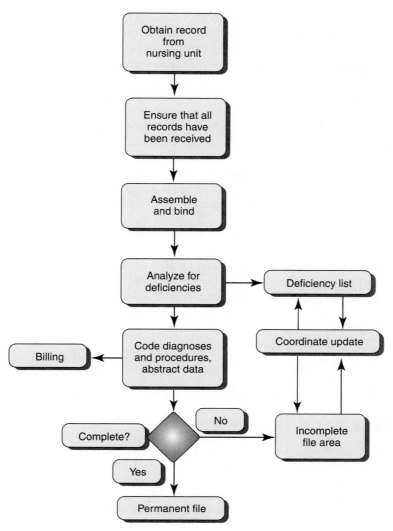

◆ Figure 5-2

Postdischarge processing in a health information management department.

Postdischarge processing is traditionally performed by the facility's HIM department. In a small physician's office or long-term care facility, the entire process may be performed by one person. In a group practice or small inpatient facility, the process may be divided into functions and distributed among several individuals. In a large facility, many individuals may perform the separate functions of the process. Even though you may never work in a health care facility, you should understand the process by which records are processed for retention because the data concepts and control issues are relevant to many other health information environments.

Chapter 2 was concerned with the clinical flow of data in a physician's office. Chapter 3 focused on the same process in an acute care facility. In those discussions, the collection of data was emphasized: what is captured, who collects it, and how it is collected. Now you are ready to consider the ways in which data are prepared for storage. The following descriptions pertain to inpatient facilities, and although the principles are similar to those related to outpatient facilities, the application of the principles may vary.

IDENTIFICATION OF RECORDS TO PROCESS

Before preparing the data for retention or storage, the HIM professional should know which records require storage. This can be accomplished by reviewing a list of the patients who have been discharged. This list is called the **discharge register** or **discharge list.** The discharge register is compiled throughout the day as patients leave the facility. It may be compiled automatically by the computer system or manually, usually by staff members on the appropriate nursing unit. Sometimes, a combination of methods is used. A corrective control in this process may involve someone physically visiting all nursing units around midnight, essentially doing a bed check to verify whether all discharges have been recorded. However it is compiled, the discharge register contains a list of the patients who have been discharged on a specific calendar day. A day is from 12:01 a.m. to 12 midnight (00:00:01 to 24:59:59), so discharges may include a patient who died at 11 pm or one who left against medical advice (AMA) at 5 p.m. Table 5-4 illustrates a discharge register.

Bear in mind that ambulatory care records are not tracked by a list of discharges but rather by a list of visits or encounters. Nevertheless, a centrally prepared document should exist that identifies patients whose records should be available for processing. For example, some kind of treatment may have to be recorded to indicate that the patient was seen; without such an entry, it may appear that the patient is still in the waiting area.

In a paper-based acute care environment, patient records move from the point of care, or patient unit, to the HIM department after completion of treatment and discharge. Once the patient has been discharged (including elopements, patients leaving against medical advice, or expirations), documentation should be nearly complete. Records are no longer needed for direct patient care after discharge. Usually, however, records remain on the patient unit until the morning of the day after discharge. This practice gives the physicians, who are not necessarily at the facility all day, time to sign off on orders and perhaps dictate the discharge summary.

Hit-Bit

Pneumatic Tube Systems

Pneumatic tube systems are widely used today at banks for drive-through customers. The customer drives up to a stand that holds a container. The checks or other documents are placed in the container, which is then transported at the press of a button, by forced air, to the teller inside the bank. Larger documents, such as health records, require larger containers. These systems are quick and generally efficient; however, the tendency of containers to get stuck in the tubes and the relatively short range of the system limit their appeal for this purpose. However, they are still used for transporting records and other purposes, such as the physical delivery of physicians' orders to the pharmacy.

TABLE 5-4	**Discharge Register**

DISCHARGE DATE: JUNE 5, 2006

ADMISSION DATE	PATIENT IDENTIFICATION NUMBER	PATIENT NAME		ATTENDING DISCHARGE	ROOM PHYSICIAN	DISPOSITION NUMBER
		LAST	FIRST			
6/2/06	234675	Johnson	Thomas	Bottoms	Transfer LTC	313A
6/4/06	234731	Kudovski	Maria	Patel	Home	303A
6/4/06	234565	Kudovski	Vladimir	Thomas	Home	Nursery
5/31/06	156785	Macey	Anna	Flint	Home	213B
6/3/06	234523	Mattingly	Richard	Johnson	Home	202A
6/5/06	274568	Ng	Charles	Kudro	Home	224A
5/15/06	234465	Rodriguez	Francisco	Benet	Deceased	ICU-4
6/1/06	198543	Rogers	Danielle	Patel	Home	226B
6/2/06	224678	Young	Rebecca	Muniz	Home	325B

The process by which the records move from the patient unit to the HIM department varies from facility to facility. Some of the considerations that determine what process is used include the distance from the patient units to the HIM department, the staffing levels on the patient unit, the staffing levels in the HIM department, and the availability of alternative personnel, such as volunteers. For example, patient unit personnel may remove the records from their binders and leave them in a pile for pickup. The records may then be picked up by any authorized person and delivered to the HIM department. Alternatively, the patient unit personnel may deliver the records. Some facilities use physical transportation systems such as pneumatic tube systems, elevators, and even transport robots.

Once the record arrives in the HIM department, postdischarge processing can begin. The first step is to ensure that all records have been received. This can be accomplished by checking the records received against the discharge register. If a patient was discharged but a record was not received, the patient unit should be contacted immediately to obtain the record. If a record was received but the patient is not listed on the discharge register, the record may have been sent in error (e.g., the patient may not actually have been discharged). Alternatively, the discharge register may be incorrect (e.g., the patient was discharged but not added to the discharge register). The patient unit should be contacted to verify the patient's status, and whatever error was made should be corrected immediately. Although the physician orders the patient's discharge and prepares a final progress note to that effect, it is the nursing staff that is usually responsible for recording the actual discharge of the patient. This is a nursing responsibility because there is often a time lag of many hours between the order to discharge the patient and the physical movement of the patient out of the facility. The use of computers greatly facilitates this process. Other departments also rely on the accuracy of the discharge register. Members of the nutritional or dietary department would not want to deliver meals to patients who are no longer at the facility. Members of the housekeeping department might not be alerted to clean a patient's room for the next patient if they are not notified that the former patient has been discharged. The nursing department must know the exact bed occupancy statistics for every unit to ensure appropriate staffing levels. The admitting department must know which beds are open for new admissions. Therefore the facility must have a procedure in place, whether telephone, fax, or Internet communication, to systematically notify the relevant departments.

ASSEMBLY

Assembly is the set of procedures by which a record is reorganized postdischarge and prepared for storage. The extent to which a record is reorganized varies among facilities and arises from the differences between the order of the sections and documents of the record as filed on the patient unit and the order of the sections and documents of the record used in postdischarge processing and eventual storage. For example, patient unit staff members may organize the documents in the record in reverse chronological order (i.e., the current document is first). Imagine a book in which the last page is the first page, and so on. The reason the patient unit organizes the documents this way is so that the health care provider does not have to waste time by searching for the latest entry. The patient unit may also place all sections pertaining to physician documentation in the front part of the record so that the physician does not have to wade through other sections first, which may be time-consuming. Although reverse chronological order makes sense while the record is on the patient unit, after the patient is discharged, this method may actually distract from and hamper record review and understanding of the hospitalization because most people are used to reading events in chronological order. Similarly, sections that were considered sufficiently important to be placed up front for ease of documentation may be shifted after the patient is discharged so that the overall record may be more easily read.

Reorganization of a paper record is done manually by staff members who are often called *assemblers*; this may take a long time, particularly in the case of large records that have to be substantially reorganized. Depending on the facility, the assembly job may be a full-time position or part of a clerical position, and many administrators question the cost-effectiveness of this function. An obvious solution to the problem is to store the record the same way as it is kept on the patient unit. This approach is called **universal chart order.** In theory, universal chart order is a practical solution. However, because the uses of the record vary dramatically among various staff members, universal chart order is not always acceptable to all parties and therefore not implemented.

It may seem obvious that in a computer-based environment, assembly is not performed because there is no paper and therefore nothing to assemble. However, even personnel in hospitals that have a high percentage of records in computer-based format still print out much of the record during the patient's hospitalization or afterwards to, for example, reply to outside requests. The assembler must be aware of which parts are received from the patient unit that are original documents and which parts are printouts (i.e., copies or duplicates) that should be destroyed to prevent confusion. Original documents may contain signatures or indicate in other ways that they are originals. Printouts of the original document should be the only copies retained because it is difficult to ensure that copies are secured and unaltered. For this reason also, printing out documents from the computer-based record should be regulated by policy and procedure.

Once the paper record has been organized, it is bound. Binding consists of affixing the pages of the record within a permanent cover, usually a manila folder. The front of the folder usually contains the name of the facility. It may also contain warnings about the confidentiality of the record and other pertinent facility record policies. (Confidentiality is discussed in Chapter 11.) The front and tabs of the folder contain the patient's name and medical record number. Sometimes, the front of the folder also shows the discharge date.

You may be familiar with file folders that have a tab on the long, open, top side of the folder. This tab enables the user to label the folder and identify the contents when the folder is placed in a file cabinet drawer. Because health records are generally stored in open shelves (or shelves that can open), the tab is on the short side of the folder. This position enables the user to identify the contents of the folder when the folder is placed on a shelf. See Chapter 8 for a complete discussion of paper file storage.

QUANTITATIVE ANALYSIS

One important detective control in place in health care facilities is **analysis.** Analysis is the process of reviewing a health record to ensure that the record is complete in every respect. You learned from the previous discussion of data concepts that *completeness* refers to the entirety of data: Are all of the data elements accounted for? Therefore this type of analysis is called **quantitative analysis.** The HIM professional who performs this function is frequently called a *medical record analyst, medical record analysis specialist, health information specialist, health information analyst,* or *analyzer* or by a similar title. This person's responsibility is to review the patient's record and determine whether any reports, notes, or necessary signatures are missing.

The extent of quantitative analysis performed in a facility depends on the type of facility and the rules of its licensure and accreditation. However, there are three guiding principles:

- The record must contain all of the elements required by the clinical services pertaining to that patient's treatment as well as the elements common to all patients.
- Each element of the record must be properly dated, including the correct time, and authenticated in accordance with the rules and regulations of state or accrediting agencies that apply to the facility, with the authors clearly identified.
- The record must contain all of the elements required by the licensure and accrediting bodies for the particular type of facility.

Elements of the Record

Different clinical services may have special forms that pertain to that service. Physical therapy may have special assessment and progress forms that differ from those used by nursing. Ambulatory surgery may use different operative record forms than inpatient surgery. The analyst must know which forms are used in each service and be able to identify any forms that are missing. The analyst must also be able to identify forms that are incomplete.

The absence of the author's authentication or of identification of authorship is easily recognized as long as the analyst is aware of when and where a signature must appear. However, the analyst must also know who *should* have authenticated the document. This knowledge becomes critical if a document has been signed but not by the correct individual. Perhaps a countersignature is required. A **countersignature** is authentication by an individual in addition to the author.

For example, an unlicensed resident may write (author) a progress note, which the attending physician must then countersign to provide evidence that the resident was supervised.

Finally, the analyst ensures that the record is complete according to licensure and accreditation rules. Sometimes, this requirement overlaps with the requirement for authentication. Again, the complete absence of the element is not as difficult to identify as the partial absence. For example, an H&P must be documented on every inpatient record. Failure to perform an H&P is a serious error. If either the history portion or the physical portion of the transcribed report is missing, it may not have been performed. More often, however, the H&P was performed, noted in the record, and dictated, but the dictated report has not yet been matched with the chart. The same is true of operative reports and consultation reports. No rule or regulation states that reports must be dictated, so on some records, depending on hospital policy, a hand-written H&P is acceptable. The analyst must know the rules and be able to identify noncompliance. Table 5-5 summarizes the major record elements for which quantitative analysis acts as a detective control.

As the analyst identifies missing elements, the pages are flagged and the missing elements are noted, along with the responsible party. Flagging consists of affixing stickers to the pages of the record. The stickers come in multiple colors so that various clinicians can be identified, each with a different color, in a single record. In many facilities, the policy is to analyze only the physician portions of the record, such as orders, progress notes, and all dictated reports. In other facilities, the policy is to analyze many sections or all of the clinical documentation, which would include nursing progress notes.

In a completely computer-based record, most of the quantitative analysis can be performed by the computer. The analyst would then receive a computer exception or error report for follow-up purposes. Analysts can then turn their attention to the qualitative analysis of other data quality issues, such as the extent of patient/family education documentation and consistency of diagnostic statements between caregivers and other departments.

Record Completion

Once the missing elements, or **deficiencies,** are identified, the responsible parties are then required to complete the record. Time limits for completing the record vary from state to state. The Joint Commission on Accreditation of Healthcare Organizations (JCAHO) requires that acute

Hit-Bit

Signatures Serve Dual Purposes

The author of a verbal order may be a registered nurse, who then authenticates the entry by initialing or signing it. The physician then authenticates the order to prove that it has been reviewed. Because both parties can be identified by their unique signatures, a signature can verify identity as well as represent an activity, such as review or approval.

TABLE 5-5 Elements of Quantitative Analysis

ELEMENT	ANALYSIS TO DETERMINE	COMMON DEFICIENCIES
Existence	Do the data exist?	Missing operative report Missing discharge summary
Completeness	Are the data entirely present, or are there missing components?	Missing reason for consultation
Authentication	Is the author's or other appropriate signature/password present?	Unsigned H&P Unsigned discharge summary Unsigned order

care records be completed within 30 days of discharge; therefore JCAHO-accredited facilities have policies that fall within that time frame. If the state requires completion in a shorter time frame (e.g., 15 days), then the facility must comply with this rule instead.

The usefulness of requiring clinical staff to authenticate records after discharge is somewhat controversial because the lack of authentication has no clinical significance for patient care. For example, if a physician forgot to sign the progress note of a patient who has already been discharged, what possible impact could the addition of the signature have on the patient 30 days later? Any control function that would have been effected by the physician's signature has been lost. A small benefit may be obtained in the event that the entry is later questioned. These arguments, of course, are not relevant as long as licensure and accrediting agencies are still reviewing postdischarge records for compliance with such standards. On the other hand, the argument has prompted some administrators to implement analysis procedures while the patient is still at the facility. This process is called **concurrent analysis,** and because it occurs concurrently with the patient's stay, it facilitates compliance with the intent of authentication rules. For example, if verbal or telephone orders are required to be signed within 24 hours, this deficiency can be captured by concurrent analysis but probably not by postdischarge analysis. In addition, concurrent analysis may speed postdischarge processing of the record.

It should be noted that an analyzer performing a concurrent analysis can look only for deficiencies that will have occurred up to that point. For example, if the chart is being reviewed 48 hours after admission, it should certainly contain an H&P, but there will not be a discharge summary because the patient is still in the facility. When the analyst reviews the chart after the patient has gone home, it is called a *retrospective* or *postdischarge analysis.*

Obtaining other data elements after the patient's discharge offers many benefits. In some cases, there may have been a delay in obtaining a particular report. Suppose, for example, that the results of a radiology examination were communicated verbally to the physician but the transcribed report did not arrive at the nursing unit before the patient's discharge. Because the record is used primarily for communication and is a legal document, the lack of a report must certainly be resolved. If an excessive amount of documentation (also known as "loose sheets" and discussed later in this chapter) is still being received by the HIM department after discharge, this may indicate organizational issues that should be resolved with the other departments involved. Filing loose reports of discharged patients is not an effective use of HIM staff members' time if these reports should have been filed by patient unit personnel while the patient was still inhouse.

Deficiency System

Once the patient's record has been reviewed and missing elements have been identified, the corrective control procedure is initiated. The responsible party—that is, the individual who was responsible for preparing the report or signing the note or report—is notified and asked to complete the record. The most common deficiencies that exist in inpatient records are lack of a discharge summary, operative report, formal consultation report, and signatures. This process of completing missing elements in a record is called the **deficiency system** or, in some facilities, the **incomplete system.** The deficiency system consists of procedures to record, report, and track identified deficiencies. This system applies to retrospective analysis. Concurrent analysis is not generally recorded and tracked because the clinician is expected to see the flag, whether manually inserted or computer-generated, the next time he or she reviews the record.

Keeping track of "who did not do what" is a classic application for computerization and was one of the first HIM department functions to become computerized in many facilities. To track deficiencies, the name of the clinician and the type of the deficiency must be captured and recorded on the record and reported to the clinician. Manual systems of tracking may require multipart forms or rewriting deficiencies on separate forms. Performance of this task with a manual system engenders a healthy appreciation for computerization. Figure 5-3 depicts a deficiency sheet, the form used to capture deficiencies.

When deficiencies are tracked manually, the analyst frequently records a separate slip for each physician, in duplicate, which can then be given to the clinician to inform him or her to complete the chart. When tracked in a computer, screens are generally organized by chart, with different lines or pages for each physician. In many cases, the deficiencies are first captured on a paper form and then transferred to the computerized tracking system. This is an example of a computer-assisted function, which we defined earlier. In either case, the analysis form is kept with the chart,

Community Hospital
City, State

Frank Bright
ID #354792
Admission Date 05/02/05
Discharge Date 05/07/05

DEFICIENCIES

PHYSICIAN:					
H&P					
Report					
Signature					
Discharge Summary					
Report					
Signature					
Face Sheet					
D/C Diagnosis & Procedures					
D/C Disposition					
Signature					
Orders					
Signature					
Operative Report					
Report					
Signature					

Partial list of deficiencies for which analysts review the record. Can you think of additional deficiencies?

◆ **Figure 5-3**
Deficiency sheet.

which enables clinicians to quickly reference their deficiencies and facilitates the distribution of the records to their colleagues.

Incomplete charts are routinely maintained in a special area of the department to allow clinicians easy access to complete the charts. The organization of this area depends on the extent to which the record has been computerized as well as the level of staffing available. If physicians are expected to retrieve their own charts, the area is typically organized alphabetically, by physician's last name. An incomplete chart is shifted from physician to physician until the chart is complete. If the HIM department is sufficiently well staffed that the charts can be gathered (pulled) for the physician, then all the charts are generally filed together. For a discussion of filing and storage methods, see Chapter 8.

When a record appears to be complete, it is analyzed again to ensure that nothing was missed. If it is indeed complete, it is transferred to permanent storage. Incomplete records are returned to the incomplete chart area.

On a regular basis, typically weekly or biweekly, clinicians are reminded of their incomplete records. This report of incomplete records must be compiled at least quarterly for accreditation purposes. JCAHO-accredited facilities must comply with rules covering the maximum allowable number of incomplete records. Because acute care records must be completed within 30 days of discharge, all records incomplete after 30 days of discharge are considered **delinquent**. The maximum number of delinquent records that acute care facilities are permitted equals 50 percent of their average monthly discharges. Therefore a facility with an average of 2000 discharges per month would be allowed to have 1000 delinquent records. Specific deficiencies, such as missing H&Ps and operative reports, are very serious. Some facilities track these deficiencies as well to ensure that the records are completed in a timely manner (e.g., within 24 hours of admission for H&Ps and immediately after surgery for operative reports).

Each facility has its own policies and procedures for ensuring that records are completed; these depend on the number of incomplete charts, the location of the HIM department, and the historical compliance of clinicians with policies governing record completion.

Computerization helps ensure the completeness of charts simply because when data are entered into a computer, they can automatically be authenticated by electronic signature (see Chapter 12). This type of authentication works best with orders, nurses' recordings of vital signs, nursing assessments, laboratory results, and admission data. Such types of data collections lend themselves to menus and short entries. A growing number of facilities are also computerizing dictation of reports, which also can be electronically authenticated. Other elements of the medical record, such as progress notes, are more difficult to capture in the database format.

CODING

More information concerning **coding** can be found in Chapter 6. Because you will have additional coursework in the coding process, it is not discussed here in detail. Coding is the representation of diagnoses and procedures as alphanumerical values in order to capture them in the database. Many codes begin with zero so that they are not captured as numerical values.

Nomenclature and Classification

There are two basic types of coding systems: nomenclature and classification. A **nomenclature** is a system of naming things. Scientific and technical professions typically have their own nomenclatures. In medicine, nomenclature is the naming of diseases and procedures. A number of different nomenclatures are used in medicine. A common nomenclature with which HIM professionals are generally familiar is the **Healthcare Common Procedure Coding System (HCPCS)** and **Current Procedural Terminology (CPT)**.

In addition to nomenclatures, **classification** systems are very important in health care. The primary classification system used in health care delivery systems is the International Classification of Diseases (ICD). ICD is used worldwide and is in its Ninth Revision. In the United States, it has been modified (Clinical Modification, CM) to increase its level of detail. We usually refer to the system as ICD-9-CM. At the time of this writing, policy makers in the health care industry and the federal government are considering the implementation of the Tenth Revision—ICD-10, which is already in use elsewhere in the world. Additional nomenclature and classification systems are discussed in detail in Chapter 6. Some coding systems are used for specialty settings, such as dental and veterinary practices. HIM professionals must be knowledgeable about the coding systems used in the setting in which they are employed.

Inpatient Coding

There are three times during a patient's encounter with the facility that coding routinely occurs, all of which relate to the physician's development of the diagnosis: on admission, during the stay, and at discharge.

When a patient is being admitted, whether it is to an acute care, rehabilitation, or mental health facility, a physician must state the reason for the admission. The physician's statement of the reason for admission is expressed as a diagnosis—in this case, an admitting diagnosis. For example, the patient may arrive in the emergency department with a complaint, be assessed by the emergency department physician, and be admitted by the emergency department physician. The emergency department form contains a section for a diagnosis, which is the reason for admission. In another scenario, a physician may see a patient in his or her office and determine that the patient requires admission, contact the hospital to make the arrangements for admission, and communicate an admitting diagnosis at that time. At the time of admission, a code is frequently assigned to the diagnosis so that computer-assisted tracking of the patient's stay can take place. If the admitting diagnosis is expressed only as words, the computer cannot match and track the patient's diagnosis with known lengths of stay and clinical treatment plans. The responsibility for coding an admitting diagnosis may rest with the patient registration department. However, if the patient registration staff member merely writes out the words, it is frequently left to the HIM department, after the patient is discharged, to assign a code to the admitting diagnosis.

Codes also may be assigned during the patient's stay in the facility. While the patient is in the facility, there are many reasons for HIM professionals to review the patient's record and assign codes to it. For example, computer matching and tracking of the patient's diagnosis is useful to help estimate the patient's length of hospital stay and thus can help control the delivery of health care. Coding that is done while the patient is still in the facility is called **concurrent coding.**

The most common point at which patient charts are coded by HIM professionals is after the patient's discharge. Coders then read the entire record and assign their codes. In acute care, rehabilitation, and mental health facilities, this postdischarge coding process generates the patient's bill. (For more information about reimbursement, see Chapter 2.) Because it is not the discharge of the patient that generates the bill to the payer but rather the coding, the function of assigning postdischarge codes has become critical. Even in a physician's office, the postvisit assignment of a code is critical in determining the reimbursement.

The importance of coding cannot be overemphasized. The capture of diagnosis and procedure codes enables facilities, payers, government agencies, researchers, and other users to analyze health data on a large scale. In the Uniform Ambulatory Care Data Set (UACDS) and the Uniform Hospital Discharge Data Set (UHDDS), the diagnoses and procedures are conveyed by code.

RETRIEVAL

Chapter 8 discusses the storage and uses of health data. It is appropriate to mention here that in a paper environment, storage is a very critical function in the facility. The storage and retention of health records, as well as the ability to retrieve those records efficiently, are traditionally the responsibility of health information technology (HIT) professionals.

Once the records are complete and filed, the need for retrieval is based on a number of factors. If no one would ever need to look at the record again after the patient has gone home, it could probably be discarded. As previously mentioned, however, the health record is a critical communication tool and will be reviewed many times after the patient leaves the facility.

The function of retrieving the health record and providing it, or parts of it, to individuals who need it is commonly called *release of information* or *correspondence*. It is extremely important that HIT professionals understand who is allowed to receive a record, who is allowed to receive a copy of a record, and how to prepare a record for review. The function of releasing a record is discussed in Chapter 11, in the section concerned with confidentiality.

ABSTRACTING

HIM professionals are uniquely suited to perform functions that require identification of the best source of data. Coding is one such function. **Abstracting** is another. The term *abstracting* refers to a number of activities in which specific data are located in the record and transferred to another document. The necessity for abstracting arises for various reasons, including data transfer, volume reduction, and analysis.

If the data in a paper-based record are to be transmitted electronically, then the data must be transferred from the paper record to the electronic medium. The data are located in the record and copied into a computer through data entry. Sometimes, an interim step is performed in which the data are transcribed to a form as they are located and then entered all at once into the computer. Diagnosis and procedure codes are often captured this way, as are surgical procedure dates and physician identification numbers.

Another reason for abstracting is to reduce the volume of data. There are often far more data in a health record than are needed for a particular user. For example, a patient keeping a file of his or her health records at home (a Personal Health Record) would not usually need an entire copy of the record. The patient may need only a copy of the discharge summary or the operative records. These data could be abstracted for the patient.

Finally, health data are frequently analyzed for research, performance improvement, and other uses. These activities are described in detail in Chapter 9; HIM professionals are well suited by their training to be involved in these functions.

TRACKING RECORDS WHILE PROCESSING

While the patient is in the facility, the responsibility for maintaining his or her record rests with clinical staff members, particularly nursing and patient unit clerical staff members. Traditionally, in a paper-based environment, the HIM department assumes control once the patient is discharged. In a computer-based environment, a number of departments may control aspects of the record. Because the record never actually moves from the computer, the physical location of the record is not in question. However, a paper-based record moves virtually every time an individual touches it. Therefore keeping track of it requires control procedures.

Batch by Days

One way to keep track of records while processing is to batch the records together by day. In this method, all records of discharges from April 15 are gathered and kept together while processing. These records are moved as a group through assembly, analysis, and coding. After coding, they are separated. Completed charts are moved to the permanent file area; incomplete charts are moved to the incomplete chart area. A **batch control form** lists the processing status of each record. This is particularly helpful if the record must be removed from the processing cycle for any reason.

Records may be removed from the processing cycle for various reasons. The patient may have been readmitted, requiring review of the previous record. The record may need to be reviewed by any number of different departments—for example, Quality Assurance. When the record is removed from the processing cycle, a batch control sheet clearly highlights the status of the record and facilitates its return to the appropriate processing step.

Loose Sheets

In a paper-based record, some reports, test results, and other data have not been compiled with the record before the patient's discharge. While the patient is in the facility, it is the responsibility of the clinical staff, usually nursing or patient unit clerks, to compile these pages into the record. This is not an issue in a completely computer-based record. Because many reports and other data are delivered to the area that requested them, a delay may occur in rerouting the data to the HIM department. These noncompiled pages are frequently called **loose sheets.**

Loose sheets may arrive in the HIM department hours, days, or weeks after the patient has been discharged. By that time, the record has been processed and must be located. Handling the volume of loose sheets arriving daily may be a full-time job in a large facility. Sometimes, considerable creativity is required to ensure that the loose sheets are properly filed. Bear in mind that in an ambulatory care facility, most reports arrive loose and must be compiled. Regular, systematic sorting and distribution of loose sheets is necessary to ensure a complete record.

Efficiency

To facilitate the many uses of the health record, related documents must be processed in a timely manner. Common sense suggests that you must obtain the record in order to assemble it, assemble the record in order to analyze it, and analyze the record in order to code it. In some facilities, all personnel perform all of the steps. In other facilities, the chart is coded before analysis. All facilities process the health record in the way that best suits their individual needs. For efficient processing, the record should be moved as little as possible, and each step should be performed in its entirety before the next step is attempted. Many facilities maintain a central staging area, where records in process are kept between steps. This approach facilitates the location of records and the movement to the next processing step. Figure 5-2 illustrates the post-discharge processing flow.

▎OTHER HEALTH INFORMATION MANAGEMENT ROLES

HIM professionals are employed various roles and settings in the health care industry. Throughout this text, you will be introduced to many activities and the professionals who perform them. As some of the traditional paper-based activities are replaced by computer-based activities, exciting new opportunities arise for well-trained professionals with an eye to the future and a willingness to learn new skills. Opportunities in pharmaceuticals, insurance, and research are increasing, along with new roles in health care. We encourage you to explore traditional as well as new avenues in planning your career in HIM.

Postdischarge Processing

1. What type of control is provided by the first processing step of receiving the records, as previously described?
2. Because physicians often are not actually employees of the facility at which they have privileges, what incentive do they have to complete their records?
3. The physician accidentally entered an order into the computer to request a cardiology consultation for the wrong patient. A staff nurse noticed the error. How should the correction be handled?
4. Health information management professionals perform a variety of internal control tasks within the context of postdischarge processing. List and describe one example of each type of control that is performed during this process.
5. In a paper environment, records must physically move from the patient care area to the health information management department for processing and storage. Give two examples of how that movement can occur.
6. Postdischarge processing follows a logical order. List the postdischarge processing steps in chronological order, beginning with obtaining control of the record.

■ SUGGESTED READING

Abdelhak, Mervat, Sara Grostick, Mary Alice Hanken, and Ellen Jacobs. *Health Information: Management of a Strategic Resource.* 2nd ed. Philadelphia: Saunders, 2001.

Andress, Alice A. *Manual of Medical Office Management.* Philadelphia: Saunders, 1996.

Buck, Carol J. *Step-by-Step Medical Coding.* 3rd ed. Philadelphia: Saunders, 2000.

WEB SITE

Joint Commission on Accreditation of Healthcare Organizations: http://www.jcaho.org

CHAPTER ACTIVITIES

CHAPTER SUMMARY

Accuracy, validity, timeliness, and completeness are important data qualities. Prevention, detection, and correction of errors promote data of the best quality. HIM professionals are traditionally responsible for the postdischarge processing of health data. The focus of postdischarge processing of a health record is the retention of health data—that is, storage, security, and access.

After the patient's discharge, records must be obtained, assembled, analyzed, coded, and completed. Some data are abstracted for data transfer, volume reduction, and analysis. Once control over the health record has been obtained, the record must be tracked and controlled throughout the processing cycle. Ultimately, control passes to the permanent file area. HIM professionals are employed in these traditional functions and also in many other functions throughout the health care industry.

Review Questions

1. List and explain the elements of data quality discussed in this chapter.
2. List, explain, and give examples of the three types of processing controls.
3. Explain the flow of postdischarge processing of health information.
4. List and explain the major functions of a health information management department.
5. Explain the principles and process flow of an incomplete record system.

Coder

My name is Shamees, and I am a coder in the health information management department at Community Medical Center. There are six coders in our department: four inpatient coders and two outpatient coders. In addition, there is a coding supervisor, who trains us and checks our work.

I started out as an assembler in the department. I assembled records for a year. I had to learn the postdischarge order of the record and how to file loose sheets. When an opening came up in the analysis section, I applied for it and was promoted. I enjoyed analysis, but I also began to understand the importance of the data contained in the records. I was really interested in the clinical data and decided to go to school to learn about coding, because coders work with the data.

Our local community college has a health information technology department, and I enrolled in their coding certificate program. I studied medical terminology, health record development and retention, anatomy and physiology, and disease pathology. I took several coding courses, learning ICD-9-CM and CPT. While I was a student, the coding supervisor allowed me to study completed records so that I could practice coding. When I finished the program, I was promoted to outpatient coder. I kept practicing inpatient coding with the completed records, and I asked a *lot* of questions. Now I code inpatient records most of the time and help out with the outpatient records.

After 2 years as an inpatient coder, I sat for and passed the Certified Coding Specialist (CCS) examination that is offered by the American Health Information Management Association. I am now a CCS! I really enjoy coding. It's challenging and interesting, and there are a lot of opportunities for me as I learn more about clinical data and how to manage health information.

Merging Expectations

You are the director of health information management at Community Hospital, a small hospital that has just merged with another hospital in your area. The facilities are roughly the same size. Approximately half of the physicians at your facility also have privileges at the other facility. With some exceptions, both facilities have similar departments and services. Both facilities are partially computer-based and, fortunately, use the same computer vendor. Full computerization will not take place for at least 5 years. The administration of the two facilities would like to standardize the data collection with the goal of reducing the cost of forms and facilitating communication between the two facilities. As the senior director, you have been asked to coordinate this effort. What issues do you think should be addressed first? Who will you ask to assist in the project? What impact does this standardization project have on the health information management department?

CODING AND REIMBURSEMENT

By the end of this chapter, the student should be able to

- Describe different coding and classification systems and their uses.
- Describe different prospective payment systems and the settings in which they are used.
- Identify and explain the major components of the CMS-1500.
- Identify and explain the major components of the UB-92.
- Explain the role of the coder in reimbursement and data quality.
- Identify unethical billing practices.

VOCABULARY

ABC	Federal Register	patient accounts
ambulatory patient classifications (APCs)	fee schedule	principal diagnosis
bar graph	fiscal intermediary (FI)	principal procedure
billing	grouper	Prospective Payment System (PPS)
case mix	ICD-9-CM	provider number
case mix index	ICD-10-CM	Quality Improvement Organization (QIO)
charge capture	ICD-10-PCS	relative weight
Chargemaster	ICD-O	reliability
charges	local medical review policy (LMRP)	Resource Utilization Groups (RUGs)
claim	Major Diagnostic Categories (MDCs)	revenue code
coding compliance plan	maximization	SNOMED-CT
comorbidity	Minimum Data Set (MDS)	superbill
complication	modifier	validity
Cooperating Parties	National Center for Health Statistics (NCHS)	working DRG
Diagnosis Related Groups (DRGs)	optimization	
DSM-IV	outlier	
encounter form		

Coding

Chapter 5 covered the two basic types of coding systems: nomenclature and classification, as well as how and where the coding function fits in with postdischarge processing of the inpatient medical record. This chapter focuses on several of the most commonly used coding systems, how and when codes are used for reimbursement or payment purposes, different types of insurance plans and government payment systems, and regulatory issues.

Although the coding function is most obviously associated with payment and reimbursement, coded data are used for other, equally important purposes. For example, coding professionals are key players in ensuring providers' compliance with official coding guidelines and government regulations. The statistical data collected from complete and accurate coding are necessary to provide a facility or health care provider with quality management and utilization information, physician profiling information, information to assist in planning and marketing objectives, research, and other administrative initiatives and activities.

On the patient level, the codes assigned for an individual patient's encounter or hospital stay may follow that patient throughout the health care delivery system and have an impact on future treatments and insurability. In the quest for fast billing turnaround time and payment (discussed in greater detail later in this chapter), it is sometimes easy to forget that the patient record is a highly personal document, one that often describes a person's last days, and therefore must be treated respectfully with regard to the coded data assigned. The American Health Information Management Association (AHIMA) has issued "Standards of Ethical Coding," guidelines that all coders, regardless of setting, should be aware of and follow (Figure 6-1).

Coding is essentially the translation of written descriptions of diagnoses (e.g., diseases, injuries, reasons for encounters and other conditions requiring an encounter or admission) into a numerical or alphanumerical code. The same can be said of translating written descriptions of procedures, services, or treatments.

Of interest to coders today are the Standards for Code Sets under the Health Insurance Portability and Accountability Act (HIPAA). HIPAA is discussed in greater detail in Chapter 11. Under HIPAA, code sets are sets of codes used to encode the diagnosis and procedure codes, data elements, and medical concepts used in electronic transactions. These code sets are mandatory for use in reporting and reimbursement under HIPAA. The current code sets are ICD-9-CM, Volumes I and II; ICD-9-CM, Volume III; National Drug Codes (NDCs); Codes on Dental Procedures and Nomenclature, 2nd edition; HCPCS; and CPT-4.

The coder encapsulates an encounter, or inpatient admission, by way of a group of codes that, together with other demographic and provider data, describe the encounter or admission in a format that then may be electronically transmitted to insurers or state or government agencies and also retained electronically, separate from a paper record within a facility or with a provider. Such coded data can also be shared within a network. Imagine attempting to share information about hundreds or thousands of patients without translating the written descriptions of diagnoses and procedures into codes, and you will begin to appreciate the complexity of coded data and the importance of those who perform the coding function.

There are many coding systems in use today throughout the United States and the world. The word *international* can be found in the titles of many of these different coding systems. Some systems are sponsored and maintained by governmental agencies and others by various medical or health associations in the United States and internationally. In the United States, the coding system used depends on the applicable HIPAA code set used in the provider setting. For example, inpatient hospital-based coders today use the ICD-9-CM system; they cannot use the ICD-10-CM system even if they prefer it to the ICD-9-CM system. ICD-10-CM is not listed as a code set, although efforts are under way to replace ICD-9-CM with ICD-10-CM.

Because this chapter concerns coding and reimbursement, it focuses on the applicable types of coding systems, which primarily are the ICD-9-CM and HCPCS/CPT-4. Some other important coding systems, including SNOMED-CT, are also discussed.

SNOMED-CT

SNOMED stands for systemized nomenclature of medicine. CT stands for clinical terms. This system is developed, maintained, and revised by the College of American Pathologists (CAP), a

In this era of payment based on diagnostic and procedural coding, the professional ethics of health information coding professionals continue to be challenged. A conscientious goal for coding and maintaining a quality database is accurate clinical and statistical data. The following standards of ethical coding, developed by AHIMA's Coding Policy and Strategy Committee and approved by AHIMA's Board of Directors, are offered to guide coding professionals in this process.

1. Coding professionals are expected to support the importance of accurate, complete, and consistent coding practices for the production of quality healthcare data.
2. Coding professionals in all healthcare settings should adhere to the ICD-9-CM (International Classification of Diseases, 9th revision, Clinical Modification) coding conventions, official coding guidelines approved by the Cooperating Parties,* the CPT (Current Procedural Terminology) rules established by the American Medical Association, and any other official coding rules and guidelines established for use with mandated standard code sets. Selection and sequencing of diagnoses and procedures must meet the definitions of required data sets for applicable healthcare settings.
3. Coding professionals should use their skills, their knowledge of currently mandated coding and classification systems, and official resources to select the appropriate diagnostic and procedural codes.
4. Coding professionals should only assign and report codes that are clearly and consistently supported by physician documentation in the health record.
5. Coding professionals should consult physicians for clarification and additional documentation prior to code assignment when there is conflicting or ambiguous data in the health record.
6. Coding professionals should not change codes or the narratives of codes on the billing abstract so that meanings are misrepresented. Diagnoses or procedures should not be inappropriately included or excluded because payment or insurance policy coverage requirements will be affected. When individual payer policies conflict with official coding rules and guidelines, these policies should be obtained in writing whenever possible. Reasonable efforts should be made to educate the payer on proper coding practices in order to influence a change in the payer's policy.
7. Coding professionals, as members of the healthcare team, should assist and educate physicians and other clinicians by advocating proper documentation practices, further specificity, and resequencing or inclusion of diagnoses or procedures when needed to more accurately reflect the acuity, severity, and the occurrence of events.
8. Coding professionals should participate in the development of institutional coding policies and should ensure that coding policies complement, not conflict with, official coding rules and guidelines.
9. Coding professionals should maintain and continually enhance their coding skills, as they have a professional responsibility to stay abreast of changes in codes, coding guidelines, and regulations.
10. Coding professionals should strive for optimal payment to which the facility is legally entitled, remembering that it is unethical and illegal to maximize payment by means that contradict regulatory guidelines.

*The Cooperating Parties are the American Health Information Management Association, American Hospital Association, Health Care Financing Administration, and National Center for Health Statistics. All rights reserved. Reprint and quote only with proper reference to AHIMA's authorship.

◆ **Figure 6-1**
Standards of ethical coding. (From the American Health Information Management Association: http://www.ahima.org/infocenter/guidelines/standards.asp)

not-for-profit medical society. It is widely used internationally (see SNOMED International at http//www.snomed.org) in more than 30 countries and is available in English and other languages. **SNOMED-CT** claims an extensive clinical vocabulary that is updated and released twice a year. The English edition of SNOMED-CT core content is available free through the National Library of Medicine's (NLM) *Unified Medical Language System (UMLS) Metathesaurus* ("Fact Sheet" 2006).

SNOMED-CT is designed for use in and support of electronic health record (EHR) systems. It is important because it provides the core general terminology for an EHR. In 2004 President George W. Bush announced an initiative to have an EHR in use in America within the next 10 years. The federal government has licensed SNOMED-CT with that goal in mind. In addition, the **National Center for Health Statistics (NCHS)** has recommended adoption of SNOMED-CT as the general terminology standard for patient medical record information. It remains to be determined whether SNOMED-CT will be used to complement or replace other coding systems currently in use (College of American Pathologists 2004).

Unlike the other coding systems discussed in this chapter, the process of assigning SNOMED-CT codes is fully automated. SNOMED-CT codes are embedded in the EHR, and codes are assigned during the course of patient care. Also unlike the previously discussed coding and classification systems, it would be both impractical and nearly impossible to manually assign SNOMED-CT codes with the degree of accuracy and complexity that the automated process achieves in the

Hit-Bit

Metathesaurus

The Metathesaurus is one of three knowledge sources developed and distributed by the National Library of Medicine as part of the Unified Medical Language System project. The Metathesaurus contains information about more than 1 million biomedical concept names from more than 100 controlled vocabularies and classifications used in patient records and administrative health data. It includes vocabularies and coding systems designated as U.S. standards for the exchange of administrative and clinical data, including SNOMED-CT (UMLS http://www.nlm.nih.gov/pubs/factsheets/factsheets.html).

EHR. Attempts at manual code assignment would defeat the purpose of SNOMED-CT's intent and design.

Classification systems such as ICD-9-CM and ICD-10-CM are designed to assign codes to patient encounters according to diseases. The "output" of the coding process is an ICD code that is not generally used during the course of, or directly for, patient care. Data generated from ICD codes are most useful when aggregated after the encounter and are necessary for reimbursement. Classification systems such as ICD-9-CM are not designed to capture all of the available data and clinical information in a health record that is used by clinicians during the course of patient care. This is true whether the record is stored on paper or electronically but especially true in a paper-based environment because clinical information is not standardized in terms of format or documentation in paper health records.

SNOMED-CT differs in that it is a nomenclature system. SNOMED-CT works behind the scenes in the EHR, using all of the available data and clinical information that the EHR contains. It is able to use all of this information because, as mentioned earlier, EHRs use standardized clinical terminology. This is the input from the EHR that SNOMED-CT uses to assign codes. Because SNOMED-CT codes are assigned during the course of patient care, these codes can be linked with other software programs that can facilitate current patient care. For example, a SNOMED-CT code may be assigned using input from a complex set of data extracted from various sections of the EHR. This SNOMED-CT code may be programmed to link to a software system to alert the clinician to a life-threatening condition.

Because classification systems and nomenclature systems are designed for different purposes and uses, one type of system cannot entirely replace the other. SNOMED-CT is designed to use very specific data and documentation to assign extremely detailed levels of codes, whereas codes in

Hit-Bit

Granularity

The level of detail that a system provides is referred to as its *granularity*. A system with a high level of granularity is able to capture more specific, detailed information than a system with a lower level of granularity. Think of the beach: If you examine it closely, you see millions of grains of sand. If you view the beach from a distance, it may appear as more of a solitary object. In terms of practical application, if you are a painter, you many need the view with less granularity to portray the beach. If you are a marine scientist, you may need to view many individual grains of sand for a research project. With regard to choosing a code system, the level of granularity will be determined by the reason that a code system is needed and for what it is being used.

ICD-9-CM and even ICD-10-CM are often more general. Where there may be one code for a disease in ICD-9-CM, several code selections may be present in SNOMED-CT based on levels of detail.

Therefore it is possible to map (or cross-walk) codes from SNOMED-CT to ICD but not from ICD to SNOMED-CT without losing the SNOMED-CT specific data.

To achieve the full benefits of the EHR and SNOMED-CT in the United States, the United States would have to adopt ICD-10-CM and ICD-10-PCS for use. A map of SNOMED-CT to ICD-9-CM has been developed; however, ICD-9-CM is 30 years old, and unlike ICD-10-CM and ICD-10-PCS, its codes do not have the capability to capture the complex current array of medical conditions and treatments.

Moving to the use of the EHR and SNOMED-CT will not eliminate the need for coders in the foreseeable future. The accuracy of the coded data still must be reviewed and verified as it pertains to each specific patient encounter. Although no computerized system is infallible, the extent to which we can depend on them will probably increase with time. Even if the coding function were somehow entirely eliminated in the future, health information professionals with that knowledge base would assume more complex and advanced roles in, for example, development and maintenance of the code mapping, quality control of individual patient and aggregate data, and sophisticated data analysis.

ICD-O-3

ICD-O stands for *International Classification of Diseases for Oncology,* currently in its third revision as of January 1, 2001. The World Health Organization (WHO) is responsible for this coding system. Its purpose is to be the standard tool for coding neoplasm, or cancer, diagnoses. In a hospital setting, ICD-O-3 is used in the pathology department and in tumor (cancer) registries to code the site (topography) and the histology (morphology) of neoplasms. Because it is an international coding system, it is available in several languages. ICD-O-3 is not used for reimbursement purposes.

DSM-IV

DSM-IV stands for *Diagnostic and Statistical Manual of Mental Disorders,* Fourth Edition. Its sponsoring organization is the American Psychiatric Association. DSM-IV codes are similar in appearance to ICD-9-CM codes, the main difference being that the DSM-IV codes may provide a higher degree of specificity for some diagnoses. DSM-IV codes are used only for data analysis of patients with psychiatric disorders, not for reimbursement purposes.

ABC

ABC stands for *alternative billing concepts* codes. This coding system is used by providers of alternative medicine to report their services when required for reimbursement or other regulatory purposes. Alternative medicine includes, and is sometimes referred to as, complementary medicine. These complementary or alternative medicine services include acupuncture, holistic

Hit-Bit

Certified Tumor Registrar

Many health information professionals choose to specialize in cancer coding and cancer registries and obtain the credential of Certified Tumor Registrar (CTR). Those professionals working in Tumor Registries use ICD-O-3 to code cancer cases similar to the way inpatient coders use ICD-9-CM. Depending on the facility, in an inpatient setting, a patient with cancer will have been coded using both ICD-O-3 and ICD, usually by different professionals in different departments, with each distinct case and code set reported electronically to entirely separate databases.

medicine, and naturopathy. These services are often provided by chiropractors and midwives as well as other practitioners more often seen in standard medicine, such as physician assistants and nurse practitioners. ABC codes were developed by Alternative Link, which also holds the copyright (see www.alternativelink.com). ABC codes have been incorporated into the *Metathesaurus*.

As you can see, different coding systems currently in use satisfy the need to capture coded data for different uses by different providers. Some systems are very specialized, whereas some systems, such as SNOMED-CT, are far more comprehensive, with a broader range of users. Each system has its own unique uses. In most provider settings today, such as physician offices and acute care hospitals, there are two important coding systems currently in use: ICD-9-CM and HCPCS/CPT.

ICD-9-CM

ICD-9-CM stands for *International Classification of Diseases*, Ninth Revision, Clinical Modification. WHO originates and is responsible for ICD, which is in use in different modifications and versions internationally. The phrase *clinical modification* refers to the adaptation of ICD for use in the United States. Interestingly, in the United States, ICD-9-CM was preceded by two different but related coding systems: ICDA-8 (*International Classification of Diseases*, Eighth Revision, Adapted for Use in the United States) and H-ICDA (*Hospital Adaptation of ICDA*), also referred to as *H-ICDA-2*. Hospital administrators could choose to use either ICDA-8 or H-ICDA-2. Each system had its own merits; however, the opportunity to select one of two options prevented the development of general comparative national data. In January 1979, the federal government required all hospitals and physicians to use ICD-9-CM.

There are three volumes within ICD-9-CM. The term *volumes* made more sense in the days when coding was not computerized and code books were not streamlined because there were originally three separate books, or volumes, published when ICD-9-CM was first used. Volume I is the tabular list of diagnosis codes and their descriptions. Volume II is the alphabetical index to Volume I. Volume III contains both the tabular list and the alphabetical index for procedure codes. You may still hear references to a particular volume when you are learning coding or when coding updates are issued.

In the United States, the **Cooperating Parties** are responsible for all volumes of ICD-9-CM. The Cooperating Parties consist of representatives of the American Hospital Association (AHA), AHIMA, the Centers for Medicare and Medicaid Services (CMS), and NCHS. The Cooperating Parties meet twice yearly, usually in April and October, to hear and discuss proposed code changes or revisions. Anyone can attend these meetings. Notices and agendas can be found on the CMS Web site in the **Federal Register** section at http://www.gpoaccess.gov/fr/. If and when proposed code changes meet final approval, they can be accessed in the Federal Register section as a Final Rule. Coding changes may be approved and issued for use twice yearly, in April and October, although most major changes are effective in October.

When ICD-9-CM was mandated for use in 1979, it really had no special purpose other than to ensure an updated and unified coding system in the United States. The coding function did not change, and coders just had to learn the new system without adhering to any particular timetable; there were no major pressures to complete coding in what we would consider a timely manner today. It may be hard to imagine now, but in 1979 coding had little or nothing to do with billing or reimbursement. In addition, although the structure and rules are the same, ICD-9-CM was considerably less complicated in 1979 than it is today. Think of the many advances in medicine and technology and the great number of newly defined diseases that have been incorporated over the years into the ICD-9-CM system used today. Coding changed nationally in 1983 with the implementation of the diagnosis related group–based hospital prospective payment system (PPS), which is discussed later in this chapter.

HCPCS/CPT-4

HCPCS stands for Health Care Common Procedure Coding System. HCPCS was developed as a standard coding system for claims processing and is therefore extremely important to physicians and other providers. HCPCS consists of two levels. Level I is *CPT*, which stands for *Current Procedural Terminology*, currently in its fourth version (CPT-4). CPT is copyrighted, developed, and maintained by the American Medical Association (AMA). CPT codes are composed of five numerical characters. CPT codes are used to report procedures and services performed by physicians and other health care professionals and in facilities or institutions for services performed in the outpatient setting (e.g., ambulatory surgery centers, emergency departments, clinics, and rehabilitation facilities). CPT-4 codes are updated and published yearly by the AMA and become effective for use each January. The code changes and new codes must be purchased from the AMA.

Additions, deletions, and revisions to CPT-4 are determined by the AMA's editorial panel. The editorial panel consists of physicians representing the AMA, the Blue Cross and Blue Shield Association (BCBSA), the Health Insurance Association of America (HIAA), the AHA, and CMS. Providing input to the panel are two advisory committees. The CPT advisory committee consists solely of physicians. The Health Care Professionals advisory committee is composed of allied health professionals, including health information management (HIM) professionals.

Level II codes are generally called *HCPCS codes.* HCPCS Level II codes consist of codes used by providers and institutions to report products, supplies, and services not included in CPT. For example, HCPCS Level II codes would be used to submit claims for durable medical equipment and ambulance services. HCPCS codes are alphanumerical: a letter followed by four numerical characters. HCPCS Level II codes are maintained jointly by America's Health Insurance Plans (AHIP), the BCBSA, and CMS. These same groups also serve on an HCPCS national panel, the functions of which include maintaining national permanent HCPCS Level II codes as well as additions, revisions, and deletions. The purpose of the permanent national codes is to provide a "standardized coding system that is managed jointly by private and public insurers. It supplies a predictable set of uniform codes that provides a stable environment for claims submission and processing" ("Level II Coding Procedures" 2005). HCPCS Level II codes are updated as needed, usually every quarter, and become effective once announced. Updates can be found on the CMS Web site: http://www.cms.hhs.gov/medicare/hcpcs.

Dental codes are a separate category of national codes called *Current Dental Terminology* (CDT). CDT, although published and copyrighted by the American Dental Association (ADA), is included in HCPCS Level II. However, any changes to CDT are made by the ADA, not the National Panel. You will recall that CDT is included as a code set under HIPAA.

ICD-10-CM

ICD-10-CM (*International Classification of Diseases and Related Health Problems,* Tenth Revision) is already in use in approximately 100 countries, including Australia and Canada; its adoption is pending in the United States at the time of this publication. As with all ICDs, it is maintained by WHO and is intended for worldwide reporting of morbidity and mortality. Once approval for adoption of ICD-10 is achieved in the United States, it will replace ICD-9-CM Volumes I and II. It is anticipated that there will be a lead time of 2 years from the notification point of final approval to the point of mandatory use. In the meantime, many HIM professionals are familiarizing themselves with ICD-10-CM because this new system is entirely different from ICD-9-CM in structure and format. Because billing and reimbursement depend on timely and accurate coding, HIM professionals and coders are learning as much as possible about ICD-10-CM now to minimize billing and reimbursement delays caused by decreases in coding productivity once the new codes become effective.

ICD-10-CM has many advantages over ICD-9-CM, which is why many organizations such as AHIMA have vigorously promoted its adoption. According to NCHS, improvements include "the addition of information relevant to ambulatory and managed care encounters; expanded injury codes; the creation of combination diagnosis/symptom codes to reduce the number of codes needed to fully describe a condition; the addition of a sixth character; incorporation of common fourth and fifth digit subclassifications; laterality (i.e., the ability to specify right or left side of the body); and greater specificity in code assignment" ("About the ICD-10-CM" 2004). A great deal of information about ICD-10-CM can be found on the NCHS Web site: http://www.cdc.gov/nchs.

ICD-10-PCS

ICD-10-PCS (*PCS* stands for procedure coding system) was developed in the United States to replace Volume III of ICD-9-CM. ICD-10-CM is also entirely different in structure and format from

ICD-9-CM Volume III in that it uses a seven-character alphanumerical code structure. The same groups responsible for ICD-9-CM Volume III are responsible for ICD-10-PCS. Information about ICD-10-PCS can be found at the CMS Web site: http://www.cms.hhs.gov/providers/ pufdownload/icd10.asp. The final draft (9/8/05) and coding manual are also available at this Web site.

It is generally thought that ICD-10-CM and ICD-10-PCS will become effective for use at the same time. In addition to the need for coders to learn entirely new classification systems, the transition to these new coding classification systems will greatly affect reimbursement systems and information systems because existing formats must be changed to accommodate the new codes.

Although the list of coding classification systems discussed in the previous sections is not exhaustive, these are the systems that most HIM professionals are most likely to encounter (Table 6-1). The following sections cover prospective payment systems and billing, with a focus on ICD-9-CM and HCPCS/CPT-4.

Exercise 6-1

Coding

1. Provide three examples for which coded data might be used in a facility.
2. What does *SNOMED* stand for?
3. Where can the English core content of SNOMED-CT be found?
4. The Cooperating Parties consist of representatives from what entities or organizations?
5. What is the purpose of the Cooperating Parties?
6. HIM professionals contribute to addition, deletions, and revisions to CPT-4 through what committee?
7. What are the main purposes of HCPCS/CPT-4 codes?

PROSPECTIVE PAYMENT SYSTEMS

Prospective payment systems, as they apply primarily to inpatient acute care, are based on **diagnosis related groups (DRGs)**. Later in this chapter, you will learn about the outpatient prospective payment system, **ambulatory patient classifications (APCs).**

DRGs classify, or group, patients by common type according to diagnosis, treatments, and resource intensity. The statistical foundation of DRGs is based on the assumption that the same diagnosis requires the same type of care for all patients. The term *resource intensity* generally refers to demands and costs associated with treating specific types of patients: how much it costs to treat a particular disease or condition, depending on what types of resources that type of patient consumes and in some instances factoring in the age and gender of the patient. For example, if a patient is being treated in the hospital for congestive heart failure and nothing else, then that patient will probably consume the same amount of resources, have the same procedures performed, require the same number of consultations, and have the same intensity of nursing care as any other patient coming into the hospital with that same diagnosis, barring complications. Statistically, on the basis of review of hundreds of thousands of records, this assumption proves to be true, which allows for the classification of the patient's stay into a DRG assignment.

Classifying types of patients into DRGs and predicting their expected resource consumption provide the basis for assigning monetary amounts for each DRG in PPS. For example, even though a normal newborn and a patient scheduled for gallbladder removal may both stay in the hospital for 3 days, the normal newborn will not consume as much in the way of resources as someone who required use of the operating room and postoperative care. Both patients, having different diagnoses and treatments, would be assigned to two different DRGs, with the amount reimbursed for the newborn's hospitalization less than the amount reimbursed for the gallbladder surgery patient.

TABLE 6-1	Comparison of Coding Systems	
ACRONYM	**FULL NAME**	**USE**
SNOMED-CT	Systemized Nomenclature of Medicine—Clinical Terms	Extensive clinical vocabulary, machine-readable terminology for potential use in an electronic health record (EHR)
ICD-O-3	International Classification of Diseases for Oncology, 3rd Revision	Coding of neoplasm/cancer diagnoses for tumor reporting
DSM-IV	Diagnostic and Statistical Manual of Mental Disorders, 4th Edition	Coding of psychiatric disorders for psychiatric patients
ABC	Alternative Billing Concepts	Complementary or alternative medicine coding
ICD-9-CM	International Classification of Diseases, 9th Revision, Clinical Modification	Volumes I&II: coding of diagnoses for inpatient, outpatient, and physician office settings Volume III: coding of procedures in inpatient settings Reporting and reimbursement in inpatient settings.
HCPCS/CPT-4	Healthcare Common Procedure Coding System and Current Procedural Terminology, 4th Version	Reporting for reimbursement in outpatient and physician office settings
ICD-10-CM	International Statistical Classification of Diseases and Related health Problems, 10th Revision	Replaces ICD-9-CM, Volumes I and II
ICD-10-PCS	Procedure Coding System	Replaces ICD-9-CM, Volume III

HISTORY OF DIAGNOSIS RELATED GROUPS AND IMPACT ON HEALTH INFORMATION MANAGEMENT AND THE CODING FUNCTION

Currently, the DRG system is known as a "patient classification scheme, which provides a means of relating the type of patients a hospital treats (i.e., its **case mix**) to the costs incurred by the hospital" (*Diagnosis Related Groups Definitions Manual* 1989). It also serves as a basis for hospital reimbursement by Medicare and certain other payers. However, DRG classifications were

Hit-Bit

Case Mix Groups

It should be noted that there are many grouper systems in use in the United States and, in fact, the world. In 1983, the Canadian Institute for Health Information developed case mix groups.

The Prospective Payment System does not apply to Canadian hospitals. Instead, hospitals in Canada operate under a global budget. Each hospital receives a sum of money according to its size and the types of services it provides. A large hospital that performs organ transplants, for example, would receive a higher monetary global budget than a small community hospital would.

originally developed by Yale University in the 1960s as a tool to ensure quality of care and appropriate utilization. DRG classifications had nothing to do with reimbursement until the late 1970s, when the New Jersey Department of Health mandated use of the system for reimbursement. In New Jersey, DRG-based methodology reimbursement applied to all patients and all payer classifications; DRG reimbursement classifications were adopted with the goal of containing overall inpatient health care costs, which were rapidly increasing. Because the DRG classification system in New Jersey applied to all inpatients and payers, even self-pay patients, it has been referred to as an "all payer" prospective payment system. (This is a historical reference, as the New Jersey systems has since changed.)

Later in this chapter, you will see in greater detail how patients are classified in groups according to the DRG classification system, with coding the main critical element needed. Without assigned codes for each patient, there cannot be a DRG assignment. Without a DRG assigned, a hospital cannot receive reimbursement. When the coding function became linked to reimbursement, coders and HIM personnel (e.g., medical records staff) made enormous gains in importance and stature. There was a saying at the time that medical records professionals came out of the basement and into the board room. For the first time ever, a national health care publication featured a medical records director on its cover when it published a feature article about DRGs. With the advent of the DRG system, HIM professionals basked in the national health care spotlight and embraced their new leadership roles and responsibilities.

Earlier in this chapter, you learned that the coding function had comparatively fewer pressures before the implementation of prospective payment systems and DRGs. The accuracy of codes was not so closely scrutinized, and coders were under less pressure to perform their task in a timely manner, although most hospital administrators would try to complete the previous month's cases no later than 2 weeks into the following month. Coding was more or less considered just another function in a medical records department, perhaps on par with the analysis function. Coders were primarily trained by their employers, and some were credentialed as either registered record administrators or accredited record technicians, which were the only two credentials offered at the time. People earning either credential did not specialize in coding but rather took one or two courses in coding. Today, coding has become a highly specialized and desirable profession in itself, with several credentials offered solely for coding by different organizations.

With the evolution of coding and the coding profession, tremendous changes occurred in hospital computer systems. In the late 1970s, most medical records departments did not have computers or even access to their hospital computer. In some instances, DRG grouping was actually done by using a large paper manual that outlined the DRG **grouper** program. In most cases, however, coders dialed into a system off-site, entered codes and other data elements for each patient, and received a DRG assignment over the telephone connection. This was not even an Internet connection but rather a telephone modem connection to an off-site computer, originally the one at Yale University, where DRGs were developed. One advantage (possibly the only one) in grouping cases this way was that the coder truly understood the software program and could therefore provide feedback and suggestions. Because all grouping is computerized, coders today may not be as familiar with all of the nuances and elements of grouping. On the other hand, computerized

Hit-Bit

History of AHIMA Credentials

Before 1978, Registered Record Administrators (RRA) were registered, or certified as Registered Record Librarians (RRL), although registration of individuals in the medical records profession goes back to 1933. In the early days, individuals could be registered as long as they qualified by being "of the full age of 21 years, ethical, and of good moral character." No formal examination was necessary. The Accredited Record Technician (ART) came later, in 1953. Both credentials changed again in 2000, with RRA becoming RHIA (Registered Health Information Administrator) and ART becoming RHIT (Registered Health Information Technician).

grouping is certainly far more accurate than grouping with a paper manual. In any event, coders not only began to take greater responsibility for timely and accurate coding because of the DRG system but also learned more about information technology and health information. Eventually, computerization and the data collection activities required to support coding, DRG assignment, and reimbursement moved facilities closer to what will eventually become an EHR.

Overall, the impact of DRGs and the prospective payment system on health care was enormous. In addition to New Jersey, a number of states soon adopted prospective payment systems, or "all payer" systems, requiring all payers, including Medicare, to use DRGs as a reimbursement methodology for hospital inpatients. Because prospective payment system was a completely new type of reimbursement, its adoption had a dramatic financial impact on facilities during the initial years. Patients were also affected as lengths of stay were gradually decreased. Before the adoption of prospective payment systems, there were no financial incentives to reduce a patient's length of stay. For example, it was once common for a new mother and baby to stay in the hospital for a week; today it would be unusual for a healthy mother and baby to stay more than 2 or 3 days.

DIAGNOSIS RELATED GROUP ASSIGNMENT

In the United States, DRGs are presently derived from ICD-9-CM codes. When the ICD-10-CM and ICD-10-PCS coding systems are adopted for use, the DRG system is expected to be adapted to accommodate the new codes. DRGs were developed with some basic characteristics in mind (Figure 6-2).

DRG assignment can proceed once all of the necessary information is abstracted into the hospital's information system. Grouper software is used to assign each DRG. Health Systems International (HSI) has had oversight of the Medicare DRG grouper software since 1983, when it received a contract from CMS. The DRG grouper software follows a process that resembles a flowchart, much like any flowchart created to track a process or procedure. This particular flowchart is referred to as a *tree diagram*. DRG grouper programs vary depending on the DRG system in use, but some generalizations may be made about the basic formats.

The process begins with examination of the **principal diagnosis** code. The principal diagnosis is defined in the Uniform Hospital Discharge Data Set (UHDDS) as the reason, after study, that

Characteristics	Explanation
"The patient characteristics used in the definition of the DRGs should be limited to information routinely collected on hospital abstract systems."	This information consists of the patient's principal diagnosis code, secondary diagnosis code or diagnoses codes, procedure code or codes, the patient's age, sex, and discharge status. In some DRG groupers, a newborn's birth weight must also be included.
"There should be a manageable number of DRGs which encompass all patients seen on an inpatient basis."	The point of this is so that meaningful comparative analyses of DRGs can be performed and patterns detected in case mix and costs.
"Each DRG should contain patients with a similar pattern of resource intensity."	Clinical coherence means that patients in a particular DRG share a common organ system or condition and/or procedures, and that typically a specific medical or surgical specialty would provide services to that patient. For example, one would expect a psychiatrist to treat all patients in DRGs created for mental diseases and disorders.
"Each DRG should contain patients who are similar from a clinical perspective (i.e., each class should be clinically coherent)."	This is so that a hospital can establish a relationship between their case mix and resource consumption.

◆ **Figure 6-2**

Characteristics of DRGs. (From Diagnosis Related Groups, *Definitions Manual*, Version 15.0. Minneapolis: 3M Health Information Systems, 1998.)

the patient was admitted to the hospital. Codes must be currently valid and accepted as a principal diagnosis code by the Medicare Code Editor (MCE). The MCE is essentially a list of codes that would not make sense if used as a principal diagnosis in an acute care facility. For example, many V codes are on this list, such as V10.3, "history of breast cancer." The codes must also, when applicable, align with the sex of the patient. For example, a patient who is abstracted as male cannot then be assigned pregnancy codes.

If you examine an ICD code book, you will see that the codes are divided into chapters or sections, primarily according to body system. In similar fashion, once the principal diagnosis code is accepted, the grouping process begins by assigning patients into basic sections called **Major Diagnostic Categories (MDCs)**. Whereas hundreds of DRGs exist, there are 25 MDCs in the Medicare DRG Grouper that resemble the chapters in ICD-9-CM, although not necessarily in the same order. Examples of MDCs are as follows:

MDC 1—Diseases and Disorders of the Nervous System
MDC 6—Diseases and Disorders of the Digestive System
MCD 14—Pregnancy, Childbirth, and the Puerperium
MDC 19—Mental Diseases and Disorders
MDC 22—Burns
(Health Systems International, 1989)

Once the patient is assigned to an MDC, the grouper then examines any procedure codes. Not all procedure codes are used for DRG assignment. For example, codes for ultrasounds are essentially ignored during the grouping process. Procedure codes that are recognized and used for grouping are categorized as either OR (operating room) or Non-OR. OR procedure codes mean that those patients have undergone a procedure requiring the use of an operating room: for example, a gastric bypass or open fracture reduction. Non-OR procedures include procedures or treatments such as chemotherapy or bedside debridements. Figure 6-3 shows an example of an MDC decision tree.

Most MDCs have two main sections, one for medical patients and one for surgical patients. The two sections are referred to as *medical partitioning* and *surgical partitioning*. Once a case is assigned to an MDC, that case is then sorted or assigned to one of these main sections. Note that in Figure 6-3 the first question is whether the patient had an operation (OR procedure). If the answer is yes, then the correct DRG is found in the surgical partitioning. If the answer is no, then the decision tree sends the user to the medical partitioning.

For cases sorted into the medical partition, the grouper looks for, depending on the MDC, the patient's age. The MCE detects instances in which a patient's age does not correspond with the principal or secondary coded diagnoses. For example, an 80-year-old woman with pregnancy codes would not pass the edit and would not be grouped until a correction was made in abstracting.

Next, depending on the MDC, the grouper will search the secondary diagnosis codes for a comorbidity or complication (CC). A **comorbidity** is a condition that was present upon admission, whereas a **complication** is a condition that arose during the hospitalization. If a secondary diagnosis code, when matched with a certain principal diagnosis code, is statistically proved to extend a patient's length of stay by at least 1 day in 75% of those cases, that secondary diagnosis is considered a CC in combination with that principal diagnosis. For example, suppose a patient has a principal diagnosis of pneumonia (486) and also has congestive heart failure (428.0). It has been statistically demonstrated that 75 % of pneumonia patients with a secondary diagnosis of congestive heart failure must remain in the hospital at least 1 day longer than patients having pneumonia alone. Therefore 428.0 is considered an applicable CC code when 486 is the principal diagnosis code.

The list of these CC codes, called the *Complication and Co-morbidity (CC) Code List*, is reviewed and revised each year by CMS and published in the Federal Register, usually at the same time as any DRG revisions. Again, not all CC codes appearing in the CC Code List apply in all instances. Sometimes, the secondary code is considered to be an inherent part of the principal diagnosis disease process or condition. For example, code 303.90 ("other and unspecified alcohol dependence, unspecified") appears on the CC Code List. Suppose that a patient's record is coded with 291.0 ("alcohol withdrawal delirium") as the principal diagnosis followed by 303.90. In this case, 303.90 is not considered a CC because alcohol dependence is considered an inherent part of alcohol withdrawal. When this concept is applied, these CC codes are said to appear on the CC Exclusion List for those particular principal diagnosis codes. If, however, the previous patient with pneumonia had the secondary diagnosis code 303.90, then 303.90 would be considered a CC code because alcohol dependence is not considered an inherent part of pneumonia.

CC codes are important to DRG assignment because the presence of a CC code can determine the final DRG assigned. The final stage in the MDC tree diagram is frequently a choice between a DRG with a CC or a DRG without a CC. For example, DRG 180 is "GI [gastrointestinal] obstruction with CC," and DRG 181 is "GI obstruction without CC." These types of closely related DRGs are called *DRG pairs.* The DRG in the pair with the CC is reimbursed at a higher rate than the DRG without the CC. Multiple CC codes do not have any impact because only one CC code is needed for the case to be assigned to the higher DRG.

Cases assigned to the surgical partitioning section of an MDC essentially follow the same format for DRG assignment as those in the medical partitioning but must account for instances when patients have more than one procedure performed (from the OR or Non-OR List) during the same admission. Only one DRG is assigned for each admission, even if multiple procedures are performed. In these cases, the grouper reviews all of the procedure codes assigned and identifies the single procedure that required the most resource intensity. Each surgical partition is sequenced according to a surgical hierarchy. When multiple procedures have been performed, the procedure code that is highest in the surgical hierarchy is selected by the grouper for DRG assignment. On the MDC tree diagram, the surgical hierarchy lists procedures in descending order, with the procedure requiring the greatest resource intensity at the top. For example, assume that a patient in MDC 8 ("diseases and disorders of the musculoskeletal system and connective tissue") undergoes a total hip replacement. This case would group to DRG 209, "major joint and limb reattachment procedures." In another case, a patient undergoes a shoulder arthroscopy. That case would group to DRG 232, "arthroscopy." Now, suppose that a patient who was admitted for and had a total hip replacement later complained of severe shoulder pain and returned to the OR for a shoulder arthroscopy. The DRG for this admission would be DRG 209 because a total hip replacement is higher on the surgical hierarchy than a shoulder arthroscopy. The arthroscopy has no influence on DRG assignment in this case because it is superseded by the total hip replacement in resource intensity. When abstracting a case, even if the arthroscopy was listed first as **principal procedure**, the *grouper* would still select the total hip replacement for DRG assignment. This is a major difference compared to cases in the medical partition, in which the principal diagnosis selected by the *coder* is used for DRG assignment.

Exceptions to the program format described in the preceding paragraphs include organ transplant cases and patients who have had a tracheostomy and a certain diagnosis. These cases are not assigned to an MDC first but rather directly assigned to each respective DRG. Examples of these DRGs include DRG 103, "heart transplant or implant of heart assist system," and DRG 482, "tracheostomy for face, mouth, and neck diagnosis." As of fiscal year (FY) 2006, there were 10 DRGs grouped without MDC assignment first.

There are other exceptions in which a case is grouped directly to a DRG without first being assigned to an MDC. Unusual, unpredictable, or unique circumstances occasionally occur during hospitalization, which make such cases exceptions to the usual rules of DRG assignment. These exceptions are categorized into the following DRGs:

- DRG 468—"extensive OR procedure unrelated to principal diagnosis." An example of this would be a patient admitted for a myocardial infarction. During the hospitalization, a breast lump is noticed, the patient is found to have breast cancer, and a mastectomy is performed. The myocardial infarction as principal diagnosis is not associated with or related to the mastectomy, so that case is grouped to DRG 468.
- DRG 469—"principal diagnosis invalid as discharge diagnosis."
- DRG 470—"ungroupable." The relative weights (RWs) of DRG 469 and DRG 470 are both 0.0000, meaning a hospital would not receive any reimbursement for cases submitted if either of these DRGs were assigned and submitted for payment. Cases in these DRGs indicate an error in coding or other data. Therefore a correction to the codes or data submitted would be made, and the case would be reassigned to a DRG for which reimbursement will be received.
- DRG 476—"prostatic OR procedure unrelated to principal diagnosis."
- DRG 477—"nonextensive OR procedure unrelated to principal diagnosis" is similar to DRG 468 except that the procedure is, as it states, nonextensive. An example of this would be if the previously mentioned patient with a myocardial infarction had a breast biopsy instead of a

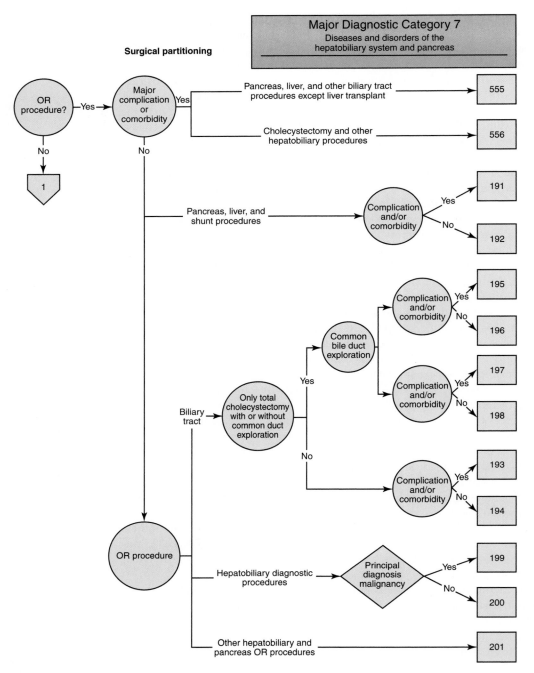

◆ **Figure 6-3**

Decision tree. Major Diagnostic Category: Surgical partitioning. (Adapted from 3M DRG Definitions Manual, 3M Health Information Systems.)

mastectomy. The myocardial infarction as principal diagnosis is not associated with or related to the breast biopsy, and the breast biopsy is a nonextensive procedure, unlike the mastectomy, so that case is grouped to DRG 477.

A complete list of DRGs and related information is published yearly, in late summer, as a Final Rule in the Federal Register on the CMS Web site in conjunction with ICD-9-CM, effective each October 1.

Understanding how DRGs are assigned helps coders to properly sequence their code assignments and focus on the correct principal diagnosis. Figure 6-4 summarizes the steps in DRG assignment.

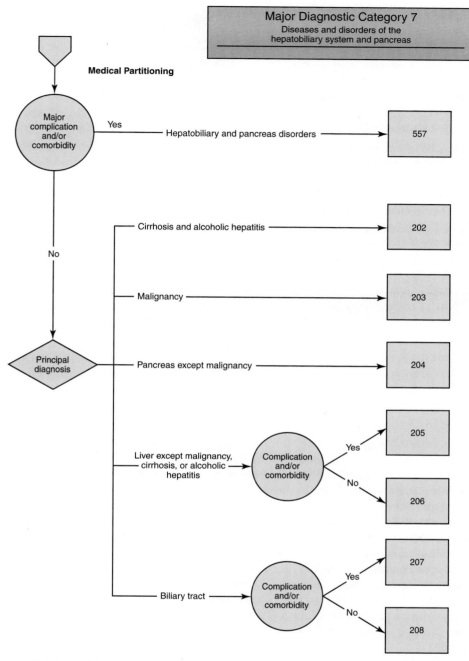

◆ **Figure 6-3 (cont'd)**

Diagnosis Related Group Reimbursement Calculation

Medicare reimbursements for DRGs are based on two components: the national numerical value or **relative weight** of each DRG and each hospital's **Prospective Payment System (PPS)** rate, sometimes referred to as the *blended rate* because it is derived from each hospital's combined operating costs, or blended, with other factors. The PPS rate is expressed in a dollar amount specific to each hospital. All hospitals are reimbursed on the basis of the same national RW for each DRG multiplied by the individual hospital's PPS rate. For example, suppose DRG 999 (fictional) has a national RW of 3.0000. Hospital A has a PPS rate of $5,000.00, and hospital B has a PPS rate of $4,500.00. Hospital A will receive $15,000.00 for each case in DRG 999 (3.0000 × $5,000.00). Hospital B will receive $13,500.00 for each case in DRG 999 (3.0000 × $4,500.00).

MOST CASES IN VARIOUS GROUPER PROGRAMS FOLLOW THE FOLLOWING FORMAT:

- Search for critical procedures: transplants, ventilators, and tracheotomies and group immediately to the appropriate DRG, if detected.

- The principal diagnosis code assigns a case to MDC.

- The grouper reviews all diagnoses and procedure codes and then assigns the case to either the medical or surgical partition of the MDC.

- The grouper, using the Medicare Code edits, makes sure that the principal diagnosis code is appropriate for an inpatient admission.

- The grouper, using the Medicare Code edits, makes sure that the patient's age and sex are appropriate for the diagnoses and procedures assigned.

- The grouper may further route the case based on the patient's age.

- The grouper reviews all secondary diagnoses codes for the presence of a comorbidity or complication and may further route the case.

- If the case is surgical the grouper reviews all procedure codes assigned and bases DRG selection on the procedure code highest in the surgical hierarchy.

◆ **Figure 6-4**
Assignment of the DRG.

There are variations to this basic calculation for cases incurring extraordinarily high costs. These cases may qualify for **outlier** payment. "To qualify for outlier payments, a case must have costs above a fixed-loss cost threshold amount (a dollar amount by which the costs of the case must exceed payments in order to qualify for outliers)" (*Acute Inpatient Prospective Payment System* 2005). There are several calculations to determine outlier payments that depend on the hospital's specific operating and capital cost factors.

Because each DRG has its own RW used to calculate reimbursement, the importance of correctly assigning codes for each case to group into the correct DRG is apparent. For example, suppose that you are a coder at Hospital A. Your fictional DRG 999 has an RW of 3.0000. DRG 999 happens to be a pair DRG (i.e., there is another similar DRG, DRG 998, that resembles DRG 999 except DRG 998 denotes that a CC code is present). Suppose DRG 998 has an RW of 4.0000. If we do *not* correctly code and *do not include* the CC code for DRG assignment, the case would group to DRG 999. If the CC code were *included*, the case would group to DRG 998. In this example, the absence or presence of the CC code would have the following effect on reimbursement with Hospital A's PPS rate of $5,000.00:

DRG 998 "With CC" RW 4.0000 × $5,000.00 = $20,000.00 reimbursement

DRG 999 "Without CC" RW 3.0000 × $5,000.00 = $15,000.00.reimbursement

Consider how the DRG grouper assigns cases to a DRG and the great importance of assigning the correct principal diagnosis. If the incorrect principal diagnosis is assigned, it is highly likely that the DRG will also be incorrect. The resultant incorrect DRG assignment may be reimbursed at either a higher or lower rate than the correct DRG assignment would have been. In either case, the hospital will not receive the appropriate reimbursement. When such errors in DRG assignment are found, the hospital must re-bill or reconcile the reimbursement amount with Medicare and other affected providers. In addition, the hospital's statistics will be negatively affected if cases are not correctly assigned. One important statistic is the hospital's **case mix index (CMI)**.

Case Mix Index

A hospital's CMI is a number derived by adding the RWs of all of the actual DRG cases and then dividing by the total number of cases discharged in a given time period.

A hospital uses the CMI to monitor its performance: the higher the number, the greater the reimbursement received. Fluctuations in CMI indicate incorrect coding, changes in patient populations, changes in physician practices and personnel, or other conditions.

For example, Hospital A discharged 54 patients in January. Each of the 54 DRG RWs is added together, with a combined total of 43.9675. To calculate its CMI for January, Hospital A divides 43.9675 by 54; the CMI for January is 0.81421. Hospital A then decides to do a 6-month comparison and calculates its CMI for June. In June, there were 47 patients discharged with a combined RW of 41.5482. The CMI for June is calculated by dividing 41.5484 by 47; the CMI for June is 0.88400. Hospital A must decide whether the difference in the CMI from January to June is significant enough to warrant further investigation. In this example, the CMI was higher in June than January, so the hospital received more reimbursement on average per patient.

The CMI for all hospitals is published yearly by CMS on its Web site in the Public Use Files. Each hospital has its own unique **provider number** that can be referenced on a chart. The chart notes the total number of Medicare cases discharged in the previous FY and CMI for that FY. The federal FY begins October 1 and ends September 30. The chart is useful in that hospitals can use it as a reference to compare their CMIs with those of other hospitals that have a similar number of cases. Because the provider number is used instead of the hospital's name, each hospital remains anonymous. For example, an employee at Hospital A checks the chart and goes to the hospital's provider number, 000099. The chart shows that Hospital A had 808 Medicare cases discharged in the previous FY and that Hospital A had a CMI of 1.023784 for that period. Next, the Hospital A employee checks the chart for hospitals that had a similar number of discharges and sees that provider number 000054 had 812 cases and a CMI of 2.371271, significantly higher than that of Hospital A. The employee reviews the chart again and in each instance notes that the CMI for similar providers is higher than the CMI for Hospital A. Hospital A administrators may elect to perform an internal investigation, such as a coding audit.

The Coder's Role in Diagnosis Related Group Assignment

The coder must be able to properly apply current coding rules and coding conventions to each case. Although this section focuses on the Medicare PPS system, all cases, regardless of payer, should be coded with equal care, even if payment is not affected, if a hospital's statistics are to be accurate and useful. As previously emphasized, complete and accurate coding is necessary to generate data and statistics beyond DRG assignment.

It is unethical and fraudulent to deliberately code a case incorrectly so that it may be placed into a DRG with a higher reimbursement rate. This practice is sometimes referred to as *upcoding, maximizing,* or *DRG creep.* Some coding software includes prompts that alert the coder that a case would group to a higher-paying DRG if a CC were added or if a different principal diagnosis were assigned. The coder may wish to review the medical record to search for a CC or confirm that there is no CC. Under no circumstances should the coder simply add a CC without confirming that the CC is documented in the medical record. Likewise, the principal diagnosis code should not be changed unless an error was made in the original assignment. The coding software prompts are intended to assist the coder in ensuring proper coding and sequencing; this is sometimes referred to as *optimizing.* The prompts should never be interpreted as directives to code or sequence a certain way simply to obtain higher reimbursement when no supporting documentation exists.

In all cases, without exception, coding and sequencing must be supported by documentation in the medical record. To code otherwise is considered fraudulent by the federal government under the Civil False Claims Act and may subject the hospital to considerable monetary penalties if a pattern of fraud and abuse is demonstrated.

Under the auspices of the Department of Health and Human Service's Office of the Inspector General (OIG), the federal government released *Compliance Program Guidance for Hospitals,* which addresses coding issues. Coders should be familiar with this publication as well as their own hospital's compliance program. The OIG publishes a Work Plan every year that includes coding projects focused on particular DRGs and patterns of DRG assignment.

Usually, medical records are coded and DRGs are assigned after the patient is discharged. The hospital cannot submit a claim for reimbursement until after the patient is discharged. To minimize the time between discharge and claims submission, some facilities perform coding concurrently —that is, while the patient is still in-house. The coder may review the medical record when the patient is admitted and every day or every other day thereafter until discharge. Temporary codes are assigned as well as a temporary DRG. This concurrently assigned DRG is often referred to as a **working DRG.** The coder has the opportunity to question the physician about documentation and potentially facilitate coding and DRG assignment accuracy; these efforts may shorten the time between discharge and claims submission. Coding concurrently does present some disadvantages, however. More coding staff may be needed, and some necessary information, such as pathology reports, may not yet be available.

AMBULATORY PAYMENT CLASSIFICATIONS

As is true for inpatient services, the costs for outpatient, or ambulatory, services has risen. In addition, many patient care services have shifted from inpatient to outpatient settings, thus increasing the amount of reimbursement from inpatient to outpatient/ambulatory services. In ambulatory health care, a number of different reimbursement methodologies apply; fee for service and discounted fee for service are most commonly used. A number of insurers are participate in capitation as well.

In the 1990s, the federal government was spending billions of dollars on outpatient services using a cost-based system. In an attempt to cut or at least control the costs of these services and as part of the Balanced Budget Act of 1997, Congress mandated that CMS (at that time the Health Care Financing Administration [HCFA]) develop a PPS for Medicare outpatient services, referred to as *OPPS (Outpatient Prospective Payment System).* Just as DRGs are used for reimbursement for Medicare inpatient services under PPS, the OPPS uses ambulatory payment classifications (APCs) to reimburse for Medicare outpatient services. Originally, this system was called *ambulatory payment groups (APGs),* but HCFA changed the name when it modified APGs in 1998. The OPPS and APCs were implemented for services provided on or after August 1, 2000. The Final Rule for implementation and subsequent updates can be found on the CMS Web site and in the Federal Register (65[68]). APCs are updated annually to include additions, deletions, and modifications. Updates occur each calendar year (CY).

The APC system uses HCPCS/CPT-4 procedure, service, or item codes to group patients. ICD-9-CM codes are used not for grouping but to indicate the medical necessity of the procedure, service, or item provided. For example, if a claim were submitted for reimbursement of an electrocardiogram, there should be a logical corresponding cardiac ICD-9-CM code that indicates the reason that the electrocardiogram was performed. ICD-9-CM procedure codes are not used in OPPS and the APC system, although they are sometimes assigned.

Under the APC classification system, patients are grouped on the basis of clinical similarities and similar costs or resource consumption. There are approximately 1000 APCs, a figure subject to change depending on the yearly modifications. APCs are categorized as follows:

- Significant procedures, therapies, or services
- Medical visits
- Ancillary tests and procedures
- Partial hospitalization
- Drugs and biologicals
- Devices

Consideration of these categories makes it easier to envision how one outpatient visit can result in the assignment of multiple APCs. That more than one APC can be assigned per visit is a major difference between APCs and DRGs, in which only one DRG is assigned per inpatient hospitalization. For example, suppose a man is found unconscious on the sidewalk and brought to the hospital's emergency department by the police. The emergency department physician performs a workup, discovers that the patient is in a diabetic coma, and gives him insulin to bring his glucose level under control. In addition, the emergency physician notes that the patient injured his arm after falling on the sidewalk and orders an x-ray to rule out a fracture. In such a scenario, there will be an APC for the emergency visit, an APC for the drug (insulin), and an APC for the x-ray. Each APC has its own payment. The facility is reimbursed in an amount equal to all three APCs added together or, in some instances, receives a reduced or discounted payment for one of the services. For example, if a patient requires the use of a minor surgery suite for multiple procedures, the patient probably uses fewer resources overall than if the procedures were performed separately at different times. Therefore a reduced payment is warranted. By the same logic, if a procedure is terminated or discontinued, the payment will be reduced or discounted depending on whether anesthesia was started.

Final payment for APCs is based on a complex set of edits and payment rules that include, for example, HCPCS/CPT-4 codes, code modifiers, and revenue codes. The coder is usually responsible only for assigning the HCPCS/CPT-4 codes and modifiers, and the other billing elements are the responsibility of other departments where charges have been incurred.

A code **modifier** is a two-digit number added to a HCPCS/CPT-4 code that provides additional information regarding the procedure or service performed. A modifier may be used, for example, to indicate a right, left, or bilateral body part; a specific appendage; extent of anesthesia; limited or reduced services; and other situations or circumstances. A **revenue code** is a three-digit code that denotes the department in which a procedure, service, or supply item was provided. Revenue codes are in the Chargemaster, which is discussed later in this chapter.

Based on the HCPCS/CPT-4 code or codes, each APC is assigned a payment status indicator (SI) that determines reimbursement under OPPS. For example, SI T indicates "significant procedure, multiple-procedure reduction applies." SI V indicates "clinic or emergency department visit," and SI X indicates "ancillary service." The entire list of APCs and each SI can be found on the CMS Web site along with the RW for each APC, each payment rate, national unadjusted co-payment, and minimum unadjusted co-payment. CPT/HCPCS codes and APCs are updated each CY; therefore it is important to note any changes because reimbursements may be affected.

PAYMENT DENIALS/CLAIMS REJECTIONS

Coding professionals in various settings, from ambulatory hospital settings to physician offices, are frequently involved in responding to payment denials or claims rejections. As noted in this brief overview of APCs, the system undergoes changes yearly and is complicated on several levels, from coding to billing. When claims are submitted through the **fiscal intermediary** (FI), the claims are subjected to a number of edits that include the outpatient code editor (OCE) and National Correct Coding Initiative (NCCI) edits. The OCE and NCCI edits flag coding errors in the claims. Until the errors are corrected, the claim is rejected and reimbursement is denied for that claim.

Avoidance of payment denials or claims rejections is of paramount concern because income is adversely affected. One way to avoid these rejections is to understand the reasons for the rejections. Each FI includes a **local medical review policy (LMRP)** that is available to providers, usually on the FI's Web site. The LMRP is extremely useful in that the policy defines covered services and details concerning exactly what diagnosis codes are needed for a service, procedure, or item to be deemed medically necessary. Coders familiar with the LMRP, as well as the OCE and NCCI edits, can be proactive in avoiding payment denials and claims rejections.

ADDITIONAL PROSPECTIVE PAYMENT SYSTEMS

Inpatient Psychiatric Facility Prospective Payment System

CMS has recognized that providing services for psychiatric patients is unique and not readily comparable to providing services for medical or surgical patients. The psychiatric setting is often more difficult to manage in terms of resources and length of stay. Many hospitals no longer have inpatient psychiatric patient units because of these difficulties, which lead to reimbursement problems. The new inpatient psychiatric facility prospective payment system (IPF PPS) was designed to address these issues beginning January 1, 2005, with an anticipated transition period of 3 years. The major change concerning reimbursement is that under IPF PPS, payment will be on a per diem rate based on a federal rate. The federal rate will be based on various factors and adjustments. There are two levels of adjustments: patient level and facility level. The patient level includes length of stay and patient age, and the facility level includes the geographical location of the facility and whether the facility is a teaching hospital.

IPF PPS will be based on ICD-9-CM coding, and, as was the case under DRGs, all of the coding rules apply. A difference that coders will notice is that CC codes play a larger role than in the psychiatric DRGs in the PPS DRG system. The addition of these CC codes under IPF PPS will cause a case to fall into additional adjustment categories. It is important for psychiatrists to fully document all secondary diagnoses, including all medical diagnoses, in addition to psychiatric diagnoses.

Inpatient Rehabilitation Facility Prospective Payment System

The Balanced Budget Act also required CMS to establish a PPS for inpatient rehabilitation facilities (IRF PPS). The Final Rule for IRF PPS was published in the *Federal Register* August 1, 2000, and became effective January 1, 2002. IFR PPS replaced a cost-based payment system. IFR PPS reimburses on a per-discharge basis and covers all costs of inpatient rehabilitation services as well as the characteristics of each patient that a facility admits. A comprehensive patient assessment instrument, called the *Inpatient Rehabilitation Facility Patient Assessment Instrument (IRF-PAI)*, is used to assess each patient with the intent that patients with greater needs be identified and that the facility receive higher payment for these individuals. IRF-PAI includes sections on, for example, bowel continence, impairments, infections, and pressure ulcers. Two sections of IRF-PAI require the use of ICD-9-CM codes. Patients are grouped into case-mix groups (CMGs). Each CMG has four possible weights; the final weight is determined by the patient's co-morbidities.

Unique to IRF PPS is that two types of coding practice are applied: one type for IRF-PAI and one type for billing. IRF-PPS requires coding the etiology diagnoses, essentially the same diagnoses that would have been coded in the acute setting even though the patient is no longer receiving acute care. For reporting purposes on the Uniform Bill (UB), standard coding rules and conventions are applied, so in most circumstances the principal diagnosis will be a V code. For example, suppose a patient admitted to the hospital was diagnosed with severe insulin dependent diabetes with peripheral vascular disease and had to have his leg amputated. The ICD-9-CM diagnosis codes would be 250.71 and 443.81. After the amputation, the patient was transferred to an inpatient rehabilitation facility to learn how to use an artificial leg. The same codes, 250.71 and 443.81, would be used for IRF-PAI, but a rehabilitation code, V57.81 ("orthotic training"), would be reported as the principal diagnosis on the UB.

Long-Term Care Hospital Prospective Payment System

The long-term care prospective payment system (LTC-PPS) became effective for cost reporting periods beginning on or after October 1, 2002. Medicare regulations define long-term care hospitals as hospitals that have an average inpatient length of stay greater than 25 days. Patients in long-term care hospitals have multiple acute and chronic complex conditions and may need, for example, comprehensive rehabilitation services, respiratory therapy, cancer treatment, and pain management. LTC-PPS is based on DRGs, but these DRGs are modified to reflect patient acuity and the greater costs involved in treating the complex conditions of these patients, which require longer lengths of stay.

Home Health Prospective Payment System

The home health prospective payment system (HH PPS) applies to reimbursement for services rendered by home health care providers. Payments are in units, each unit being a 60-day episode, and are distributed to the provider in two split payments. The case mix system used is called Home Health Resources Groups (HHRGs), and the level of the HHRGs determines the payment. A comprehensive patient assessment tool, OASIS (Outcomes and Assessment Information Set), is used with ICD-9-CM codes to group these patients into HHRGs.

Skilled Nursing Facility Prospective Payment System and Resource Utilization Groups

Resource Utilization Groups (RUGs) are the basis for payment for skilled nursing facility (SNF) services for Medicare patients. RUGs are currently in their third version and referred to as *RUG-III*. Unlike DRGs and APCs, RUGs are not a retrospective reimbursement system for an entire stay or visit. Reimbursement based on RUGs is a daily, or per diem, rate based on the admission assessment of the patient. A review of data sets may help you understand this concept.

As discussed in Chapters 2, 3, and 4, specific data sets are abstracted and reported retrospectively for both ambulatory and hospital care: the Uniform Ambulatory Care Data Set (UACDS) and the Uniform Hospital Discharge Data Set (UHDDS), respectively. In long-term care, the **Minimum Data Set** (MDS) is collected as part of the Resident Assessment Instrument (RAI). The MDS, currently in version 2.0, contains far more data than the UHDDS or the UACDS. It includes the patient's cognitive and medical condition as well as his or her ability to perform self-care and other activities of daily living. Assessment therefore is performed at the beginning of the patient's stay, not at the end. Reimbursement is then based on the patient's care needs, consisting of one of 44 groups within seven broad categories: rehabilitation, extensive services, special care, clinically complex, impaired cognition, behavior problems, or reduced physical function. Although there are other RUG systems in existence, Medicare reimbursement is determined using the RUG-III system.

In most SNF settings, much of the information collected has been under the domain of the nursing department. Nursing staff members usually collect and record the MDS data, largely composed of diagnostic statements and including the ICD-9-CM codes associated with the patient's medical condition. This is not to imply that health information professionals are incapable of performing this task.

PPSs continue to evolve and expand into various patient settings, primarily as a result of legislation and instruction from Congress. Although these PPSs are initiated and developed for reimbursing services for Medicare patients, other payers and insurers often use or modify these systems for their patients as well. To code accurately and in compliance with regulations, all coding professionals should be aware of what PPSs apply, and to whom, in the setting in which they are employed. Table 6-2 contains a summary of the previously discussed PPS systems.

Resource-Based Relative Value System

The resource-based relative value system (RBRVS) is the basis of reimbursement to physicians for services rendered to Medicare patients. Because the reimbursement is for physician services, the location where services were provided can be the physician's office, a hospital, or a nursing home—essentially anywhere that a patient can be treated. Physicians submit claims for reimbursement using HCPCS/CPT-4 codes. Each HCPCS/CPT-4 code has three relative value units (RVUs). Each RVU corresponds to the complexity of the service provided, the consumption of resources incurred by the service provided, and the relation of the service provided in comparison with other services provided. Physicians receive reimbursement on the basis of a national Medicare physician **fee schedule** that is adjusted according to the physician's geographical location. Physicians located in different areas of the United States receive varying reimbursement amounts for identical services because Medicare recognizes that operating costs vary by location.

TABLE 6-2	**Summary of PPS Systems**		
SYSTEM	**SETTING**	**CODE SYSTEM**	**BASIS OF REIMBURSEMENT**
DRG	Short-stay facility, inpatient acute care	ICD-9-CM diagnosis and procedure codes	Diagnoses and procedures Single DRG assignment Retrospective
APC	Ambulatory care, outpatient services, emergency departments	CPT-4 HCPCS ICD-9-CM diagnosis codes	Procedures Diagnoses used for validation May have multiple APCs Retrospective
IPF-PPS	Inpatient psychiatric	ICD-9-CM	Per diem and federal rate
IRF-PPS	Inpatient rehabilitation facilities	ICD-9-CM	Per discharge IRF-PAI CMGs
LTC-PPS	Hospitals with average length of stay > 25 days	ICD-9-CM	DRGs Patient acuity
HH-PPS	Home health care providers	ICD-9-CM	HHRGs Payment units OASIS
RUG-III	Medicare CNF services	ICD-9-CM	Per diem rate Not retrospective MDS data

Exercise 6-2

Prospective Payment System

1. If patients are grouped into the same Diagnosis Related Group (DRG), it is because they have what three criteria in common?
2. What is meant by the phrase *resource intensity*?
3. Describe how a case is assigned to a major diagnostic category (MDC).
4. After assignment of the MDC, what occurs next in the grouping process?
5. What patient attributes are important to grouper assignment?
6. What is a CC code, and why is it significant?
7. What is the difference between a comorbidity and a complication?
8. What does the Medicare Code Editor do?
9. Describe two types of coding errors that may affect DRG assignment.
10. What coding classification or nomenclature system is used to indicate medical necessity?
11. What is a modifier, and for what is it used?

BILLING

To be reimbursed for services rendered to a patient, a facility must alert the payer that payment is due. This is accomplished by **billing.** To the insurer, this bill is a **claim.** In an acute care facility, the billing function is performed in a department that is often called **patient accounts.**

PATIENT ACCOUNTS

The patient accounts department is responsible for ensuring that accurate bills are sent for each patient's account, that they are sent to the correct payers, and that the facility receives the correct payment. Most billing is done electronically. A patient's bill includes a compilation of charges for items and services rendered. Each patient is assigned an account number for items received and services rendered during a particular visit or stay. The account number, unlike the patient's medical record number, changes for each encounter. In this way, charges can be accurately assigned, or "posted," to each specific encounter so that the bill reflects the charges for each individual account. For example, a patient may visit a hospital three times in one month: once as a clinic patient, once as an emergency department patient, and once as an inpatient. The hospital does not lump all three visits into one monthly bill. Instead, a different account number is assigned for each encounter, and a separate bill is sent for each account that reflects the charges incurred for each individual visit. A bill that is produced and sent is called a "dropped," or final, bill. A bill that has been dropped is pending payment. Once the dropped bill has been paid, the account is closed to any further activity.

To use an acute care inpatient as an example, there are three key steps that must happen in order to produce and drop a bill: (1) The patient's charges must be entered into, or posted to, the account; (2) the patient must have been discharged so that the account reflects the charges accumulated for the patient's entire length of stay; (3) the medical record must be coded. Whether or not payers use DRGs as a method of reimbursement, they still want to see the ICD-9-CM codes related to the clinical stay, and these codes must appear on the UB. It is through the coding of the diagnoses and procedures that the payer often gets the first impression of what actually should have happened in terms of services rendered.

When Steps 1 and 2 have occurred but not Step 3, hospitals monitor this by creating a list that tracks each unbilled account. This list of undropped bills is called by a variety of names depending on the facility, but it is most often referred to as the *unbilled list* or the *DNFB* ("discharged no final bill" or "discharged not final billed"). Regardless of the name used, this list of delayed payments can add up to millions of dollars. Because the delays are due to the fact that coding has not occurred on the medical records representing these outstanding accounts, the HIM department proactively and aggressively monitors the DNFB on a regular basis. Management of the coding function and the DNFB is often complex, with many factors contributing to uncoded medical records that then result in unbilled accounts. Because the patient accounts and HIM departments both have the same goal of reducing or eliminating unbilled accounts, one may assist the other in reducing the factors contributing to payment delays.

CHARGEMASTER (CHARGE DESCRIPTION MASTER)

Whether a facility is reimbursed using PPS or another system, a variety of procedures must be in place to ensure the accurate accumulation of charges and the accurate coding of the clinical data. **Charges** are the facility's individual fees, or the dollar amount for items or services provided to a patient and owed to the facility. Each item or service is assigned a charge, which is usually reviewed and adjusted or changed annually. Charges may be set on the basis of fee schedules or contractual arrangements with certain payers or determined internally using the facility's cost-accounting system. The actual charges are not always equal to the amount that the payer reimburses a facility; the payment received depends on contractual agreements and may be discounted accordingly. A facility compares its charges to actual reimbursements to determine the impact of contractual arrangements and whether they allow the facility to operate profitably (i.e., earn more money than it spends).

The report of the data fields that contain a facility's charges or costs for services and items is called a **Chargemaster**. Other terms that are sometimes used include *Charge Data Master* and *Charge Description Master (CDM)*. Table 6-3 illustrates key data fields that usually appear in a Chargemaster. The Chargemaster must be updated regularly so that fees and costs are accurate. Because HCPCS/CPT-4 codes are included in the Chargemaster, these codes must also be updated when changes or revisions occur. All the services that a facility provides, from adhesive bandages to intravenous drips and room and board, must appear on the Chargemaster, or they are not subject to billing. Coding professionals often initiate or assist in making the updates to the CDM and informing departments about changes.

CHARGE CAPTURE

As previously discussed, charges must be posted to a patient's account in order for proper billing to occur. This process is called **charge capture**. The Chargemaster can be thought of as an à la carte menu. When you go to a restaurant, the server takes your order and indicates, often electronically, the items of food and beverage that you have ordered. These items are part of a much larger list of food and beverages offered by the restaurant. When you are finished, your food and beverages are matched with their costs, these costs are tallied, and you are presented with a check. The restaurant check is analogous to a hospital bill, or the UB, which is discussed in more detail later in this chapter.

In an inpatient hospital setting, charges are usually posted to the patient's account electronically, using order-entry software, each time a service or item is provided. Most of the time, these charges are accumulated daily for each account and then grouped together, or "batched." The order-entry program then sends these batches on to the hospital's accounting or billing system,

TABLE 6-3	Sample Fields in a Charge Description Master
FIELD	**DESCRIPTION**
General ledger code	Internal code used by the facility's accounting department to track revenue and expenses
CPT/HCPCS code	Billing code for transmission to the insurer
Cost basis	The cost of the item to the facility
Charge	The amount that the facility charges for the item or service
Description	Definition or description of the item or service
Date	Date of the most recent update of the aforementioned fields for the item or service

usually at midnight. If the hospital does not use order-entry software or does not use the software for all types of charges, these charges still must be captured; in this case, they are captured manually on a paper form called a *charge ticket*. All charge tickets must be forwarded to the accounting or billing department at the end of each business day and manually posted to the correct account. As you can imagine, manual charge capture is extremely laborious and vulnerable to human error.

Depending on factors such as length of stay, each account may have hundreds of posted charges. Most facilities allow time between discharge and submission of the bill so that all charges can be posted. In smaller facilities, posting delays may occur because of reduced staff on weekends. This period is called the *bill-hold period* and usually ranges from 1 to 5 days after discharge, perhaps longer for outpatient or ambulatory services. If charges are still not posted during the bill-hold period and the bill is dropped, these charges are considered late. Because late charges must be submitted separately and some insurers do not pay late charges at all or only after a certain time, it is essential that charges be posted no later than the end of the bill-hold period.

In an ambulatory setting, charges are often captured, by service, on an **encounter form,** or **superbill.** An encounter form is usually a single sheet of paper, sometimes double-sided, that contains a list of the most common patient complaints, diagnoses, procedures, and services provided by the facility. Some insurers provide their own encounter forms. A comprehensive encounter form includes ICD-9-CM diagnoses codes and HCPCS/CPT-4 procedure codes. Encounter forms facilitate communication between the physician or other health care provider and the administrative personnel who are responsible for coding and billing. Because it is not the encounter form but the health record that supports the reimbursement claim, care must be taken to ensure that the health record indicates all services provided. Figure 6-5 is an example of an encounter form (superbill).

In a physician's office, the process of obtaining reimbursement may rest with the administrative personnel (e.g., the medical secretary, medical assistant, or practice manager). The role of these employees is to determine which services were provided for which patient and which insurer or insurers should receive a bill and to ensure that all services provided are billed correctly.

In some situations, such as in a solo practitioner's office, the physician may file the claims. Because the insurance industry is so complex and there are many different types of providers, all with their own rules, many physicians rely on billing services to perform the administrative tasks of charge capture and billing. Performing all of these tasks is critical to accurate and timely reimbursement.

THE UNIFORM BILL

The National Uniform Billing Committee (NUBC) is responsible for developing and implementing a single billing form and standard data set to be used nationwide by providers/hospitals and payers/insurers for handling inpatient health care claims. The NUBC comprises representatives from all the major provider and payer organizations, including the AHA and Medicare, the public health sector, and electronic standards development organizations.

The first standard UB appeared in 1982 and was referred to as the *UB-82*. Representatives from across the country were surveyed to seek improvements on the UB-82, and the UB-92 was the result of their efforts. At this time, more than 98% of hospital claims are submitted electronically to Medicare using the UB-92. Although the UB was originally used for claims reimbursement only, the NUBC has recognized that it contains a wealth of data that can be used for additional purposes. The data captured on the UB is now also used by health researchers to gauge the delivery of health care services to patients and to set future policy.

Changes to the UB-92 form have been implemented. The new UB is called the UB-04. Figure 6-6 shows a UB-04 form. Coding professionals should be aware that fields on the UB-04 form have been expanded from the UB-92 to include the diagnoses code on admission, distinct fields for the patient's reason for visit, and expanded diagnosis and procedure fields to accommodate ICD-10-CM and ICD-10-PCS codes (NUBC 1999).

CMS-1500

The CMS-1500 form is the data collection form used for transmittal of billing information for ambulatory/outpatient claims and physician's office claims. The CMS-1500 form has fewer fields that the UB-92, but it contains much of the same information. Figure 6-7 shows a CMS-1500 form.

X	PATIENT VISITS DESCRIPTION	CODE	AMOUNT
	NEW PATIENT		
	Problem focused Hx	99201	
	Expanded prob/Focused Hx	99202	
	Detailed Hx	99203	
	Comp Hx/Moderate complex	99204	
	Comp Hx/High complex	99205	
	ESTABLISHED PATIENT		
	Minimal	99211	
	Problem focused Hx	99212	
	Expanded prob/Focused Hx	99213	
	Detailed Hx	99214	
	Comprehensive Hx	99215	
	CONSULTATION		
	Problem focused Hx	99241	
	Expanded prob/Focused Hx	99242	
	Detailed Hx	99243	
	Comp Hx/Moderate complex	99244	
	Comp Hx/High complex	99245	
	NURSE SPECIALIST		
	Computer analysis	99090	
	Group health ed	99078	
	Skills management (15 min.)	97535	
	PROCEDURES		
	Accucheck/One Touch	7182948	
	EKG w/interpretation	93000	
	IV infusion, up to 1 hr.	90780	
	IV infusion, each add'l hr.	90781	
	Immunization administration	90471	
	Two or more vaccines/toxoids	90472	
	Therapeutic/diagnostic injection	90782	
	Specify: med/dose		
	Injection of antibiotic	90788	
	Specify: med/dose		
	Occult blood (guaiac)	82270	
	ANS	95937	
	24 hour cardiac monitor	93230	
	Pap smear	88150	
	Thyroid fine needle asp. (proc.)	7190357	
	Group counseling, 30 min.	99411	
	Group counseling, 60 min.	99412	

X	PROCEDURES cont. DESCRIPTION	CODE	ALPHA	AMOUNT
	Preventive counseling, 15 min.	99401		
	Preventive counseling, 30 min.	99402		
	Preventive counseling, 45 min.	99403		
	Preventive counseling, 60 min.	99404		
	DIABETES/LIPID			
	Cholesterol, HDL	7190053	HDL	
	C-peptide	7190219	CPEP	
	Glucose serum	7182947	GLU	
	HGB A1 C	7190057	HA1	
	Insulin	7190343	INS	
	Lipoprotein panel A	7175004		
	Micral, random	7190335	MLBU	
	Protein, urine 24 hr.	7195011	PROU	
	GONADAL			
	Estradiol	7190044	ESD	
	FSH	7190048	FSH	
	LH	7190069	LH	
	Progesterone	7190078	PROG	
	PSA	7190079	PSA	
	SHBG	7190622	SHBG	
	Testosterone	7190086	TEST	
	Testosterone, Free	7190322	FTES	
	PSA, Free	7184999		
	PROFILES			
	Basic metabolic panel	7180049	CH7	
	Comp. metabolic panel	7180054	CMP	
	Electrolyte panel	7180051	ELEC	
	Hepatic function panel	7180058	HFPA	
	Hepatitis panel	7180059		
	Lipid profile 2	7190257	LPP2	
	THYROID			
	Antimicrosomal antibody	7190213	TM	
	TSI	7190476	TSIG	
	Thyroglobulin	7190584	THY	
	T4 - Thyroxine	7190047	FT4	
	T3 uptake	7190292	TU	
	Total T3	7190095	T3 C	
	T3-Free	7190595	FT3	
	TSH (Thyroid stim hormone)	7190253	TSH	

X	CALCIUM/BONE/KIDNEY DESCRIPTION	CODE	ALPHA	AMOUNT
	Calcium, ionized	7190821	ICAL	
	Calcium, serum	7190311	CAL	
	Calcium, urine 24 hr.	7190222	CALU	
	Creatinine, clearance ht. ___	7194754	CRCP	
	wt. ___			
	Microalbumin, urine 24 hr.	7190335	MLBT	
	Magnesium, serum	7190317	MAG	
	Parathyroid hormo	7190387	PTH	

X	ADRENAL/PITUITARY DESCRIPTION	CODE	ALPHA	AMOUNT
	ACTH	7190005	ACTH	
	Aldosterone, serum	7190204	ALD	
	Androstenedione	7190336	AND	
	Cortisol, serum	7190032	COR	
	DHEA	7190341	DHEA	
	DHEA S serum	7190312	DHES	
	Human growth hormone	7190379	HGH	
	Prolactin	7190316	PRL	
	17OH Progesterone	7190479	HY17	
	17OH Pregnegalone	7190480	LONE	
	Urine catecholimine 24 hr.	7190021	CATU	
	Urine cortisol 24 hr.	7190033	CORU	
	Urine metanephrines 24 hr.	7190475	METU	
	Urine potassium 24 hr.	7190077	POTU	
	Urine sodium 24 hr.	7190261	SODU	
	Urine VMA 24 hr.	7190534	VMAU	

X	CHEMISTRY/HEMATOLOGY DESCRIPTION	CODE	ALPHA	AMOUNT
	CBC w/diff & platelets	7190327	CBC1	
	Erthrocyte sed rate	7190330	ESR	
	Potassium, serum	7184813	POT	
	Urine culture	7190041	BACTI	
	Urinalysis, routine	7190334	URTN	
	Urinalysis, dipstick	7190384	URCH	
	Venipuncture	7190323	VENI	
	GGI	7184773		
	HCE	7190329		

AUTHORIZATION #			
DIAGNOSIS	**REFERRING MD**	Tax ID #	62-1162462
SPECIAL INSTRUCTIONS		Previous bal.	
		Amount paid	
		Today's chrg	
		Amount paid	
Physician signature:	Date:	Total rec'd	

I authorize release of any medical information necessary to process this claim. I also authorize the direct payment of any benefits due me for the described services to _____ I understand I am financially responsible for paying any unpaid balance and will be responsible for the entire bill if this claim is not covered. **Medicare Patients:** The Medicare program requires that all diagnosis be ICD 9 coded. We are unable to provide this service to you at the time of your visit, and therefore, require that you permit us to file an insurance claim with your Medicare carrier.

Balance due	
Check one:	
☐ Cash	
☐ Check, M.O.# _____	
☐ MC ☐ VISA	
☐ Care Card # _____	

Patient (Beneficiary) signature: _____ Date: _____

98381 7/99

◆ **Figure 6-5**
Ambulatory care encounter form/superbill. (From Mervat Abdelhak, Sara Grostick, Mary Alice Hanken, and Ellen Jacobs. *Health Information: Management of a Strategic Resource.* 2nd ed. Philadelphia: Saunders, 2001, p 244.)

Exercise 6-3

Billing

1. What are some possible reasons that a bill has not been dropped?
2. What management tool is used to track unbilled accounts?
3. How would someone use the tool described in Question 2?
4. The charges or costs for a vaccination are listed in a facility's _____.
5. For the vaccination charge to appear on a patient's bill, how does the charge get to the patient's account?
6. In an ambulatory setting, an encounter form is often used for charge capture. Name three items that would be on an encounter form.

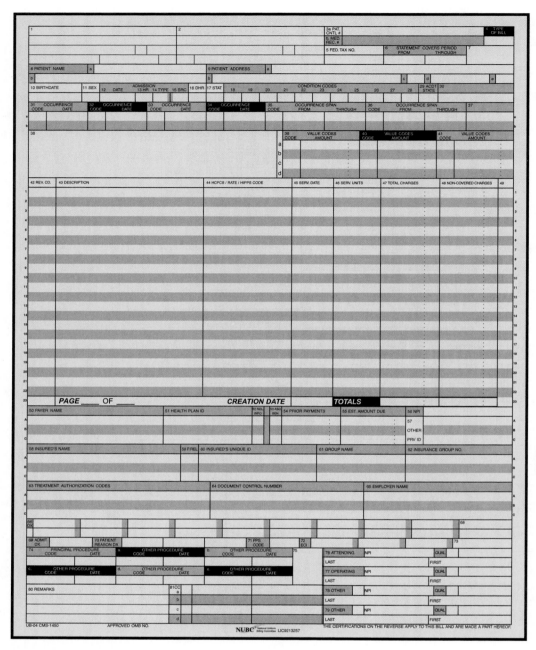

◆ **Figure 6-6**
UB-04.

IMPACT OF CODING

In any discussion of the various reimbursement methodologies, the importance of accurate ICD-9-CM and HCPCS/CPT-4 coding cannot be overstated. Because the codes determine the payment and facilitate the claim, the accuracy and timeliness of the coding function are critical.

CODING QUALITY

The timeliness and completeness of the postdischarge processing of a record are important. In addition to charge capture, all pertinent medical record data must have been collected for correct assignment of codes, and the processing cycle must facilitate efficient, timely coding. For exam-

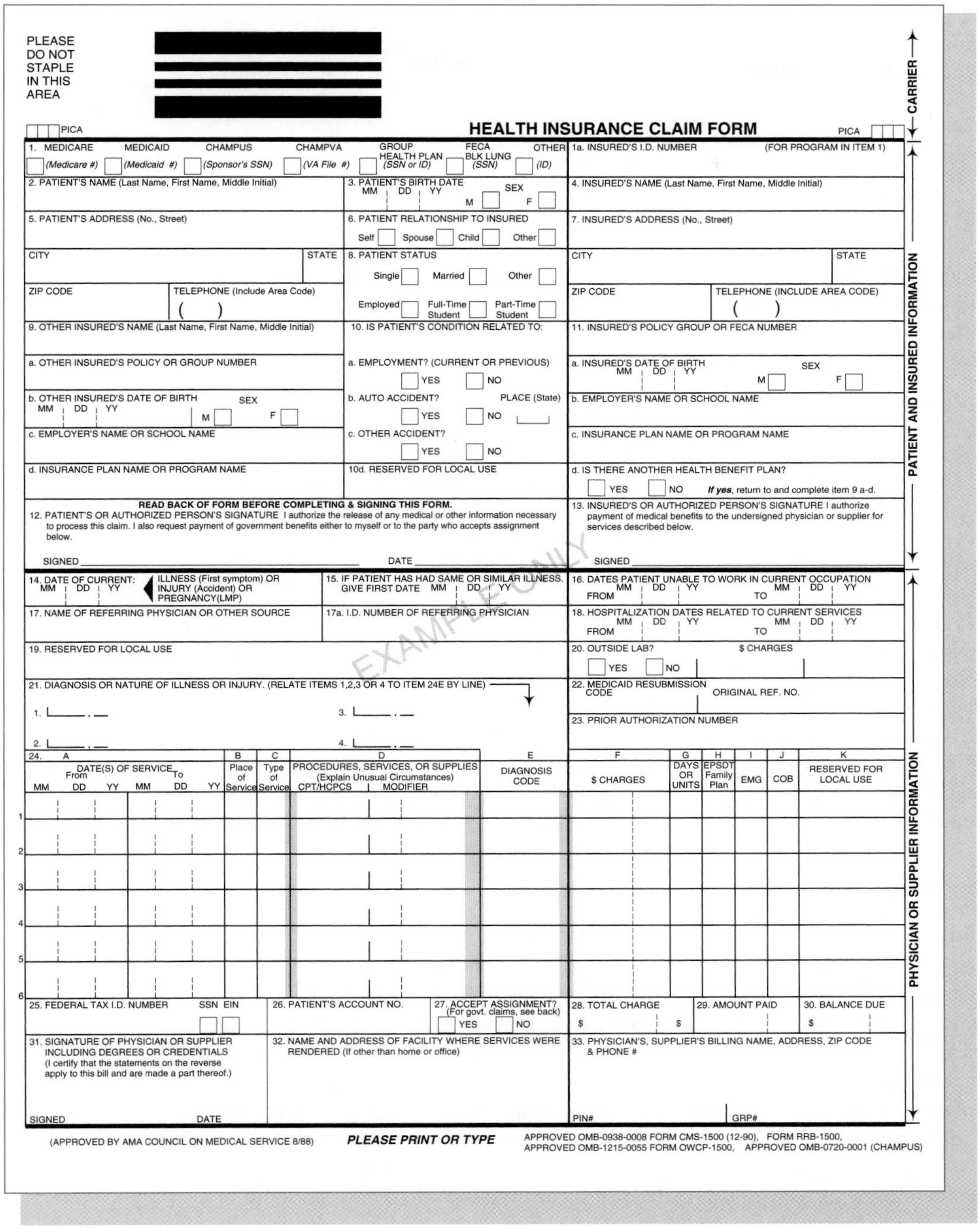

◆ Figure 6-7
CMS-1500 health insurance claim form.

ple, if a paper-based medical record must be assembled and analyzed before it is given to a coder, and if the assembly and analysis sections are 5 or 6 days behind the current discharge date, then medical records may not be coded until the 7 days after the discharge date. Even factoring in the bill-hold period, a week is a long time for a facility to go without dropping a bill for a patient's stay. Facilities sometimes choose to code the record before it is assembled or analyzed so that the bill may be dropped more quickly. Although this sequence expedites payment, it can also lead to coding errors if the medical record is incomplete because missing elements are not clearly identified or if important reports are hidden in the wrong sections of the medical record.

Coding also must be reliable and valid, both individually and collectively within a facility or group. A coder or group of coders is said to demonstrate **reliability** when codes are consistently assigned for similar or identical cases. **Validity** of coding refers to the degree of accuracy of the codes assigned.

REGULATORY ISSUES

Effective April 1, 2005, an updated version of *ICD-9-CM Official Guidelines for Coding and Reporting* was issued by CMS and NCHS and approved by the Cooperating Parties. This document can be found in its entirety at http://www.cdc.gov/nchs/data/icd9/icdguide.pdf. Adherence to these guidelines is required under HIPAA (see Chapter 11). The following statement is made regarding coding from incomplete medical records:

> A joint effort between the health care provider and the coder is essential to achieve complete and accurate documentation, code assignment, and reporting of diagnoses and procedures. These guidelines have been developed to assist both the health care provider and coder in identifying those diagnoses and procedures that are to be reported. The importance of consistent, complete documentation in the medical record cannot be overem-phasized. Without such documentation, accurate coding cannot be achieved. The entire record should be reviewed to determine the specific reason for the encounter and the conditions treated.

Accurate coding is necessary for **optimization** of reimbursement, particularly in a PPS, and is best achieved through coding from a complete medical record. Optimization occurs when the coding results in the DRG that most accurately represents the facility's utilization of resources, based on the diagnoses and procedures, and is completely substantiated by documentation. **Maximization**, on the other hand, is simply assigning and sequencing codes to obtain the highest-paying DRG. Optimization is highly desirable; maximization is illegal and unethical. Under the U.S. federal government's National Correct Coding Initiative (NCCI), as well as fraud and abuse audits, patterns of maximization, if proved, can result in the criminal prosecution of facility administrators.

CODING COMPLIANCE

A comprehensive **coding compliance plan** is an important part of a facility's corporate compliance plan (see Chapter 11). The coding compliance plan should include regular internal audits and audits performed by objective external reviewers who have no vested interest in the facility's profit margin. Coding audits performed by payers are not necessarily useful in determining coding accuracy because their overall goal is to find only those coding errors that adversely affect the payer. In any type of audit, however, results should be shared and discussed with the coding staff.

There are two fundamentally different approaches to coding audits: general reviews of all records of all payer types to identify potential problems and targeted reviews of known or potential problem areas. In general reviews, records are selected by a statistical method or by any method that captures a representative sample of records. All coders, all record types, and all payers should be included in a general review. The audit results can be used to determine coding error rates by coder or more generally.

Targeted reviews may be aimed at specific coders, codes, DRGs, or other factors or elements of coding. For example, the OIG develops a list of so-called targeted DRGs, which are DRGs that have a history of aberrant coding (i.e., inaccurate coding leading to Medicare overpayments). **Quality Improvement Organization**s (QIOs) monitor and assess facility data and may perform reviews of cases assigned to these targeted DRGs. Regardless of audit findings, coding error rates are not applicable to targeted reviews because such audits are not based on a random selection.

Throughout this chapter, the importance of the coding function and reimbursement has been emphasized. By now you should understand the essence of what being a professional coder entails: training and development; continuous education; knowledge and application of current rules, regulations, and guidelines; and ethical conduct, even in the face of daily challenges and pressures. Performing the coding function well makes the professional coder a valuable member of the health care team.

Exercise 6-4

Impact of Coding

1. Why is the timing of postdischarge processing important to a coder?
2. What is a coding compliance plan?
3. Explain the difference between optimization and maximization.
4. Compare and contrast two different approaches to coding high-quality audits.

■ WORKS CITED

"Acute Inpatient Prospective Payment System – Outlier Payments." 2005. Center for Medicare and Medicaid Services, 12 July 2006 <http://cms.gov>.

College of American Pathologists. 6 May 2004. News release, 12 July 2006 <http://www.cap.org/apps/docs/media_resources/newsrel_snomednlmannouncement.htm 12>.

"Diagnosis Related Groups Definitions Manual (6th revision)." Number 89-009 Rev.00. New Haven, CN: Health Systems International, 1989.

"Fact Sheet." *UMLS Metathesaurus.* 28 March 2006. National Library of Medicine Fact Sheet, 6 July 2006 <http://www.nlm.nih.gov/pubs/factsheets/umlsmeta.html>.

Federal Register 65(68): 18433-18820.

"HCPCS Level II Codes." *Level II Coding Procedures – 11/30/05.* 2005. Center for Medicare and Medicaid Services, 16 July 2006 <http://www.cms.hhs.gov/MedHCPCSGenInfo/02_HCPCS_LEVEL_II_CODES.asp#TopOfPage>.

National Uniform Billing Committee. "The History of the NUBC." 1999. American Hospital Association, 11 October 2005 <http://www.nubc.org/history.html>.

■ SUGGESTED READING

AHIMA Coding Practice Team. "Internet Resources for Accurate Coding and Reimbursement Practices" (AHIMA Practice Brief). *Journal of AHIMA* 75.7 (2004): 48A-G.

American Hospital Association. *Coding Clinic for ICD-9-CM.* Chicago: American Hospital Association, published quarterly.

Averill, Richard F., Thelma M. Grant, and Barbara A. Steinbeck. "Preparing for the Outpatient Prospective Payment System." *Journal of AHIMA* 71.7 (2000): 35-43.

Bowman, Sue. "Coordination of SNOMED-CT and ICD-10: Getting the Most out of Electronic Health Record Systems." *Perspectives in Health Information Management* 25 May 2005.

Brown, Faye. *ICD-9-CM Coding Handbook, with Answers.* Chicago, American Hospital Association, 2006.

Cade, Toni. "A Comparison of Current Prospective Payment System Methodologies in the United States" Washington, D.C.: 2004 IFHRO Congress & AHIMA Convention Proceedings, October 2004.

CPT Assistant. Chicago: American Medical Association, 2006.

Schraffenberger, Lou Ann and Lynn Keuhn, eds. *Effective Management of Coding Services,* 3rd edition. Chicago: American Health Information Management Association, 2007.

Scichilone, Rita. "Getting Ready for APCs." *Journal of AHIMA* 70.8 (1999): 84-92.

WEB SITES

Alternative Link: http://www.alternativelink.com

Center for Medicare and Medicaid Services: http://www.cms.gov; see Federal Register section at http://www.gpoaccess.gov/fr/;see ICD-10-PCS section at http://www.cms.hhs.gov/providers/pufdownload/icd10.asp

Department of Health and Human Services: http://www.dhhs.gov

JustCoding.com, a service of HP3: http://www.justcoding.com/

National Center for Vital and Health Statistics: http://www.ncvhs.hhs.gov

National Uniform Billing Committee: http://www.nubc.org

SNOMED-CT: http://www.snomed.org

CHAPTER ACTIVITIES

CHAPTER SUMMARY

Coding is an increasingly important function in health care. Guided by a strict code of ethics, coders in a variety of settings use different nomenclature and classification systems to facilitate communication among providers, payers, and other users of health care data. These systems include SNOMED, ICD-O, DSM-IV, ABC, ICD-9-CM, HCPCS/CPT-4, ICD-10-CM, and ICD-10-PCS. As these coded data become more widely used, the role of the coder becomes more important.

One of the key uses for coded data is reimbursement. Medicare prospective payment systems arose out of cost-control measures and are based on code systems originally designed for other purposes. Inpatient hospitals are reimbursed using Diagnosis Related Groups. Medicare outpatient services are reimbursed under Ambulatory Patient Classifications. Additional Prospective Payment Systems include Inpatient Psychiatric Facility Prospective Payment System (IPF PPS), Inpatient Rehabilitation Facility Prospective Payment System (IRF PPS), Long-Term Care Hospital Prospective Payment System, Home Health Prospective Payment System, and Skilled Nursing Facility Prospective Payment System and Resource Utilization Groups.

Billing in a hospital is generally the responsibility of the patient accounts department. Charges are posted to the patient's account on the basis of data maintained in the facility's Chargemaster, or Charge Description Master. Hospital-based services are submitted for payment using a Uniform Bill, currently UB-92. Outpatient services are billed using the CMS-1500 form. Because of the importance of the coded data in correct billing and collections, health information professionals must maintain a strong working relationship with the patient accounts professionals.

Coders are an integral part of maintaining the quality of a facility's coded clinical data, ensuring compliance with regulatory mandates, and facilitating optimal reimbursement.

Review Questions

1. Discuss how SNOMED-CT, a nomenclature system, differs from ICD, a classification system.

2. Why is SNOMED-CT used in the electronic health record?

3. Discuss the impact of the prospective payment system on the coding function.

4. Discuss the significance of a hospital's case mix index and reasons that it should be monitored.

5. What are the major differences between DRGs and ambulatory patient classifications?

6. Provide an example of how incorrect inpatient coding would financially affect a hospital.

7. Distinguish between the UB-92 and the CMS-1500.

8. List three prospective payment systems, and describe how reimbursement is obtained in each.

9. Describe and discuss an example of an unethical coding practice.

10. Name two types of coding audits. When would you use each?

11. Discuss the relationship between the HIM department and the patient accounts department with regard to unbilled accounts in an acute care hospital.

12. Describe how charges are captured in an inpatient setting, and compare this to charge capture in an ambulatory setting.

13. What is the difference between optimization and maximization?

DRG Audit Specialist

My name is Robin, and I am a DRG audit specialist for a small consulting firm. My firm performs a number of services for hospitals, physicians' offices, and physician group practices. We code records, abstract and enter data, and perform coding quality and compliance audits. My specialty is auditing records to ensure that the optimal DRG was obtained by the coding.

To audit records, I needed to have excellent coding skills. I developed these skills as a coder for an acute care facility, where I coded both outpatient and inpatient records. I later went to work for this consulting firm as a coder, and now I spend most of my time auditing. In addition to my work experience, I am also a Registered Health Information Technician (RHIT) and a Certified Coding Specialist (CCS).

I can perform several types of audits, depending on what the client needs. Sometimes, I take a random sample of records and review them just to see whether there are any coding problems. I think all facilities should do this on a regular basis because sometimes coders make mistakes. If you catch the errors quickly, the facility can re-bill with the new codes. Also, the coders need to know if they are doing something wrong. My firm performs these audits periodically, not just on client coders' records but also on our own employees' work.

My favorite audits are DRG audits. To do a DRG audit, I review a computer report of all of the records that have been coded in a given time period. I pay particular attention to records that are grouped to an uncomplicated DRG and those that are grouped to a problem DRG. Then, I review some of the records to determine whether I can recommend any coding changes. I discuss my recommendations with the coding supervisor, and she meets with the coders separately to help them keep from making these errors in the future. The facility sometimes asks me to give training to the coders on particularly difficult issues.

Auditing of cases that are reimbursed on the basis of DRGs are especially important because changes in coding may affect reimbursement. Facilities that routinely code incorrectly— and therefore routinely bill the wrong amount for the stay—are subject to penalties from the government or the private insurer. By performing these audits, I really feel as though I'm helping the facility maintain high-quality coding and billing standards. That's a good feeling.

APPLICATION

Implementing ICD-10

Since 1979, ICD-9-CM has been the classification system used by U. S. health care providers to collect diagnosis and some procedure data for reporting and, more recently, reimbursement purposes. If and when the Centers for Medicare and Medicaid Services adopt ICD-10, the industry will follow. Implementation of ICD-10 will involve a massive effort on the part of health industry professionals throughout the country. Based on your knowledge of health care data, coding, and reimbursement, what do you think the impact of ICD-10 will be? Imagine that ICD-10 will be implemented in 2 years. If you were the director of HIM at an acute care facility, what steps would you take to ensure a smooth transition?

Timely Billing and Quality Coding

HIM departments are frequently under intense pressure to code medical records as soon as possible after patient discharge so that the hospital may be reimbursed. Pressure may come from patient accounts department staff members, who may not completely understand the myriad reasons that all medical records cannot be accurately coded or even coded at all immediately after discharge. If you were the coding supervisor at a hospital, how would you describe the reasons for delays in coding with patient accounts department staff members? How would you discuss the DNFB (discharged , no final bill) and coding requirements under HIPAA with patient accounts staff members in a collaborative, rather than adversarial, way? Can you identify ways in which patient accounts staff members might assist HIM employees in decreasing delays?

Chapter 7

HEALTH INFORMATION MANAGEMENT ISSUES IN ALTERNATIVE SETTINGS

CHAPTER OUTLINE

CHAPTER OBJECTIVES

By the end of this chapter, the student should be able to

- List and describe non-acute care facilities.

- List and describe the services provided by non-acute care facilities.

- Compare and contrast the data collected in acute care facilities with data collected in non-acute care facilities.

- List and describe the data sets unique to non-acute care facilities.

VOCABULARY

Accreditation Association for Ambulatory Health Care (AAAHC)

ambulatory surgery

baseline

clinic

Commission on Accreditation of Rehabilitation Facilities (CARF)

Community Health Accreditation Program (CHAP)

Data Elements for Emergency Department Systems (DEEDS)

dialysis

dialysis centers

encounter

group practice

home health care

hospice

laboratory

National Center for Injury Prevention and Control (NCIPC)

Outcome and Assessment Information Set (OASIS)

palliative care

physiatrist

physician's office

primary care physician

primary caregiver

radiology

respite care

triage

Uniform Ambulatory Care Data Set (UACDS)

visit

t this point, you should have a clear idea of what occurs in an acute care facility, including how data are collected and by whom. We have touched briefly on the special data requirements of certain diagnoses and other health care facilities. The most important thing to remember is that the skills and the knowledge that you have acquired so far in this text are applicable to any health care delivery setting. Demographic, financial, socioeconomic, and clinical data are collected in all settings. The volume and types of physician data, nursing data, and data from therapy, social services, and psychology vary significantly depending on the diagnosis and the setting. In addition to discipline-specific data requirements, health care facilities must also comply with the licensure regulations of the state in which they operate. The regulations may include very specific documentation requirements. Further, all facilities seeking Medicare reimbursement must comply with the Medicare Conditions of Participation. The Center for Medicare and Medicaid Services (CMS) Web site should be consulted for detailed information about those requirements. Health information management (HIM) professionals who are employed in special health care settings should become familiar with the unique data requirements of those settings. The Joint Commission on Accreditation of Healthcare Organizations (JCAHO) offers accreditation of all providers discussed in this chapter, either independently or in conjunction with the host facility.

AMBULATORY CARE

Ambulatory, or outpatient, care is that which is provided in a brief period, typically in one day or in less than 24 hours. This distinguishes it from inpatient care, in which the patient is expected to stay overnight. As discussed in Chapter 1, a physician's office is only one type of ambulatory care setting. Although other ambulatory care settings provide different services than does a physician's office, the basic clinical flow of events is similar.

MEASURING QUANTITY OF SERVICES

The term *ambulatory care* refers to a wide range of services provided at a variety of facilities. Patients receive those services in a relatively short amount of time. Facilities render services on the same day that the patient arrives for treatment or, in some cases, within 24 hours. Therefore the terms *admission* and *discharge* have little or no relevance in ambulatory care. In the ambulatory care environment, the interaction between patient and provider is referred to as an **encounter** or a **visit**.

To determine the quantity of services rendered, we count the number of visits or encounters. *Visits* and *encounters* may mean the same thing. For example, think of a patient who goes to a physician's office to see the doctor and has a chest x-ray done at the same time in the same facility. The patient interacted with the facility in two ways: an examination by the doctor and a chest x-ray. Think of it another way: The patient *visited* the facility and *encountered* the doctor and the radiology technician. Thus the visit represents the number of times that the patient interacted with the facility as a whole. The encounter represents the number of different areas of the facility

---

Hit-Bit

Ambulatory Care

Ambulatory literally means the "process of walking." Therefore an ambulatory care patient is theoretically walking in and out. However, the name is a little misleading. Ambulatory care patients are not always ambulatory. *Ambulatory* also refers to a patient who is *able* to walk. However, patients in wheelchairs can visit physicians at the office. Some patients are driven to the physician's office in special vans that resemble ambulances. Clearly, in neither case do the patients actually walk into the office, but they are nonetheless ambulatory care patients.

that were used. As you explore different ambulatory care settings, think about how you would count the quantity of services rendered.

Beyond the time frame stated above, the services rendered in ambulatory care facilities vary widely. Each type of facility has its own specific data collection, retention, and analysis needs. However, the general flow of patient care is similar. The patient initiates the interaction, gives demographic and financial data to the facility, meets with the provider, and takes any needed follow-up action.

AMBULATORY CARE SETTINGS

Physician's Office

A **physician's office** is one type of ambulatory care facility. Most of us have been to a physician's office, so this is a good place to start our discussion. Most physicians maintain an office where patients can visit. There are many different types of physicians, as you learned in Chapter 1. Some physicians have offices attached to their homes; others have space in office buildings. Still others are associated with different types of facilities and, as employees, maintain offices in those facilities. Some physicians do not see patients at all. For example, a pathologist examines tissue samples in a laboratory. Some radiologists examine only x-rays and other types of tests. In general, these physicians give the results of those examinations to another physician to discuss with the patient. For the purposes of this section, only physicians who see patients in their offices are discussed.

Group Practice

Sometimes, physicians share office space and personnel with other physicians to reduce the cost of maintaining an office. For example, several physicians working together may need only one receptionist. Sharing office space and personnel also provides increased opportunities for professional collaboration among physicians. This sharing by physicians is called a **group practice.**

Group practices may have only one type of physician, such as a group of family practitioners. Frequently, these physicians not only share office space and personnel but also see one another's patients. To help one another with their patient loads, the physicians must also collaborate in developing and maintaining relationships with pertinent insurance companies.

Another combination of physicians may consist of several different specialties; this arrangement is called a *multispecialty group.* A family practice physician may be in a group with a pediatrician and a gynecologist, for example. One of the advantages of a multispecialty group practice is the convenience of centralized care that it provides for the patient.

Another administrative advantage of a group practice is the ability to centralize record-keeping. Whether the patient records are maintained in paper or electronic form, centralization offers substantial cost savings and efficiency.

Clinic

A **clinic** is a facility-based ambulatory care department that provides general or specialized services such as those provided in a physician's office. Clinics may be funded or established by charitable organizations, the government, or different types of health care facilities. For example, a

---

Hit-Bit

Open Access Physician Offices

Some physicians rely solely on appointments for scheduling office time. Other physicians employ open-access techniques. In open access, some appointments are made, but time is allowed for patients who call for a same-day appointment. Scheduling appointments requires knowledge of time budgeting, and implementation of open-access methods requires a firm understanding of the demand for time in relation to the number of patients per doctor.

community health center is a type of clinic that provides primary care in a specific geographical area. Many of these centers are located in areas accessible to economically depressed populations. Many acute care facilities have developed clinics that resemble physicians' office services. A hospital may have clinics that serve particular patient populations, such as an infectious disease clinic or an orthopedic clinic. Clinics may also closely resemble multispecialty group practices. Large teaching facilities may be affiliated with many clinics. The clinic may be part of the physicians' general practice, the physicians may be employees of the parent facility, or they may donate their time.

Emergency Department

Emergency departments are unique to hospitals, usually acute care facilities. They are designed to handle patients in crisis and are considered ambulatory care. Acutely ill patients who are admitted to the hospital are reclassified as inpatients. This reclassification also occurs for Medicare patients who are admitted to the hospital within 72 hours of being treated for the same condition. For example, consider a patient who is treated for congestive heart failure in the emergency department who is admitted to that hospital 2 days later—also for congestive heart failure. Because it is within 72 hours, Medicare will not pay separately for the emergency department visit (CMS 72-Hour Rule, 1998).

Emergency department services vary dramatically. Broken legs and heart attacks are typical cases. Trauma patients often are treated first in the emergency department and are stabilized there before being admitted. Because the services vary so much, the facility must determine the order in which to treat the patients. The policy of "first come, first served" does not make much sense when the first patient strained a ligament and the second patient is experiencing a myocardial infarction. Therefore patients are screened as part of the registration process to determine the priority with which they will be treated. This prioritization process is called **triage** and is generally performed by a registered or advanced practice nurse. In some emergency departments, a separate section of the department is set aside for noncritical services. Noncritical services in this scenario may include minor wound repair, for example.

Because the pace in the emergency department is fast, data collection must be equally fast. In a paper-based environment, menu-based forms have long been the standard for data collection (Figure 7-1). This menu-driven data collection has facilitated the implementation of computer-based data collection in the emergency department environment. Data collection unique to the emergency department includes the method and time of arrival.

An emergency department is licensed and accredited under the umbrella of its host facility.

Other Settings

The settings mentioned above are exclusively ambulatory care. However, many specialty services are offered on both an inpatient and an outpatient basis. These are included below in their specialty categories.

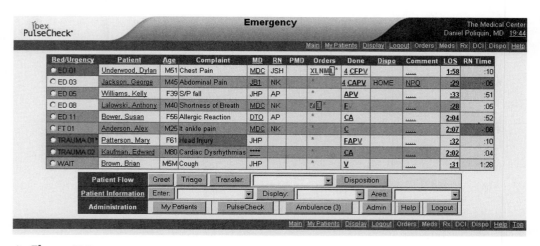

◆ **Figure 7-1**

Example of an emergency department form.

SERVICES

The following sections illustrate a hypothetical visit to a physician's office to trace the clinical flow of a patient's data through the office and list the data that are collected. Figure 7-2 shows the flow of activities in a typical physician's office. Obviously, different combinations of personnel and procedures are seen. Our visit is a general guide to the events so that you can understand the flow of information.

Patients can generally choose the physician whom they will visit as long as the physician they choose is accepting new patients. However, patients with certain types of health insurance will not always be reimbursed for the cost of that visit. If payment is an issue, the first step in selecting a physician is to determine whether that physician participates in the patient's insurance plan.

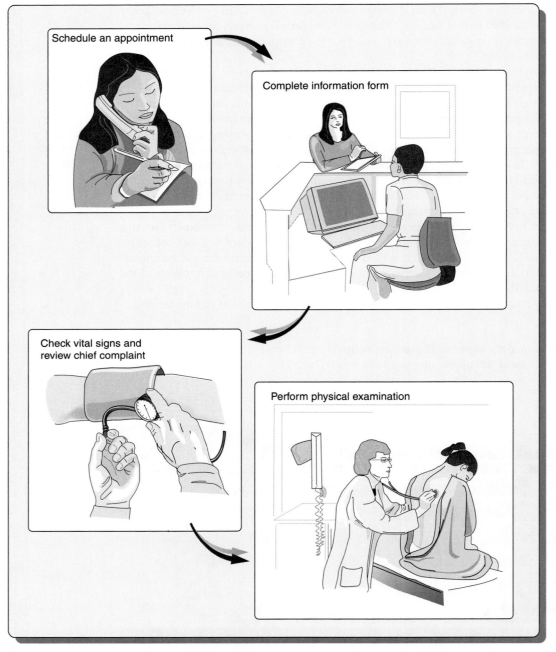

◆ **Figure 7-2**
Flow of activities in a physician's office.

Patients may also ask friends and family members for recommendations. If the patient needs to see a specialist, such as a cardiologist, the **primary care physician** may refer the patient to a specific physician. Some specialists, such as thoracic surgeons, see only those patients who have been referred by other physicians. Thus the visit is initiated either by the patient or by referral and may be influenced by the patient's insurance plan.

CARE PROVIDERS

After choosing a physician, the patient calls the office for an appointment. Very likely, the patient will speak to someone who works with the physician. The individual who answers the telephone and handles the appointments may be any one of a number of different allied health workers, such as a receptionist, a medical secretary, or a medical assistant. A *receptionist* usually handles the telephones, does some filing, and schedules appointments. A *medical secretary* has a more detailed knowledge of office procedures, scheduling, filing, and billing. A *medical assistant* has all of that knowledge and some basic clinical knowledge, such as taking blood pressure and temperature. Medical secretaries and medical assistants have generally received formal training, particularly if they are certified in their fields.

Other personnel who support the physician include physician's assistants, nurses, and nurse practitioners. A physician's assistant (PA) is a highly trained clinical professional who can take the medical history and assist the physician in diagnosing and treating patients. PAs undergo at least 2 years of training, including rotations through multiple specialties ("Information about PA's" 2006). A PA nurse is a highly trained clinician who can collect a variety of information and assist in treating patients. A nurse practitioner is an advanced practice nurse with extensive additional training. Nurse practitioners often work in areas where there are not enough physicians. Figure 7-3 shows some employees common in a physician's office.

DATA COLLECTION ISSUES

Suppose that a physician's office has a number of different staff members and employs a receptionist to handle telephone calls and appointments. When the patient calls for an appointment, the receptionist asks for the patient's name and telephone number and inquires whether he or she is a current patient. It is very important to know whether the patient is a current patient because a new patient requires more data collection, which takes more of the staff's time. The receptionist

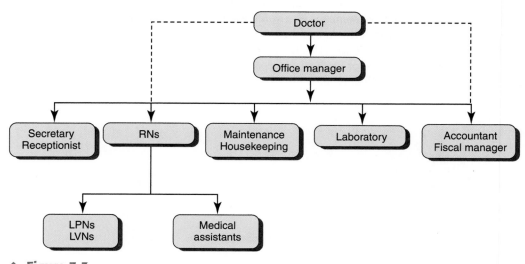

◆ **Figure 7-3**
Sample of employees in a physician's office. (From Louise Simmers. *Diversified Health Occupations*. 4th ed. Albany, NY: Delmar Publishers, Inc., 1998.)

also asks why the patient wants to see the physician, which also aids in scheduling. A regular patient coming in for a flu shot takes far less of the physician's time than does a new patient who complains of stomach pains. Identification of a new versus an established patient is also important for billing physician services.

When the patient gets to the office, the receptionist asks the patient to fill out some forms. On these forms, the patient provides personal information: name and address, past medical history, and who is responsible for paying the bill. The receptionist or a medical secretary may then enter some or all of this information into the computer. A folder is created for new patients, labeled by name, and used to hold the personal information form as well as any other papers containing necessary data. For a current patient, an existing folder would be retrieved. This folder of information is also called the patient's *record*. Historically, the folder has been the only record; however, keeping the data in the computer instead of on paper is becoming increasingly common. Patients also sign forms that authorize the physician to treat them, to release information to their insurance company, and to acknowledge their receipt of the physician's statement of privacy policies. Chapter 11 discusses this authorization and other types of consents and releases.

Once the administrative record-keeping processes are completed, a medical assistant or nurse takes the patient's temperature, blood pressure, height, and weight—all data that develop a profile of information about the patient and the visit. If this is the patient's first visit, this profile is called the **baseline.** It is the information against which all future visits will be compared.

Eventually, the physician sees the patient and performs and documents the appropriate level of history and physical. Perhaps the physician recommends tests to determine the extent of disease or to help determine the diagnosis. If the diagnosis is clear, the physician prescribes treatment at this visit. Before the patient leaves the physician's office, he or she either remits payment for the visit or signs a release for the insurance company. For managed care patients, a co-pay may be required (see Chapter 2).

LICENSURE AND ACCREDITATION

Practitioners are licensed in the state in which they operate. Ambulatory care accreditation is offered by the JCAHO and the **Accreditation Association for Ambulatory Health Care (AAAHC).**

DATA SETS

In ambulatory care, the minimum data set is called the **Uniform Ambulatory Care Data Set (UACDS).** The UACDS was developed in 1989 by committees working under the auspices of the Department of Health and Human Services.

Minimum data sets are easy to understand if you think about the key data elements you want to know about a patient and then think about what someone else would want to know about the health care given to the patient. Figure 7-4 lists the elements of the UACDS.

The National Center for Injury Prevention and Control (NCIPC) is developing a uniform data set for emergency departments. The Data Elements for Emergency Department Systems (DEEDS) apply to hospital-based emergency departments (Figure 7-5).

Exercise 7-1

Ambulatory Care Facilities

1. Describe the experiences of a patient in a physician's office.
2. What professionals is the patient likely to encounter in a physician's office?
3. What role do those professionals play in caring for the patient?
4. List and describe the elements of the UACDS.

UNIFORM AMBULATORY CARE DATA SET

Section I: Patient Data Items

1. Personal identification (including name and facility reference number)
2. Residence
3. Date of birth
4. Sex
5. Race and ethnicity
6. Living arrangements and marital status (optional)

Section II: Provider Data Items

1. Provider identification
2. Location or address
3. Profession

Section III: Encounter Data Items

1. Date, place or site, and address of encounter
2. Patient's reason for encounter (optional — problem, diagnosis, or assessment)
3. Services
4. Disposition
5. Patient's expected sources of payment
6. Total charges

◆ **Figure 7-4**

Sections I, II, and III from the Uniform Ambulatory Care Data Set. (Modified from Mervat Abdelhak, Sara Grostick, Mary Alice Hanken, and Ellen Jacobs. *Health Information: Management of a Strategic Resource.* 2nd ed. Philadelphia: Saunders, 2001, pp 108–110.)

AMBULATORY CARE: RADIOLOGY AND LABORATORY

Radiology and **laboratory** facilities serve both the inpatient and outpatient settings with a variety of services. Virtually all of those services are performed on an ambulatory basis, regardless of the patient's actual status. Diagnostic radiology and laboratory services are almost always offered on an ambulatory basis. Patients are not admitted; they are tested and sent back to their rooms or their residences. Therapeutic radiology may be a reason for admission in and of itself, and the length of stay depends on the procedure being performed.

SETTINGS

Radiology and laboratory services are maintained in acute care facilities and many inpatient rehabilitation facilities. These services are often available to the general public and can be obtained through a physician's order. Some of these hospitals do not maintain the services on an employee basis but rather lease the space to organizations that agree to provide the services to the facility. Radiology and laboratory services may also be offered in freestanding facilities.

SERVICES

Diagnostic radiology services include x-rays, computerized tomography (CT) scans, magnetic resonance imaging (MRIs), and positron emission tomography (PET) scans. Three-dimensional

Section 1:
Patient Identification

Internal ID
Name
Alias
Date of Birth
Sex
Race
Ethnicity
Address
Telephone Number
Account Number
Social Security Number
Occupation
Industry
Emergency Contact Name
Emergency Contact Address
Emergency Contact
   Telephone Number
Emergency Contact
   Relationship

Section 2: Facility and
Practitioner Identification

ED Facility ID
Primary Practitioner Name
Primary Practitioner ID
Primary Practitioner Type
Primary Practitioner Address
Primary Practitioner
   Telephone Number
Primary Practitioner
   Organization
ED Practitioner ID
ED Practitioner Type
ED Practitioner Current Role
ED Consultant Practitioner ID
ED Consultant Practitioner
   Type
Date/Time ED Consult
   Request Initiated
Date/Time ED Consult Starts

Section 3: ED Payment

Insurance Coverage or Other
   Expected Source of
   Payment
Insurance Company
Insurance Company Address
Insurance Plan Type
Insurance Policy ID
ED Payment Authorization
   Requirement
Status of ED Payment
   Authorization Attempt
Date/Time of ED Payment
   Authorization Attempt
ED Payment Authorization
   Decision
Entity Contacted to Authorize
   ED Payment
ED Payment Authorization
   Code
Person Contacted to
   Authorize ED Payment
Telephone Number of Entity of
   Person Contacted to
   Authorize ED Payment
Total ED Facility Charges
Total ED Professional Fees

Section 4: ED Arrival and
First Assessment

Date/Time First Documented
   in ED
Mode of Transport to ED
EMS Unit that Transported
   ED Patient
EMS Agency that
   Transported ED Patient
Source of Referral to ED
Chief Complaint
Initial Encounter for Current
   Instance of Chief Complaint
First ED Acuity Assessment
Date/Time of First ED Acuity
   Assessment
First ED Acuity Assessment
   Practitioner ID
First ED Acuity Assessment
   Practitioner type
First ED Responsiveness
   Assessment
First ED Glasgow Eye Open-
   ing Component Assessment
First ED Glasgow Verbal
   Component Assessment
First ED Glasgow Motor
   Component Assessment
Date/Time of First ED
   Glasgow Coma Scale
   Assessment
First ED Systolic Blood
   Pressure
Date/Time of First ED
   Systolic Blood Pressure
First ED Diastolic Blood
   Pressure
First ED Heart Rate
First ED Heart Rate Method
Date/Time of First ED Heart
   Rate
First ED Respiratory Rate
Date/Time of First ED
   Respiratory Rate
First ED Temperature
   Reading
First ED Temperature
   Reading Route
Date/Time of First ED
   Temperature Reading
Measured Weight in ED
Pregnancy Status Reported
   in ED
Date of Last Tetanus
   Immunization
Medication Allergy Reported
   in ED

◆ **Figure 7-5**
Data elements for emergency department systems. (DEEDs). From *Data Elements for Emergency Department Systems, Release 1.0 (DEEDS)*. 1997. (From Centers for Disease Control and Prevention: http://www.cdc.gov/ncipc/pub-res/pdf/deeds.pdf)

Section 5: H&P Exam Data

Date/Time of First Ed
   Practitioner Evaluation
Date/Time of Illness or Injury
   Onset
Injury Incident Description
Coded Cause of Injury
Injury Incident Location type
Injury Activity
Injury Intent
Safety Equipment Use
Current Therapeutic
   Medication
Current Therapeutic
   Medication Dose
Current Therapeutic
   Medication Dose Units
Current Therapeutic
   Medication Schedule
Current Therapeutic
   Medication Route
ED Clinical Finding Type
ED Clinical Finding
Date/Time ED Clinical
   Finding Obtained
ED Clinical Finding Practitio-
   ner ID
ED Clinical Finding Practitio-
   ner Type
ED Clinical Finding Data
   Source

**Section 6: ED Procedure
and Result Data**

ED Procedure Indication
ED Procedure
Date/Time ED Procedure
   Ordered
Date/Time ED Procedure
   Starts
Date/Time ED Procedure
   Ends
ED Procedure Practitioner ID
ED Procedure Practitioner
   Type
Date/Time ED Diagnostic
   Procedure Result Reported
ED Diagnostic Procedure
   Result Type
ED Diagnostic Procedure
   Result

**Section 7: ED Medication
Data**

Date/Time ED Medication
   Ordered
ED Medication Ordering
   Practitioner ID
ED Medication Ordering
   Practitioner Type
ED Medication
ED Medication Dose
ED Medication Dose Units
ED Medication Schedule
ED Medication Route
Date/Time ED Medication
   Starts
Date/Time ED Medication
   Stops
ED Medication Administering
   Practitioner ID
ED Medication Administering
   Practitioner Type

**Section 8: Disposition and
Diagnosis Data**

Date/Time of Recorded ED
   Disposition
ED Disposition
Inpatient Practitioner ID
Inpatient Practitioner Type
Facility Receiving ED Patient
Date/Time Patient Departs ED
ED Follow-Up Care
   Assistance
Referral at ED Disposition
ED Referral Practitioner
   Name
ED Referral Practitioner ID
ED Referral Practitioner Type
ED Referral Organization
ED Discharge Medication
   Order Type
ED Discharge Medication
   Ordering Practitioner ID
ED Discharge Medication
   Ordering Practitioner Type
ED Discharge Medication
ED Discharge Medication
   Dose
ED Discharge Medication
   Dose Units
ED Discharge Medication
   Schedule
Ed Discharge Medication
   Route
Amount of ED Discharge
   Medication to be Dispensed
Number of ED Discharge
   Medication Refills
ED Disposition Diagnosis
   Description
ED Disposition Diagnosis
   Code
ED Disposition Diagnosis
   Practitioner ID
ED Disposition Diagnosis
   Practitioner Type
ED Service Level
ED Service Level Practitioner
   ID
ED Service Level Practitioner
   Type
Patient Problem Assessed in
   ED outcome Observation
ED Outcome Observation
Date/Time of ED Outcome
   Observation
ED Outcome Observation
   Practitioner ID
ED Outcome Observation
   Practitioner Type
ED Patient Satisfaction
   Report Type
ED Patient Satisfaction
   Report

◆ **Figure 7-5** (*cont'd*)

ultrasounds may be used to visualize a fetus in utero. Increasingly, radiological images are captured in digital format. These digital images can be given to patients and their physicians on computer disk, along with the software to read them. Therapeutic radiology (also known as *radiation*) is most closely association with the treatment of certain types of cancers.

Services are provided on the order of a physician. An interesting recent phenomenon, though, is the increasing marketing of radiology services to the general public as a prophylactic diagnostic measure. For example, a PET scan may be advertised to provide the patient with peace of mind.

Laboratory services include examinations of blood, urine, and other bodily fluids.

CARE PROVIDERS

Radiology technicians capture the images. Technicians are typically trained in trade schools or hospital-based training programs to operate the equipment and obtain the clearest images. Associate degree programs are also available for radiology technicians. Physicians called *radiologists* interpret the images and write or dictate the reports associated with the interpretation.

Laboratories are staffed with a variety of personnel, including medical technicians.

DATA COLLECTION ISSUES

Radiology and laboratory services generate different but parallel documentations. The original material (x-ray film, computer image, or fluid sample) is retained in the testing department or facility. The report of the analysis of the material is maintained in the testing department. A copy is sent to the requesting physician and to the facility that ordered the test. The report will become a part of the health record in the facility that ordered the test.

Radiology services typically handle their own release of information because copies of films are often required. As digital imagery becomes more common, the stored images can be easily linked to the patient's electronic health record. Some facilities download the image to disk along with the program to view the image. This facilitates communication with the physician and provides the patient with a valuable tool for developing and maintaining a personal health record.

LICENSURE AND ACCREDITATION

Facilities are licensed by the states in which they operate. Accreditation is available through the JCAHO and the AAAHC. Services maintained in other facilities come under the accreditation umbrella of their parent organization.

Clinical laboratories are regulated by the CMS under the Clinical Laboratories Improvement Amendments (CLIA). For current information about this program, refer to the CMS Web site: http://www.cms.hhs.gov/clia.

Exercise 7-2

Ambulatory Care: Radiology and Laboratory

1. What services are provided by radiology and laboratory facilities?
2. Describe the unique data collection issues in radiology and laboratory facilities.

AMBULATORY CARE: AMBULATORY SURGERY

As health care costs rise, providers are under increasing pressure to offer services on an ambulatory basis. Also contributing to the rise in ambulatory services is improved technology that allows for less postsurgical recovery time.

LENGTH OF STAY

Ambulatory surgery patients technically have a length of stay of 1 day. In other words, they are admitted and discharged on the same day. Patients being treated in an acute care facility whose stay exceeds 24 hours are generally reclassified as inpatients.

SETTINGS

Ambulatory surgery may take place in an acute care facility or a freestanding ambulatory surgery center. Certain minimally invasive procedures, generally those requiring local anesthetic (such as some minor skin procedures), may be performed in the physician's office.

SERVICES

Ambulatory surgery is just that: surgery. The type of procedures performed in this environment is limited only by the postsurgical care required. Cataract removal, endoscopies, removal of skin lesions, and carpal tunnel release are examples of procedures that are typically performed on an ambulatory basis.

CARE PROVIDERS

Care providers in this setting are generally limited to physicians, nurses, and general medical office personnel. Surgical technicians may also be employed in this area.

DATA COLLECTION ISSUES

The volume of data collected for an ambulatory surgery case is relatively low compared with that of other surgeries. Preadmission testing may include lab work and radiological services as well as an anesthesia consultation. The history and physical must be completed. The surgical report may be brief and contain substantial menu-based data.

LICENSURE AND ACCREDITATION

Ambulatory surgery centers are licensed by the state in which they operate. Accreditation is offered by the JCAHO, the American Osteopathic Association (AOA), and the AAAHC.

DATA SETS

In ambulatory surgery, the UACDS applies (see Figure 7-4).

Exercise 7-3

Ambulatory Care: Ambulatory Surgery
1. Define and give examples of ambulatory surgery.
2. Describe the unique data collection issues in ambulatory surgery.
3. Who accredits ambulatory surgery facilities?

■ LONG-TERM CARE

In addition to length of stay, there are other fundamental differences between long-term care facilities and acute care facilities. Although both care for inpatients, their focus and delivery are significantly different. Long-term care patients are considered residents of the facility: In other words, they are not only being treated there—they actually live there. Thus there is a greater emphasis on comfort, activities of daily living (ADL), and recreational activities such as games and crafts. Group activities are common ways to facilitate residents' interaction and socialization.

LENGTH OF STAY

Many state licensure documents define a long-term care facility as one in which the average length of stay exceeds 30 days.

SETTINGS

A wide variety of facilities are considered long-term care. Some of these facilities, such as assisted living facilities, are not as strictly regulated as others. Table 7-1 contains a brief description of long-term care facilities.

TABLE 7-1	Examples of Long-Term Care Facilities
TYPE OF CARE	**DESCRIPTION**
Independent living	Residents are housed in apartment setting. Health care is provided on-site; however, residents are independent in their activities of daily living and do not require medical supervision on a 24-hour basis. Some meals may be provided in a cafeteria or restaurant atmosphere.
Assisted living facility	Residents are housed in apartment-like setting, often with limited food preparation equipment, or in dormitory rooms—usually with private bath. Health care is provided on-site. Residents have varying degrees of independence in their activities of daily living and need for medical supervision. Some or all meals may be provided in a communal or restaurant atmosphere. Ancillary services may include computer labs, chapel, spa services, entertainment and activity rooms, and laundry facilities.
Subacute care	This is usually a transitional level of care between acute care and either home care or other long-term care. Subacute care may be offered in acute care facilities or in long-term care facilities. Patients require substantial treatment but no longer need the 24-hour supervision of an acute care facility.
Transitional	Generally offered in an acute care facility, patients require up to 8 hours of nursing care per day. Average length of stay is within acute care definition.
General	Patients require up to 5 hours of care per day and typically stay from 10 to 40 days in a long-term care facility.
Chronic	Patients require up to 5 hours of care per day and typically stay from 60 to 90 days in a long-term care facility.
Long-term transitional	Patients require up to 9 hours of care per day and typically stay more than 25 days in an acute care facility.
Intermediate care	Patients do not require 24-hour supervision. Cognitive or motor impairment contraindicates independent living.
Skilled nursing	Residents require substantial assistance with activities of daily living. Frequent therapies from a variety of professionals are needed to maintain status.
Long-term acute care	Patients require an acute level of care over an extended period. The average length of stay is more than 25 days. Services may be provided in an acute care, long-term care, or rehabilitation hospital. Medicare considers this long-term care.

These are general categories of care provided to help the reader understand the environment of long-term care. Facility, licensure, and regional differences in terminology exist. Many facilities offer multiple levels of care and are not distinguishable as a specific type of facility. For example, some organizations offer lifetime care that transitions from independent to assisted to intermediate to skilled care as the patient deteriorates.

SERVICES

Long-term care facilities typically offer rehabilitation services, such as occupational therapy and physical therapy, in addition to nursing care.

CARE PROVIDERS

Patients entering a long-term care facility are evaluated by a physician to ensure that the facility is appropriate for the patient's optimal care. Once admitted, the physician plays a small role in the patient's daily life. Unless there is a change in the patient's medical condition, the physician routinely sees the patient only once every month.

The level of nursing care required by the patient is the key to determining what type of facility the patient needs. In a skilled nursing facility, the patient typically needs 24-hour supervision. In an assisted living facility, a patient may need only a nurse on call.

DATA COLLECTION ISSUES

Long-term care facilities generate voluminous data on their patients. Much of the data consists of nursing notes and medication sheets. Therapies also add to the volume. In a paper-based environment, the records must be periodically thinned. Older documentation is transferred to storage, leaving relevant and current documentation at the nursing unit.

LICENSURE AND ACCREDITATION

Long-term care facilities are licensed in the states in which they operate.

DATA SETS

Long-term care facilities seeking reimbursement from Medicare must complete the Minimum Data Set (MDS) for long-term care patients. This lengthy data set is initiated upon admission and contains detailed clinical data about the patient. It must be submitted within 14 days of admission and resubmitted at least annually. Appendix C contains the most recent version of the MDS, as of the preparation of this text. The MDS is one component of a series of data collections required for long-term care called the *Resident Assessment Instrument (RAI)*. The MDS is of interest because it illustrates the volume and type of data that are collected in long-term care, which is mirrored in other non-acute care settings as well.

Exercise 7-4

Long-Term Care Facilities

1. When does a patient require long-term care?
2. What services are provided by long-term care workers?
3. Describe the unique data collection issues in a long-term care environment.
4. What minimum data set is associated with long-term care?
5. Who accredits long-term care facilities?

BEHAVIORAL HEALTH FACILITIES

Behavioral health facilities and behavioral health services housed in other types of facilities focus on the diagnosis and treatment of psychological disorders.

Hit-Bit

Outpatient

When ambulatory services are offered by an otherwise inpatient facility, those patients are also called *outpatients*.

LENGTH OF STAY

The length of stay for behavioral health services offered on an inpatient basis depends on the diagnosis and the patient's response to treatment. It is also sometimes partly dependent on reimbursement. Behavioral health services are also offered on an outpatient basis.

SETTINGS

Behavioral health services are offered in virtually all health care settings. In acute care, services may be by consultation; there are also likely to be psychiatrists on staff. In rehabilitation, behavioral health services are vital for cognitive remediation (discussed in more detail later in this chapter). Behavioral health services are also offered in psychiatric hospitals, freestanding outpatient clinics, and physician office settings.

BEHAVIORAL HEALTH SERVICES

Behavioral health services address a wide range of issues and disorders. Services include counseling, psychological testing, therapy, and pharmaceutical interventions.

DRUG AND ALCOHOL REHABILITATION

Although treatment is referred to as *rehabilitation,* drug and alcohol abuse or dependence is considered a psychological condition. There are two phases of treatment: detoxification and rehabilitation. *Detoxification* refers to the treatment of a patient who is going through withdrawal of substances from his or her body. This withdrawal may take 3 or 4 days. Rehabilitation is the treatment of the patient by psychiatrists, psychologists, drug and alcohol counselors, and social workers that teaches the patient ways to resist drugs and alcohol in the future. Although treatment varies, initial rehabilitation may take weeks or months, with continuing treatment throughout the patient's life. Drug and alcohol rehabilitation facilities may be freestanding or connected with another facility, such as a psychiatric hospital or an acute care facility.

CARE PROVIDERS

Although some patients in behavioral health facilities may have additional medical conditions that require treatment, the primary thrust of care is delivered by psychiatrists (physicians), psychologists (nonphysician specialists), and social services personnel. Particularly in an inpatient facility, there may also be on staff a physician known as an *internist.* The internist is responsible for treating any medical conditions that patients may have.

DATA COLLECTION ISSUES

Much of the data collection in behavioral health is free text. Psychology notes tend to be voluminous and detailed and do not lend themselves to menu-driven data collection. Of particular concern are psychology notes and documentation of restraints.

Psychology notes may include testing instruments and extensive interview notes. Many of these notes are retained in the psychology department and do not become part of the patient's legal health record. The facility must have a policy specifically dealing with the storage, retention, and access to these notes.

The use of restraints requires a physician order. Restraints include not only physical restraints but also confinement in protective enclosures. Documentation of the order, the application of restraints, the monitoring of a restrained patient, and the timely release from restraints are all required.

Release of information is strictly protected by law and requires special authorization (see Chapter 11).

LICENSURE AND ACCREDITATION

Behavioral health facilities are licensed by the states in which they operate. In addition to JCAHO, accreditation is available from the **Commission on Accreditation of Rehabilitation Facilities (CARF)** and the National Committee for Quality Assurance (NCQA).

DATA SETS

There is no specific data set unique to behavioral health, so the data collected reflects the setting in which the services are provided. However, the new CMS inpatient psychiatric facility prospective payment system (PPS) does propose a Case Mix Assessment Tool (CMAT). The CMAT includes detailed information about the patient (Medicare Program, 2004).

Exercise 7-5

Behavioral Health Facilities
1. Describe conditions that would require behavioral health treatment.
2. What services are provided by behavioral health workers?
3. Describe the unique data collection issues in a behavioral health environment.
4. What minimum data set is associated with behavioral health?
5. Who accredits behavioral health facilities?

REHABILITATION FACILITIES

Rehabilitation facilities offer care to patients who need specific therapies as a result of illness or injury. Patients recovering from cerebrovascular accident, joint replacement surgery, traumatic head injury, or spinal cord injury are examples of typical rehabilitation patients. Therapies include physical therapy, occupational therapy, speech therapy, and cognitive remediation.

LENGTH OF STAY

Rehabilitation is offered on an inpatient or outpatient basis depending on the needs of the patient. Rehabilitation services may also be offered in acute care facilities and long-term care facilities.

SETTINGS

Rehabilitation facilities may offer service on an inpatient (also called *acute rehabilitation*) basis. To qualify for reimbursement at this level of service, patients must participate in a specific number of hours of therapy. For Medicare patients, 3 hours of therapy daily is required.

Outpatient services may be housed in an inpatient facility, a stand-alone outpatient facility, or in a related facility. For example, an increasing number of outpatient rehabilitation services are associated with exercise facilities.

SERVICES

Occupational therapy, physical therapy, speech therapy, and cognitive remediation are common services available for rehabilitation patients. Social services are important in helping patients find the additional services that they may need. In inpatient facilities, recreation therapy may play a role in helping patients increase their ability to accomplish their ADL.

A unique aspect of rehabilitation, as compared to acute care, is the ability of the care providers to focus on preparing the patient to return to the workplace. Industrial rehabilitation, a holistic program of multiple therapies and evaluation techniques, plays an important role in this process. Further, the patient may need to be redirected in his or her employment goals as a result of the sequelae of the illness or injury.

CARE PROVIDERS

As with behavioral health patients, rehabilitation patients may have medical conditions that require treatment while they are in therapy. There is an internist on staff at inpatient facilities to treat these conditions. However, the thrust of treatment is the therapy. Rehabilitation therapy occurs under the direction of a **physiatrist,** a physician who specializes in physical medicine and rehabilitation. Physical therapists (PTs), occupational therapists (OTs), speech language pathologists (SLPs), social workers, and psychologists play major roles, to varying degrees, in the rehabilitation of individual patients.

DATA COLLECTION ISSUES

In a paper-based inpatient environment, the patient's record may travel with the patient from one therapy to the next; this may be accomplished by transporting the charts on a cart or with the patient's transporter. Many rehabilitation patients are moved from place to place by wheelchair, and the chart can be placed on the back of the chair.

With a large number of patients and little time between appointments, therapists may have insufficient time to adequately document treatments. Delays in charting may increase errors in documentation. A moving chart also exposes the facility to the risk of the documentation being lost. Incomplete documentation may result in decreased reimbursement or denial of reimbursement.

Some facilities leave the medical portion of the paper record (physician orders, progress notes, medication administration records) at the nursing unit for physician and nursing documentation. In that case, only the therapy notes travel with the patient. This strategy hampers communication among the care team.

An electronic health record solves the logistical problem of the moving chart. Therapists log all notes directly into the computer. However, the time allotted to do so must be sufficient to accommodate the documentation requirements.

LICENSURE AND ACCREDITATION

Rehabilitation facilities are licensed by the states in which they operate. Accreditation is available from the JCAHO and CARF. Some facilities choose to seek accreditation from both organizations.

DATA SETS

Facilities seeking reimbursement from Medicare must complete the MDS 2.0 data set. This data set is composed of detailed clinical data about the patient similar to those required by long-term care.

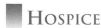

HOSPICE

As discussed in Chapter 1, **hospice** care is focused on the terminally ill and their friends and family members. The focus of hospice is to provide **palliative care:** aid and comfort rather than curative treatment. According to the National Hospice and Palliative Care Organization (NHPCO), the

> ### Exercise 7-6
>
> ### Rehabilitation Facilities
> 1. When is a patient eligible for rehabilitation?
> 2. What services are provided by rehabilitation workers?
> 3. Describe the unique data collection issues in a rehabilitation environment.
> 4. What minimum data set is associated with home health care?
> 5. Who accredits rehabilitation facilities?

number of hospice providers has more than doubled between 1985 and 2002, with over 3200 organizations currently. In that same period, the number of patients served has grown from about 158,000 to 885,000 ("NHPCO Facts and Figures" 2004; "Patients Served 1885 to 2002" 2003; "885,000 Terminally Ill Americans" 2003).

LENGTH OF STAY

The duration of hospice care varies depending on the life expectancy of the patient and the friends' and family's need for support after death. The patients themselves are in the end stage of illness and have a life expectancy of less than 6 months. (Although care could be rendered to patients with a longer expected life, reimbursement entities typically look to the 6-month rule, as certified by the physician.) Friends and family members may receive bereavement services during the illness and for up to a year after the patient's death. The NHPCO states that in 2003, the average length of service for a hospice patient was 50.6 days, with a more representative median of 20.9 days (*NHPCO Facts and Figures* 2004).

SETTINGS

Hospice services may be provided at the patient's residence or in an inpatient setting. Hospice inpatient facilities may resemble group homes because they are specifically designed to give comfort rather than to render acute treatment.

SERVICES

Hospice staff members are on call 24 hours a day. Services include medical services, nursing, counseling, pharmaceuticals, and bereavement services.

CARE PROVIDERS

Volunteers play a major role in attending to patients. Physicians, nurses, and therapists are involved to the extent needed to make the patient comfortable. Virtually any care may be rendered that is needed by the patient. Medicare benefits cover the following therapies to covered individuals:
- Physician services for the medical direction of the patient's care
- Regular home visits by registered nurses and licensed practical nurses
- Home health aides and homemakers for services such as dressing and bathing
- Social work and counseling
- Medical equipment such as hospital beds
- Medical supplies such as bandages and catheters
- Drugs for symptom control and pain relief
- Volunteer support to assist patients and loved ones
- Physical therapy, speech therapy, occupational therapy, and dietary counseling ("How Does Hospice Work" 2006)

DATA COLLECTION ISSUES

The initial plan of treatment is required within 48 hours of admission. Continuous nursing care, when provided, must be documented to facilitate reimbursement.

LICENSURE AND ACCREDITATION

Licensure requirements vary by state, and not all states license hospice providers. The NHPCO offers accreditation.

Exercise 7-7

Hospice
1. Who receives hospice care?
2. When is a patient eligible for hospice care?
3. What role do volunteers play in hospice care?
4. Who accredits hospice organizations?

HOME HEALTH CARE

An increasingly important segment of health care is focused on delivery of services in the home. **Home health care** is significantly less expensive than inpatient care.

As with ambulatory care, length of stay has no significance in home health. Patients receive services at their residence. Patients may reside at home or in a health care facility, such an assisted living or other long-term care facility. The duration of home health care is usually measured in visits by specific therapies (such as two visits per week by physical therapist for 14 weeks) or by specific dates (such as 4 weeks of assistance from a live-in home health aide).

SETTINGS

Home health care is generally rendered by an agency that provides multiple services. Services may be rendered by employees of the organization or by subcontractors. For Medicare reimbursement, the providing organization must offer nursing and at least one additional therapy, the patient must be confined to the place of residence, and the patient must be under the care of a physician who determines what services are needed.

SERVICES

Most services available on an outpatient/ambulatory care basis can be offered as home health care. Rehabilitation services, nursing care, and even physician visits can be accomplished in the home. Table 7-2 lists the types of services provided under home health care.

CARE PROVIDERS

In addition to nursing and therapies, home health providers also render assistance to the patient for a variety of ADL. Care providers include housekeepers and companions.

DATA COLLECTION ISSUES

In the home health care environment, data collection and documentation should be completed at the time of service. This poses a problem because care providers are with the patient and not at the agency that is responsible for the record. Multiple care providers for the same patient have competing needs to review the patient record. In a paper environment, agencies should have policies that require all documentation for a patient's record to be returned to the agency within a short time frame, such as 24 hours after service is rendered. However, a patient may need multiple visits from other caregivers in that time frame. For that reason, a copy of the documentation of service provided is often left at the patient's residence for reference by other caregivers.

It is this logistical problem that drives the development of electronic record-keeping in home health care. Increasingly, agencies are requiring real-time data entry at the time of service to facilitate communication among care providers.

All orders for home health care must be given by a physician. The physician must review the plan of care every 62 days or whenever there is a significant change in patient status.

LICENSURE AND ACCREDITATION

Home health agencies must be licensed in the state in which they operate. The **Community Health Accreditation Program (CHAP)** and the JCAHO both offer accreditation opportunities for home health agencies.

DATA SETS

The **Outcome and Assessment Information Set (OASIS)** applies in home health care. A copy of this data set can be obtained from the Center for Health Services Research, in Denver, Colorado. Table 7-3 contains a summary of the minimum data sets discussed in Chapters 4 and 7.

Exercise 7-8

Home Health Care
1. What services are provided by home health care workers?
2. Describe the unique data collection issues in a home health environment.
3. What minimum data set is associated with home health care?
4. Who accredits home health agencies?

☐ OTHER SPECIALTY FACILITIES

Other types of facilities are defined by medical specialty or by the types of patients that they treat. Some specific issues are adult day care, respite care, dialysis centers, and children's hospitals. Adult day care is usually rendered on an outpatient basis in a rehabilitation or long-term care facility. It provides care for adults who need supervision during the day when their primary caregiver is not available— for example, when the primary caregiver has a full-time job. Adult day care provides activities, social interaction, some therapies, and some medical treatment. Medical treatment usually consists of ensuring that the patient takes the proper medication at the appropriate time.

Respite care is any care that is provided to give relief to the **primary caregiver**. Caring for the chronically ill can be stressful and exhausting. **Respite care** allows the primary caregiver to go on vacation or just to take a break.

Dialysis centers provide renal dialysis services to patients with chronic renal failure. Dialysis may also be accomplished on an inpatient basis; however, that is often in conjunction with admission for an acute episode.

Children's hospitals provide a variety of inpatient and outpatient services, specifically to children. Accommodations may be made for parental participation and presence in the care process.

TABLE 7-2	Home Health Services
CAREGIVER	**ROLE IN HOME HEALTH**
Home care providers	These caregivers deliver a wide variety of health care and supportive services, ranging from professional nursing and HCA care to physical, occupational, respiratory, and speech therapies. They also may provide social work and nutritional care, as well as laboratory, dental, optical, pharmacy, podiatry, x-ray, and medical equipment and supply services. Services for the treatment of medical conditions usually are prescribed by an individual's physician. Supportive services, however, do not require a physician's orders. An individual may receive a single type of care or a combination of services depending on the complexity of his or her needs. Home care services can be provided by the following professionals, paraprofessionals, and volunteers.
Physicians	Physicians visit patients in their homes to diagnose and treat illnesses just as they do in hospitals and private offices. They also work with home care providers to determine which services are needed by patients, which specialists are most suitable to render these services, and how often these services need to be provided. With this information, physicians prescribe and oversee patient plans of care. Under Medicare, physicians and home health agency personnel review these plans of care as often as required by the severity of patient medical conditions or at least once every 62 days. The interdisciplinary team reviews the care plans for hospice patients and their families at least once a month or as frequently as patient conditions or family circumstances require.
Registered nurses (RNs) and licensed practical nurses (LPNs)	RNs and LPNs provide skilled services that cannot be performed safely and effectively by nonprofessional personnel. Some of these services include injections and intravenous therapy, wound care, education on disease treatment and prevention, and patient assessments. RNs may also provide case management services. RNs have received 2 or more years of specialized education and are licensed to practice by the state. LPNs have 1 year of specialized training and are licensed to work under the supervision of registered nurses. The intricacy of a patient's medical condition and required course of treatment determine whether care should be provided by an RN or can be provided by an LPN.
Physical therapists (PTs)	PTs work to restore the mobility and strength of patients who are limited or disabled by physical injuries through the use of exercise, massage, and other methods. PTs often alleviate pain and restore injured muscles with specialized equipment. They also teach patients and caregivers special techniques for walking and transfer.
Social workers	Social workers evaluate the social and emotional factors affecting ill and disabled individuals and provide counseling. They also help patients and their family members identify available community resources. Social workers often serve as case managers when patients' conditions are so complex that professionals need to assess medical and supportive needs and coordinate a variety of services.
Speech language pathologists (SLPs)	Speech language pathologists work to develop and restore the speech of individuals with communication disorders; usually these disorders are the result of traumas such as surgery or stroke. Speech therapists also help retrain patients in breathing, swallowing, and muscle control.
Occupational therapists (OTs)	OTs help individuals who have physical, developmental, social, or emotional problems that prevent them from performing the general activities of daily living. OTs instruct patients on using specialized rehabilitation techniques and equipment to improve their function in tasks such as eating, bathing, dressing, and basic household routines.
Dietitians	Dietitians provide counseling services to individuals who need professional dietary assessment and guidance to properly manage an illness or disability.

TABLE 7-2	*(cont'd)*

CAREGIVER	ROLE IN HOME HEALTH
HCAs/home health aides	These caregivers assist patients with ADLs such as getting in and out of bed, walking, bathing, toileting, and dressing. Some aides have received special training and are qualified to provide more complex services under the supervision of a nursing professional.
Homemaker and chore workers	These caregivers perform light household duties such as laundry, meal preparation, general housekeeping, and shopping. Their services are directed at maintaining patient households rather than providing hands-on assistance with personal care.
Companions	These caregivers provide companionship and comfort to individuals who, for medical and/or safety reasons, cannot be left at home alone. Some companions may assist clients with household tasks, but most are limited to providing sitter services.
Volunteers	Volunteers meet a variety of patient needs. The scope of a volunteer's services depends on his or her level of training and experience. Volunteer activities include, but are not limited to, providing companionship, emotional support, and counseling and helping with personal care, paperwork, and transportation.

From National Association for Home Care, 1996: http://www.nahc.org/famcar_types.html.
HCA, Home care aide.

TABLE 7-3	**Summary of Minimum Data Sets**

DATA SET	SETTING
UHDDS	Acute care
UACDS	Ambulatory care
MDS	Long-term care
OASIS	Home health care
DEEDS	Emergency departments

Exercise 7-9

Other Specialty Facilities

1. List and describe three types of specialty facilities.
2. List the data sets discussed in this chapter and the settings to which they apply.
3. Compare and contrast the UHDDS with the UACDS.

■ WORKS CITED

"885,000 Terminally Ill Americans Served by Hospice in 2002." 2003. National Hospice and Palliative Care Association, 7 July 2006 <http://www.nhpco.org/i4a/pages/index.cfm?pageid=3795>.

"How Does Hospice Work?" 2006. National Hospice and Palliative Care Association, 7 July 2006 <http://www.caringinfo.org/i4a/pages/index.cfm?pageid=3467>.

"Information about PA's and the PA Profession." 2006. American Academy of Physician Assistants, 6 July 2006 <http://www.aapa.org/geninfo1.html>.

Medicare Program: Prospective Payment System for Inpatient Psychiatric Facilities; Final Rule. 2004. 69 C.F.R. § 66967.

"NHPCO Facts and Figures." 2004. National Hospice and Palliative Care Association, 12 July 2006 <http://www.nhpco.org/files/public/facts%20figures%20feb04.pdf>.

"Patients served 1985 to 2002." 2003. National Hospice and Palliative Care Association, 12 July 2006 <http://www.nhpco.org/files/public/Patients_Served_1985_2002.pdf>.

■ SUGGESTED READING

Abraham, Prinny Rose. *Documentation and Reimbursement for Home Care and Hospice Programs.* Chicago: American Health Information Management Association, 2001.

"Ambulatory Care." *Documentation for Ambulatory Care.* 2nd edition. Chicago: American Health Information Management Association, 2001.

Clark, Jean S. *Documentation for Acute Care,* Revised Edition. Chicago: American Health Information Management Association, 2004.

Documentation and Reimbursement for Behavioral Health. Chicago: American Health Information Management Association, 2005.

James, Ella. *Documentation and Reimbursement for Long-Term Care.* Chicago: American Health Information Management Association, 2004.

Manger, Barbara J. *Documentation Requirements in Non-Acute Care Facilities & Organizations.* Pearl River, NY: Parthenon Publishing Group, Inc., 2001.

Peden, Ann H. *Comparative Health Information Management.* 2nd edition. Clifton Park, New York: Thompson Delmar Learning, 2005.

WEB SITES

Accreditation Association for Ambulatory Health Care: http://www.AAAHC.org

Commission on Accreditation of Rehabilitation Facilities: http://www.carf.org

Community Health Accreditation Program: http://www.chapinc.org/

Centers for Medicare and Medicaid Services: http://www.cms.gov; see Clinical Laboratory Improvement Amendments: http://www.cms.hhs.gov/clia

Hospice and Palliative Care: http://www.nhpco.org

Joint Commission on Accreditation of Healthcare Organizations: http://www.JCAHO.org

National Center for Injury Prevention and Control (Data Elements for Emergency Department Systems): http://www.cdc.gov/ ncipc/pub-res/deedspage.htm

National Committee for Quality Assurance: http://www.ncqa.org

"OASIS Overview." U.S. Department of Health and Human Services: http://www.cms.hhs.gov/apps/hha/hhoview.asp

CHAPTER ACTIVITIES

CHAPTER SUMMARY

Health care is delivered in a multitude of settings. Ambulatory care is rendered in physicians' offices as well as emergency departments, surgery centers, radiology and laboratory facilities, rehabilitation facilities, and in the home. Specialty services are offered both in hospitals and also on an outpatient basis, including physical, occupational, and psychological therapies.

In general, health care facilities are licensed in the states in which they operate. Accreditation is offered by the JCAHO, AOA, AAAHC, CHAP, and CARF.

Important data sets include UACDS, DEEDS, OASIS, and MDS.

All facilities seeking Medicare reimbursement are regulated by CMS. The CMS Web site should be consulted for detailed information on those regulations. HIM professionals who are employed in special health care settings must become familiar with the unique data requirements of those settings.

Review Questions

1. List and describe hospital-based ambulatory care settings.
2. Compare rehabilitation facilities to long-term care facilities.
3. What services are available on a home health basis?

APPLICATION

New Challenges

Fred has been working in acute care facilities for the past 5 years in progressively responsible positions. After he graduated from his HIT program and passed the RHIT exam, he was offered a position as the HIM manager in his organization's new long-term care center, which was recently purchased. Fred has heard through the grapevine that the center's records have not been strictly maintained and that the new manager will be expected to organize the records and to ensure that the facility's documentation policies are in compliance with all regulatory and accrediting bodies.

If Fred decides to accept this position, what can he do to ensure that he is prepared for the challenges of his new position?

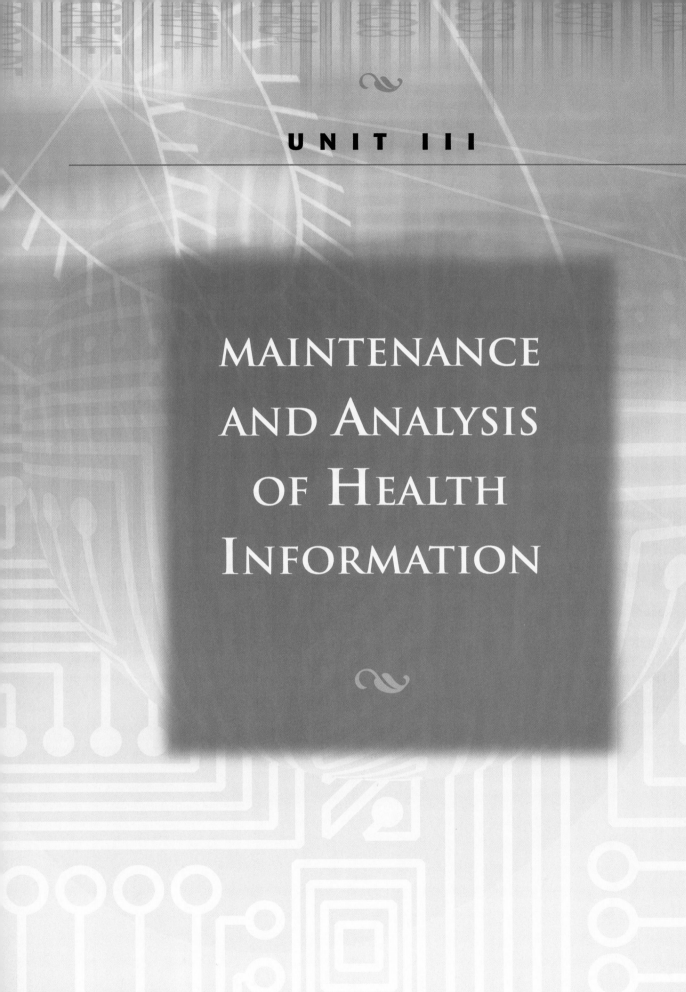

UNIT III

MAINTENANCE AND ANALYSIS OF HEALTH INFORMATION

Chapter 8

∽

STORAGE

By the end of this chapter, the student should be able to

- Explain the use of the master patient index.
- Determine whether a patient has a previous health record at the facility.
- Compare and contrast numbering systems for identification of patient records.
- Compare and contrast filing systems for patient records.
- File health records appropriately according to the file system used by the facility.
- Maintain accuracy of filing methods.
- Identify the alternative storage system best suited for a particular health care facility when it is running out of file space for records.
- Determine the appropriate file space for a given set of circumstances.
- Determine the retention schedule for specific health care records.
- Identify ways to ensure the physical security of health information.
- Explain a chart locator system.

VOCABULARY

chart locator system	microfiche	scanner
computer-based patient record	microfilm	serial numbering
family unit numbering	middle-digit filing	serial-unit numbering
file folder	optical disk	straight numerical filing
index	outguide	terminal-digit filing
master patient index (MPI)	record retention schedule	unit numbering

lthough many facilities have transitioned (or are transitioning) to an electronic health record (EHR), it remains important for health information management (HIM) professionals to understand the issues associated with storage of the paper health record. Storage of paper health records continues to be an important function in the management of health information because many facilities will have to maintain dual systems, paper and electronic, and at least maintain filing of the older paper health records until they are transitioned to electronic format. Because an entire chapter of this text is devoted to the EHR, much of our discussion (but not all) in this chapter will focus on the management of the paper health records.

HIM professionals systematically collect and organize each patient's health information to create a timely, accurate, and complete record. Health information is vital to the patient, health care provider, and community; therefore it must be stored in a secure, accessible, organized environment. The patient's health record must be retained for the continuation of patient care, for reimbursement, accreditation, potential litigation, research, and education purposes. HIM departments demonstrate excellence by providing health information on request to authorized users. To provide health information, you must first be able to locate the information requested. To locate patient health information, you must ensure the systematic organization of all health record files.

The health data (collected on hospital-approved forms) for each patient are organized in the patient's health record. The record may be in a paper or electronic file. This chapter explores the issues of health record storage, including file identification, filing systems, filing furniture, and security of the file environment.

◼ THE PAPER PERSPECTIVE

Physicians, clinics, hospitals, and other health care facilities provide health care to hundreds or even thousands of patients each week. The number of health records that can accumulate is staggering. For example, consider the information in the Hit Bit below.

How many records would this facility have in storage after 2 years? The answer, of course, is 39,000 records (19,500 × 2). How would you locate a record for a patient who was seen in the clinic last year and is coming for a return visit, if you had to look through 39,000 records?

In Chapter 3, you learned about the necessity of recording patient data for communication. Previous patient data may communicate to a physician important information that is necessary for a patient's current treatment. What happens if the physician cannot locate the patient's health record from the last visit? What if the notes from the previous visit compared with the present information reflect a significant weight loss for the patient? This information may be important in the care and treatment of the patient. For example, it could change the patient's dosage of a particular medication or indicate a new diagnosis. A patient's health care may depend on the review of the patient's previous health records. Therefore it is important to make sure the patient's health data are recorded, organized, and analyzed in the health record and stored in a way that allows the information to be retrieved when the patient returns to the facility for follow-up care. Organized storage of health records begins with appropriate identification of each patient's record. Let's begin with a discussion of health record identification.

Hit-Bit

The Paper Explosion

Imagine that a busy clinic sees 75 patients each day and is open just 5 days a week.
5 days × 75 patients = 375 records per week
375 records per week × 52 weeks = 19,500 records annually
If each record is only one sheet of paper, then 19,500 records could amount to approximately four cases of paper.

Hit-Bit

Retrieval of Health Information

Other reasons that a health record may be retrieved include the following:
- A physician specialist may review a patient's record before providing care.
- Insurance companies request copies of reports before paying the claim (reimbursement).
- Facilities review their own records to assess quality of care.
- Accrediting bodies review records to evaluate compliance with standards.
- Litigation: Lawyers present a health record during a lawsuit to represent their client.
- Research: Health records may be used to investigate disease trends.

MASTER PATIENT INDEX

The **master patient index (MPI)** is the key to locating a health record in the HIM department. The MPI contains information on every patient admitted to the facility. The MPI is the primary tool for identifying each file for all patients who have been seen at a particular facility. HIM departments use the MPI as the source of information correlating the patient to his or her health record file. An MPI may be a manual system maintained on index cards organized in a file cabinet in alphabetical order, or it may be a computerized system.

The information contained in the MPI is first collected during the patient registration process. During registration, the patient provides demographic information to the facility (see Chapter 3). This information is used to individually identify each patient within that health care facility and initiates the patient's health record. An identification number is assigned (the *medical record number [MR#])* and correlated to the patient's health record in the process of creating the patient record.

To envision an MPI, think of the catalog index at your local library. To locate a book in your library, you must first access the catalog to determine whether the book is available in the library. If it is available, then you must know the book's catalog number to locate it on the library shelf. The library catalog index correlates the book to its catalog number, allowing you to locate the book on the shelf in the library, which organizes books by catalog number (Figure 8-1).

To relate this example to health information, each health care facility has an MPI. The MPI is a list of all patients who have had encounters at the facility. When looking for the health record of a particular patient, you must first find out whether that the patient was previously seen at the facility and then find out the patient's file identification (medical record) number. You must use the MPI to obtain this information. The MPI correlates the patient to the facility's medical record number to identify the patient's health record. Figure 8-2 lists the recommended and optional contents of an MPI. The information contained in the MPI is a combination of the demographic, financial, and clinical data.

Each patient is entered only once in the MPI. All visits for a particular patient are listed in the MPI under the patient's name. You must be very careful to prevent duplication of patients within the MPI because it may cause confusion and delay when retrieving patient files.

MANUAL MASTER PATIENT INDEX

In a manual MPI system (an outdated method), each patient who is registered in the health care facility has an index card in the MPI located in the HIM department. As patients are registered in the facility, the HIM department is notified of the admission. The notification may be a copy of the face sheet, a computer printout of the admission, or the admit log. To locate a record for the patient, the HIM clerk researches the MPI to see whether the patient has been treated at the facility before.

An MPI card is created for each new patient registered. If the patient has been treated at the facility on a previous occasion, the patient's MPI card is retrieved from the card file. The MPI card is reviewed to make sure the patient's information is correct, and the new admission information

A

B

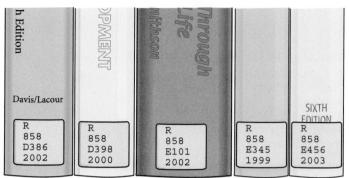
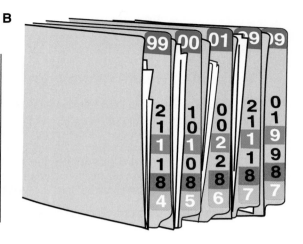

◆ **Figure 8-1**
Books with catalog numbers (**A**) and file folders with medical record numbers (**B**).

CONTENTS OF A MASTER PATIENT INDEX

RECOMMENDED DATA ELEMENTS

- Patient's name
- Alias/previous name
- Address
- Date of birth*
- Social Security number
- Gender
- Race
- Ethnicity
- Medical record number, hospital identification number
- Patient's account number
- Admission date(s)*
- Discharge date(s)*
- Type of service for the encounter
- Patient disposition

OPTIONAL DATA ELEMENTS

- Marital status
- Physician
- Telephone number
- Mother's maiden name
- Place of birth
- Advance directive and surrogate decision making
- Organ donor status
- Emergency contact
- Allergies/reactions
- Problem list

When capturing dates, it is important to record the year as four numbers, i.e., MMDDYYYY or YYYYMMDD.

◆ **Figure 8-2**
Contents of a master patient index. (From AHIMA Practice Brief No. 433.)

Hit-Bit

Duplicate Master Patient Index Entries/Medical Record Number

In a unit numbering system, extra care must be taken to identify whether the patient already has a medical record number from a previous admission. Failure to identify a previously assigned number results in duplicate entries into the master patient index for the same patient (i.e., more than one medical record number for the same patient). This redundancy will create problems when you are trying to locate the patient's medical record.

Hit-Bit

New versus Old records

Do you know how a facility distinguishes a new patient from an old patient?
- *New:* new to the facility as a patient; not registered or treated at the facility on a prior occasion
- *Old:* returning patient; has an MPI card or entry and has been registered or treated previously in the facility; new visit added to patient's existing MPI card or entry

Hit-Bit

The Master Patient Index

By now, you are probably thinking, how antiquated is this manual master patient index (MPI) system? Answer: very antiquated. Today, it is rare for a facility to have a manual MPI system. This system does not allow you to capture all of the recommended data elements because it is limited by the size of the index card. The manual system will not typically have all of the items listed in Figure 8-2. Likewise, because the index cards are filed alphabetically, it is possible for cards to be misfiled and problems to occur, as they do in alphabetical filing.

is added (date of admission, type of service, account number for that visit, attending physician, discharge date). The MPI must be updated each time the patient is admitted to the health care facility. Figure 8-3 illustrates a manual MPI card.

The advantages of a manual MPI system are that it can be inexpensive, implemented quickly, and accessible regardless of energy supply to the facility, unless the MPI cards are stored in a revolving file system (discussed later in this chapter, in the section on filing furniture). One disadvantage of the manual MPI system is that the amount of information for each patient is limited by the size of the index card. The manual index is also inefficient if the index cards are labeled incorrectly or if they are misfiled, and it can be accessed only from the HIM department.

COMPUTERIZED MASTER PATIENT INDEX

A computerized MPI is often more flexible than a manual system. It captures more patient information and can be accessed from areas outside the HIM department, such as the emergency room or patient registration. A computerized MPI system uses computer software to capture and store patient identification and admission information. The computerized MPI software is typically one

Last Name, First Name, Middle Initial	Date of Birth ___ / ___ / ___	Medical Record # _____
Address	Phone # (___) ___ - ___	Married _____ Death _____
City, State _____ Zip Code _____	Social Security # ___ - ___ - ___	
Gender _____		
Race _____ Financial Class _____		

Admit Date	Discharge Date	Service	Physician	Patient Account #

◆ **Figure 8-3**
MPI card in a manual system.

Hit-Bit

Master Patient Index Purge

It is important to note that when the master patient index (MPI) file cabinet is full, the HIM department may need to remove, or purge, MPI cards and store them in another location or format (discussed later in the chapter). How does a purge begin? The department must set criteria to determine which MPI cards should be removed from the file cabinet. For example, the decision may be made to remove all cards for patients who are deceased. It is important to inform all facility employees and to update the department's policy and procedure manual (discussed in Chapter 13) when an alternative storage site exists for MPI cards. Employees will need to know the criteria used for MPI card removal. This facilitates locating old charts and ensures that new numbers are not assigned to patients who are readmitted to the facility.

Hit-Bit

Computer Interface

A computer *interface* allows two different computer systems or software products to exchange information.

feature of a larger computer system or is interfaced with other computer systems in the health care facility.

As stated previously, the facility begins collecting identification information on the patient at the time of registration. Information entered into a computerized MPI creates a demographic history for each patient. At registration, the admitting clerk searches the MPI history files to determine whether the patient has been treated at the facility on a previous occasion. If the patient is new, a new history is created by entering the information (as prompted by the system) listed in

Figure 8-2. If the patient has been treated at the facility on a previous occasion, the admitting clerk identifies the patient's history and reviews it to ensure the accuracy of all of the information. For example, if the patient's address has changed, this information must be updated in the patient's MPI history file. If his or her insurance company has changed, this information is also updated. The new admission information is also entered into the MPI—that is, the date of admission, type of service, account number for that visit, and name of the attending physician are recorded.

Figure 8-4 shows computerized MPI screens. The first screen shows the results of a search for patient Mary Davidson. Notice that there are three results. The example shown is an MPI for a multihospital system in which all of the facilities share an MPI. This system is commonly called an Enterprise MPI (EMPI). This particular MPI indicates that that Mary Davidson has been a patient in three different health care facilities within the multihospital system. The EMPI improves access to records and allows for easy retrieval of the patient's health information when authorized. There is also an option in the computerized MPI in which you are able to view AKA (also known as) and "merges" for a particular patient (the buttons at the bottom of the small window). The AKA feature helps you link any other names for this patient (e.g., maiden name). The merge feature allows you to identify whether any duplicate numbers have been assigned to this patient; this can be helpful if a chart was incorrectly filed under a duplicate patient number.

There are advantages and disadvantages to a computerized MPI. The computerized MPI provides the opportunity to store more patient identification information for each admission—for example, patient financial class, marital status, social security number, and "also known as" (AKA) functions, which link the patient to another name resulting from divorce or marriage or to a pseudonym. More information is stored in a smaller space combined with greater search capabilities to access possible matches for a name using phonetics, date of birth (DOB), Social Security number (SS#), or age. Computerization also allows the MPI to be linked to other departments within the facility (e.g., the emergency department or the patient registration area). A computerized MPI system may be more expensive than a manual system, and uninterrupted access to the MPI requires a connection to an emergency power supply. However, after consideration, most HIM departments find that the benefits of a computerized MPI far outweigh the disadvantages.

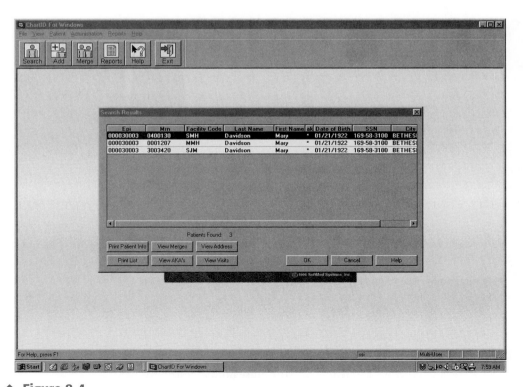

◆ **Figure 8-4**

MPI screens in a computerized system. (Courtesy SoftMed Systems, Inc., Bethesda, MD.)

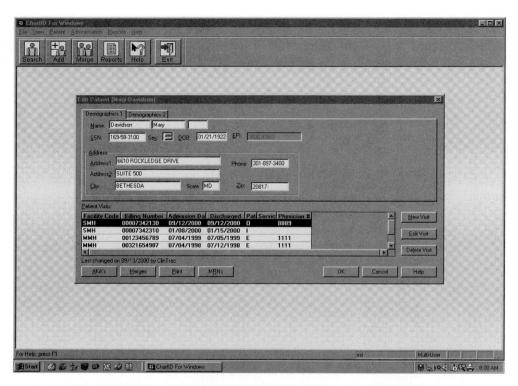

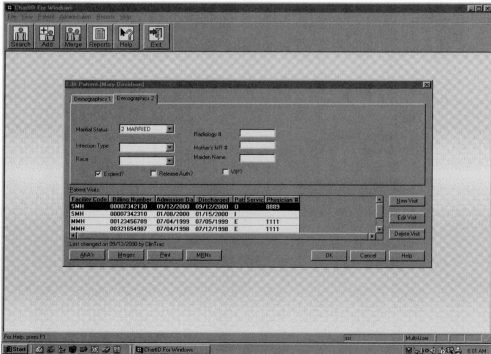

◆ **Figure 8-4,** *cont'd*

RETENTION OF MASTER PATIENT INDEX

The MPI must be retained permanently. This index is extremely important in the everyday operations of a health care facility and the HIM department. The MPI must not be destroyed. In a numerical filing system, you must know the medical record number to retrieve the patient's health record. The MPI is the easiest way to access the patient's medical record number.

Hit-Bit

Phonetic Search

Phonetic searching is the function in a computer system that queries the database for all names that sound like the name that has been entered. For example, all forms of the name Steven sound the same, even though they are spelled differently. With a phonetic feature, the computer can search for all sound-alike spellings of the name, such as Stephen, Stefan, Stephan, and Steven.

Hit-Bit

Master Patient Index Conversion

During or following a conversion from a manual master patient index (MPI) to a computerized MPI, if the manual MPI information is not entered into the computerized system, then the manual card index must be checked each time a patient is admitted to ensure that the patient does not have a previous record.

When a facility implements a computerized MPI, it must decide what to do with the manual system. Because the information in an MPI is never destroyed, the facility must devise a way to convert the information from the manual file into the computerized system. When a computerized MPI is installed, the data on the manual MPI cards are entered into the computerized system, which allows computer access to all MPI information. HIM professionals should monitor the accuracy of the manual MPI conversion. If the information on even one patient or encounter is omitted or entered incorrectly, the MPI is not accurate. The omission or error may cause great difficulty when accessing patient records. Maintenance of the original MPI information secures the validity of the data in the computerized MPI and provides a reference if a discrepancy arises in a patient's file that originated before the conversion. The ability to reference the original MPI cards allows the correction of any discrepancies caused by an error or omission. In this type of conversion, the facility should consider storing the manual MPI in the original format or microfilming the original MPI cards for future reference. The minor inconvenience caused by storing the manual system can prevent serious problems with record discrepancies in the future.

FILING

ELECTRONIC FILES

In the electronic record environment (see Chapter 12), health records may be kept by way of a hybrid-type system in which paper records still exist and are converted to electronic images, are entirely electronic, or are a combination of both. In the electronic format, when the paper record is scanned into a computer system so that the data on the paper documents are digitally stored in the computer for future use, there is a need to identify the files. In this file format, the patient's health record can be located by searching the patient's name, medical record number, and encounter number and by various other methods, as discussed earlier in the electronic MPI scenario. When the paper record is scanned into the computer system, the images are indexed or named so they can be retrieved at a later date. The creation of an accurate **index** facilitates future retrieval of the images. Through the correct identification (indexing or naming) of the document for each patient, the computer system is able to locate the correct image when you perform a

Exercise 8-1

Master Patient Index

1. The _____ contains patient and encounter information, which is often used to correlate the patient to the file identification.
2. The MPI is especially useful in a facility that uses a numerical system to identify patient records because the MPI _____ the patient to the MR# for the patient file.
   a. maps
   b. correlates
   c. copies
   d. registers
3. List the uses of the MPI.
4. The _____ is a tool in the health care facility used to store unique identifiable information on each patient who has been registered in that facility.
5. The emergency room calls the health information management department for the old chart on Mr. Tom Jones. What is the first step in locating Mr. Jones's old record from a previous admission?
6. When you receive a request for an old patient health record (from a previous visit), what is the first step to take in locating the record?

search. For example, when you scan a document into a computer using a standard flatbed scanner, you must name the file to identify the information stored. Because you name the file when you save it, the next time you access the file index, you are able to identify the contents without opening each file. Therefore indexing in the computer environment facilitates future retrieval.

What happens if the image is indexed by the wrong patient's name? How do you find the missing images of a record in the computer? All computer systems have various search methods to aid in the retrieval of the images. Additional methods to locate missing files require searching the discharge list to identify other patient records indexed on the same day. When records are scanned into a computer system, they are typically scanned in groups or batches. A typical group or batch of records would be 1 day of discharges. Therefore by looking through the images of all the patients' records scanned the same day, you may be able to retrieve the missing image. Once the missing image is identified, it is renamed or indexed appropriately.

PHYSICAL FILES

In the paper record environment, health data captured during the patient's stay are organized on appropriate hospital-approved forms (e.g., the face sheet, history and physical [H&P], nursing admission assessment, laboratory reports, and progress notes). To file these forms in the correct patient file folder, you must label each form with the patient's name and identifying medical record number. This can be accomplished in several ways: by using an addressograph, by affixing printed labels, or by writing the data by hand.

All of the forms for each patient are assembled (see Chapter 4) in a file folder. The **file folder** is the container used to store the forms that document the patient's health information. A few housekeeping rules and recommendations apply to the file folder and its design and labeling.

The file folder must be durable to protect the forms containing the patient's health information. File folders are available in many different weights and sizes, varying from very thin (onionskin) to thick (card stock). The heavier the weight, the more durable the folder. HIM personnel must be sure the file folders are strong enough to handle daily use. A file folder that is used repeatedly shows wear over time. The file folder must also expand in width enough to allow for the thickness of the patient's record. In an acute care environment for a patient stay of 5 days, the record may be 1-inch thick. Therefore the folder should be heavier than the standard manila weight to with-

Hit-Bit

The Addressograph

Before computerized technology, health care forms were manually stamped with the patient's name, medical record number, account number, and room number by using an addressograph. The addressograph is a machine that uses a plastic card imprinted with the patient's identification information. The imprint on the card resembles the name imprinted on a credit card. The plastic card is put into the addressograph machine, the patient's forms are placed one at a time on top of the card, and an ink roller is passed over the paper and card to mark the patient's information on each piece of the record. The addressograph card contains enough information to identify the patient so that the forms can be placed in the correct patient record. Although this system is still used, technology has replaced it in many facilities with printed labels, computer-generated forms, and bar codes.

stand the weight of the forms and the frequency of use. Thin files, typically used for physicians' office records, may be adequately stored in lighter-weight folders.

A fastener on the inside of the folder is used to secure the forms in the folder. The fastener usually has two prongs and may be positioned in several different places within the folder (e.g., on the top right side or on the inside right (see Figure 8-17). The fastener keeps the record assembled in the appropriate order and prevents pages from falling out of the folder.

Health record folders commonly have a tab that protrudes from the edge of the folder. The tab may be on the top or on the side of the file folder. The tab is used to label the folder for easy recognition within the file cabinet or on the shelf. Top tabs are used for folders filed in a file cabinet (i.e., for alphabetic filing). Side tabs, also known as *end tabs,* are used to label folders filed on shelves, and they may even include a bar code, the patient's name, date of service, volume numbers, year-band labels, and other data. The medical record number labeled on the side tab of a folder may also be color coded. Normally, colors are assigned to each alphabetical or numerical character. This method easily identifies a section of files by the colors associated with the number or alphabetical character. Color coding aids in accurate filing because misfiled folders are easily recognized. Figure 8-5 shows the different labeling styles for file folders.

Health record file folders must be clearly labeled with appropriate patient identification information, such as the patient's name and medical record number, if applicable. Clear labeling of the patient's file folder is important for accurate filing and storage. Use ink or marker, not pencil. The patient's name should be printed on the outside of the folder; do *not* use script or fancy handwriting. If applicable, the medical record number should also be printed on the outside of the folder.

When a patient's record is too thick to fit into the file folder, or when the patient has multiple visits, several file folders may exist for that one patient. Labeling each of the patient's folders by the volume number identifies the number of file folders that exist for the patient.

HIM professionals also use colored file folders to differentiate one type of file from another. Color coding of a patient's file folder can identify the type of documents contained in the file folder; for example, outpatient records may be in a folder of a color different from the inpatient files. The color of file folders may also indicate the record type, such as skilled nursing facility, acute care, same-day surgery, or rehabilitation, or it can be coordinated in some way with the medical record number.

File folders can also contain information about the facility to which the files belong (e.g., "Property of Southern Hospital, CONFIDENTIAL. If found please return this record to Southern Hospital, 615 Medical Center Blvd., Orange, TX 77777").

The following is a list of factors to consider when choosing file folders for a health care facility:

■ How often will the folder be accessed and handled by file clerks? For example, do many of the patients make repeated visits, requiring retrieval of the old record for patient care?

A

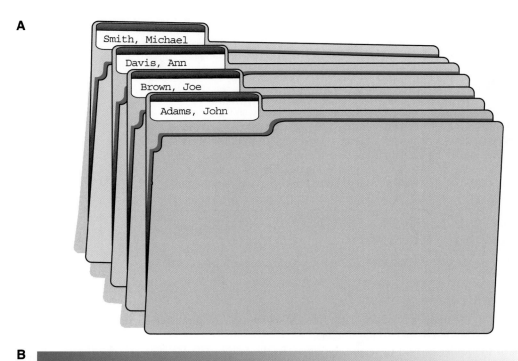

B

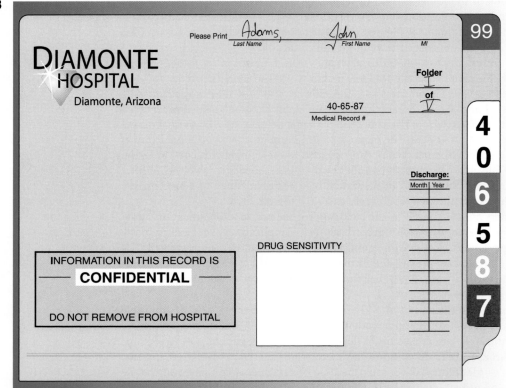

◆ **Figure 8-5**
File folder labeling showing top (**A**) and side (**B**) tabs.

Hit-Bit

File Folders

Some health care environments may retain patient health records in manila folders, binders, envelopes, or pocket expandable files.

◾ Are the records in the facility thick or thin? For thick files, be sure to purchase a file folder that expands enough to contain and cover the documents in the record.

◾ Choose a fastener to secure the forms inside the folder. Be sure to have the fastener in the correct position for the documents within the folder. Make sure the fastener does not require holes to be punched through the patient information.

◾ Consider identifying the facility to which the file belongs on the cover of the file. Other information can be printed on the file folder, such as the address of the facility, a confidentiality statement, and a place to highlight patient allergies.

◾ The folder should accommodate labeling for the file system used in the facility—for example, patient's name, discharge date, and medical record number.

◾ Check the placement of the tab. Is it in the correct place? Side or end tabs are used in shelf filing, and top tabs are used in cabinet filing. Also, is the tab large enough to accommodate the medical record number or the patient's name?

IDENTIFICATION OF PHYSICAL FILES

For easy identification and filing, the file folder containing the patient's health information is labeled with alphabetical or numerical characters. In a small health care facility or a physician's office, the file folder may be identified alphabetically with the patient's name. In a large health care facility, the medical record number is used to identify the patient's health record file. Medical record numbers vary in length: Some are only six digits, others are eight or nine digits, and some may even be longer. Currently, the number of digits or type of number used by a facility is not mandated. However, accreditation agencies such as the Joint Commission on Accreditation of Healthcare Organizations (JCAHO) require facilities to use a system that ensures timely access to patient information when requested for patient care or other authorized use. Additionally, the facility chooses the system (alphabetical or numerical) that best suits its purpose for identification and storage of patient files. Five types of health record identification are discussed here: alphabetical filing, unit numbering, serial numbering, serial–unit numbering, and family unit numbering. As you read about these identification methods, keep in mind that, except for alphabetic filing, a numbering (identification) system is not the same as a filing method (discussed later in the chapter).

Alphabetical Filing

A typical setting for the filing of patient records in alphabetical order is a small physician's office, clinic, home health care facility, or nursing home. The patient's file folders are labeled using the patient's name with the last name followed by the first name. The name *John Adams* becomes *Adams, John.* File folders are arranged on the shelf in alphabetical order, beginning with the patient's last name (Figure 8-6). For those records stored on a shelf, the patient's name is color coded on the side tab, often using the first three letters of the patient's last name. The records are still filed alphabetically, but the labeling is different. In the alphabetical system in which records are filed in a cabinet, the folder is labeled with the patient's name, preferably on the top tab.

Alphabetical filing works well in health care environments where the number of patient visits or records is relatively low. The file folders are easy to label, and pulling a patient's file can be accomplished if the patient's name is known. Alphabetical filing does not require an additional system, such as the MPI, to correlate patient names and numbers to identify the file folder.

Hit-Bit

Medical Record Number

Medical record numbers are assigned by the facility in which the patient is registered to receive health care. Patients do not have the same medical record number for their files when receiving care at another facility. However, if a patient receives care in a large multifacility health care system, one that is owned and operated by the same organization, patients may be assigned a system-wide medical record number that is used in all the facilities.

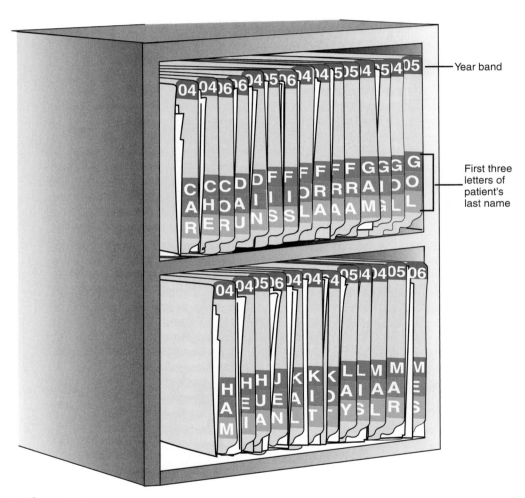

◆ **Figure 8-6**
File folders in alphabetical order.

Problems can arise when two patients have the same name. Common names, such as Michael Smith, José Cruz, and Ann Davis, require careful attention to be certain that the correct patient record is found. Think about the names Michael, Joe, and Ann. How many other ways may these names be identified? Mike, Michael, Jo, Joe, Joseph, José, Josef, Ann, Anne, Annie, and Annette are common versions of Michael, José, and Ann. When duplicate names occur in an alphabetical filing system, procedures must be specified to further organize the records by the patient's middle name, by titles (Jr., Sr., III), or by the patient's date of birth (DOB). Common rules for alphabetical filing are as follows:

TABLE 8-1	Advantages and Disadvantages of Alphabetical Filing

ADVANTAGES	DISADVANTAGES
Easy to learn	Illegible handwriting may cause problems with filing.
Does not require additional cross-reference to locate a patient chart	Space within the popular letters of the alphabet can fill quickly.
Works well in smaller facilities	It can be inefficient for a large facility with a large patient population.
	Many alternative spellings of names exist.

- Personal names are filed last name first; for example, the name John Adams is filed by *Adams* first, followed by *John*: Adams, John. The first name is followed by the middle initial (e.g., *E*) or name if necessary: Adams, John E.
- All punctuation and possessives are ignored. Disregard commas, hyphens, and apostrophes. In the last name, prefixes, foreign articles, and particles are combined with the name following it, omitting spaces (e.g., *De Witt* is filed as *dewitt*).
- Abbreviations, nicknames, and shortened names are filed as written (e.g., *Wm, Bud, Rob*).
- Suffixes are considered after the middle name or initial. Titles are considered after suffixes. Royal or religious titles follow the given name and surname; the title is indexed last.
- When identical names occur, consider the DOB for filing order and proceed chronologically.

Patients' files must be clearly labeled. It is important to print clearly when labeling the patient's file folder. This is not an occasion for fancy script or calligraphy. Illegible or fancy handwriting may cause a file folder to be misfiled. Table 8-1 lists the advantages and disadvantages of alphabetical filing.

Space is a common problem in the alphabetical filing system. The shelves or cabinets holding the files of patients' names beginning with common letters become full very quickly, so be sure to allow adequate file space for these letters of the alphabet. Filing in a section that is full of records is difficult and requires shifting of the records for further filing. Alphabetical filing systems can become inefficient in a facility that serves a large population with a high volume of patient records.

Another consideration with this system is the spelling of patient names. Sometimes even the easiest names are misspelled. In an alphabetical file system, a folder labeled incorrectly because of misspelling will not be filed correctly on the shelf. When the HIM employee attempts to locate the patient's folder, efforts will involve searching for a misspelled, misfiled record. If you are unsure of the spelling of the patient's name, ask for identification (driver's license) to clarify the spelling.

Unit Numbering

In a **unit numbering** system, a patient receives the same medical record number for each admission to the facility. Therefore the numerical identification of each individual patient is always patient specific. For example, if a person is born in a facility that uses unit numbering, at birth (admission) the patient is assigned a number (e.g., MR# 001234). Any subsequent admissions of this patient to the facility would use the same medical record number. In a unit numbering identification system, the patient's medical record number remains the same, within the facility, throughout the lifetime of the patient. Medical record numbers are not shared and are not reused after a patient dies.

Consider the following scenario: Molly Brabant was born at Diamonte Hospital on January 1, 2001. At birth, Molly is assigned the number MR# 001234. Her birth record is filed in a folder identified with MR# 001234. At age 7, Molly returns to the same facility to have a tonsillectomy. Molly's new records are stored in the same folder identified as MR# 001234. Any subsequent admissions (e.g., for a hip replacement later in life) are filed under the same identification number (Figure 8-7).

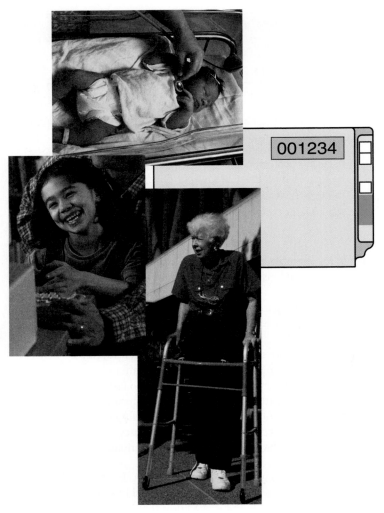

◆ **Figure 8-7**
Unit medical record number.

Serial Numbering

In a **serial-numbering** system, a new medical record number is assigned each time a patient has an encounter at the facility. In this type of system, the patient's file folders containing the health record for each encounter are not filed in the same folder. Therefore the records are not located together on the file shelf.

Using the previous scenario in a serial numbering system, Molly is assigned MR# 001234 at birth. However, when she returns at age 7 for a tonsillectomy, a new number, MR# 112233, is assigned (Figure 8-8). In this system, Molly's records are not stored in the same folder, and they are not located near each other on the file shelf. Molly now has two separate folders containing her health record, and she receives a third medical record number and a new folder when she visits the facility for a hip replacement in later years.

Serial-Unit Numbering

A **serial-unit numbering** system is a combination of the previous two numbering systems. In this system, the patient receives a new medical record number each time he or she comes into a facility. The difference is that each time the patient receives health care, the old records are brought forward and filed with the most recent visit, under a new medical record number. This system requires a cross-reference system from the old medical record number to the new number so that records

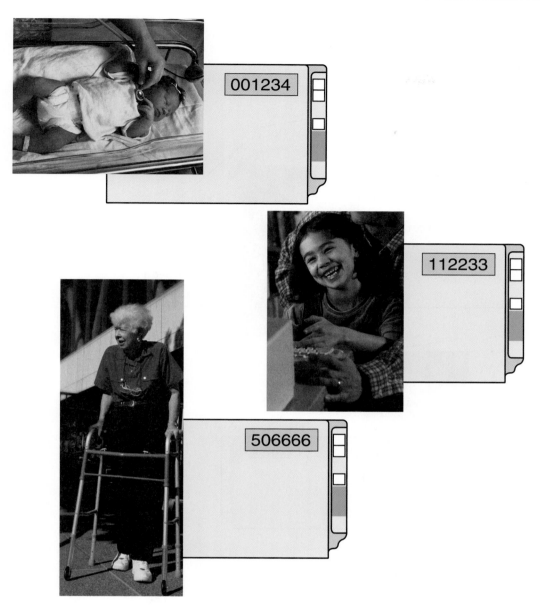

◆ **Figure 8-8**
Serial medical record number.

can be located. To cross-reference, the MPI must be updated so each encounter reflects the corresponding medical record number, and a file guide is placed in the old file location alerting HIM employees to look for the current medical record number to locate the patient's health record.

In the serial-unit numbering system, Molly is assigned MR# 001234 at birth, and on return 7 years later for a tonsillectomy, she is assigned a new number, MR# 112233. When Molly returns for the tonsillectomy, the birth record (MR# 001234) is retrieved from its place in the files and combined with the file folder numbered MR# 112233. A cross-reference should be set up by placing an outguide (see Figure 8-19) in place of the old MR# 001234 to indicate that the record is now filed at MR# 112233 (Figure 8-9). Molly's records are transferred and cross-referenced a third time when Molly has a hip replacement later in life.

Family Unit Numbering

In health care settings where it is common for an entire family to visit a physician or clinic, an entire family's records may be contained in one file folder. This family file is then identified by

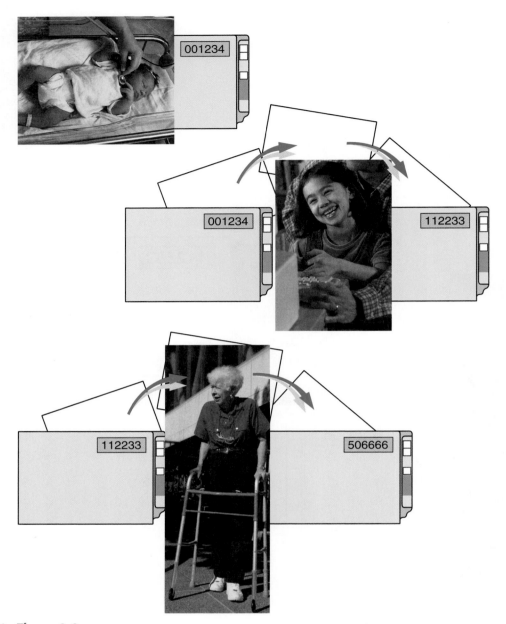

◆ **Figure 8-9**
Serial-unit medical record number.

assigning one medical record number to the entire family (father/husband, mother/wife, and children). This system is called **family unit numbering.** The family unit number requires a modifier at the end of the family unit number unique to each member of the family. The modifier is a number attached to the MR# using a hyphen. Each member of the family can be identified by a modifier associated with his or her position in the family: head of household, 01; spouse, 02; first born, 03; second born, 04; and so on. With this system, all of the family members' records may be contained in one file folder. If you think about all members of a family having the same last name and then being identified individually by their first names, you may see the similarity to family unit numbering.

In our example, Molly's family unit number is MR# 123456. At birth, Molly, being the first-born child, is assigned MR# 123456-03. Molly's mother has MR# 123456-02. The last two numbers after the hyphen indicate to which family member the record belongs. Table 8-2 provides an example of family unit numbering.

This system is beneficial in a small clinic or physician's office setting where clinical and financial records are combined for claims processing. There are potential problems with this numbering system. Families change, couples divorce, and grown children marry and adopt other names. When members of the family divorce, die, marry, or remarry, the medical records for those patients must be renumbered. This process can be quite tedious. Even in a family unit numbering system, the facility is responsible for maintaining the confidentiality of each patient's health information. Safeguards must be taken to ensure that husbands and wives are allowed access to each other's information only with appropriate authorization (see Chapter 11). Likewise, procedures should exist to safeguard the confidentiality of a child's information after the legal age of majority.

Each facility should examine the positive as well as negative aspects of each numbering identification system to choose the system that allows efficient delivery of health care for the patient. The system should have a positive impact on both employee and facility productivity. Table 8-3 summarizes the advantages and disadvantages of each numbering system.

FILING METHODS

Now that you know how medical records are numbered, you are ready to learn how those numbers are used to file the records. Filing is the process of organizing the health record folders on a shelf, in a file cabinet, or in a computer system. There are three methods for organizing paper-based health records in a file area: alphabetical, straight numerical, and terminal digit. In a computer system, patient health information is indexed, as discussed previously.

TABLE 8-2	Family Unit Numbering		
FAMILY MEMBER	**FAMILY NUMBER**	**MODIFIER**	**PATIENT NUMBER**
John Smith	123456	01	123456-01
Mary Smith	123456	02	123456-02
Molly Smith	123456	03	123456-03
Tommy Smith	123456	04	123456-04

TABLE 8-3	Advantages and Disadvantages of Numbering Systems	
SYSTEM	**ADVANTAGES**	**DISADVANTAGES**
Unit	All patient records can be located under one number.	Filing of all encounters in one folder can cause problems with incomplete records.
Serial	Each admission is filed in a single folder.	Retrieving all the records for one patient involves going to multiple places in the files.
Serial-unit	Each admission has a unique number, but they are all filed with the most recent.	This method is time consuming.
Family unit	Records are combined for clinical and financial processing of claims.	Confidentiality can be compromised; divorce, remarriage, and other factors can create complications.

Alphabetical Filing

Alphabetical filing has already been discussed under identification of files.

Straight Numerical Filing

Straight numerical filing involves placing the folders on the shelf in numerical order (e.g., MR# 001234, MR# 001235, MR# 001522). This filing system is easy for HIM staff to understand. Straight numerical filing is best used in a system in which there is minimal activity in the records once they are filed in the permanent file area.

Straight numerical methods usually work well in long-term care facilities. In this filing method, the activity is concentrated at the end of the file shelf. The filing shelves are filled as records are added. Increased filing in the older records (lower numbers) will cause growth in shelves that may already be full, which causes a need to shift records. Shifting records involves the systematic physical relocation of files so that they are more evenly distributed on the shelves. In large file rooms, this is a time-consuming task.

Terminal-Digit Filing

Terminal-digit filing is a system in which the patient's medical record number is divided into sets of digits for filing purposes. Each set of digits is used to file the health record numerically within sections of the files, beginning with the last set. Terminal-digit filing, and other variations of digit filing, is very common in health care facilities. The easiest example of terminal-digit filing uses a six-digit medical record number. The six-digit number is separated into three sets of two numbers before filing. For example, for MR# 012345, the sets would look like this: 01-23-45. The sets of digits have names: The first two numbers are called the *tertiary digits,* the second two numbers are called the *secondary digits,* and the last two numbers are called the *primary digits* (Table 8-4). To file in terminal-digit (TD) order, you must locate the section of files that correspond with the sets, beginning with the primary digits, then within the primary section locate the secondary digits, and finally file the record in numerical order by the tertiary digits. Filing in TD order is easy once you understand how to separate the digits in the medical record number and then which digit set to use first.

In this example, you begin by using the last two numbers of the medical record number, the primary digits.

Step 1. Separate the medical record number into the necessary sections. This example uses a six-digit number separated into three sections with two numbers each: MR# 012345 converts to 01-23-45. To file this health record (#01-23-45), you would begin with the primary digits 45, the last two digits of MR# 01-23-45. In the file area, you must locate the primary section 45. All files in primary section 45 will end with the number 45.

Step 2. In primary section 45, you then search for the middle digits, 23. Remain in section 45, where the bottom two numbers are all the same, and be sure not to venture into another primary section on the shelf. Find middle digits 22 to 24 because 23 is going to be filed between middle digits 22–45 and 24–45.

TABLE 8-4	Terminal-Digit Sorting of Medical Record Number 01-23-45	
MEDICAL RECORD NUMBER	**NUMBER IN SECTION**	**FILING**
0 1	Tertiary	Finally, file in numerical order by this number.
2 3	Secondary	Then find number 23 in section 45.
4 5	Primary	First, find section 45 in the files.

Step 3. Once you have located the appropriate middle-digit section, file the record numerically by the first two digits.

TD filing can be modified in several different ways. Some facilities use a larger nine-digit medical record number or the SS#. There are several ways to separate a nine-digit medical record number for filing:

- One method is to have three sections with three numbers each; for example, MR# 111222333 converts to 111-222-333 for filing.
- Another method is to separate the number as you would an SS#; for example, MR# 012345678 converts to 012-34-5678.

In a six-digit filing scenario, there are 100 primary sections of record, 00 through 99. In a nine-digit filing system, there are 1000 primary sections, 000 through 999. Primary sections reaching 1000 require a tremendous file area.

Middle-Digit Filing

TD filing can be modified into another filing method, **middle-digit filing.** As in TD filing, the six-digit number is separated into three sets of two numbers before filing; MR# 012345 sets would look like this: 01-23-45. The sets of digits, however, have been renamed (Figure 8-10); the first two numbers are the secondary digits, the second two numbers are the primary digits, and the last two numbers are the tertiary digits (Table 8-5).

The following shows middle-digit filing for MR# 012345.

Step 1. Separate the medical record number into three sections with two numbers each. MR# 012345 converts to 01-23-45. In middle-digit filing, begin with the middle set of digits and use that set as the primary digits; in our example, it is number 23. Locate the primary section 23 in the file area. All files in primary section 23 will have middle sets with the number 23.

Step 2. Remain in section 23. Be sure not to move into another primary section on the shelf. Find the second set of digits, 01.

Step 3. Remain in section 01-23, and then file the record numerically by the tertiary digits 45.

Figure 8-10 shows an example of terminal-digit filing and of middle-digit filing.

Each facility should examine both the positive and the negative aspects of each filing method. An organized filing system allows you to efficiently retrieve patient health records. Quick retrieval of health records can improve the quality of patient care. A good system should have a positive impact on both employee and facility productivity. Table 8-6 lists the advantages and disadvantages of each filing method.

COMPUTER INDEXING

Some health care facilities store patient health records in an electronic system. These files may be in several different formats (discussed in Chapter 12) and saved on optical disk, CD, or a computer hard drive.

TABLE 8-5	**Middle-Digit Sorting of Medical Record Number 01-23-45**	
MEDICAL RECORD NUMBER	NUMBER IN SECTION	FILING
0 1	Secondary	Then, find number 01 in section 23.
2 3	Primary	First, find 23 in the files.
4 5	Tertiary	Finally, file in numerical order by this number.

TABLE 8-6	Advantages and Disadvantages of Filing Methods	
FILING METHOD	**ADVANTAGES**	**DISADVANTAGES**
Alphabetical	+ Easy to learn; does not require additional cross-reference to identify a file number.	Illegible handwriting can cause problems; space requirements for popular letters also problematic.
Straight numerical	+ Easy to learn.	File activity is concentrated.
Terminal-digit	+ Equalizes filing activity throughout the filing sections. + It can be a security feature because those who are unfamiliar with terminal digit filing will be unable to identify a patient's record.	– Challenging for some file clerks to learn. – Misfiles are often difficult to locate.
Middle-digit	+ Equalizes filing activity throughout the filing sections.	– Even more challenging for some file clerks to learn; misfiles are often difficult to locate.

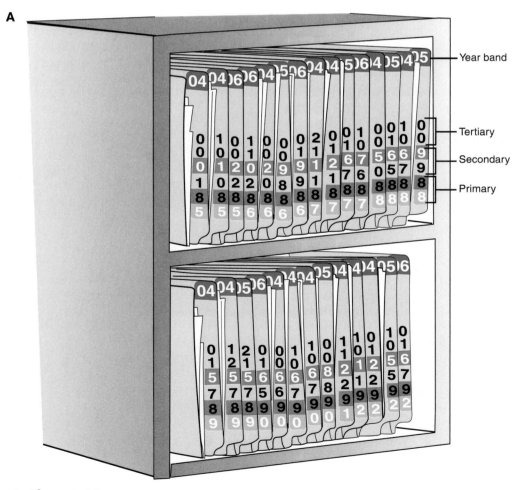

◆ **Figure 8-10**
Filing by terminal digit (**A**) and middle digit (**B**).

Document imaging of patient health records allows a facility to scan original pages of patient records into a computer to save the image on a compact disk (CD), optical disk, platter, or magnetic tape. Using these methods of storage can significantly decrease the amount of storage space necessary to file paper records. This type of system does not require the physical filing of patient records, but it requires indexing. Indexing, as previously discussed, is the naming of an image so that the computer can identify the file. HIM employees index the patient information so that the computer system recognizes the patient's record and attaches the location of the images for that patient.

An example of indexing is the creation of a file in a word processing software application. When you finish, you must save the work so that you can find it on the system later. To differentiate it from other saved work, you must name your work. Indexing allows future retrieval of the images, without a lengthy search. Another example of indexing is a music CD on which the songs are listed with a corresponding number; this is the order in which each song can be found on the disk. To locate a song on the CD, you look at the cover and find the corresponding number. After putting the CD in the player, you forward through the songs until the song is reached or simply press the number on the keypad for the song.

Indexing—attaching specific numbers to the images on the optical disk—allows an employee to go directly to the appropriate patient record. To retrieve information stored on an optical disk, the disk is placed in the computer, and the HIM employee enters the patient's name or identifying information into the computer. The computer software will then reference the index to locate the appropriate point on the individual disk storing the patient's record. The patient's record may then be printed or sent to another station for viewing.

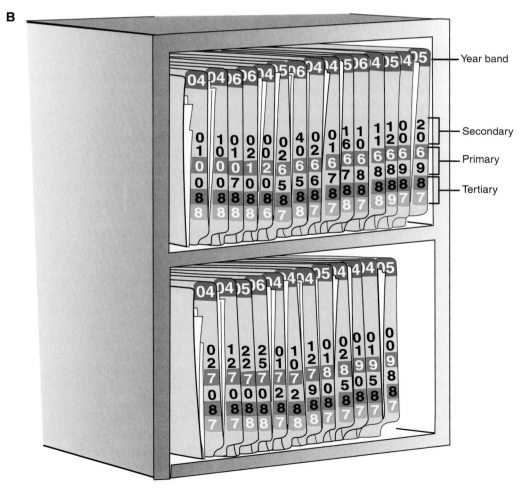

◆ **Figure 8-10,** *cont'd*

Indexing reinforces the importance of organized maintenance of patient health records. Patient files, images, and information must all be linked by the correct identifying information. Failure to accurately index a patient's information results in what we call a *misfile* in a paper-based system. When the patient's electronic records are retrieved, they will not be in the appropriate location. The employee then searches the electronic files for the patient information, just as in a search for physical paper files. When the information is found, it must be relocated (re-indexed) to the appropriate patient or patient visit.

RECORD RETENTION

Now that you have learned the methods of record storage, you should know how long a health care facility must keep health records. The length of time a record is kept by a facility is the **record retention schedule.** Health records must be maintained by a facility to support patient care; meet legal and regulatory requirements; achieve accreditation; allow research, education, and reimbursement; and support facility administration. The duration of record retention differs for the various types of records kept (e.g., laboratory data, radiology reports and films, fetal monitor strips, birth certificates, MPIs) and for different facilities (e.g., physicians' offices, hospitals). Most states have laws mandating how long a facility must maintain health information. In the absence of state law, the facility must follow the federal requirements stipulated by the Centers for Medicare and Medicaid Services (CMS), which is to save them for 5 years. A facility should also consider extending retention time to allow for cases in which malpractice, patient age, or research activity requires review of the record.

The retention time for patient health records (stipulated by law or regulation) may be a specific number of years, or it can be counted from the date of the patient's last encounter. For example, if the retention schedule in a state is 10 years and includes all previous records, when Jane Ryan has an appendectomy at age 20, a broken ankle with repair at age 25, and a motor vehicle accident (MVA) at age 29, the appendectomy record—a previous visit within the 10-year limit—cannot be destroyed until 10 years have passed from the patient's last encounter. On admission for the ankle repair, the appendectomy record would be retained for another 10 years, and the same for the MVA. Jane's records are maintained until the retention time of 10 years has lapsed from her last visit. However, if the retention schedule does not include previous visits, then the appendectomy can be destroyed when the retention period expires. Refer to Figure 8-11 for the retention schedule for health information suggested by the American Health Information Management Association (AHIMA).

Retention Policy

Each HIM department must have a policy explaining how the medical records within the facility are stored. The policy describes which health records are maintained in the department, how each type of record is organized (by number, filing system, or both), the storage medium used (optical disk, microfilm, paper, hard drive), and the length of time each record is to be retained. The retention policy is very important to a facility with many records that may be stored in different locations. The policy must state that a record is maintained on all patients registered to the facility; provide the retention schedule; indicate how the records are identified, organized, or filed; state their location; and document alternative locations or media, if necessary.

Facility Closure

What happens when a facility, physician's office, or clinic closes its operation? Where do the records go? In the event of a facility's closing, the retention schedule remains in effect. The facility must investigate the applicable laws to determine the best method for retaining the records. If the facility or practice is purchased, the records are managed by the new owner. However, if the practice or facility closes, the records must be maintained for the duration of the retention schedule in an appropriate, secure, confidential location.

The facility must notify its patients when it is closing. There are several excellent methods to inform patients of closure. One method is to run an advertisement in the local newspaper explaining the closure and what will happen to the patient records (Figure 8-12). Another method is to notify patients of the closure through letters or notices mailed directly to the patients'

RETENTION SCHEDULE OF HEALTH CARE RECORDS

Type of Health Information	Retention Schedule	
Acute care facility records	Adults	10 years
	Minors	Age of majority + 10 years (or statute of limitations)
Birth, death, surgical procedure registers	Permanently	
X-ray films	5 years	
Fetal monitor strips	10 years after the patient reaches the age of majority	
Master patient index	Permanently	
Diseases index	10 years	
Emergency room register/log	Permanently	
Employee health records	30 years	

◆ **Figure 8-11**

Retention schedule for health care records. Medicare Condition of Participation (MCOP) requires retention of records, films, and scans for at least 5 years. Each provider should develop a retention schedule for records in that facility. (Modified from AHIMA Practice Brief: Retention of Health Information.)

homes. It is also important to post similar notices in and around the facility to notify patients of the closure. Because patient information is critical in the continuity of care, it is important to maintain patient access to the records even after the facility is closed. This may be accomplished by transferring the records to another local facility or physician's office, as appropriate.

FILING FURNITURE

Now that you can identify and file health records, it is time to review the different furniture found in file areas of health care facilities. These include file cabinets, open shelving, revolving systems, and movable shelves.

File Cabinets

A file cabinet (Figure 8-13) can be a vertical or lateral drawer system for filing records. This type of furniture is secure in many ways because it is easily locked, keeps records out of plain sight, and is typically a good way to secure records from fire or water damage. The disadvantages associated with this type of filing furniture are as follows:

■ File cabinets are bulky and require more space than shelving systems.

ince April was $6543 that the Spro
anufacturing Company spent in
e for Rep. Alphonse Traubin, D-NH.
if Thacburn, and his wife Shakira,
comlass to Vancouver, British Co-
BIA for a speech at a two day con-
ence. Traubin spokesman, Kevin
th, also traveled to the conference
an additional $1643 in travel, lodg-
and meals.

Smith said that because Traubin
he conference for the entire time,
the expenses are legally buisness

ut they aren't allowed to pay for the
ips. Atttendence at events is not
mandatory. Some staffers submit
tdated forms that don't indicate, as
e new ones require, whether they
ok their spouses or children along

hat all legal channels will be pro-
ly contacted.

When the Nuclear Energy Inst-
te took Galveston and the other
gressional staffers to France, in
see BUSINESS, B-13

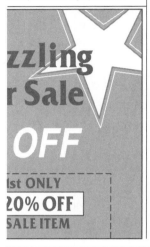

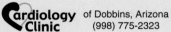

Dr. Fred Davenport

announces the transfer of his practice,
Diamonte Cardiology, to the Cardiology
Clinic of Dobbins, Arizona.

Patients of Dr. Davenport's have had their
records transferred to the offices ot the
Cardiology Clinic of Dobbins, Arizona.

Dr. Davenport thanks the community and
patients who have entrusted their care to
him over the years. Patients are urged to
continue their care at the Cardiology Clinic
of Dobbins, Arizona.

Cardiology Clinic of Dobbins, Arizona
(998) 775-2323

Out-of-town referrals and consultations accepted

Answering Service and 24-Hour #
(998) 775-2323

BLUE CROSS • PRIVATE INSURANCE • MEDICARE
(PARTICIPATING) • HMO and PPO PLANS ACCEPTED

◆ **Figure 8-12**
Newspaper advertisement of facility closure.

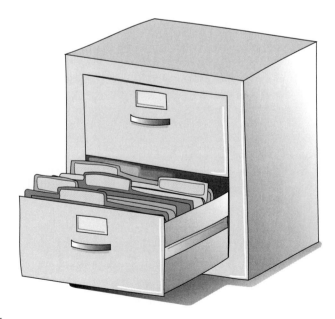

◆ **Figure 8-13**
File cabinet.

- They are not efficient if the department has a large number of records that need to be accessed frequently.
- Only one drawer of records in each file cabinet can be accessed at a time.

When file cabinets face one another in rows, always leave enough room for facing drawers to open. Approximately 5 feet between rows is necessary unless aisle space is not required.

Open Shelves

This type of filing furniture is simply a shelf that is always open to the file area (Figure 8-14). Open shelves allow the filing of many health records on shelves with open access to all records at all times. Open shelves require less space than filing cabinets; they may be 16 inches deep and require an aisle space of only 4 feet. Therefore two shelves can face each other and allow good access with only a 4-foot aisle. The disadvantages are that the records are always visible to visitors in the file area, and they are exposed to potential fire or water damage.

Compressible Shelves

Compressible or movable shelves allow storage of files on shelves that can be compressed so that more shelves will fit in a smaller file space (Figure 8-15). This type of shelving can move back and forth or side to side. This file furniture works well in a file room where space is limited and there are numerous patient files. The problem encountered with this filing furniture is that it provides access only to those sections of the files that are open. If a file area is very busy, compressible units may hinder filing productivity. This furniture also allows some visibility of records to visitors in the file area and potential exposure of the records to fire or water damage.

Revolving File System

A revolving file system looks like a Ferris wheel (Figure 8-16). This system can revolve laterally or horizontally. On a revolving file shelf, a record cannot be retrieved until the relevant file shelf rolls

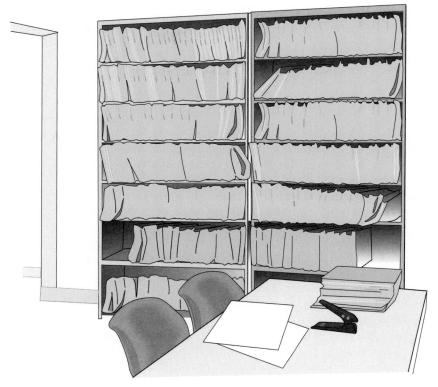

◆ **Figure 8-14**
Open shelves.

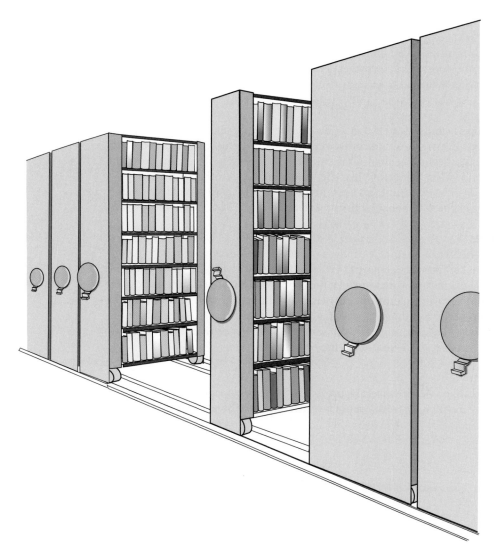

◆ **Figure 8-15**
Compressible shelves.

around to the opening. The system may use a computer to correlate the medical record numbers to a file. When a record is needed, the file identification (MR#) is entered into the system. The revolving system presents the shelf on which the record is located so that it may be pulled from the shelf. This system provides a secure environment for storing records; however, access is limited to only one shelf at a time. In a horizontal revolving system, if the power supply is out, only one shelf can be accessed.

There are many types of file furniture capable of storing health records. Table 8-7 compares the advantages and disadvantages of each type of filing furniture and describes the most appropriate setting for each.

FILE ROOMS

Although there are many types of file furniture for storage of health records, it is important to consider the Occupational Safety and Health Administration (OSHA) space requirements for filing areas. The OSHA requirements specify the appropriate space to provide a safe environment for employees working in the file area. OSHA mandates an aisle at least 3 feet wide between filing units or shelves, and the exit aisle must be at least 5 feet wide. Other requirements specify the amount of space required between the top shelf and the ceiling of the file room (i.e., there should

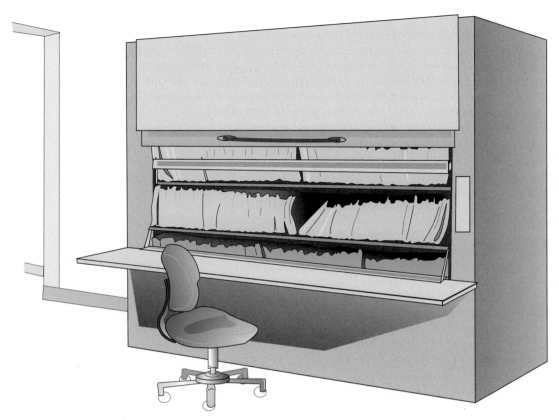

◆ **Figure 8-16**
Revolving file system.

TABLE 8-7	**Advantages and Disadvantages of Filing Equipment**	
FILING EQUIPMENT	**ADVANTAGES**	**DISADVANTAGES**
File cabinets	Protects information from exposure to the environment Conceals information from public view Typically provides ability to lock/secure information	Allows access to only one drawer of information at a time Requires additional space to open for access to information
Open shelves	Allows easy access to records	Open to environment Requires space for aisle access to each shelf
Compressible shelves	Increases file space in small area	Limits access to information
Revolving file system	Accommodates file personnel, reducing time spent looking for file on shelf	Limits access to files

be 18 inches between the top shelf and the ceiling to allow sprinkler systems to function properly if they are used as a security feature).

When you are designing a file area, the first item of business is to measure the file space. Before you can consider cost for filing furniture and other supplies, you must ensure that the area has adequate space to comply with OSHA guidelines to store the files. Do you have a room by itself for files, or will you be using part of the space in the department? If you are relocating a file room, you should measure your existing file area to determine whether the files will fit into the new space. If you plan to order new file furniture, be sure that the new furniture will accommodate all of your files and includes room for growth. When ordering shelves or file cabinets, be sure to calculate the filing space within each shelf unit (see Figures 8-14 and 8-15). Count the number of shelves per unit. This will be important later when you are trying to calculate the correct number of shelves to purchase. If each shelving unit has 8 shelves at a width of 36 inches, you will have 288 inches (8 shelves × 36 inches = 288 inches, or 24 feet) of file space on each shelving unit.

Calculation of file space is equally important if you plan to enlarge or reorganize an existing file area. It may be inaccurate to assume that each record will occupy 1 inch. It is best to measure a sample of files to estimate the number of files that will fit on a shelf. Rather than counting an entire shelf, count the files in several 1-foot sections. For each sample section, note how many records you counted. Then average the total number.

Once you know the average number of records occupying 1 foot of file space, you can calculate the file space needed for the entire room. We can use the answer to the Test Your HI-Q example: Marcus calculated an average of 12.3 records per 1 foot of file space. The next information necessary to determine is the number of years of records that are stored in this location. Assume that at Marcus's facility the file area contains 3 years of files. Knowing the facility's average number of discharges (12,000) allows an approximate calculation of 36,000 files in the file area. Knowing 1 foot equals 12.3 records, you will divide 36,000 by 12.3 to determine 2926.8 or 2927 feet of file space is needed to accommodate 3 years of records at Marcus's facility.

Before ordering furniture, you must determine how many shelves are necessary to store 2927 feet of files. Measure your current file space to determine whether you can use the current furniture. Using the eight-shelf unit that contains 36 inches of file space on each shelf, we know that one shelf unit (eight shelves) can hold 288 inches, or 24 feet of records. For 2927 feet of files, you will need 122 shelving units to accommodate these files (2927 divided by 24 feet for one eight-shelf unit equals 121.95, or 122 shelving units). This calculation is adequate for current files, but it does not allow room for expansion in the future. The facility should plan for an increase in the number of patient files. Planning for an increase by overestimating the necessary space may prevent overcrowding of records in the future. To determine an appropriate amount of growing space, recall how much the files have grown over the past several years. This will help you project space needed for the future storage of records. Sometimes, a facility has a strategic plan for growth, and the financial planners in the facility can provide you with information on expected growth of discharges for the coming years.

If you are planning file space in a new facility, you will need to work with estimations. An easy method for estimating is to contact the HIM professional at facilities in your area providing a similar type of health care. The HIM professional should be able to provide information regarding the facility's chart size, which you can use in your calculations. If another facility does not exist in your area, create a mock chart. A mock chart is a made-up record including an example of each document that could exist in the patient's health record. Keep in mind whether you will require one or more pages for a specific document, such as progress notes, operative reports, and so on. Remember, the length of stay has an impact on the size of a record. After you create a mock chart, measure it. How thick is the record? Multiply this measurement by the number of patient records estimated, and allow enough space in the file area for a specific time period. If you have a space shortage, you will need to evaluate alternative storage methods, which are discussed next.

ALTERNATIVE STORAGE METHODS

It is common for HIM departments to store health records in an alternative site or format, either because of limited space or because the records are inactive. The phrase *activity of patient records* refers to the facility's need to retrieve the record. A record is considered active as long as it is needed within the facility or for patient care. In the paper environment, a patient's health record may be termed *inactive* after it is complete and a specified number of years have passed since it was last needed.

The most common reason that HIM departments need alternative storage is a shortage of filing space in the department. In the paper-record environment, health records can quickly fill all of the filing space available in the HIM department. Health care facilities maintain increasing

Exercise 8-2

Filing

1. The numerical file identification system used to identify an entire family's health record using one number and modifiers is called _____.

2. The physical container used to store the paper-based health record is a _____.

3. An _____ is used to identify or name a file or record so that it can be located in the computer-based health record.

4. _____ and _____ are an alternative storage method for paper records using plastic film.

5. A physical file called an _____ is used to identify an alternate location of a file in the paper-based health care record system.

6. The length of time that a record must be retained is called the record _____ _____.

7. A numerical patient record identification system, which gives the patient a new number for each encounter, is called _____ numbering.

8. A numerical patient record identification system, in which the patient is given a new number for each visit and with each new admission, the previous record is retrieved and filed in the folder with the most recent visit, is called _____ numbering.

9. The filing method of organizing folders in numerical order is _____ _____ filing.

10. A filing method in which the patient's medical record number is separated into sets for filing and the first set of numbers are tertiary, the second set is secondary, and the last set is primary is called _____ _____ filing.

11. In a _____ _____ system, the patient record is filed under the same number for all visits.

12. In the absence of state laws regarding retention of health care records, CMS requires that records be maintained for
    a. 10 years
    b. 21 years
    c. 30 years
    d. 5 years

13. Identify which of the following is not an alphabetical filing rule:
    a. Suffixes are considered after the middle name or initial.
    b. All punctuation and possessives are ignored.
    c. Abbreviations and shortened names are ignored.
    d. Personal names are filed last name, followed by first name, then middle initial.

14. Color coding of the numerical identification on the end tab of a file folder
    a. prevents messy files
    b. aids the identification of misfiles
    c. is mandatory under JCHAO standards
    d. warrants approval form the safety committee

15. If a shelf unit is 36 inches wide and has eight shelves, how many linear inches of filing space are available?
    a. 36
    b. 288
    c. 240
    d. 272

16. On a shelving unit that is 30 inches wide with 8 shelves, how many linear inches of file space are available?
    a. 240
    b. 288
    c. 24
    d. 300

(continued)

Exercise 8-2

17. If the average thickness of a record is 1.5 inches, how many records can you store on a shelving unit that is 30 inches wide with eight shelves?
    a. 240
    b. 288
    c. 160
    d. 80

18. As the new supervisor of Diamonte Hospital, you must order new filing furniture to store 12,000 annual outpatient charts. After measuring, you determine that four charts equal 1 inch of linear file space. How many 36-inch wide, eight-shelf units must you buy to store these records?
    a. 288 shelving units
    b. 10 shelving units
    c. 11 shelving units
    d. 42 shelving units

19. Shelley is the new health information management file room supervisor at Diamonte Hospital. Upon entering the file room, she notices that the files are cramped and there is no room on the shelves to file any new charts. Shelley determines that it is critically necessary to order additional shelving to increase the file shelf space to store all of Diamonte's records. The facility has approximately 15,000 discharges each year. They keep 2 years of paper records on site. The average thickness of a record is 1 inch. They currently have 30 shelving units that each have eight shelves and are 36 inches wide. How many records can they currently store in this filing furniture?
    a. 288 records
    b. 2880 records
    c. 8640 records
    d. 15,000 records

20. Shelley is the new health information management file room supervisor at Diamonte Hospital. Upon entering the file room she notices that the files are cramped and there is no room on the shelves to file any new charts. Shelley determines that it is critically necessary to order additional shelving to increase the file shelf space to store all of Diamonte's records. The facility has approximately 15,000 discharges each year. They keep 2 years of paper records on site. The average thickness of a record is 1 inch. They currently have 30 shelving units that each have eight shelves and are 36 inches wide. How many additional filing units should Shelley order?
    a. 22
    b. 23
    c. 52
    d. 53

21. Compare the following file numbering or identification systems listing the pros and cons of each: alphabetical, unit MR#, serial MR#, serial-unit MR#, or family medical record number.

22. Explain how to locate a record using terminal-digit filing.

23. The file room in a recently acquired clinic (which filed records alphabetically) must be converted to terminal digit. List the steps involved in the conversion.

24. Given the file space area of 25 feet × 40 feet with a ceiling height of 10 feet (use grid paper; each block equals 1 foot), determine which filing furniture is best to store 40,000 records, averaging 1-inch thickness. Keep in mind OSHA requirements for aisle and exit space.

25. File the following names in alphabetical order:

P. B. Josh	Lauren McIntyre
Drew B. LaPeu	Amanda Modelle
Hannah Curelle	Beth Katerina Von Amberg
Cecelia Lower	Aubrey Bartolo, III
Ginger Dugas	Sister Gabrielle Brown
Wm. Bill Matata	Brett Thomasse, Jr.

(continued)

Using your knowledge of how numbers/identifiers are assigned to patient files in each of the following numbering systems, answer the questions below.

Numbering System	Next MR# Assigned
Unit	123456
Serial	234567
Serial-unit	345678
Family unit	456789

Scenario: Green Oak Hospital uses a serial numbering system to identify patient health records. Jane Creason is admitted to Green Oak facility for repair of a broken ankle. On a previous admission to Green Oak for a tonsillectomy, Jane was assigned MR# 012345.

26. What number will be assigned to Jane for the broken ankle admission, using a serial numbering system?

27. If Green Oak used a unit numbering system, what medical record number would be assigned for the broken ankle admission?

amounts of patient health information. Remember, the patient health record must be retained for several reasons: state and federal laws, the continuation of patient care, reimbursement, accreditation, potential litigation, research, and education.

A likely solution that provides a significant amount of room for new files is to store the patient records in a new location or in a format that takes up less space. When space is limited within a facility, sometimes even active records are relocated. Microfilm, optical imaging, and on-site and off-site storage are alternative storage choices available to health care facilities.

MICROFILM

Microfilm, simply described, is the reproduction of the original paper record into miniature pictures stored on plastic film, either on reels or on sheets. To microfilm patient records, each page must be carefully prepared. The pages in each record must be free of staples, tears, and adhesives. Failure to prepare the documents before scanning the images to microfilm can cause the document to become jammed in the machine or torn, or it may obscure the image. The prepared pages are scanned, both back and front as necessary, into the microfilm machine, much like a copy machine. The image of each page is stored on film, and the film is developed to produce the final microfilm product (Figure 8-17).

At first glance, microfilm looks like a negative from pictures taken with a camera. Further study reveals that the image is a small picture of the original document that was scanned through the machine. After processing, the images are assembled on roll film or sliced into small strips of

Hit-Bit

Active Versus Inactive Records

Active records are regularly accessed for patient care. *Inactive records* are those that are rarely accessed for patient care or other activity.

film and put into a jacket. The film that is sliced and put into jackets is also known as **microfiche.** Careful attention is required to ensure that each page in the patient record is scanned. Loss of one page of a record could eliminate valuable patient information and ultimately affect the completeness of the patient's record or compromise future care provided to the patient. Likewise, once the image is processed onto microfilm, the image cannot be updated or altered. A facility should microfilm only complete patient records. Like other formats, microfilmed records are carefully labeled with the patient's identifying name or number. Each roll or sheet of film is labeled so that HIM employees are able to determine which patient records are stored on that roll or sheet. In the file cabinet, microfiche records are filed in the same way that files were stored in their original format, using either alphabetical, straight numerical, or TD filing systems. When microfilm is stored on roll film, the rolls may be numbered and additional methods are necessary to correlate the records to the roll film. Also, when roll film is used, a facility may choose to have two copies of each roll available at the facility, and possibly even one master copy stored off-site, as back-up in case one of the rolls is spliced or splits as it is processed through the microfilm reader machine.

Microfilm Equipment

When microfilm is used to store records, some equipment is necessary to maintain access to the files. A printer is needed to reproduce a paper copy of the patient's record for release to another

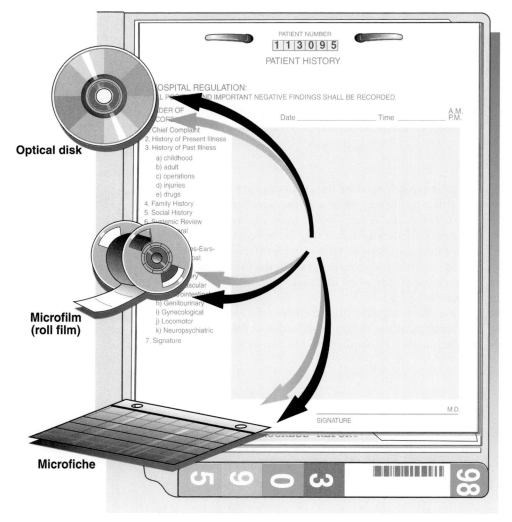

◆ **Figure 8-17**
Microfilm and microfiche.

facility or authorized individual. The microfilm or microfiche health record must be maintained in appropriate storage equipment. Microfilm should be stored in a file cabinet or drawer capable of being locked or kept enclosed in a locked room. The cabinets should also protect the records from the environment and from temperature and water damage.

It is important to remember the following:

- Microfilming can be performed at an on-site or off-site location.
- If an off-site contractor is chosen, the company is responsible for maintaining the confidentiality of the information while it is being processed.
- The contracted company must also allow the necessary access to the information in a timely manner should it be required.
- The quality of the microfilm must be checked before any of the original records are destroyed.

Document Imaging

Document imaging is the reproduction of the original paper record into miniature pictures stored on **optical disk.** As with microfilm, each page (front and back) of the original health record must be prepared for scanning. When the original pages of the patient health record are scanned into a computer system, the record may be saved on a disk similar to a computer CD. The actual scanning process is analogous to sending a piece of paper through a copy machine. In this format, the machine, called a **scanner,** does not produce the image onto another piece of paper or plastic; instead, the image is digitally stored in a computer system, on magnetic tape, or on optical disk. This method of storage saves a significant amount of space because it eliminates the need for paper storage (Figure 8-18).

Interestingly, this form of storage does not typically require a separate MPI system to locate the patient's health record. Patient identification by name or number is still a very important factor in the indexing of the patient information. The medical record number is still used to name or identify the records; however, an optical imaging system is capable of searching for the patient's health information by patient name, discharge date, or any other identifying data known to the system. Likewise, if one page of the record was not scanned with the original record, it can be added later and remain identifiable by the system as a part of the patient's original record within the system. This system allows for the scanning of records before they are complete. Loose work, transcription, and sometimes signatures can be added at a later date.

This format requires the use of a reader and printer to reproduce a paper copy of the patient's health record. However, some systems are capable of electronically sending the image to another authorized location for reproducing a paper copy.

ONSITE STORAGE

Space may limit the number of records that can be stored in the HIM department. Therefore some facilities maintain their records in storage space in a separate room or building owned by the facility. This concept is called *onsite storage.* Storing medical records on site allows a facility to maintain security, confidentiality, and timely access to its health care records. The HIM department simply relocates specified records to the new location, ensuring that the records are in a secure environment and organized as they were in the HIM department. The new location of the files should be updated in the MPI and in the department policy and procedure manual.

Onsite storage of health records is usually the least expensive method for alternative storage. It is also the alternative allowing the HIM custodian to maintain direct control over the files. Costs associated with this type of storage include additional filing furniture, improvements to the environment, employee time, and filing supplies. If a facility chooses onsite storage, it is very important that a plan of action be developed so that the transferring of the records happens in a secure, timely, and organized manner.

OFFSITE STORAGE

Offsite storage is a system in which the original health records are stored at a separate location outside the facility that may be owned and operated by some party other than the facility. The offsite company or storage location operates much like the file room in the health care facility. Patient

Computer Storage

On the shelves pictured here (4 units, 7 shelves per unit, 36 inches wide), let's assume there are approximately 100,000 sheets of paper in the stored records.

100,000 pages can be stored on 3.2 gigabytes.
  1 gigabyte = 1,073,741,824 bytes
  Therefore 3.2 × 1,073,741,824 = 3,435,973,836.8 bytes
  ÷ 1 MB (1,048,576 bytes) = 3276.8 MB
  For ZIP drive, divide by 250 MB.
  For CD, divide by 750 MB.

As technology continues to improve, storage options will change and more information will be stored on smaller devices. One example of this is the USB drive that can store from 128 MB to 4 to 6 GB

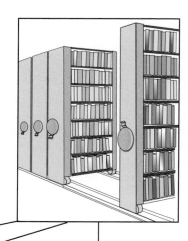

It would take 14 ZIP disks to store this information.

A ZIP disk can hold up to 250 MB.

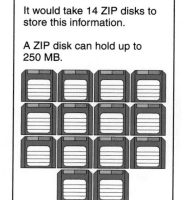

It would take 5 CDs to store this information.

A CD can hold up to 750 MB.

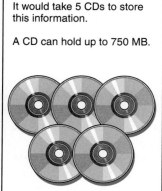

It would take one 12″ optical disk to store this information.

One 12″ optical disk can hold up to 3.2 gigs.

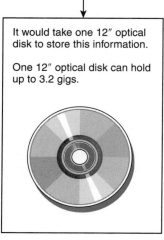

◆ **Figure 8-18**
Computer storage.

health records can be requested when needed for patient care, release of information, record review, billing, or any other appropriate reason, whereupon they are brought to the facility. The records no longer take up space at the facility. The records are no longer under the direct control of the facility's HIM custodian but are relocated to another secure environment. Within this new environment, the facility HIM custodian must ensure that appropriate measures are taken to secure and organize the patient records.

There are many things to consider before choosing to store records off site. The offsite storage facility signs a contract with the health care facility to maintain its health care records. All of the

Hit-Bit

Centralized Versus Decentralized Files

In a health care facility, centralized and decentralized file areas reflect the number of separate locations within or outside the facility that store health records.

A *centralized file area* describes a file room where *all* health records for the facility are in one location.

A *decentralized file* area describes one or more locations outside the HIM department or outside the facility that are used to store the health records of a facility.

facility's concerns should be addressed in the contract. The contract must be reviewed thoroughly and clarified if anything is unclear. The following is a list of issues to consider before choosing an offsite facility:

- Be sure that the site has appropriate security for the storage of health information.
- Personally go to the site, and examine the security system.
- What are the operating hours?
- How will you request a record in an emergency, for patient care, or for other review? Do you have to telephone an employee or fax a request, or can you order the chart on-line via a secure site?
- How often will the requested records be delivered to your facility?
- How will records be transported from the off-site facility to yours and back again? In secure vehicles, taxi, fax only, courier?
- Is there a charge for immediate delivery of a record in case of emergency?
- How will the company charge your facility—by linear foot of storage space or by record storage type?
- How will the company store your records: in boxes or open shelving? Do they have a computerized chart locator system?
- Is the storage facility climate controlled?
- What are the training procedures for their employees?
- What are the safety and confidentiality procedures?
- Does the facility have online access to track a request or to view the history of a particular file as it moves back and forth between the off-site storage and the health care facility?
- What is the vendor's policy for inadvertent disclosures? How soon will you be notified if one of your charts is inadvertently delivered to another facility?
- Does the storage company have a disaster recovery plan?

SELECTION OF STORAGE METHOD

Before choosing an alternative storage method, analyze the amount of records that you plan to store and the length of time that you plan to store the records. This analysis should focus on the initial cost of storing the records and include maintenance of the records in the storage site. For example, if you choose microfilm or optical imaging, you will have to consider the cost of converting the records, storing the records in the new format, and purchasing reader-printer machines (including maintenance contracts) to produce paper images of the records. Onsite storage is ideal if your facility has adequate space. With offsite storage, the length of time that you will have to pay the offsite storage company to maintain the records is a factor. The annual cost to store 1 year's worth of health records in an offsite storage company over the length of the retention period may eventually be more than the original price of microfilming or optical imaging. This concept is called the *pay-back period*.

CHART LOCATOR SYSTEMS

Health information is useful only if it is available for review. A **chart locator system** keeps track of the location of all records in the health care facility. Many people in the health care facility have authorized need of and access to patient records. As a result, records are not always on the shelf in the permanent file location. Records may be signed out to a health care unit when a patient is readmitted. Records may be requested for research or for patient follow-up care. The quality management (QM) department may need to review records to ensure that the care provided to the patient was appropriate. Copies of records may be requested for litigation, which requires removing the health record file from the file system in order to copy it for authorized users. Because all of this use is necessary to the function of the facility, it is important that the HIM department be able to locate and retrieve patient records.

A chart locator system allows the HIM department to keep track of the facility's patient health records. Records that are removed from the department or from the normal processing flow in the department are "signed out" to the location to which they are being sent. Once the records are

Exercise 8-3

Alternative Storage Methods

1. A copier-like machine called a _____ is used to convert paper-based records into digital images for a computerized health care record.
2. The machine used to input a paper document into a computerized imaging system is called a
   a. copier
   b. indexer
   c. mapper
   d. scanner
3. Images stored in a document imaging system must be _____ for identification and future retrieval.
   a. copied
   b. indexed
   c. mapped
   d. e-mailed
4. Compare the following alternative storage methods, listing the pros and cons of each: microfilm, document imaging, onsite storage, offsite storage.
5. List important things to consider before choosing an alternative storage method.

returned, they must be "signed in" to the department. This allows anyone in the HIM department to easily determine when a record is available for review and when it is out of the department. A chart locator system also allows faster retrieval of a record from another location in an urgent time of need—for example, for a patient care emergency. It has been said that the HIM department is only as good as the information it can provide. If the HIM department can easily access and retrieve information, then the department is functioning productively.

MANUAL SYSTEMS

Manual systems for chart location of the paper record use an **outguide** and a log or index card box to identify that a patient's health record file folder has been removed and sent to a new location. An outguide is a physical file card or jacket identifying that the record is away from its expected location (Figure 8-19).

The log or index card box is used as a quick alphabetical reference of all records that are signed out of the HIM department. When a patient's health record is needed in another location, the HIM file clerk completes an outguide slip as shown in Figure 8-19 to put in place of the file when it is removed. The outguide informs anyone who looks for the patient's file that it has been moved

Hit-Bit

Audit Trail

Chart locator systems apply primarily to the paper health record. In a computerized or computer-based environment, records are tracked using an *audit trail*. The computer system keeps a log (known as the *audit trail*) of all transactions by recording the name of the employee performing the task, what information is sent and to which location, the recipient, the date, the time, and other pertinent facts. This audit trail is an important tool in the computer environment for tracking the use of patient health records and information.

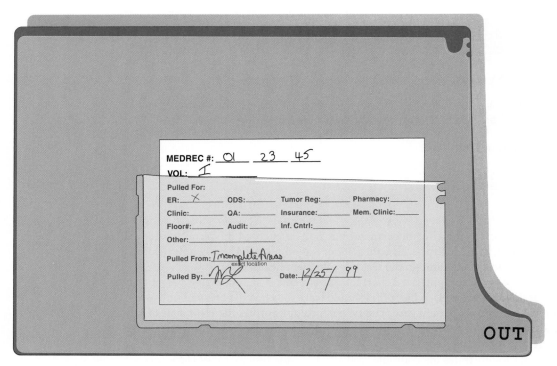

◆ **Figure 8-19**
Outguide identifies a record removed from its usual location.

to a new location. Outguides prevent HIM employees from spending unnecessary time searching for a file.

How does the manual system operate? When the HIM department receives a request for a health record, the clerk retrieves the patient's medical record number by looking up the patient's name in the MPI. The clerk locates the health record in the department. This may be the clerk's thought process: Is the record old enough to be in the permanent files? Is it just a week old, in which case it is probably in the incomplete record area? Is it a recent discharge and possibly in the coding area? Once the record is located and pulled, the clerk will sign the record out to the new location, meaning the clerk notes where the record is going. In a manual chart locator system, duplicate outguide forms are completed with the following information: medical record number, discharge date(s), the location to which the record is being sent, and the date the record was sent. The duplicate copy of the outguide is filed alphabetically in a box (or card file) for reference. The department may also require that the person requesting the records sign for them on pickup.

COMPUTERIZED SYSTEMS

Computerized chart locator systems can eliminate the need for physical outguides and cards, although some HIM departments simultaneously use the manual chart locator system and the computer system. In a computerized chart locator system, the new location to which the record is being signed out is entered into the computer system. Therefore if a chart is pulled from the permanent file location and sent to a clinic, in the computerized chart locator system that record is signed out to the clinic. The chart locator system must accurately reflect the current location of each patient record at all times.

Sign-in is done to check records back into the department, which involves updating the computerized chart locator system to note that the record has been returned. On a daily basis, records returned to the department must be signed in and placed back into their appropriate location. It is also very important to perform a regular (e.g., weekly) audit of the health records that are checked out to each location. For example, if 10 records are signed out to the clinic and, upon inspection of the clinic, you do not locate all 10 records, it is necessary to search for the missing

Hit-Bit

Chart Locator System

As a rule of thumb, in a large HIM department, all records should be listed in the chart locator system as the record progresses through each function in the HIM department. When a record moves from one location, it must be "signed out" of that location and "signed in" to the new location. This method allows personnel to determine the location of a patient file without spending time searching through the various sections of the HIM department.

records. Did they come back to the HIM department but not get checked in? Were the records transferred to a unit within your facility because the patient was admitted? Always know the location of your records to ensure and maintain the security of patient health records.

A beneficial feature of some computerized chart locator systems is an automated prompt for the return of patient files. For example, patient files should leave the HIM department only when they are needed for continuity of patient care. The system prompt notifies the HIM staff of any files that were due back in the department but not yet signed in on the chart locator system. This prompt cues the clerk to locate the record.

The following scenario illustrates the computerized chart locator system. Mary Davidson has been a patient at the Diamonte facility several times over the past 5 years. In the course of her treatment, physicians have noted that Ms. Davidson is allergic to penicillin. On one particular evening in October, Mary is brought to the emergency room (ER) unconscious. Review of her personal belongings alerted health care workers to her name and DOB. The ER makes a routine call to the HIM department for her old records. The HIM department clerk enters "Mary Davidson" into the MPI system, and several patients with that name appear on the screen. Because the clerk has the DOB, she can easily check the MPI to find the correct patient file. With the medical record number for Mary Davidson, the clerk goes to the file room to look for the old record. She goes to the appropriate shelf in the terminal-digit order, but the record is not there. The clerk then returns to the computer to enter Ms. Davidson's medical record number in the chart locator system (Figure 8-20).

On doing so, the clerk learns that this record is signed out to the QM department for review. Knowing the routine of the facility, the clerk can go directly to the section of records set aside for the QM staff and retrieve Mary Davidson's record. The clerk then makes an entry into the chart locator system indicating that the record is being sent to the ER and on return to the HIM department should be returned to the QM staff record section. Appropriate notes should also be made to tell the QM section that this record has been removed.

Hit-Bit

Electronic Health Record Security

In a **computer-based patient record** environment, HIM file clerks are able to send a copy, a viewable image, of the patient's record while maintaining the original in the computer system. Once a patient's record is in the system, it can be shared by many users simultaneously. HIM professionals should be aware of the security concerns in the computer environment. Patients' health records must be secure from potential for loss, computer tampering, deletion, and unauthorized access.

Exercise 8-4

Chart Locator Systems

1. A _____ is used to identify the location of records within a facility.
2. A manual chart locater system must use _____ to hold the place of the original record.
   a. spacers
   b. outguides
   c. indexers
   d. blank files
3. A manual chart locator system maintains more information about a charts location(s) than a computerized system.
   a. True
   b. False
4. Diamonte Hospital uses a computerized chart locator system. The ER has requested an old (paper) chart on Mr. Tom Jones. Prior to bringing the chart to the ER, the HIM clerk must
   a. initial the chart.
   b. request verification form Mr. Jones previous attending physician.
   c. sign the chart out of the HIM department to the ER.
   d. call the Diamonte attorney.
5. When Mr. Jones is discharged form the ER and his old (paper) chart is returned to the HIM department,
   a. the record must be signed back into the HIM department.
   b. the record must be initialed.
   c. the facility attorney must be contacted.
   d. the record should be shredded.

SECURITY OF HEALTH INFORMATION

Storage of health information involves its security. HIM professionals are considered custodians of patients' health information. They are responsible for ensuring that the information is complete, timely, accurate, and secure. HIM practitioners also ensure the physical security of health information. Security issues related to the storage of health records include damage of records by fire, water, theft, tampering, and destruction. Every HIM department has policies to safeguard records from these hazards. It is the specific responsibility of HIM practitioners and all delegated employees to safeguard this information. Careful forethought and preparation for security of health records can prevent every HIM practitioner's worst nightmare.

DISASTER PLANNING

Unfortunately, there are few solutions for a nightmare once it occurs. However, careful forethought and policies can be established by facilities to protect health information. This is called *disaster planning*. Disaster planning is a method for dealing with catastrophes and other emergencies that can adversely affect the normal performance of the health care environment. For example, a disaster can be a large number of patients' requiring medical attention as a result of an explosion or a plane crash. In this situation, the increased number of patients requiring treatment would require implementation of a plan to handle their care and processing in a timely manner. Disasters include explosion and bomb threats, power failures, earthquakes, hurricanes, tornadoes, flooding, fires, patient abduction, and theft. All JCAHO-accredited facilities are required to maintain a disaster plan. Facilities must also educate HIM employees on the security procedures and make sure that they are prepared to follow procedure if a disaster occurs.

Security of health records is mandated by regulatory and accreditation agencies. HIM practitioners must protect all health information, including records; diagnosis, procedure, and physician

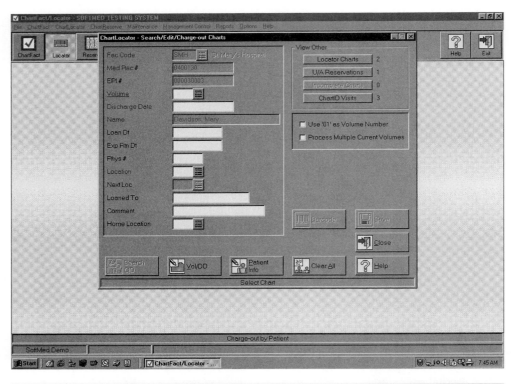

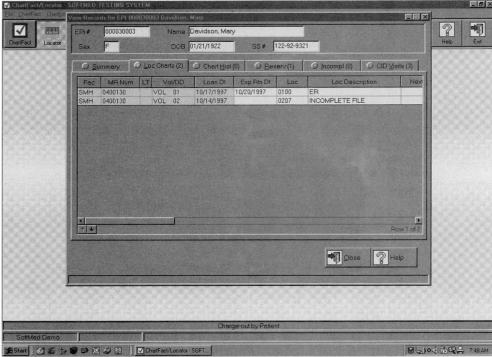

◆ **Figure 8-20**
Chart locator screens. (Courtesy SoftMed Systems, Inc., Bethesda, MD.)

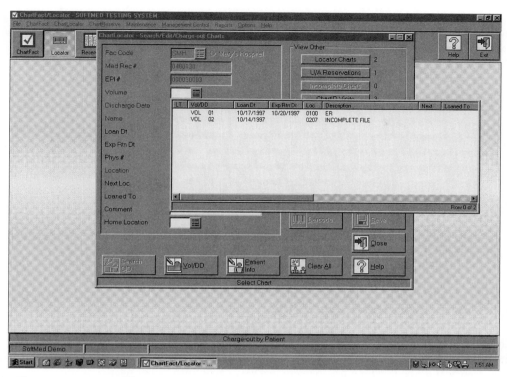

◆ **Figure 8-20,** *cont'd*

Hit-Bit

Health Information Management Nightmares

Read these two health information management (HIM) nightmare scenarios, and you can see the importance of taking precautions with patient records.

Case 1. Your facility is caught unprepared during an unexpected torrential rainstorm, on a Sunday afternoon. While entering the HIM department Monday morning, you notice puddles of water on the floor in the file room. Further inspection reveals that the file room had been flooded with 16 inches of water.

Case 2. The HIM department receives a request for a patient record from the emergency room. After thorough search of the files, department, and facility, the HIM practitioner is unable to locate the requested patient record. Furthermore, failure to provide this patient record in a timely manner results in the patient's being treated with a medication to which the patient is allergic. The patient dies as a result of this treatment. When it is finally located, the patient's previous record documented the patient's allergy.

---

indices; the MPI; computerized health information databases; x-ray films; and admission, discharge, and transfer logs.

SECURITY FROM FIRE

Providing protection from fire for the health information environment can prevent irreversible damage to the facility's health records. Some of the systems and barriers that can assist in the protection from fire are chemical systems, sprinkler systems, fire walls, fire compartments, and fire extinguishers.

Chemical systems deplete the oxygen from the air in an area where a fire exists. File rooms and computer facilities may be equipped with this type of system. The chemical system is designed to sense fire and release a chemical that removes oxygen from the air in the room. Removing the oxygen smothers the fire to prevent further damage to files or facility. (All personnel need to leave the area immediately when the alarm sounds.)

Building structures such as fire walls or fire compartments are designed to contain a fire within a facility. Fire walls prevent a fire from moving in a parallel direction on a particular floor of the building. Recall your last visit to a health care facility: As you were walking down the hallway, you may have passed through double doors in which the doors were held open by magnets on each wall. When the fire alarm is triggered in a health care facility with fire walls, those double doors close to seal the fire and prevent it from spreading to other areas of the facility. A fire compartment is a structure in a building in which all sides of a room or area are protected by fire barriers. In other words, the walls, ceiling, and floor are all fire resistant. If a fire begins in a fire compartment, the compartment contains the fire; likewise, if the fire is outside the compartment, the contents within the compartment are protected from the fire. A fire compartment is the ideal solution to protect the permanent file area or your central computer system if a fire occurs in another part of the facility.

Sprinkler systems release water to extinguish fire when activated by heat or smoke. When a sprinkler system is used to safeguard files, it is important to have at least 18 inches of clearance between the top of the file space and the ceiling. Failure to keep these areas clear prevents the water sprinklers from extinguishing the fire at a lower level. In the event of a fire, sprinkler systems may extinguish the fire and cause minimal water damage to your records.

All health care facilities are equipped with fire extinguishers. HIM employees must be familiar with the location of the nearest fire extinguisher. Employees must be able to operate the fire extinguishers in case of emergency. It is possible for a fire to begin in a very small trash can or near an electrical outlet. Using a fire extinguisher, the fire can easily be controlled without activating a sprinkler system or chemical system.

SECURITY FROM WATER DAMAGE

Water damage to health records, whether paper based or computerized, can occur because of flooding, storms, or fire control. A plan must be established to protect health information from water damage. For example, is your facility in an area where flooding is common? Some options for this scenario may be to relocate the file area to a higher floor of the facility, elevate the file room a few feet, or, if the need arises, be capable of activating an emergency plan to move records on low shelves to a higher location in the facility. Health records maintained in file cabinets or on shelves that are closed or covered also must be considered for protection from flooding. Although damage to file cabinets from a sprinkler system is usually minimal, sprinkler systems cause damage to open shelving. In case of flooding, the bottom drawers in file cabinets are likely to flood. Evaluate the health record environment and the potential for flood or water damage. Remember to protect computer terminals and to have a plan in case of emergency.

On a positive note, processes exist to assist in the restoration of paper health records that are damaged by water. If paper records are soaked with water or other fluid, be sure to act immediately to restore and protect the information. Once the paper records dry, the opportunity to salvage them may be lost. Remember wet paper may be salvaged, but records destroyed by fire are gone forever. Be proactive; contact some disaster-recovery companies. Meeting with these companies before disaster strikes provides information for the department that you might not have considered otherwise. The companies can supply references to other facilities that have used their services. Proactive conversations can be very useful to your facility in a disaster. You will know whom to contact, how long it will take them to arrive at your facility, and other helpful information to secure or preserve your health records.

SECURITY FROM THEFT OR TAMPERING

The issues to consider when protecting health records from theft or tampering are the location of the health records, access to health records, and security. Health information, both paper and electronic, must be protected from theft or tampering by parties both within and outside the facility. Within a facility, only authorized, appropriate personnel should have access to patient health information. Paper documents are secured by allowing release of the original record from the HIM department only if it is needed for the patient's treatment. The HIM department maintains appropriate measures to track the location of patient records (discussed earlier in the section on the chart locator system). Other review of a patient's record must occur within the HIM department and is allowed only if the person reviewing the record is authorized to do so.

How do you maintain the security of the paper record when it leaves the HIM department? HIM professionals cannot follow every patient record checked out to every location in a facility. Therefore it is important to have policies and procedures in place to secure the information to the best of your ability. This security may be achieved by notifying others of the policy and procedure for security of information, by performing regular in-service training for facility employees to inform them of the rules governing health information, and by restricting the reasons for which a patient's health record is allowed to leave the department. Inservice training and policies are discussed under training and development (see Chapter 14).

Additional security measures include

- After office hours, the HIM department is closed and all access doors locked, and only those people authorized to enter the department are allowed entrance. Anyone with a key to your area must be aware of all HIM policies and procedures regarding the appropriate use of health information.
- Areas may also be protected by a key code entry system. Access codes are assigned only to appropriate employees or physicians. After hours, an authorized physician can gain access to any incomplete health records with this code.
- A swipe badge security feature allows entry to the HIM department only with the appropriate access card, which is assigned to authorized physicians or employees.
- Computer passwords assigned to authorized users allow the facility to limit and monitor the persons who access health information.
- Biometric technology, such as fingerprinting and retinal scanning, is also a means for limiting access to health records. With this technology, the system scans a person's fingerprint or retina to evaluate his or her authority to enter an area or gain access to a system.
- Cameras are another security feature found in health care facilities. In areas where there is increased need for security, cameras monitored by the facility's security personnel guard against unauthorized entry.

For computerized health information, a facility must secure records when transferring files from one system to another within or outside of the facility. When upgrading or changing computer software or systems, patient health information is transferred from one system to another. Copying of records from one system to another is acceptable; however, the HIM department must supervise this type of data transfer. Additionally, the department must validate that patient information is not deleted in the transfer. Failure to maintain complete patient information may affect future patient care. Likewise, an incomplete medical record may not be admissible in court as evidence in the event of litigation. Maintain an index of the old system to verify accuracy of the new.

Computerized health information must be protected from sabotage (e.g., attack by a computer virus). Equipment should be secure, and precautions should be taken to prevent others from accessing the system. It is also important to ensure that the facility can update current systems and still retrieve information from obsolete systems. Otherwise, much time and energy are spent converting information from one system to another.

DESTRUCTION OF HEALTH INFORMATION

There are circumstances in which it is appropriate to destroy health information. For example, records (stored on paper, microfilm, or electronic formats) may be destroyed at the completion of the retention period or when paper-based records are successfully transferred to another medium, such as microfilm, diskette, or optical disk. However, HIM employees must prevent negligent destruction. In a paper-record environment, a common method of destroying health information is the shredding or incineration of the paper document. The destruction must occur in a confidential manner. It should be done in the presence of a credentialed custodian of the HIM department or the delegate. Do not leave health information to be destroyed without the proper supervision. If a vendor is chosen, do they use a third party for shredding? Is the third party a business associate (Health Insurance Portability and Accountability Act [HIPAA] rule)? Do you have a choice to recycle? What is their procedure for destruction? How and when will you receive written confirmation or a destruction certificate (HIPAA rule)?

In the computerized environment, destruction of health information may include entering a virus into the computer software system, destroying the equipment or software used to retrieve the health information, or removing the information from the system.

To prevent premature destruction of health information in the paper environment, several measures must be taken. Employees should be aware of the appropriate content of the health record, so the pertinent and valuable patient information is not inadvertently thrown out. Likewise, the employees should be aware of the record retention schedule for all materials in the HIM department. If the facility has chosen to store records in an alternative format, the finished product—microfilm, diskette, or optical images—must be reviewed to ensure that all of the information is intact before the original paper record is destroyed. Once a paper record is destroyed, it cannot be recovered.

For computerized health information, a backup file of all health information in all systems must be completed daily. The backup copy allows information to be restored up to the time that the backup was created. For instance, if you are typing a 10-page report, it is wise to save the report each time you step away from the computer or at certain intervals in the report. By saving the information, you will be able to retrieve it when you return to the system. A procedure called *backup* is performed daily in health care facilities. The backup file copies the information from the computer systems in the facility. If the system crashes, at least the facility will have all of the information necessary to restore the system to the previous day's business.

Computerized health information should be maintained in an environment that supports the use of computers. The HIM department must maintain the computerized equipment so that it is free from harm by temperature, water, and other environmental effects. These considerations also apply to microfilm and optical disk storage. Microfilm and optical disks can be damaged by intense heat. Computers are affected by temperatures as well. Water can damage a computer and cause loss of function and information. Falling objects can damage computer equipment and disks, and liquids spilled on keyboards or hard drives can impair or destroy a system.

RESTORING INFORMATION LOST INADVERTENTLY

What can be done when health records are lost or destroyed inadvertently? It is important to have a plan of action. In a computerized record system, daily backups of the information in the system should allow full recovery of all patient information (prior to backup). In the event of inadvertent destruction of paper records, the only information that can be reproduced is the duplicate paper documents maintained by allied health departments within the facility. For example, the laboratory and radiology departments usually maintain a duplicate copy of reports, the transcription department or service may be able to recover transcription of any dictated reports, and in some instances the billing office may maintain a file including patient information. As a last-resort effort, a facility may also find information in the attending physician's office. Often, the attending physician needs copies of patient information for follow-up care or to bill for services. Obtaining a copy of information sent to the physician can assist in the effort to recover this information.

Exercise 8-5

Security of Health Information

1. To prepare for unexpected events such as a bomb threat, hurricane, or flood, a facility should routinely exercise which of the following policies?

(continued)

Exercise 8-5

  a. Confidentiality
  b. Release of information
  c. Disaster planning
  d. Code blue
2. Which of the following methods assist security of records on a computerized system?
  a. Microfilm
  b. Data dictionary
  c. Scanning
  d. Routine backups
3. Medical records should never be destroyed.
  a. True
  b. False
4. List some of the ways water can be a threat to medical records.
5. List three methods used to protect records from fire.

Matching

6. ___ computer-based patient records
7. ___ computerized records
8. ___ serial
9. ___ unit
10. ___ serial unit
11. ___ family unit
12. ___ index
13. ___ scanner
14. ___ retention schedule
15. ___ microfilm

A. an alternative method for storing records
B. a file identification system in which patients receive the same number for all admissions
C. a file identification system in which the patient receives a new number for each subsequent admission
D. a file identification system that assigns the same number to an entire family, uniquely identifying each member with a modifier
E. a file identification system in which the patient receives a new number for each subsequent admission; however, each previous admission is brought forward and filed with the most recent visit.
F. a method of identifying patient records in a computer-based system
G. the length of time required for maintenance of records
H. a copier-like piece of equipment used to input paper records in a document imaging system
I. a document imaging system
J. a system of patient health records that uses a database

■ SUGGESTED READING

Abdelhak, Mervat, Sara Grostick, Mary Alice Hanken, and Ellen Jacobs. *Health Information: Management of a Strategic Resource.* 2nd ed. Philadelphia: Saunders, 2001.

Brandt, Mary and Harry Rhodes. "Protecting Patient Information after Facility Closure" (updated). AHIMA Practice Brief. *Journal of AHIMA* 70.3 (1999 March) <http://library.ahima.org/xpedio/groups/public/documents/ahima/pub_bok2_000585.html>.

Claeys, Therese. *Medical Filing,* 2nd ed. Albany, NY: Delmar, 1997.

Huffman, Edna K. *Health Information Management.* 10th ed. Berwyn, IL.: Physicians' Record Company, 1994.

CHAPTER ACTIVITIES

CHAPTER SUMMARY

By maintaining health records in a neat and orderly manner, HIM departments provide a valuable service to the health care facility. Health records are valuable only insofar as they are available for access. Maintenance of an organized storage area facilitates timely retrieval of records for all authorized users. Records can be identified alphabetically or numerically. When numerical identification is chosen, the master patient index is the key tool to correlate the patient to his or her medical record number. Medical record (identification) numbers can be assigned as unit, serial, serial-unit, or family numbering systems. Filing methods use either the patient's name or the medical record number to organize the health record in the filing system. These filing methods are alphabetical, straight numerical, and terminal-digit order. The chart locator system allows the HIM department to keep track of the location of health records. HIM practitioners must consider the physical security issues of storing health records safely to prevent damage by fire, water, theft, tampering, destruction, and loss of confidentiality.

It is critical to secure all health information within a facility. HIM professionals must pay special attention to the storage details so that all authorized users in the facility have efficient and effective access to health information. Storage of health records is a function that many take for granted in the health care facility. After reading this chapter, you should recognize the importance of this function and its impact on the entire health care facility.

Review Questions

1. Compare and contrast the different record identification systems.
2. Compare and contrast the various filing systems.
3. Explain the use of a master patient index.
4. Describe a chart locator system.

Document Imaging Manager

My name is Melissa, and I am the document imaging manager at Foster Community Hospital, a 150-bed acute care facility. I am responsible for the document imaging of all emergency room (ER) and outpatient records. Before accepting this position, I was the supervisor of the clerical and release-of-information functions in this department. As the document imaging manager, I oversee the preparation, scanning, indexing, and quality of the document imaging.

Every day, ER and outpatient records are prepared for scanning. Pages are smoothed, staples removed, and edges cleaned. Records are batched and scanned, and the images must be reviewed and indexed. HIM staff members verify each scanned image on the computer system to identify the document for each patient record. This process tells the system the identity of an image; for example, the image is identified as a patient's history and physical (H&P) as opposed to the face sheet or consent form.

To maintain this system, I must keep a current list to identify every document in the health record. The document list (something like the chart order in a paper environment) allows the record to be indexed appropriately for document identification within each patient record.

My facility no longer uses the paper record. All staff members use the images in the computer system to reference the records, including coding, release of information, and patient care areas.

APPLICATION

File System Conversion

Diamonte Hospital is preparing to convert its current filing system. The old system uses a six-digit medical record number for file identification, and the records are stored in straight numerical order on the file shelf. The new system will maintain the six-digit medical record number, but it will use terminal-digit filing because of high volume of filing activity. The facility will also get rid of the compressible shelves and use open shelving.

Develop a plan for converting the straight numeric file system to terminal-digit filing. Remember that the medical record numbers will remain the same. The change will occur in the organization of the files on the shelves.

Determine how many shelf units and how much space will be needed to store the current records in an open-shelf system. Remember to allow for aisle space as necessary.

The current records of Diamonte occupy 3000 linear feet.

Open-shelf units contain eight shelves, and each unit is 38 inches wide (allowing for 36 inches of file space per shelf).

CHAPTER OUTLINE

Organized Collection of Data

Primary and Secondary Data
Data Set
Creation of a Database
Data Review and Abstracting
Data Quality Check

Data Retrieval

Retrieval of Aggregate Data
Indices
Identification of a Population
Optimal Source of Data

Reporting of Data

Reporting to Individual Departments
Reporting to Outside Agencies
Registries
Vital Statistics

Statistical Analysis of Patient Information

Analysis and Interpretation
Mean
Median
Adjusted Mean

Mode
Frequency Distribution
Percentages
Presentation
Bar Graph
Line Graph
Histogram
Pie Chart

Routine Institutional Statistics

Admissions
Discharges
Length of Stay
Average Length of Stay
Transfers
Census
Hospital Rates and Percentages

Chapter Activities

Chapter Summary
Review Questions
Professional Profile
Application

By the end of this chapter, the student should be able to

- Identify the required data elements of the patient's abstract.
- Identify appropriate methods for capturing useful patient data.
- Calculate the length of stay for a patient, given the admission and discharge dates.
- Perform data quality analysis of the health information database.
- Report information to individual departments.
- Report information to outside agencies.
- Retrieve appropriate data according to the request.
- Query a database by using report generation tools.
- Identify the optimal source for retrieval of information.
- Understand statistical analysis of patient information.
- Describe and state the uses for statistical tools.
- Compute routine institutional statistics.

VOCABULARY

abstract	indices	primary data
aggregate data	length of stay (LOS)	query
average length of stay (ALOS)	line graph	registry
bar graph	mean	report
census	median	sample
data set	mode	secondary data
database	percentage	statistics
frequency distribution	pie chart	
histogram	population	

*I*n earlier chapters, you learned about the collection of health data for documentation in the health record. The health record is used to gather health data for storage in a physical location or database to provide a meaningful method for retrieval of the information for future use. Organizing specific data elements for each patient allows reporting of health information as it is mandated by law, accreditation, policy, or necessity.

Other important reasons to collect specific health data are statistical analysis, outcome analysis, and quality improvement. Data analysis is a critical function in all health care facilities. To analyze data within one record or among multiple records, the data elements must be collected in the same way. An important function of the health information management (HIM) department is the organized retrieval and reporting of these data. In previous chapters, the collection of health data was discussed in the context of providing proper patient care and following health care professional guidelines. The data were categorized into reports, such as the history and physical (H&P), laboratory reports, and nurses' notes. In this chapter, you will learn about the importance of collecting specific data in an organized format—such as a database—so that the health information can be analyzed and reported as necessary.

ORGANIZED COLLECTION OF DATA

To analyze data in a meaningful way, you must first collect the data appropriately. Appropriate data collection was the subject of several previous chapters. In this chapter, you will look at the data as a user would.

PRIMARY AND SECONDARY DATA

Health data can be categorized as primary or secondary. **Primary data** are those data taken directly from the patient or the original source. Primary data also describe a caregiver's observations of the patient. Examples of primary data are the history given by the patient to the nurse (Figure 9-1) and the patient's blood pressure or temperature reading as recorded by the monitor or the nurse. These data elements are documented in the patient's health record in a format that helps to transform the raw data into usable information. Therefore the patient's health record contains primary data.

Data taken from the primary-source document for use elsewhere becomes **secondary data** (Figure 9-2). In Chapter 5, you learned about the abstracting of data from a record. Abstracted

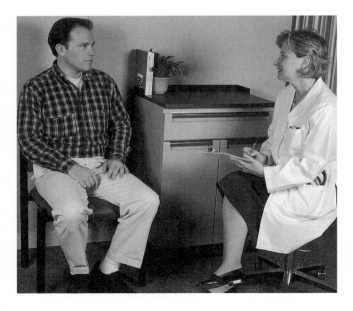

◆ **Figure 9-1**
Primary data are collected when the nurse talks to the patient to obtain his health history. (From Jarvis C. *Physical Examination and Health Assessment.* 24th ed. Philadelphia: Saunders, 2004, p 54.)

Hit-Bit

Data Versus Information

Remember the difference between data and information: The *data* collected during patient care become health *information* only after careful organization and compilation. Data are raw elements. Information results from the interpretation of that data.

data can be sorted and made available in a variety of formats. For example, a list of discharges sorted by physician is a physician index.

DATA SET

A **data set** is a group of elements collected for a specific purpose. A data set requires a standard method for collecting data elements so that they can be compared. To compare data, you must be sure that everyone is collecting the data in the same way or in a manner that is readily converted. For example, we collect certain data on all patients regardless of the health care services needed— name, address, phone number, and age. This data set is for the patient's personal identification. It allows the facility to distinguish one patient among other patients, to distinguish between men and women, mothers and babies. Each facility must make sure that its data sets are designed to comply with federal requirements as well as the internal needs of the facility.

As previously discussed, specific requirements mandate data sets for various health care organizations according to the services provided. Table 7-3 shows the data sets required by various types of facilities. The federal government, as a payer, has an interest in the services that are provided to its beneficiaries. Collection of specific data, as required by the Uniform Hospital Discharge Data Set (UHDDS) for acute care, allows the Centers for Medicare and Medicaid Services (CMS) to analyze patients, the health care provider, and services. (Figure 9-3 provides a summary of the UHDDS elements.) The analysis is possible because each data element is being collected the same way for every patient in the United States.

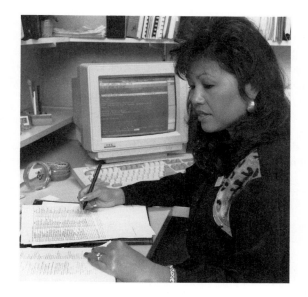

◆ **Figure 9-2**
As the HIM clerk reviews a health record and enters data into the abstract, she is creating secondary data. (From Madeline A. Clark and Virginia S. Mazza. *Health Unit Coordinating: Expanding the Scope of Practice.* Philadelphia: Saunders, 1999, p 60.)

UHDDS SUMMARY OF DATA ELEMENTS

Person/enrollment data

1. Personal/unique identifier
2. Date of birth
3. Gender
4. Race and ethnicity
5. Residence

Encounter Data

6. Health care facility identification number
7. Admission date
8. Type of admission
9. Discharge date
10. Attending physician's identification number
11. Surgeon's identification number
12. Principal diagnosis
13. Other diagnoses
14. Qualifier for other diagnoses
15. External cause-of-injury code
16. Birth weight of neonate
17. Significant procedure(s) and date(s) of procedure(s)
18. Disposition of the patient at discharge
19. Expected source of payment
20. Total charges

◆ **Figure 9-3**
UHDDS Summary of Data Elements.

Notice that CMS has requested information to identify the patient, provider, and services. The specific manner in which this information is collected allows CMS to compare Medicare patients regardless of where they receive health care services. The definition provided for each data element specifies what should be captured for that data element (e.g., the attending physician is the "clinician primarily responsible for the care of the patient from the beginning of the hospital episode") (http://www.cms.hhs.gov/manuals/downloads/clm104c25.pdf).

Throughout the course of the patient's care, data are collected by many health care professionals. The mandated data set is typically a summary of that information collected in a specific manner. Without a specific requirement for data, some facilities might not include data elements that are helpful to users when performing an analysis. For example, the patient's gender is a data element that is always helpful. However, if there were no specific requirement governing the way in which gender is captured, some facilities might not capture the data, and others might capture the data in different ways. Realistically, without a requirement, the field that captures the patient's gender could read *F, 1, or A,* for female; and *M, 2, or B,* for male (Figure 9-4).

If each health care facility determined its own method for collecting the patient's gender data, users would have to interpret each facility's method for classifying this information. By defining a specific data set and the method in which the information should be shared with the federal government on the UB-92 form (see Chapter 6), the government has mandated a data set for patients. Ultimately, this information is collected on all patients in an acute care facility regardless of who is paying and therefore allows for the comparison of the information internally and externally.

CREATION OF A DATABASE

The data collected for each patient create a **database.** This database is a collection of data elements organized in a manner that allows efficient retrieval of information. The data collection can occur

Hit-Bit

Gender Categories

In rare cases, it is necessary to use the classification of "unknown" for gender. Some health care applications have an "unknown" category for gender that may be recognized as *U, 3, or C.*

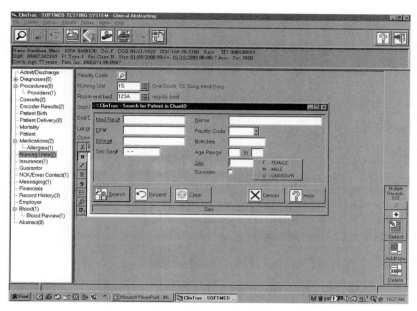

◆ **Figure 9-4**

Data set for patient gender. (Courtesy SoftMed Systems, Inc., Bethesda, MD.)

on paper or in a computer software program. For our discussion, we will consider the electronic health record; however, keep in mind that any collection of data elements can be considered a database.

Computer software is designed for health care facilities to organize patient health information in a systematic, defined format. The program requires collection of data in a special format, alphabetical or numerical, as discussed in Chapter 3.

Because each data element is defined before it is collected, the database is a useful source of information. For example, "attending physician" is one of the data elements that is collected. This data element can be collected in the admission record by entering the identification number for the physician who matches the description of the attending physician (see Table 4-1). This information (which is contained in the physician index) is collected for each patient discharged. The collection of this data element on all patients in the database makes it possible to **query,** or ask, the database for information specific to the attending physician. For example, facilities should review records on a representative sample of all physicians on the medical staff at the facility. To do so, the user must be able to run a **report** that lists records for each physician. The physician identification data element allows the user to query the database for a report and sort the information by physician. The user can then be sure that a representative sample of physicians is reviewed during the record review process.

We know that some data are required by the federal government. However, other data elements are retrieved only as specified by the facility. These types of data must be collected in the way they are going to be useful in the future. For example, in some cases, the type and frequency of a patient's consulting services, such as physical therapy, occupational therapy, or respiratory therapy, may influence the patient's outcomes. To collect this type of information, each consulting discipline may be given a number (*1,* physical therapy; *2,* occupational therapy; *3,* respiratory therapy; *0,* no therapy), and then as each patient record is abstracted, consulting services are identified and the corresponding numbers for the services provided to that patient are entered into the abstract. Later, the user can access that information in the database in the way that he or she prefers; for example, the user might look at consulting services associated with a specific diagnosis or procedure or with a physician. An example of other data that may be collected is advance directive acknowledgments. Facilities can include a field to capture whether a patient has signed the advance directive acknowledgement statement.

Hit-Bit

HL-7

Federal laws and standard-setting organizations exist to ensure that the health information contained in the databases of health care organizations and related entities is maintained in a defined, standardized format that allows comparison and sharing through an electronic or computerized format. They also strive to ensure the confidentiality and security of health information in the electronic and computer-based environment.

The Health Insurance Portability and Accountability Act (HIPAA) is a broad law that includes requirements for electronic health information to be stored in a standard transferable format that is confidential and secure.

Health Level Seven (HL-7) standards allow computer systems to exchange clinical and administrative data.

DATA REVIEW AND ABSTRACTING

Patient health data are gathered at admission and throughout the course of the patient's care. In an electronic health record, most of the data are already captured, and the HIM employee verifies the abstract. In the paper environment, once the patient is discharged, the HIM employee must correlate the information in the computer system with the patient record. The employee verifies the information to be sure that an abstract is created for the correct patient. Verification of the abstract is a detective control. Fixing any noted errors is a corrective control (see Chapter 5). The **abstract** can be defined as a summary of the patient's encounter. It provides a brief synopsis of the patient's care that would otherwise require a thorough review of the entire patient record. The abstract is a set of data elements, including those previously discussed in this chapter. At a minimum, each facility collects those data elements required by CMS; it determines additional data elements for internal analysis of patient information.

The process of summarizing the patient's information in a database by data entry of specific data elements is called *abstracting*. To complete an abstract, the HIM clerk must review the health record. The review is necessary to determine the appropriate data element for each field. As previously discussed, the HIM coder must review the record to determine the accurate code (ICD-9-CM or Current Procedural Terminology <CPT>) to represent the patient's diagnosis and procedures. To make this determination, the coder relies on the documentation in the record and his or her knowledge of coding. The other information that is captured as part of the abstract is the patient's disposition, the place the patient goes after discharge from the facility—home, nursing home, or another acute care facility. This information is usually entered in the form of a code (e.g., *1* for home, *2* for nursing home, *3* for home with home health, *8* for death). If you look at Figure 9-3, you can see that in an acute care facility, this is the minimum information that must be collected. Examples of additional information that is typically captured are type of anesthesia, length of surgery, and consent. By collecting this information in the abstract, the facility is able to query the system (run reports) for information related to these topics.

The patient's abstract is a common source of secondary data, and its creation or validation is a major function of the HIM department. Figure 9-5 is an example of patient abstract screens. Figure 9-6 contains the forms that were used to retrieve the data elements for this abstract. Note the information required in the abstract: patient's name, address, diagnosis, procedure, date, and length of procedure (Figure 9-7). As you review Figures 9-4 and 9-5, you can see how the clerk was able to determine the correct data to enter in this abstract.

When all required elements of the patient's data have been captured, the abstract is considered complete. All patient records must be abstracted as required to satisfy payer and facility guidelines for specific information. Each patient receiving services in a health care setting has an abstract. However, the abstract differs according to the setting (e.g., ambulatory care, long-term care).

Hit-Bit

Query

Query is the term used to describe the searching of a database for specific elements.

Some of the typical queries of the abstract database include the following:
- List of patients for a physician
- List of patients by diagnosis, diagnosis related group (DRG), or procedure
- List of patients by patient financial class
- List of patients by age
- List of patients with consulting physicians

DATA QUALITY CHECK

It is always necessary to ensure the quality of the abstract information. In previous chapters, you learned about the data quality concepts of validity, accuracy, completeness, and timeliness.

To maintain a functional database, abstracted data must be audited for quality. To do so, someone other than the initial clerk, usually a supervisor, routinely checks the abstracts by pulling the patient health record, retrieving the abstract from the database, and verifying the data elements. In general, only a sample of the abstracts is reviewed. However, the supervisor must be sure to choose a random sample of abstracts that includes all of the employee's work. Errors are corrected, documented, analyzed, and tracked to improve the quality of the database. The quality of the data is extremely important because of the high volume of information that the database provides for the health care facility.

The quality of the database enables performance improvement activities and appropriate decisions about the facility or about individual patients. Remember that data quality audits must be recorded for future comparison. It is important to document compliance or noncompliance with a set standard of quality for data. Over time, this information provides support for improvement efforts, indicates a need for improvement, or demonstrates quality. Discussion of database quality in the context of an electronic health record is continued in Chapter 12.

Exercise 9-1

Organized Collection of Data
1. What is primary data? Give an example.
2. What is secondary data? Give an example.
3. What is the purpose of abstracting?

DATA RETRIEVAL

You have learned about data collection, development of the database, all of the various elements that data contain, and storage of data as a paper or electronic record. Once a database exists, the data can be used for analysis or comparison. When health information is needed for utilization review, quality assurance, performance improvement, routine compilation, or patient care, the

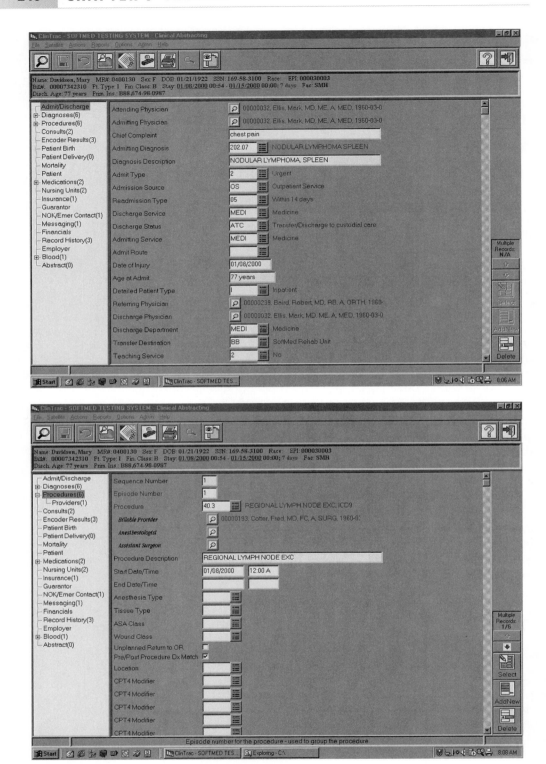

◆ **Figure 9-5**
Patient abstract screens. (Courtesy SoftMed Systems, Inc., Bethesda, MD.)

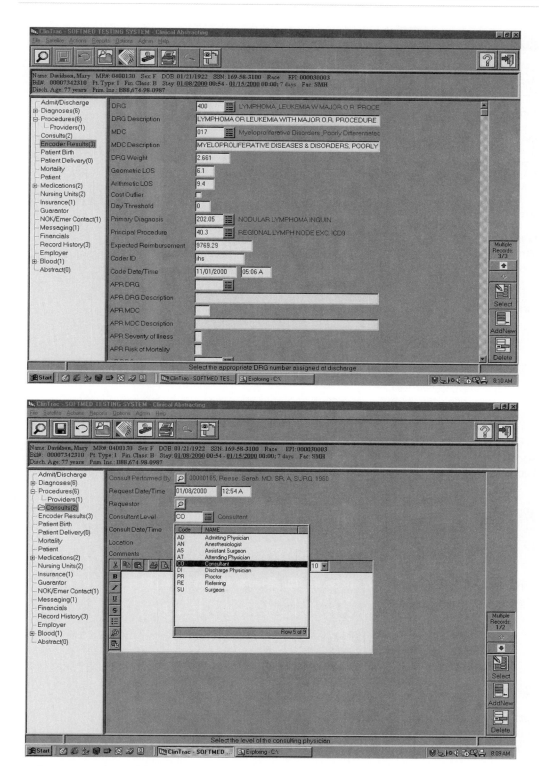

◆ **Figure 9-5, (cont'd)**

HIM department is asked to retrieve the relevant data. Through the abstract function, HIM personnel have stored this information in a systematic method for this type of retrieval. Therefore with the right instructions on the type of information needed and its intended use, HIM personnel can provide high-quality health information. Compilation of all or part of health data for groups of patients is called *aggregate data.*

OPERATIVE REPORT

Patient's name: Mary Davidson

Hospital no.: 400130

Date of surgery: 01/08/2000

Admitting Physician: Mark Ellis, MD

Surgeon: Fred Cotter, MD

Preoperative diagnosis: Nodular lymphoma
Postoperative diagnosis: Nodular lymphoma
Operative procedure: Regional lymph node excision

PROCEDURE AND GROSS FINDINGS: Under general anesthesia, after usual sterile preparation and draping, the patient was . . .

The patient tolerated the procedure well.
Approximate blood loss 200 mL.

Fred Cotter, MD

DD: 01/08/2000
DT: 01/09/2000

◆ **Figure 9-6**

The operative report from the patient's record was used to retrieve the data elements required in the patient abstract shown in Figure 9-4.

RETRIEVAL OF AGGREGATE DATA

Aggregate data comprise like data elements compiled to provide information about a group. For example, a collection of the length of stay (LOS) for all patients with the diagnosis of congestive heart failure (CHF) would be aggregate data (Figure 9-8). Further review of the report shows that the LOS data element for each patient has been retrieved. This report can be analyzed to determine average LOS and most common LOS. Sorting by any single data element for each of these patients produces a meaningful list of aggregate data.

A HIM professional needs the following information to identify the appropriate information needed by the person requesting the report: the name and contact phone number of the person making the request, the date of the request as well as the date parameters for the information requested, the specific information requested, and the reason for the request. This information will aid the person querying the database to ensure that the most appropriate information is retrieved from the database.

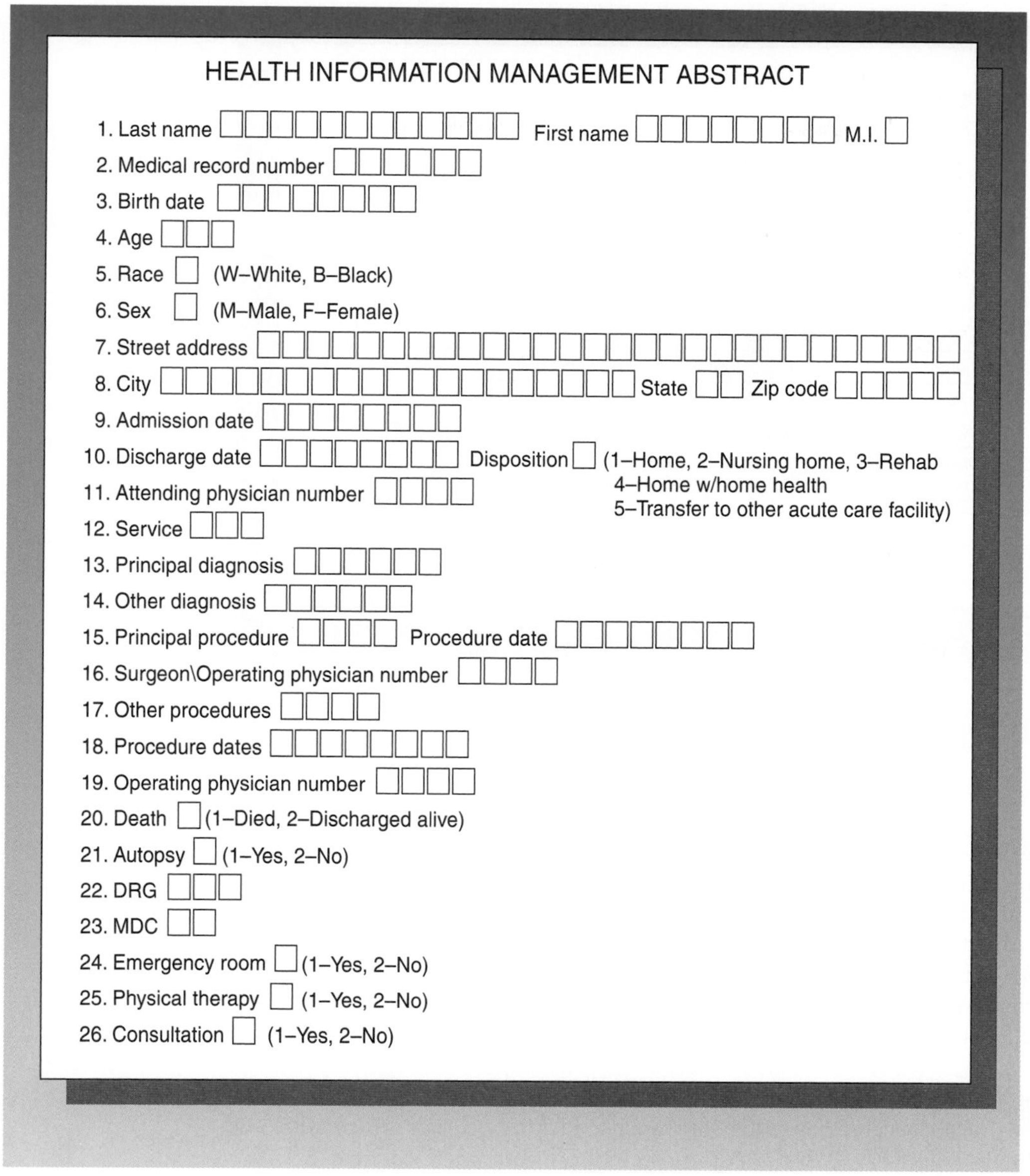

HEALTH INFORMATION MANAGEMENT ABSTRACT

1. Last name ☐☐☐☐☐☐☐☐☐☐☐ First name ☐☐☐☐☐☐☐ M.I. ☐

2. Medical record number ☐☐☐☐☐☐

3. Birth date ☐☐☐☐☐☐☐

4. Age ☐☐☐

5. Race ☐ (W–White, B–Black)

6. Sex ☐ (M–Male, F–Female)

7. Street address ☐☐☐☐☐☐☐☐☐☐☐☐☐☐☐☐☐☐☐☐☐☐☐☐☐☐☐☐

8. City ☐☐☐☐☐☐☐☐☐☐☐☐☐☐☐☐☐☐ State ☐☐ Zip code ☐☐☐☐☐

9. Admission date ☐☐☐☐☐☐☐

10. Discharge date ☐☐☐☐☐☐☐ Disposition ☐ (1–Home, 2–Nursing home, 3–Rehab
    4–Home w/home health
    5–Transfer to other acute care facility)

11. Attending physician number ☐☐☐☐

12. Service ☐☐☐

13. Principal diagnosis ☐☐☐☐☐☐

14. Other diagnosis ☐☐☐☐☐☐

15. Principal procedure ☐☐☐☐ Procedure date ☐☐☐☐☐☐☐☐

16. Surgeon\Operating physician number ☐☐☐☐

17. Other procedures ☐☐☐☐

18. Procedure dates ☐☐☐☐☐☐☐☐

19. Operating physician number ☐☐☐☐

20. Death ☐ (1–Died, 2–Discharged alive)

21. Autopsy ☐ (1–Yes, 2–No)

22. DRG ☐☐☐

23. MDC ☐☐

24. Emergency room ☐ (1–Yes, 2–No)

25. Physical therapy ☐ (1–Yes, 2–No)

26. Consultation ☐ (1–Yes, 2–No)

◆ **Figure 9-7**

Paper abstract data collection form. (Modified from Mervat Abdelhak, Sara Grostick, Mary Alice Hanken, and Ellen Jacobs. *Health Information: Management of a Strategic Resource.* 2nd ed. Philadelphia: Saunders, 2001, p 219.)

INDICES

The abstracting process has enabled facilities to create indices for diagnoses, procedures, and physicians. The database can also provide information about any group of patients according to the instructions given by the person requesting the information to HIM personnel and further refined by HIM personnel queries to the database. For example, it is common to identify all of a physician's patients for a particular time period. The easiest way to obtain a list of all of a physician's patients is to have already systematically identified on each patient record during the abstract process the name of the attending physician, as previously discussed. This listing of patients by physician creates what we have historically called the *physician index*.

The **indices** in the HIM department are vital in the organized collection of patient data according to the patient's diagnosis, any procedures performed, and the physicians who cared for

Report of patients w/DRG 127

MR #	Patient	D/C Date	LOS	Physician	DRG
056023	Austin, Dallas	02/27/2006	5	Angel, M.	127
197808	Bixby, Helena	02/12/2006	3	Kobob, L.	127
945780	China, Dollie	02/14/2006	6	Chow, A.	127
348477	Combeaux, Plato	02/02/2006	4	Thomas, B.	127
403385	Dimaro, Cheri	02/28/2006	5	Angel, M.	127
471416	Dondi, Mac	02/04/2006	3	Thomas, B.	127
362156	Foster, Dan	02/22/2006	4	Chow, A.	127
483443	Lates, Ricky	02/10/2006	6	Kobob, L.	127
483441	Smeadow, Shane	02/01/2006	5	Thomas, B.	127
201801	Titan, Tami	02/14/2006	4	Thomas, B.	127

◆ **Figure 9-8**
List of congestive heart failure patients shows aggregate data retrieval.

them. The indices are used to obtain patient information or aggregate data according to the diagnosis, procedure, or physician.

Historically, manual indices were maintained on index cards (Figure 9-9, *A*) or ledger books. HIM personnel recorded the patient's information on index cards according to the diagnosis, procedure, and attending physician. For example, each diagnosis would have an index card, and the HIM employee would record each patient with that diagnosis on the card. Therefore if a list of all patients with a particular diagnosis was needed, the HIM employee would pull the appropriate diagnosis card.

The automation of health information now allows HIM personnel to capture this information during the abstracting process because computer software can identify fields of information and create reports accordingly. Figure 9-9, *B* shows a diagnosis index in computerized format.

IDENTIFICATION OF A POPULATION

To retrieve appropriate useful information, you must be able to identify the population of interest. Identifying the population and being able to retrieve that population efficiently are extremely important characteristics of data retrieval. How is the population identified? For example, in health care a **population** can be defined as a group of people aggregated according to their race, age, gender, diagnosis, procedure, service, or financial class. A **sample** is a small representation of the entire population. A sample is often used when the population is too large to study in its entirety.

Another common reason to pull information through the identification of a population is for surgical case review or utilization review. For these studies, the population of patients is based on a diagnosis or the operation they had. The clinical data are recorded in the process of caring for the patient. Therefore when abstracting the patient health record, the HIM professional can easily determine and enter the diagnosis and procedure codes. In a paper record, the diagnoses and procedures are typically found on the face sheet after coding, and this information is also entered into the computer database.

Therefore identifying a group or population of patients for analysis is assisted by good database structure, which is supported by creating proper data dictionaries (see Chapter 3).

A

Diagnosis code: `486`

Description: Pneumonia, organism unspecified

Patient name	MR #	Admit date	D/C date	Physician
Barbara, Vinnie	216690	02/08/90	02/12/90	Strong, J.

Diagnosis code: `487.0`

Description: Influenza w/ pneumonia

Patient name	MR #	Admit date	D/C date	Physician
Angel, Florence	300455	05/18/90	05/20/90	Robin, C.
Cherub, Michael	010209	06/09/90	06/16/90	Anthony, R.

Diagnosis code: `487.1`

Description: Influenza w/ other respiratory manifestations

Patient name	MR #	Admit date	D/C date	Physician
Gabe, Beth	112245	01/10/90	01/16/90	Thomas, R.

B

06/16/2006

Diagnosis Index   Discharges: 01/01/06 – 03/31/06

Diagnosis Code	Description	Medical Record #	Admit Date	D/C Date	LOS	Physician
650		010111	12/30/05	01/01/06	2	Oscar, D.
		125544	12/31/05	01/01/06	1	Jons, J.
		098805	01/02/06	01/04/06	2	Vida, E.
		112096	01/05/06	01/06/06	1	Oscar, D.
		113095	01/09/06	01/12/06	3	Jons, J.

◆ **Figure 9-9**
Diagnosis index shown in a manual format (**A**) and a computerized format (**B**).

OPTIMAL SOURCE OF DATA

The next matter to discuss with regard to data retrieval is how to ascertain the optimal source of the data. In a well-constructed database, with unique data dictionary definitions, the computer program will have stored the data in only one place. Therefore the data will always be recorded at the best time by the best person. For example, if you want to retrieve a population of all of the patients with pneumonia, the computer knows that there is only one place that the patient's diagnosis is recorded, it will go to that location to review each patient record and determine which patients have the diagnosis of pneumonia, and then it will retrieve all the appropriate records for a report.

However, in a paper record, understanding what is an optimal source of data becomes critical. In many paper environments, the same information is recorded multiple times. The patient's admitting diagnosis, for example, is recorded on the face sheet by the admitting clerk; it is recorded on the nursing assessment by the nurse; and it is recorded on the admitting notes by the physician. What is the optimal, most reliable place to determine the patient's admitting diagnosis? It depends on the reason that you want the information. If you want to know why the patient thought he or she was admitted, then the admitting record is probably the most important place to look. However, if you want to know the physician's clinical reason for admitting the patient, then you are going to retrieve the admitting notes.

Another example of how important it is to identify the optimal source of data is during a Joint Commission on Accreditation of Healthcare Organizations (JCAHO) survey. JCAHO surveyors may ask to review specific records (e.g., records of patients who were restrained). This information is not normally identified in the patient abstract. From the HIM perspective, several different data elements in the database can indicate that a patient may have been restrained. In a computerized system, a special data field can be added to indicate (*Yes* or *No*) whether a patient was restrained. If a special data field does not exist, other information in the abstract may help identify patients who were restrained. For example, certain diagnoses indicate that a patient may have required restraints (e.g., patients with organic brain syndrome or delirium).

Trying to find the optimal source of data requires knowing your database and knowing how to query it and relate the data elements, as well as being a bit of a detective. Sometimes you have to begin with data that you know you did not collect and work backward. For instance, if the chief financial officer wants to know how many fertility treatments your facility performed, where would you go to get that information? Would you query physicians, diagnoses, or procedures? You would look up procedure codes for fertility treatments and then query your system for all of those procedures. The result should be a list of patients, their health record numbers, and the fertility procedures performed.

Exercise 9-2

Data Retrieval

1. What are aggregate data?
2. What is an index? Give an example.
3. What type of information could you obtain from indexes?
4. How does one determine the optimal source of data?
5. How do you determine the optimal source for the following data in an inpatient record?
   a. Medications that the patient has already received
   b. Possible diagnosis after 2 days in the hospital
   c. Patient's temperature

REPORTING OF DATA

REPORTING TO INDIVIDUAL DEPARTMENTS

The health data collected in the HIM department are used by various departments in the health care facility. The quality management department uses the database to retrieve specific cases and review the documentation found in the health records to determine compliance with accreditation standards, perform quality improvement studies, or study patients outcomes. The finance department may use the information in the HIM department to verify or prepare financial reports and budgets.

REPORTING TO OUTSIDE AGENCIES

Various agencies associated with health care facilities routinely require information. Some states gather information from facilities to create a state health information network. The information in the database is shared (without patient identifiers) so that facilities can compare themselves with other facilities. Organ procurement agencies may request information on deaths for a certain period to assess the facility's compliance with state regulations for organ procurement. Certain statistics must be reported to the Centers for Disease Control and Prevention so that disease prevalence, incidence, morbidity, and mortality can be studied.

Registries

A **registry** is a collection of data specific to a disease, diagnosis, or procedure. Common registries are the Tumor or Cancer Registry, Trauma Registry, AIDS Registry, Birth Defect Registry, and Implant Registry. The purpose of a registry is to study or improve patient care. The data are collected specific to the diagnosis, disease, or implant so that users can compare, analyze, or study these groups of patients.

Tumor or Cancer Registry

The study of the causes and treatments of cancers is of importance to us individually and also as a public health issue. Many cancers, such as some types of lung cancer, are thought to be of environmental origin; others seem to have a genetic component. It is only by studying these cancers that researchers can begin to identify the actual causes with the hope of finding preventive measures and effective treatments.

The investigation of cancers is facilitated by the data collected by health care providers about their patients with cancer. Although the requirements for reporting vary by state, the purpose is the same: to identify all cancer cases and gather as much relevant data about them as possible. Detailed data about specific cancers help researchers compare the efficacy of treatments, particularly in terms of survival rates.

Detailed data collection includes demographic data (name, address, identification number) and clinical data (diagnoses, procedures, pathology). Pathology data include grading (classifying the growth of the tumor), staging (describing whether the tumor has spread and how far), and other specific details about the tumor. Many providers complete the basic registry reporting; however, a certified cancer registry also requires patient follow-up.

Individuals who specialize in collecting data for this registry may become Certified Tumor Registrars (CTR) through the National Cancer Registry Association (http://www.ncra-usa.org/certification).

Trauma Registry

Researchers can identify trauma (injury) victims by the ICD-9 codes associated with the episode of care. These data are available through a variety of databases maintained by health care providers and payers. However, for study of the severity of the injury and the effectiveness of specific treatments, a trauma registry provides more data.

Trauma registries maintain data on the severity of the injury. Facilities that have a trauma registry do not rely on the coding to identify cases but also search other diagnoses to determine potential cases. As with tumor data, the users of trauma registry data are concerned about preventing trauma and providing the most effective treatment.

The American Trauma Society (ATS) offers a certification process for Certified Specialist Trauma Registry (CSTR; http://www.amtrauma.org/index.html).

Other Registries

Birth defects and transplants are examples of other registries that may be maintained. Varying degrees of detail are collected. Birth defects may not be detected at birth, and later reporting may be acceptable. Transplant registries match potential donors with recipients and follow those patients after the transplant.

Vital Statistics

Vital statistics refers to the number of births, deaths, and marriages and to statistics on health and disease. In the health care facility, specific information regarding patient births and deaths is reported to the state's Department of Vital Statistics, also known as *Vital Records*. Newborns must be registered with the Department of Vital Statistics within a specific time frame after birth. Within the health care facility, the HIM department is sometimes responsible for recording newborns' demographics, parents, and clinical information to submit to Vital Records.

Death certificates must also be submitted to Vital Records after a patient's death. The death certificate records the patient's demographic information and the cause and place of death. In some states, this information is initiated by the nursing staff and completed by the funeral home; in others, the HIM staff may be required to participate in the submission of this information to the Department of Vital Statistics.

Exercise 9-3

Reporting of Data

1. List two departments that use health databases. Why do they need the data?
2. What is a registry?
3. What is the difference between a registry and an index?

STATISTICAL ANALYSIS OF PATIENT INFORMATION

Determining which report to run is sometimes only the first step in providing information to a user or committee. Once a report has been run, further review of that report may be necessary to provide truly useful information for decision making or interpretation. For example, refer to Figure 9-8, which was used to illustrate patient LOS in the aggregate data explanation. That report could be useful in determining average LOS (ALOS). Facilities typically review the ALOS for specific patient diagnoses. The facility's average is then compared to a national, corporate, or local average. This further analysis can determine whether a facility is within the acceptable LOS limits for that diagnosis. The utilization review department analyzes patient LOS for each DRG and diagnosis. To provide this information, a report must be run and then formatted in an appropriate list or graph to represent the information for presentation at a meeting.

All of the examples involve simple arithmetic. Use a calculator or spreadsheet program to follow along as you read and reproduce the example figures.

ANALYSIS AND INTERPRETATION

Once patient data have been collected and stored in a database, reports can be run and the data can be analyzed, interpreted, or presented with various tools. The simplest methods for analyzing patient data involve the statistical evaluations of mean, median, and mode. Interpretation is an explanation of the data. Exercise 9-4 contains a set of practice data. As you read this section, use this data to ensure that you understand each concept as it is discussed.

Mean

The arithmetic **mean** describes what is commonly called the average of a group of numbers. Add the sum of the group of numbers, and divide the sum by the number of items in the group. The mean is used to compute a wide variety of averages: LOS, cost per case, or patient age. For example, to determine the average age of patients receiving a coronary artery bypass graft (CABG), you

Report of CABG patients

MR #	Patient	D/C Date	LOS	Physician	Age
560230	Bianco, Helena	02/07/2006	7	Angelo, R.	50
978081	Chowski, Shane	02/10/2006	8	Kobob, L.	53
045780	Gombeaux, Glenn	02/04/2006	12	Chi, A.	53
748473	Phoster, Dodi	02/12/2006	14	Houmas, C.	56
005338	Sondi, Mac	02/08/2006	8	Angelo, R.	59
671414	Stephens, Henri	02/14/2006	9	Houmas, C.	61
062150	White, Jean	02/20/2006	8	Chi, A.	62

◆ **Figure 9-10**

A list of coronary artery bypass graft (CABG) patients can provide data to find the mean age of this group. If you add all the ages in column 6 and divide by 7, the mean age of this group is 56 years.

MR#	Pt Age
560230	50
978081	53
045780	53
748473	56
005338	59
671414	61
062150	62
Total	394
Total divided by 7	56.286

Average age of patients in Figure 9-10

◆ **Figure 9-11**

Calculation of the mean.

would add the sum of the ages of the group of patients and then divide by the total number of patients in the group. Figure 9-10 provides a list of seven patients who had a CABG. To find the mean age, we add all of the ages (50, 53, 53, 56, 59, 61, 62 = 394), then divide by 7 (394/7 = 56.29, which rounds to 56). The average, or mean, age of patients in this group is 56 years. Calculate this easily in Excel using the AVERAGE formula: =AVERAGE(cell range). Figure 9-11 provides an illustration.

The arithmetic mean is a useful and widely understood measure. However, it is sensitive to outliers: values that are very different from most of the other values in the sample or population. Going back to the example in Figure 9-10, assume that the youngest CABG patient was 20 (rather than 50; see Figure 9-12). In this case, the average is 52. There aren't any patients younger than 53

Hit-Bit

Rounding Rules

Calculations often result in more decimal places than is necessary or appropriate. For example, the average of 3, 5, 8, and 11 is 6.75: two decimal places more than the source numbers. Sometimes this is appropriate, such as in calculations of average length of stay. At other times, the additional decimal places reflect more detail than is needed.

To reduce the number of decimal places, the number can be truncated. To truncate, just remove the unwanted digits. To truncate 6.75 to one decimal place leaves 6.7. However, truncating does not always result in appropriate accuracy. For statistical purposed, we round the numbers.

To round a number, identify the digit immediately to the right of the desired place. In this example, 5 is immediately to the right of 7. To round digits that are 5, 6, 7, 8, or 9, add one to the digit on the left. In our example, 6.75 rounds to 6.8. If we wanted only a whole number, 6.75 rounds to 7. This is called *rounding up* because the resulting rounded number is numerically higher than the original number.

To round digits that are 0, 1, 2, 3, or 4, merely truncate. The number 5.34 rounds to 5.3 or 5. This is called *rounding down* because the resulting rounded number is numerically lower than the original number.

MR#	Pt Age
[if pt 560230 were much younger]	20
978081	53
045780	53
748473	56
005338	59
671414	61
062150	62
Total	364
Total divided by 7	52.00

Average age of patients in Figure 9-10
if patients #560230 were 20 instead of 50

◆ **Figure 9-12**
Calculation of the mean with outlier.

in the group, except for the patient who is 20. Therefore the average of 52 gives an incorrect impression of the CABG patients. One way to help the user of the information to understand the underlying data is to calculate the median and report it along with the mean.

Median

The **median** describes the midpoint of the data. Arrange the data in numerical order from lowest to highest and then count toward the midpoint to obtain the median. The median is often used to help describe groups of data that contain values that are significantly different from the rest of the group. Using the same group of data from Figure 9-10, we can analyze the median. To begin this analysis, first arrange the data in order: 50, 53, 53, 56, 59, 61, 62. Because there are seven numbers, it is easy to determine the midpoint. Which number is halfway between one and seven? The answer is 4. So beginning with the first patient's age (50), count to the fourth patient's age (56). The median age in this group of patients is 56. In this group of patients, the mean and the median are the same. This means that the data are equally distributed on both sides of the mean: half of the observations are lower, and half of them are higher. If there is an even number of observations, take the middle two and average them to determine the median. For example, the median of the series 50, 53, 56, and 58 is 54.5 (53 + 56/2).

In the example in Figure 9-12, the mean is 52; however, the median is 56. Without looking at the data, you can tell that the data are unequally distributed around the mean because the middle observation is higher than the mean. In a small example such as this, these values hold no great significance. However, in a set of 300 observations, the data may be so unequally distributed that the mean must be adjusted to describe the data in a meaningful way.

Adjusted Mean

One way to adjust the mean is to remove the highest and lowest observations. In a set of observations containing outliers, this adjustment disregards the outliers and focuses on the observations that are most representative of the group under study. Try this with the Figure 9-12 example. Remove the observations 20 and 62. This results in a mean of 56 and a median of 56. When this group is being reported, the source of the calculations must be stated so that the user knows what was done with the data to make it meaningful. In a larger group of observations, removing the highest and lowest observations may have no impact if there are multiple outliers. In that case, remove a percentage of the highest and lowest observations. Up to 5% of the highest and 5% of the lowest is generally acceptable. In the absence of policies or conventions, it is up to the presenter (the analyzer of the data) to determine what percentage should be adjusted. However, a clear explanation of the adjustment must accompany the report. Compare the two reports in Figure 9-13.

Mode

Mode describes the number that occurs most often in a group of data. The mode is helpful in the study of the most common observation or observations. Unlike the mean and the median, which have a single value, there can be multiple modes in a group of data. In the list of CABG patients in Figure 9-10, the mode is 53. All of the other ages are observed only once. In a large group of observations, a mode with many observations may indicate a strong preference or tendency of the group. Because the mode is not a numerical calculation, it is possible that the group will have no mode. The lack of a mode is not inherently important.

Frequency Distribution

Another useful way to analyze data is to prepare a **frequency distribution.** A frequency distribution is a way of organizing data into mutually exclusive class intervals (groups, categories, or tiers that are meaningful to the user). In Figure 9-10, all of the patients are in their 50s and 60s: two class intervals that might be useful in identifying at-risk patients. Five patients are in their 50s; two are in their 60s. This gives us a frequency distribution as follows:

AGE	NUMBER OF PATIENTS
50 to 59	5
60 to 69	2

To construct a frequency distribution, organize the data into mutually exclusive equal groups or class intervals (so that no observation can belong in more than one group). Notice that in this example, only two groups are necessary. The example data could also have been grouped as follows:

AGE	NUMBER OF PATIENTS
50 to 54	3
55 to 59	2
60 to 64	2

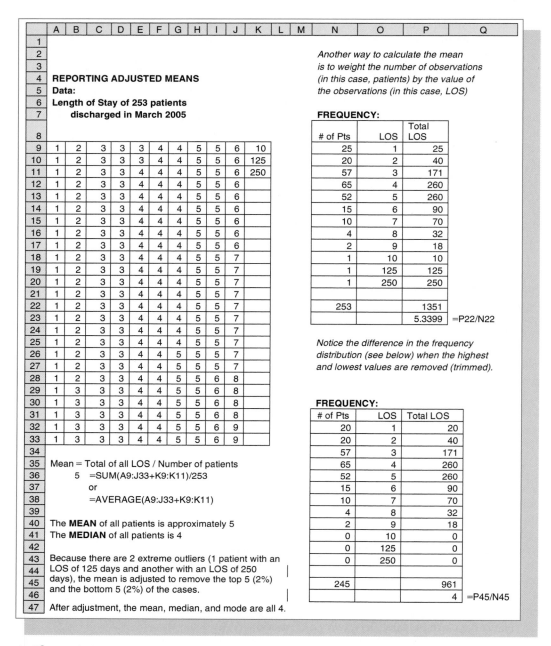

REPORTING ADJUSTED MEANS
Data:
Length of Stay of 253 patients
discharged in March 2005

A	B	C	D	E	F	G	H	I	J	K
1	2	3	3	3	4	4	5	5	6	10
1	2	3	3	3	4	4	5	5	6	125
1	2	3	3	4	4	4	5	5	6	250
1	2	3	3	4	4	4	5	5	6	
1	2	3	3	4	4	4	5	5	6	
1	2	3	3	4	4	4	5	5	6	
1	2	3	3	4	4	4	5	5	6	
1	2	3	3	4	4	4	5	5	6	
1	2	3	3	4	4	4	5	5	6	
1	2	3	3	4	4	4	5	5	7	
1	2	3	3	4	4	4	5	5	7	
1	2	3	3	4	4	4	5	5	7	
1	2	3	3	4	4	4	5	5	7	
1	2	3	3	4	4	4	5	5	7	
1	2	3	3	4	4	4	5	5	7	
1	2	3	3	4	4	4	5	5	7	
1	2	3	3	4	4	4	5	5	7	
1	2	3	3	4	4	5	5	5	7	
1	2	3	3	4	4	5	5	5	7	
1	2	3	3	4	4	5	5	6	8	
1	3	3	3	4	4	5	5	6	8	
1	3	3	3	4	4	5	5	6	8	
1	3	3	3	4	4	5	5	6	8	
1	3	3	3	4	4	5	5	6	9	
1	3	3	3	4	4	5	5	6	9	

Mean = Total of all LOS / Number of patients
5   =SUM(A9:J33+K9:K11)/253
     or
     =AVERAGE(A9:J33+K9:K11)

The **MEAN** of all patients is approximately 5
The **MEDIAN** of all patients is 4

Because there are 2 extreme outliers (1 patient with an LOS of 125 days and another with an LOS of 250 days), the mean is adjusted to remove the top 5 (2%) and the bottom 5 (2%) of the cases.

After adjustment, the mean, median, and mode are all 4.

Another way to calculate the mean is to weight the number of observations (in this case, patients) by the value of the observations (in this case, LOS)

FREQUENCY:

# of Pts	LOS	Total LOS
25	1	25
20	2	40
57	3	171
65	4	260
52	5	260
15	6	90
10	7	70
4	8	32
2	9	18
1	10	10
1	125	125
1	250	250
253		1351
		5.3399 =P22/N22

Notice the difference in the frequency distribution (see below) when the highest and lowest values are removed (trimmed).

FREQUENCY:

# of Pts	LOS	Total LOS
20	1	20
20	2	40
57	3	171
65	4	260
52	5	260
15	6	90
10	7	70
4	8	32
2	9	18
0	10	0
0	125	0
0	250	0
245		961
		4 =P45/N45

◆ **Figure 9-13**
Reporting adjusted means data: length of stay of 253 patients discharged in March 2005.

This second grouping conveys the same data. However, the second grouping is more informative because it shows that the values are spread fairly evenly across the groups. Note that the groups are equal. Each group has five consecutive values. A frequency distribution should have the lowest number of groups or categories that can present the data informatively. When the number of groups or categories is too large, it is difficult for the user to absorb the information.

Percentages

Often, the actual number of observations is confusing to the user. In that case, it is useful to also provide the **percentage** of observations. Presentation of the percentage standardizes the data so that unlike groups can be compared. To calculate a percentage, divide the observations in the category by the total observations, and multiple by 100. In the Figure 9-10 example, the percentages in each group are as follows:

AGE	NUMBER OF PATIENTS	PERCENTAGE	
50 to 54	3	3/7*100=	42.86%
55 to 59	2	2/7*100=	28.57%
60 to 64	2	2/7*100=	28.57%
Total	7	100%	

Percentages help the user compare observations between time periods and when the group under study varies in size from the group to which it is being compared. For example, look at Figure 9-14 to compare the number of Medicare patients in Hospital A to the number in Hospital B. The actual number of patients is meaningless; however, the percentages show that the hospitals are very similar in the mix of payers.

PRESENTATION

After analysis and interpretation, the data can be presented as information. To present data in a meaningful yet simple manner, tools are used to illustrate the information. Although there are many tools, the most common are the bar graph, pie chart, and line graph. Table 9-1 explains how these presentation tools are used.

	Number of discharges	
Payer	Hospital A	Hospital B
Medicare	5,000	13,229
Medicaid	2,300	6,032
Blue Cross/Blue Shield	1,500	3,975
Commercial carriers	950	2,453
Charity care	500	1,423
Self-pay	125	367
Other payers	90	325
Total discharges	10,465	27,804
	Percentage of discharges	
Payer	Hospital A	Hospital B
Medicare	48%	48%
Medicaid	22%	22%
Blue Cross/Blue Shield	14%	14%
Commercial carriers	9%	9%
Charity care	5%	5%
Self-pay	1%	1%
Other payers	1%	1%
Total	100%	100%

◆ **Figure 9-14**
Comparing payer mix.

TABLE 9-1	Presentation Tools and Their Uses	
PRESENTATION TOOL	**CONSTRUCTION**	**PURPOSE**
Table	Column and rows. Construction depends on the items being compared.	Used to compare characteristics of items. Notice in this table that the items are listed in the first column and the two characteristics (construction and purpose) head the comparison columns.
Bar graph	Bars are drawn to represent the frequency of items in the specified categories of a variable. One axis represents the category. The other axis represents the frequency.	Used to compare categories with each other, the same category in different time periods, or both.
Line graph	The horizontal axis represents the observation. The vertical axis represents the value of the observation. A point is made that corresponds to each observation, and a line is drawn to connect the points.	Used to represent data over a period of time; information is plotted along the x and y axes
Pie chart	In a circle, the percentage of each category is represented by a wedge of the circle that corresponds to the percentage of the circle.	Used to compare categories with one another in relation to the whole group
Histogram	Like a bar graph, but the sides of the bars are touching. Horizontally, each bar represents a class interval. Vertically, the height of the bar represents the frequency of the class interval.	Used to illustrate a frequency distribution.

Bar Graph

A **bar graph** is used to present the frequency of observations within specific categories. Each bar can represent the number of observations in the category. Bar graphs are also used to represent frequencies or values attached to specific events or causes. Bar graphs can be drawn either vertically or horizontally. In a vertical graph, the horizontal axis represents the categories, events, or causes. The vertical axis represents the value or number of observations, with the lowest value (often zero) at the bottom. Figure 9-15 provides an example of bar graph construction. Note that the bars for each category are separate from one another but the bars for subcategories can be adjacent. The values on vertical axis are expressed in equal increments.

Bar graphs are easy to read and interpret. Color presentation also helps the user, particularly when there are subcategories. Bar graphs can also be used to present a portion of the data to highlight a specific point, such as top ten DRGs. Bar graphs are not particularly helpful when the data have a very wide range of values. For example, if one category has two occurrences and another has 30,000, the vertical axis might be difficult to draw in a meaningful way. Also, when there are many categories, including all of the appropriate descriptions can be difficult.

Line Graph

A **line graph** is best used to present observations over time. As with the vertical bar graph, the vertical axis represents the value or number of observations. The horizontal axis in a line graph represents the time periods. Figure 9-16 provides an example of line graph construction. Note that the line graph is constructed by connecting the individual points that represent the observations.

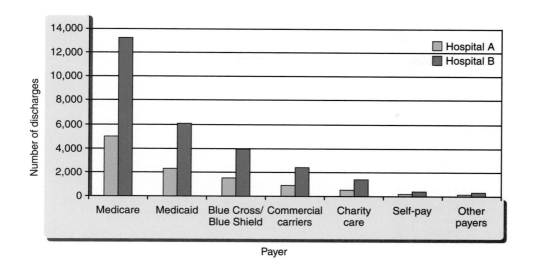

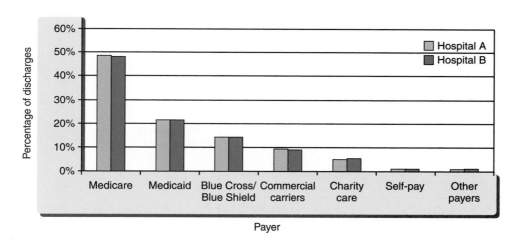

◆ **Figure 9-15**

Bar graph construction using data from Figure 9-14 to compare Hospital A and Hospital B by payer.

Line graphs are also easy to read and interpret. Color presentation facilitates interpretation when multiple time periods are superimposed on one another. For example, 3 years of data could be drawn on the same graph with each year represented by a different color. In black-and-white presentation, the line for each year could be drawn using different patterns; however, that is not as clear as using color.

Line graphs are also used to compare two variables. Figure 9-17 shows a line graph that compares LOS with age. Each patient is represented on the horizontal axis. The patients are presented in order of age. In this example, there is no relationship between two variables.

Histogram

A **histogram** is a combination of a vertical bar graph whose sides are touching. Horizontally, each bar represents a class interval. Vertically, the height of the bar represents the frequency of the class interval. A line graph may be drawn to connect the midpoints of each class interval. Histograms are used only to draw frequency distributions. Note that the bars are adjacent and a line approximates the curve created by the data (Figure 9-18).

	Number of discharges	
	Hospital A	Hospital B
2000	7,846	32,451
2001	7,998	30,675
2002	8,432	31,246
2003	9,054	29,945
2004	9,578	28,435
2005	10,465	27,804

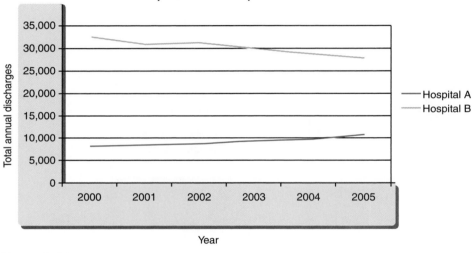

◆ Figure 9-16
Line graph construction.

Pie Chart

A **pie chart** is used to express the percentage of observations in each category of a variable. To use a pie chart, the number of observations must be converted to a percentage. All of the observations (100%) must be included in the chart. Pie charts are drawn in a circle. Each slice of the pie represents a category. The size of the slice corresponds to the percentage of observations. A complete circle is 360 degrees in circumference. To create an accurate drawing, multiply the percentages of observations by 360 to determine the number of degrees to draw the angle for the slice. To estimate the size of the slice, remember that a right angle is 90 degrees. Four 90-degree angles make a circle: 360 degrees. Therefore 25% of a circle is a quarter of the pie.

Pie charts have limited application and can be difficult to read if there are many categories. If there are many small categories, it is sometimes useful to combine them in a meaningful way. However, pie charts can make a dramatic and easily understood statement. They are particularly useful when illustrating a variable with one or two dramatically large numbers of observations. Figure 9-19 shows the percentage of discharges, by payer, for Hospital A (see Figure 9-15).

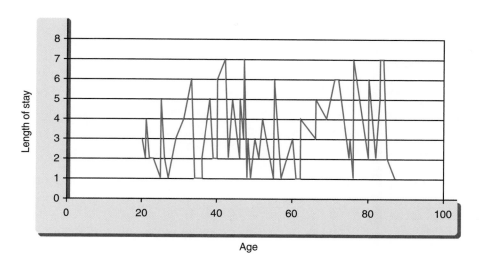

◆ **Figure 9-17**
Line graph comparing length of stay (LOS) with patient age.

Drawing charts and graphs by hand is time consuming, and the results are not always attractive. Using a spreadsheet program, such as Microsoft Excel, allows the user to experiment efficiently with the graph-making process and is best for professional-looking results.

Exercise 9-4

Statistical Analysis of Patient Information

AGE	LOS	AGE	LOS	AGE	LOS	AGE	LOS
20	3	34	1	49	1	71	6
21	2	36	1	50	3	72	6
21	4	36	2	51	2	73	5
22	2	38	5	52	4	75	2
22	2	39	2	55	1	75	3
23	2	40	2	55	6	76	1
25	1	40	6	57	1	76	7
25	3	42	11	60	3	80	2
25	4	43	2	61	1	80	5
25	8	44	5	62	1	80	11
26	2	46	2	62	2	82	2
27	1	46	5	62	4	83	5
28	2	47	7	66	3	83	7
29	3	47	3	66	4	84	14
33	4	48	3	66	5	85	2
33	11	48	1	69	4	87	1

1. Calculate:
   a. Mean age
   b. Mean length of stay
   c. Median age
   d. Mode of the length of stay
2. Prepare a frequency distribution of the patients, by age.

Ages of patients discharged in Quarter I

Age	# of D/Cs	%
Under 20	2	.4
21–30	64	12.7
31–40	118	23.4
41–50	196	38.8
51–60	93	18.4
61–70	27	5.3
Over 70	5	1
Total	505	100

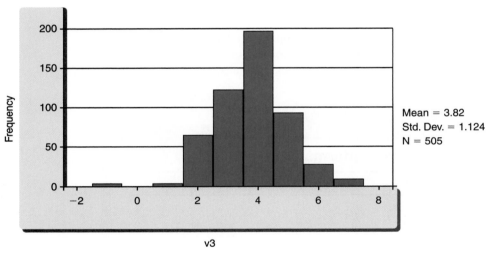

Mean = 3.82
Std. Dev. = 1.124
N = 505

◆ **Figure 9-18**
Histogram.

ROUTINE INSTITUTIONAL STATISTICS

As discussed in Chapter 1, there are a number of ways to describe and distinguish among health care facilities. Analysis, interpretation, and presentation of data provide **statistics** that further identify a facility and its activities. Figure 9-20 contains a list of important statistics for Community Hospital for the year 2004.

ADMISSIONS

Health care organizations always maintain statistics on the number of patients who are admitted to the facility. Review Figure 9-20 to identify the number of patients admitted to Community Hospital during 2004: 14,400 adults and children. The number of adults and children (14,400) does not include the number of newborn (NB) patients admitted (960). Unless otherwise specified, NB statistics are recorded separately from those of adults and children because the NB is admitted to the facility for the purpose of being born. Even though the NB may be ill, that is not

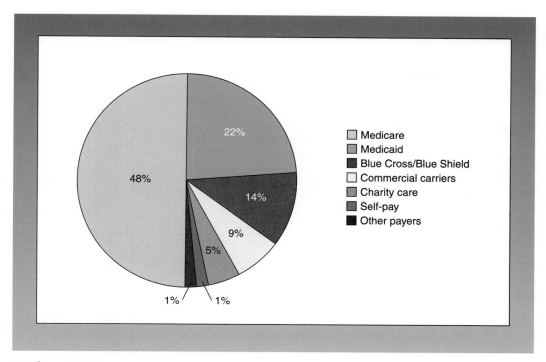

◆ **Figure 9-19**
Pie chart construction using data from Figure 9-15.

the reason for his or her admission. A birth is an admission, and a health record is created for each NB at birth.

DISCHARGES

Health care facilities also maintain statistics on the number of patients leaving the facility. The second item in Figure 9-20 is discharges. Once again, we separate the NBs from the adults and children. Note that the discharges include deaths because death is, effectively, a discharge. We still need to know the number of deaths for statistical purposes, so we also list them separately. Other discharges include the patient's release by discharge order from the physician, leaving against medical advice (AMA), and transfer to another facility.

LENGTH OF STAY

The time that a patient spends in a facility is called the **length of stay (LOS).** LOS is the measurement, in whole days, of the time between admission and discharge. Figure 9-21 illustrates how to calculate a patient's LOS. For example: A patient enters the facility on Monday, July 1, and is discharged on Thursday, July 4. The easiest way to calculate the LOS is to subtract the dates. Four minus one is three; therefore the LOS is 3 days.

It is important to note that when counting the LOS, *count the day of admission but not the day of discharge.* The times of admission and discharge are irrelevant when calculating inpatient LOS. In the previous example, the patient is considered to have stayed in the hospital on 3 days: July 1, July 2, and July 3. On July 4, the patient is no longer there. This is a fairly easy calculation when the patient enters and leaves the facility during the same month because you can just subtract the days in the month.

LOS is more difficult to determine if the patient enters and leaves the facility in different months. For example, if the patient enters the hospital in July and leaves in August, three calculations are required:
Step 1: Calculate how many days the patient was there in July.
Step 2: Calculate how many days the patient was there in August.
Step 3: Add the two together.

ADMISSIONS		
Adults & children	14,400	Total number of adults and children admitted during the year
Newborns	960	Total number of babies born in the hospital during the year
DISCHARGES (including deaths)		
Adults & children	14,545	Total number of adults and children discharged during the year
Newborns	950	Total number of newborns discharged during the year
INPATIENT SERVICE DAYS		Number of days of service rendered by the hospital
Adults & children	75,696	to adults and children
Newborns	1993	to newborns
TOTAL LENGTH OF STAY		Sum of all the individual lengths of stay of
Adults & children	72,107	all adults and children discharged during the year
Newborns	1974	all newborns discharged during the year
BED COUNT		
Adults & children	220	Number of beds staffed, equipped, and available
Bassinets	20	Number of bassinets staffed, equipped, and available
MORTALITY DATA		Deaths (these numbers are included in Discharges, above)
Total adults & children		
Under 48 hours	20	Total adult and child deaths within 48 hours of admission
Over 48 hours	138	Total adult and child deaths 48 hours after admission
Total newborns		
Under 48 hours	3	Total newborn deaths within 48 hours of admission
Over 48 hours	2	Total newborn deaths 48 hours after admission
Anesthesia deaths	1	Number of patients who died after receiving anesthesia
OPERATIONS		
Number of patients operated on	1200	Number of patients on whom operations were performed
Surgical operations performed	1312	Number of individual surgical procedures performed
Anesthesia administered	1200	Number of individual administrations of anesthesia
Postoperative infections	30	Number of patients who developed infections as a result of their surgical procedures
OTHER DATA		
Nosocomial infections	231	Number of patients who developed infections in the hospital
Cesarean sections	303	Number of deliveries performed by cesarean section
Deliveries	1304	Number of women who gave birth in the hospital

◆ **Figure 9-20**
Community Hospital 2004 year-end statistics.

Figure 9-22 gives an example of this calculation. The patient is admitted on July 26 and discharged on August 6.

Step 1: The patient is in the hospital in July for 6 days. Remember to count the day of admission.

Step 2: The stay in August is only 5 days because the day of discharge does not count.

Step 3: Add the 6 days in July to the 5 days in August.

Result: The LOS for this patient is 11 days.

If you want to do this arithmetically without actually listing the days in the month, you can subtract the days in July and add back one for the admission date and subtract the days in August and then add the July and August days.

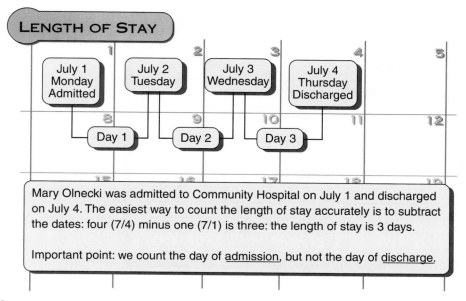

◆ **Figure 9-21**
Calculation of length of stay within a calendar month.

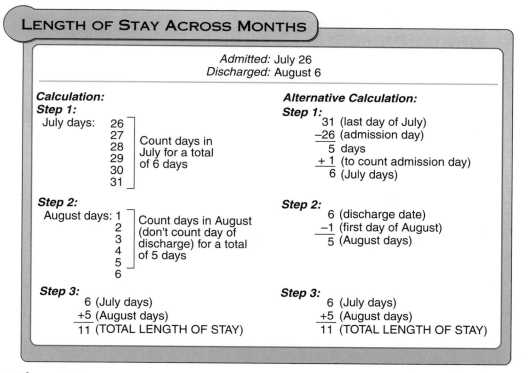

◆ **Figure 9-22**
Calculation of length of stay across calendar months.

In an electronic environment, the computer very nicely calculates this type of information for you. However, it sometimes is necessary to calculate LOS manually. If you need to calculate a patient's LOS and you happen to be sitting at a computer that has a spreadsheet program, you can use the spreadsheet to calculate the LOS by subtracting the dates. Figure 9-23 show the formula for subtracting two dates in Microsoft Excel.

	A	B	C	D	E	F
1						
2						
3						
4		**Length of Stay Using Microsoft Excel**				
5						
6		Admission date		9/15/2006		
7						
8		Discharge date		11/4/2006		
9						
10		Length of stay		= D8-D6		
11						
12						
13						
14						

◆ **Figure 9-23**
Length of stay using Microsoft Excel.

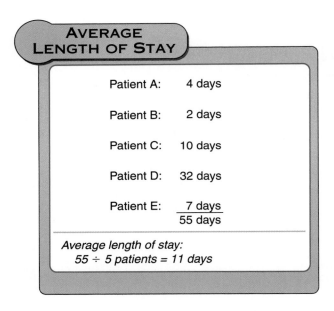

◆ **Figure 9-24**
Calculation of average length of stay.

AVERAGE LENGTH OF STAY

LOS is very important in defining the type of facility and in analyzing its patient population. **Average length of stay (ALOS)** is calculated by adding up the LOSs for a group of patients and dividing by the number of patients in the group. Figure 9-24 illustrates the ALOS of patients in an acute care facility using patients who were discharged in July as an example. In the example, the total LOS of all the patients combined is 55 days. Fifty-five days divided by five patients gives the average number of days, 11 days. This type of an average is called the *arithmetic mean.*

ALOS refers to the arithmetic mean of all the patients' LOSs within a certain period. Usually, ALOS is calculated monthly or annually or in some relevant time period. ALOS might also be calculated by medical specialty, and it can even be calculated in terms of a specific physician's

Hit-Bit

Number of Days in a Month

To calculate length of stay from one month to the next, it is important to know how many days there are in a month. There are four months that have 30 days: April, June, September, and November. February has 28 days, except in leap years (every 4 years), when it has 29 days. All of the other months have 31 days.

If you have trouble remembering how many days there are in a particular month, try creating a mnemonic. Using the first letters of each of the 30-day months, create a silly sentence that will help you associate them. You will want to use April and June in the sentence, because there are other months that begin with those letters. For example: "April and June are *N*ot *S*ummer" or "April's *S*ister is *N*ot June." As a child, you may have learned the jingle "Thirty days hath September, April, June, and November; all the rest have 31, except February alone, which has 28 in time, and each leap year 29."

practice. These calculations are useful in determining whether a physician or a particular medical specialty conforms to the average in a particular hospital or whether the physician or specialty is higher or lower in terms of ALOS.

One of the characteristics of an acute care facility is that the ALOS of its patient population is less than 30 days. In reality, the ALOS of an acute care facility may be significantly less than that, depending on what type of patients are treated there. For example, a community hospital with a large number of mothers and NBs, whose stay in the facility is generally 1 to 3 days, will tend to have a very low ALOS—perhaps only 4 or 5 days. On the other hand, a trauma center hospital with a large number of patients with serious trauma, burns, and transplants might have an ALOS closer to 12 or 13 days.

TRANSFERS

Patients can be transferred from one unit to another inside a facility, or they can be discharged and transferred to another facility (Figure 9-25). When a patient is transferred to another facility, the discharged disposition may be one of the following:

- Transfer to rehabilitation facility
- Transfer to skilled nursing facility (internal to the facility)
- Transfer to skilled nursing facility (external to the facility)
- Transfer to another acute care facility
- Transfer to long-term acute care facility
- Transfer to nursing home

Hit-Bit

Transfer Data

The transfer of a patient to another facility requires the transfer of sufficient information to support effective continuity of care. A special *transfer form* is generally used, and copies of all or part of the health record may accompany the patient. The receiving hospital (the hospital to which the patient is transferred) counts the patient as an admission. *Interhospital transfer* describes this movement of a patient from one facility to another. *Intrahospital transfer* reflects movement of a patient between nursing units and therefore has no overall impact on census. Figure 7–11 shows the transfer of patients between two nursing units on May 31, 2000.

INTRAHOSPITAL TRANSFERS

	Unit A	Unit B	Total
5/31/04 midnight census	3	2	5
Transfers in	+1	+2	+3
Transfers out	-2	-1	-3
6/1/04 midnight census	2	3	5

Transfers between Units A and B have no impact on census

Here is a table that reflects the same information:

	Unit A	Unit B	Total
6/1/04 midnight census	3	2	5
Admissions	+2	0	+2
Discharges	-2	-1	-3
6/2/04 midnight census	3	1	4

◆ **Figure 9-25**
Intrahospital transfers.

CENSUS

	Total
6/1/04 midnight census	5
Admissions	+2
Discharges	-3
6/2/04 midnight census	4

Because the number of discharges (decrease) was more than the number of admissions (increase), the inpatient census decreased.

◆ **Figure 9-26**
Census.

CENSUS

The total number of patients in the hospital is called the **census.** The term *census* describes both the physical activity of counting (or confirming a computer-generated list of) the patients as well as the resultant total. Admissions increase the census; discharges decrease the census (Figure 9-26).

The census is taken at the same time every day, usually midnight, so that the facility can compare the census from day to day over time. This census number is also called the *midnight census.* For practical purposes, a computer database allows the patient registration department to view the census at any time.

In Chapter 1, you learned that hospitals are licensed for a specific number of beds. This means that the hospital is not permitted, under normal circumstances, to admit more patients than the number of beds allowed by the state license. Because of this rule, the facility must always know how many patients are occupying beds. The patient registration department, also known as the *admissions department,* is responsible for assigning a patient to a room.

Hospital administrators like to review the census by nursing unit, wing, or floor. This view enables administrators to identify underutilized areas for planning purposes. It also allows nursing managers to plan and control staffing. The impact of the two admissions and three discharges on the census taken between June 1 and June 2, 2004 (see Figure 9-25) is detailed by nursing unit (see Table 9-2).

For statistical purposes, we record the midnight census for comparison over time. A census, however, does not measure all of the services provided by the hospital. What about the patient who is admitted at 10:40 a.m. and dies before midnight? That patient would not be present for the counting of the midnight census. The facility counts these patients in the service days for the facility called *inpatient service days (IPSDs).*

Can you tell from the census report in Figure 9-26 how many patients received services on June 2, 2004? Actually, we do not have enough information. Table 9-3 shows the admission and discharge detailed by patient. We can see that the two patients who were admitted on June 2 were also discharged the same day. Table 9-3 analyzes the service days received by those patients. From our analysis, we can see that there were actually 6 days of service (IPSDs) rendered by the hospital.

At the end of 2003, there were 325 patients in Community Hospital. At the end of 2004, the adults and children census was 180 (see Figure 9-20). There were 145 fewer adults and children in

TABLE 9-2	**Number of Patients Who Received Services Detailed by Patient**	
	INPATIENTS	**TOTAL**
6/1/03 midnight census	M. Brown	5
	S. Crevecoeur	
	F. Perez	
	P. Smith	
	R. Wooley	
Admissions	C. Estevez	2
	B. Mooney	
Discharges	S. Crevecoeur	3
	C. Estevez	
	B. Mooney	
6/2/03 midnight census	M. Brown	4
	F. Perez	
	P. Smith	
	R. Wooley	

TABLE 9-3	Analysis of Patients Who Received a Day of Service on June 2, 2003	
INPATIENTS	**ANALYSIS**	**6/2 DAY OF SERVICE**
M. Brown	Inpatient on 6/1 and 6/2	1
S. Crevecoeur	Discharged 6/2	0
C. Estevez	Admitted and discharged 6/2	1
B. Mooney	Admitted and discharged 6/2	1
F. Perez	Inpatient on 6/1 and 6/2	1
P. Smith	Inpatient on 6/1 and 6/2	1
R. Wooley	Inpatient on 6/1 and 6/2	1
Total days of service		6

Hit-Bit

Calculating Length of Stay

In counting days of service, as in length of stay, we count the day of admission but not the day of discharge. This makes sense because if the hospital counted the day of discharge as well, it would conceivably charge twice for the same bed on the same day. The same principle allows the facility to count 1 day of service for a patient who is admitted and discharged on the same day.

the hospital at the end of the year 2004 than there were at the beginning. How did that happen? Look at the admissions and discharges. There were more discharges than admissions during the year: 145, to be exact.

Understanding the relationship among the statistics helps us to use these data effectively. For example, in Chapter 1 you learned about LOS and ALOS. Looking at Figure 9-20, you know that there were 14,545 adults and children discharged in 2004. The total LOS for all of those patients combined was 72,107 days. Therefore the ALOS for adults and children in 2004 was 4.96 days (72,107 / 14,545 = 4.96).

All health care facilities keep track of their statistics according to the fiscal year, which is a 12-month reporting period. A facility's reporting period can be the calendar year (January 1 through December 31), or it can be July 1 through June 30, or October 1 through September 30. Figure 9-27 is organized into fiscal periods. To understand this, think of how a year is organized into days, weeks, and months. When we calculate and report statistics, we do so by the relevant fiscal period. In addition to days, weeks, and months, we also group the months into quarters. Each quarter represents 3 months, or approximately one fourth of the year. Health care statistics are frequently organized in this manner.

In Chapter 1, you also learned about occupancy. Occupancy is calculated by dividing the number of days that patients used beds by the number of beds available. The number of days that patients used beds is called the IPSDs. IPSDs are calculated daily by adding the admissions to the census, subtracting the discharges, then adding back the patients who were admitted and discharged on the same day. Patients who were admitted and discharged on the same day used beds, but they do not appear in the midnight census.

The census need not be analyzed patient by patient to calculate IPSDs. You can obtain the total number of patients admitted and discharged on the same day from census reports (Table 9-4). Once IPSDs have been calculated, the data can be added, averaged, graphed, and trended over time. It is also a means to calculate occupancy, as mentioned, because it includes all patients who were admitted and discharged the same day. Because the census counts only patients in beds at a

THE FISCAL YEAR

QUARTER	Month	# of Days	Admissions	Discharges	Census	
					325	**12/31/03**
I	January	31	1125	1148	302	
	February	29	1543	1555	290	
	March	31	1445	1430	305	
II	April	30	1406	1398	313	
	May	31	1242	1247	308	
	June	30	1004	994	318	
III	July	31	1254	1248	324	
	August	31	1145	1148	321	
	September	30	1212	1224	309	
IV	October	31	1478	1502	285	
	November	30	1567	1598	254	
	December	31	1229	1303	180	
Total		**366**	**15,650**	**15,795**		**12/31/04**

2004 was a leap year. In non-leap years, February has 28 days, for a total of 365 days in the year. How many weeks are there in a year?

◆ **Figure 9-27**
The fiscal year.

TABLE 9-4	**Inpatient Service Days Calculated from Census**

	TOTAL
6/1/00 midnight census	5
Admissions	+2
Discharges	−3
6/2/00 midnight census	4
Patients admitted and discharged on 6/2	+2
6/2/00 inpatient service days	6

point in time, calculating IPSDs is a better measure of the use of hospital facilities. Figure 9-28 illustrates all the IPSD concepts discussed so far.

HOSPITAL RATES AND PERCENTAGES

There are many ways to look at hospital statistics. One very common method is to look at the number of times something occurred compared with (divided by) the number of times it could have occurred.

This basic calculation provides a rate of occurrence. Multiplied by 100, the rate is expressed as a percentage. Figure 9-29 provides an example of rates versus percentages.

Once you know how to calculate percentages, you can look at occurrences in a facility as rates and percentages. For example, you may want to know the percentage of hospital patients who

CENSUS STATISTICS

A&C = Adults and children   Adm. = Admissions
N/B = Newborn   D/C = Discharges
NICU = Neonatal ICU   IPSD = Inpatient service days

| | Adults & Children | | | Newborns | | |
	UNIT A	UNIT B	TOTAL A&C	N/B nursery	NICU	TOTAL N/B
6/1/04 midnight census	15	17	32	3	1	4
Admissions/births	+4	+2	+6	2	0	2
Discharges/deaths	-5	-4	-9	0	0	0
Transfers in	+2	+1	+3	0	+1	+1
Transfers out	-1	-2	-3	-1	0	-1
6/2/04 midnight census	15	14	29	4	2	6
Adm. & D/C 6/2/04	+2	+1	+3	0	0	0
6/2/04 IPSD	17	15	32	4	2	6

In the past, spreadsheets like this were prepared daily, by hand. Imagine how complicated that could get with 500 patients spread over 16 nursing units! Fortunately, computers do the majority of work for us. Even if the main system doesn't present the information the way we want to see it, computerized spreadsheet programs help us to reorganize it. However, there is a very important rule you need to learn about computer reports: Just because something comes from a computer doesn't mean it's correct!

◆ **Figure 9-28**
Census statistics.

RATES AND PERCENTAGES

RATE:

$$\frac{67 \text{ female patients}}{134 \text{ total patients}} = \frac{1}{2}$$

One out of every two patients is female.

PERCENTAGE:

$$\frac{67 \text{ female patients}}{134 \text{ total patients}} = .50 \ (\times 100) = 50\%$$

Fifty percent of patients are female.

◆ **Figure 9-29**
Rates and percentages.

Exercise 9-5

Routine Institutional Statistics

FIRST QUARTER DATA
DIAMONTE HOSPITAL
10/1/06 - 12/31/06

ADMISSIONS
Adults and children	9218
Newborns	290

DISCHARGES (including deaths)
Adults and children	9014
Newborns	303

INPATIENT SERVICE DAYS
Adults and children	35,421
Newborns	432

TOTAL LENGTH OF STAY
Adults and children	32,542
Newborns	608

BED COUNT
Adults and children	450
Newborns	30

MORTALITY DATA
Total adults and children	
Under 48 hours	12
48 hours or over	132
Total newborns	
Under 48 hours	2
48 hours or over	1
Anesthesia deaths	1
Fetal deaths	
Early	3
Intermediate and late	9
Maternal deaths	1
Postoperative deaths	
Under 10 days	45
10 days or over	5

OPERATIONS
Number of patients operated on	836
Surgical operations performed	889
Anesthesia administered	856
Postoperative infections	12

MISCELLANEOUS
Cesarean sections	69
Deliveries	349
Nosocomial infections	13
Consultations	2,756

1. What is the hospital's fiscal year?
2. Calculate the following:
   a. Average inpatient service days
   b. Average newborn inpatient service days
   c. Average length of stay
   d. Bed occupancy
   e. Consultation rate
   f. Nosocomial infection rate

HEALTH CARE STATISTICS FORMULAS

Average Inpatient Service Days:

$$\frac{\text{Total inpatient service days for a period (excluding newborns)}}{\text{Total number of days in the period}}$$

Average Newborn Inpatient Service Days:

$$\frac{\text{Total newborn inpatient service days for a period}}{\text{Total number of days in the period}}$$

Average Length of Stay:

$$\frac{\text{Total length of stay (discharge days)}}{\text{Total discharges (including deaths)}}$$

Bed Occupancy Rate:

$$\frac{\text{Total inpatient service days in a period} \times 100}{\text{Total bed count days in the period (bed count} \times \text{number of days in the period)}}$$

Newborn Bassinet Occupancy Ratio Formula:

$$\frac{\text{Total newborn inpatient service days for a period} \times 100}{\text{Total newborn bassinet count} \times \text{number of days in the period}}$$

Other Rates Formula:

$$\frac{\text{Number of times something occurred} \times 100}{\text{Number of times something could have occurred}}$$

◆ **Figure 9-30**
Health care statistics formulas.

acquired nosocomial infections. (Nosocomial infections are infections acquired in the hospital, as opposed to infections that were present on admission.) Looking at Figure 9-20, you can see that there were 231 occurrences of nosocomial infections at Community Hospital in 2004. Because 15,495 (14,545 + 950) patients were treated (discharged), 15,495 is the number of possible occurrences of nosocomial infections. The percentage of nosocomial infections is 1.5%:

The key to understanding hospital rates and percentages is to understand the underlying data and how those data elements relate to one another. Some of the most common types of calculations are shown in Figure 9-30.

Thus there are many ways to report data. The way in which they are reported depends on the needs of the user. It is important for the HIM professional to understand the needs of the user to help identify the data for meaningful reporting and presentation.

■ SUGGESTED READING

Abdelhak, Mervat, Sara Grostick, Mary Alice Hanken, and Ellen Jacobs. *Health Information: Management of a Strategic Resource.* 2nd ed. Philadelphia: Saunders, 2001.
Quinn, John. "An HL7 Overview." *Journal of AHIMA, 70*(1999): 32-34.

■ WEB SITES

Centers for Disease Control: http://www.cdc.gov
Center for Medicare and Medicaid Services: http://www.cms.hhs.gov
National Center for Health Statistics: http://www.cdc.gov/nchs/nvss.htm

CHAPTER ACTIVITIES

CHAPTER SUMMARY

Health information must be collected in a systematic, defined format known as *data sets*. This collection of data is then stored in a database for future use. The data sets and database must comply with law, accreditation, policy, and the needs of the organization. The database is then a source of information for departments within the organization as well as agencies external to the facility.

The data can be analyzed, interpreted, and presented to appropriate users by using the following tools: statistical mean, median, and mode, as well as bar graphs, pie charts, and line graphs. The analysis of a facility's data is also referred to as the facility's *statistics*, which describes the services and activities of the facility.

Review Questions

1. Identify the minimal required data elements of a patient health information abstract.
2. List individual departments and outside agencies to which you might report information.
3. List the statistical tools, and explain their use.
4. What is the formula for computing the average length of stay?
5. The following patients were discharged from pediatrics for the week 7/16/01 to 7/22/01:

PATIENT NAME	ADMISSION DATE	DISCHARGE DATE
Groot	7/13/01	7/15/01
Smith	7/12/01	7/15/01
Brown	7/11/01	7/16/01
Kowalski	7/10/01	7/20/01
Zhong	7/09/01	7/19/01
Frank	6/29/01	7/18/01

   What is the average length of stay of these patients?

6. The time that an inpatient stays in the hospital is referred to as *length of stay*. How does one calculate length of stay? Average length of stay?

Coding Supervisor

My name is Maggie, and I am the coding supervisor at Woodlawn Memorial Hospital, a medium-sized facility. Woodlawn has 250 inpatient beds, 30 bassinets, a skilled nursing unit with 25 beds, a rehabilitation unit with 20 beds, and one unit leased to a long-term acute care facility. In addition, we have a same-day surgery wing, a pain management clinic, and a physician's clinic located within our facility. I am responsible for the daily operations of the coding staff in the facility: I supervise six coders—four full-time and two part-time employees.

My supervision of the daily routine includes the following:
- Ensuring that accounts are coded within 72 hours of the patient's discharge
- Assisting case management with questions regarding patient diagnosis related groups (DRGs)
- Handling business office issues
- Coordinating questions to physicians regarding documentation

I also oversee the quality of the data contained in the health information management (HIM) database.

During a recent conversion of our software, I participated on the team that developed a data dictionary. During this process, I became the contact person for all matters concerning the HIM database. In this new role, I process all requests for reports from the HIM database. When quality management, administration, physician, or case management staff members need information from our database, they come to me. I make sure I know the following:
- What information they want
- Why they need it
- The time frame for the information
- When they need the report

This information helps me run the correct report so that employees may use the information as necessary in their presentation, decision making, or investigation.

I find this part of my job very rewarding. I enjoy receiving a request that people think is impossible because I know that our HIM database contains the information that they need. Providing those reports is really exciting.

Making Data Informative

Health information professionals are commonly asked to analyze data for presentation. The presentation may be a simple table or report, or it may include graphs.

Using the Internet, locate a database of patient information for query of a diagnosis related group assigned by your instructor. Prepare a report with a graph for presentation to your instructor.

Using the coronary artery bypass graft report in Figure 9-10, prepare a presentation for your instructor demonstrating the average length of stay for the patients of each physician.

Chapter 10

QUALITY AND USES OF HEALTH INFORMATION

CHAPTER OBJECTIVES

By the end of this chapter, the student should be able to

- Identify various uses of health information.
- Review health records for documentation in compliance with accreditation agency standards.
- Review records to obtain information specific to a request for committee review.
- Participate in a quality improvement project using health information to improve patient care.
- Identify appropriate requests for health information to be used within and outside the health care facility.
- Identify the uses of health information related to the quality of patient care.
- Provide examples of the types of record reviews conducted by health information technologists to assist in the quality of care for patients and documentation in the health record.
- Identify the steps in the quality assurance process.
- Understand the intent of various health care regulations and standards.

VOCABULARY

American College of Surgeons (ACS)

benchmarking

brainstorming

case management

certification

clinical pathway

clinical pertinence

concurrent review

decision matrix

graph

incidence

interdepartmental

intradepartmental

litigation

marketing

morbidity

mortality

performance improvement (PI)

placebo

potentially compensable event (PCE)

prevalence

qualitative analysis

quality assurance (QA)

reimbursement

research

retrospective review

risk management

survey

table

tracer methodology

utilization management (UM)

nce you have collected a patient's health information, what can you do with it? For the data to be useful, you must ensure that the information is timely, accurate, and complete. In this chapter, you will learn the methods used to evaluate and ensure data quality and how health information is used for reimbursement, litigation, accreditation, marketing, research, education, and quality management.

THE QUALITY OF HEALTH CARE

For health information to be used effectively, it must reflect high-quality data. In Chapter 5, you learned about data quality characteristics (see Table 5-1). Now you are ready to think about the meaning of quality. Common sense suggests that quality is a good thing. However, in health care, quality is determined by the person or agency that is evaluating the product or service. Some people define *quality* as "something that is excellent," whereas others may judge quality by the outcome of the service.

Customers are typically the people who judge quality. In health care, there are many customers—patients, physicians, insurance companies, attorneys, accreditation agencies, and employees. Each of these customers analyzes quality from a different perspective. Therefore a discussion of quality management in health care can lead in many different directions. Patients determine quality according to their perception of the services and care they receive. Physicians perceive the facility through the eyes of their patients, their office staff, and their professional and personal interactions with employees in the facility. Insurance companies perceive the quality of a facility through the cost and outcome of the services provided to their beneficiaries. Employees may perceive the facility's quality through the competence of the staff and administration. Accreditation agencies perceive quality in terms of the facility's compliance with set standards. These examples are only a few of the methods by which a facility's quality is assessed, but you can see that a facility is judged from many different perspectives. The facility itself measures quality on the basis of its priorities. The next section provides a simple explanation of quality theories and the use of health information in quality activities. However they assess quality, the facility must use a formal method for measuring and improving it.

Hit-Bit

Quality

Quality is perceived through the eyes of the patient according to the patient's priorities. For some patients, a prolonged life far outweighs the pain caused by a medical procedure. For example, a patient who suffers from persistent heart attacks requires bypass surgery to correct his heart dynamics and improve his chances for a longer life. The patient experiences tremendous pain from the surgery; however, if he no longer has heart attacks after the operation, his condition is improved. The patient is probably pleased with the outcome despite the intense pain that he experienced during the procedure. Therefore quality was not determined by the amount of pain experienced by the patient.

For another patient, the health care experience may end with a healthy new baby. However, during the course of the patient's stay, the nurses and employees of the facility were rude, uncooperative, and of little help to the new mother. Although the experience ended well, this patient perceived the quality as poor because of her interaction with the staff.

Note that each circumstance is different, but in each case the quality of the service is determined by the customer.

■ QUALITY MANAGEMENT THEORIES

Typically, in the health care industry, quality is not consistent unless it is managed. Therefore health care facilities have a quality management department, usually staffed by health information management (HIM) and nursing professionals. It is the primary responsibility of this department to ensure quality for all customers throughout the facility. This department performs a significant number of record reviews, participates in and often coordinates medical staff and facility committees, and oversees performance improvement.

A sensible approach to quality includes the following:

1. The facility has a procedure or process in place that ensures quality. (Do things correctly.)
2. Employees periodically review the procedure or process and the product. (Check to make sure the facility is doing things correctly.)
3. Review of the procedures, processes, and product is always documented. (When you check the procedure or process, write down your findings.)
4. Any corrections required to guarantee quality in the procedure or process are made promptly. (If you find an error, fix it!)

Common sense prompts the development of methods to prevent, detect, or correct flaws in a product or service to improve the quality. These methods are referred to as *preventive controls*, *detective controls*, or *corrective controls*, respectively (see Chapter 5). To control something, you must be able to affect or change it in some way.

To understand quality management methods, you should know something about those who are credited with the founding theories: Deming, Juran, and Crosby. Their theories contain very similar and yet sometimes contradictory rules for managing quality. Each author has influenced the way the health care industry monitors quality. Therefore it would be correct to say they have inadvertently influenced the necessity to use health information to monitor quality and, in doing so, have promoted the improvement of the quality of health information.

DEMING

Of the three quality management pioneers, W. Edwards Deming was the first and is perhaps the most widely known. Deming established his reputation when the Japanese used his philosophy to rebuild their industry after World War II. As consumers increasingly chose products that were made in Japan, American industry realized the value of adopting a quality management philosophy.

Deming's philosophy is process oriented, which means that an emphasis is placed on *how* a task is performed or a product is produced. (This is different from the evaluation of the end product that occurs only once, at the end of production.) A product that does not meet company standards must be identified before it is completed. If the problem is noted after the production is completed, the company may not be able to correct it. However, if a company inspects the process as the product is being developed, problems are more likely to be addressed and corrected before it is too late. Deming developed 14 principles to implement a successful quality management program and identified seven deadly diseases that would harm a quality management program. Deming's quality principles (consolidated in Rudman 1997, p. 10) are as follows:

■ Change plus innovation equals stability and organizational survival.
■ Organizations have a responsibility to provide employees with appropriate education and resources.
■ Organizations must foster employee empowerment and pride in work.
■ Organizations should emphasize process and eliminate benchmark standards and performance evaluation.
■ Quality is emphasized constantly.

JURAN

Another pivotal approach to quality management is Joseph M. Juran's "quality trilogy." According to Juran, every quality management program should have a strong yet balanced infrastructure (foundation) of quality planning, control, and improvement. He also defined a successful program as one that is acceptable to the entire organization; the program should be as important to the employees as it is to the administrators. Finally, Juran emphasized the value of documentation and data in the quality management program.

CROSBY

Philip Crosby is best known for the term *zero defects*. The Crosby quality management philosophy requires education of the *entire* organization. Education of the entire organization requires that everyone—staff employees, supervisors, managers, and administrators—be knowledgeable about the program and motivated to participate.

For a health care facility to effectively improve the quality of its care and services, it needs to adopt some method or philosophy similar to the three mentioned here. The idea of checking the quality of health care provided in the United States is not new. Quality, however, has evolved into a major focus for the health care industry.

Exercise 10-1

Quality Management Theories

1. What is quality? Take a moment to define *quality*, and then discuss your thoughts with another person. Is that person's perception of quality the same as yours?
2. According to Juran's quality management philosophy, a quality management program should have a strong and balanced infrastructure of quality:
   a. planning, doing, and acting
   b. planning, control, and improvement
   c. management philosophy
   d. with zero defects
3. Your health care facility is embarking on a new quality effort. For weeks now, administrators, managers, and supervisors have been involved in meetings and training to ensure that everyone in the organization has a clear understanding of the new quality initiative message. The board has announced that this new effort will involve everyone in the organization. At the very core of this initiative is the motto "zero defects." This organization is being guided by the philosophy of which of the following thinkers?
   a. Deming
   b. Juran
   c. Crosby
   d. Shewhart
4. Which of the following philosophies is process oriented?
   a. Deming
   b. Juran
   c. Crosby
   d. Shewhart
5. Diamonte Hospital is committed to their continuous quality improvement (CQI) philosophy. They currently have several quality improvement (QI) teams organized to address the processes associated with the delivery of patient care. This facility is most likely being guided by the theories of which of the following philosophers?
   a. Deming
   b. Juran
   c. Crosby
   d. Shewhart

◼ HISTORY AND EVOLUTION OF QUALITY IN HEALTH CARE

In the eighteenth century, hospitals had a high incidence of deadly epidemics and relatively high death rates. The poor received health care in hospitals, whereas the wealthy were visited in their homes. The concept of quality in health care can be traced to the late nineteenth century, when, hospitals finally became known as places where people could go to get well. During this time, two

Hit-Bit

American Medical Association and American Hospital Association

The American Medical Association (AMA) was founded in 1847.

The American Hospital Association began as the Association of Hospital Superintendents in 1899. In 1910, the name was changed to the AHA (http://www.aha.org/about/history.html).

important associations were founded: the American Medical Association (AMA) and the American Hospital Association (AHA). These two associations worked diligently to promote high-quality health care through standardized medical education and hospital functions. Figure 10-1 provides a time line of the evolution of quality in health care.

MEDICAL EDUCATION

Before the existence of formal medical education, early physicians were trained through an apprenticeship. By the early twentieth century, many medical institutions existed to educate physicians. As the health care profession increased in size and number of physicians, the quality of patient care was compromised. Although having more physicians seemed like a good solution to an ailing population, the facts suggested that more needed to be done to improve the quality of health care. Even after the establishment of the AMA in 1847, the medical education provided by many institutions remained questionable. Medical institutions needed a standardized mechanism to guide the training of physicians.

Abner Flexner studied the quality of medical education in the United States. His report in 1910 documented critical issues and discrepancies in medical education. The findings in the Flexner Report prompted the closing of many institutions, revisions of the curriculum in those that remained, and implementation by the AMA of a mechanism for accreditation of medical education institutions.

STANDARDIZATION AND ACCREDITATION

Not long after the Flexner Report, in 1913 the **American College of Surgeons (ACS)** was founded as an association of surgeons "to improve the quality of care for the surgical patient by setting high standards for surgical education and practice" (http://www.facs.org). The ACS assumed responsibility for reviewing the quality of health care provided to patients in hospitals. Its efforts to analyze quality involved review of information from patient medical records, which revealed insufficient documentation of patient care.

18th Century	19th Century			20th Century					21st Century
Deadly epidemics Hospitals unpopular	AMA est. 1847	AOA est. 1897	AHA est. 1899	Flexner Report 1910	Club of Record Clerks 1912	ACS est. 1913	JCAHO est. 1950s	Medicare est. 1965	

◆ **Figure 10-1**

Time line of the evolution of quality in health care.

Hit-Bit

"If It Isn't Documented, It Didn't Happen"

The proof is in the documentation. The old saying "If it isn't documented, it didn't happen" had an effect on the history of health care. The lack of documentation prohibited the effective study of quality to improve health care.

In an attempt to standardize contents of the patient health record so that future reviews could provide useful information, the ACS developed the *Hospital Standardization Program.* This program established standards, or rules, by which the ACS would survey hospitals to assess quality of care. The first survey after the establishment of the Hospital Standardization Program revealed that only 13% of the hospitals surveyed (with 100 beds or more) met the standards. The ACS then determined that for a facility to be considered a hospital it must meet a set of minimum standards. These required health records to be maintained in a timely, accurate fashion and specified the minimum content or required documentation for a health record (Figure 10-2).

By the 1950s, the ACS was overwhelmed by the demand of hospitals for surveys. The establishment of the Joint Commission on the Accreditation of Hospitals (JCAH) was a collaborative effort supported by the AMA, AHA, and ACS. The JCAH was established to relieve the ACS of the responsibility of surveying hospitals. Over time, JCAH accreditation became popular in alternative health care settings, and in 1987 the organization was renamed the Joint Commission on Accreditation of Healthcare Organizations (JCAHO). Current accreditation under JCAHO requires compliance with standards found in the JCAHO accreditation manuals for the various health care settings (Table 10-1). Because JCAHO has a significant presence in health care (even though the accreditation is voluntary), many JCAHO requirements for compliance are discussed throughout this chapter.

TABLE 10-1	**List of JCAHO Accreditation Manuals**
SETTING	**MANUAL**
Health care networks	*2005 to 2006 Comprehensive Accreditation Manual for Integrated Delivery Systems* (CAMIDS)
	2005 to 2006 Comprehensive Accreditation Manual for Managed Care Organizations (CAMMCO)
	Accreditation Manual for Preferred Provider Organizations, 3rd edition (AMPPO)
Behavioral health	*Comprehensive Accreditation Manual for Behavioral Health Centers*
Home health	*Comprehensive Accreditation Manual for Home Care*
Hospitals	*Comprehensive Accreditation Manual for Hospitals*
Long-term care	*Comprehensive Accreditation Manual for Long-term Care*
Laboratories and point of care testing	*2005–2006 Comprehensive Accreditation Manual for Laboratory and Point-of-Care Testing* (CAMLAB)
Ambulatory	*Comprehensive Accreditation Manual for Ambulatory Care*
Critical access hospitals	*Accreditation Manual for Critical Access Hospitals,* 2nd edition (AMCAH)
Disease-specific care	*Disease-Specific Care Certification Manual,* 2nd edition
Health care staffing	*Health Care Staffing Services Certification Manual*
Office-based surgery	*Accreditation Manual for Office-Based Surgery Practices,* 2nd edition

Modified from "Manuals," Joint Commission on Accreditation of Healthcare Organizations: http://www.jcrinc.com/publications.asp?durki=77#aclink.

MEDICAL RECORD SPECIFICATIONS — MINIMUM STANDARDS

A complete case record should be developed, including the following:

- Patient identification data
- Complaint
- Personal and family history
- History of current illness
- Physical examination
- Special examinations (consultations, radiography, clinical laboratory)
- Provisional or working diagnosis
- Medical and surgical treatments
- Progress notes
- Gross and microscopic findings
- Final diagnosis
- Condition on discharge
- Follow-up
- Autopsy findings in the event of death

◆ **Figure 10-2**
Minimum standards for medical record specifications.

ACCREDITATION AGENCIES

Accreditation is a common indicator of quality and compliance with predetermined standards in today's health care industry. JCAHO is no longer the only accreditation agency. Other examples of accreditation bodies are the Commission on Accreditation of Rehabilitation Facilities (CARF), which accredits rehabilitation facilities; the American Osteopathic Association (AOA), which accredits osteopathic facilities; the Accreditation Association for Ambulatory Health Care, which accredits ambulatory care facilities; and the National Committee for Quality Assurance (NCQA), which accredits managed care organizations. Table 1-6 provides a list of major accreditation agencies.

FEDERAL GOVERNMENT

In 1965, the federal government established the Medicare (Title XVIII) and Medicaid (Title XIX) programs. Medicare is federally funded health insurance for the elderly and some disabled people. Medicaid is health insurance for the poor that is funded by both federal and state government.

When the federal government began paying for health care, the quality and cost of care for the beneficiaries became a concern. Thus the federal government began performing reviews of the actual care received by Medicare patients through audits of patient health records. Reviewers traveled to health care facilities and looked at the health record documentation to be certain that Medicare patients were receiving appropriate care. If the documentation did not reflect high-quality care, the facility was cited and its administrators asked to explain why the services did not meet minimal standards; in some cases, the administrators were forced to return reimbursements.

In the twenty-first century, the health care industry is still heavily regulated and surveyed for compliance with standards and quality. Today, aforementioned reviews are performed by a Quality Improvement Organization (QIO). As stated on the CMS Web site, "QIOs work with consumers, physicians, hospitals, and other caregivers to refine care delivery systems to make sure patients get the right care at the right time, particularly among underserved populations. The program also safeguards the integrity of the Medicare trust fund by ensuring payment is made only for

Hit-Bit

History of the American Health Information Management Association

The history of the American Health Information Management Association (AHIMA) can be traced back to the Club of Record Clerks, which was organized in 1912 by a small group of women known as medical record librarians. The group officially initiated the Association of Record Librarians of North America (ARLNA), which included members from both the United States and Canada. The first president of this organization was Grace Whiting Myers. Eventually, the members from Canada and the United States separated, and the U.S. organization became known as the American Association of Medical Record Librarians (AAMRL). In 1970, the association changed its name to the American Medical Record Association (AMRA). AMRA conferred the following credentials: Accredited Record Technician (ART) and Registered Record Administrator (RRA). Over the next 20 years, the roles and responsibilities of the ART and the RRA reflected more diverse areas. By 1991, the association voted to change the name of the AMRA to the American Health Information Management Association (AHIMA). Since that time, the credentials have also changed from ART to Registered Health Information Technician (RHIT) and from RRA to Registered Health Information Administrator (RHIA). The change from medical records to health information was motivated by the changing health care environment and the responsibilities of the association's members. HIM professionals hold positions in various roles, health care settings, and associated areas, such as hospitals, alternative health care settings, consulting, accreditation agencies, managed care companies, case management , quality management, insurance agencies, and attorneys offices.

AHIMA is a membership organization with offices in Chicago and Washington, D.C.

medically necessary services and investigates beneficiary complaints about quality of care" (http://www.cms.hhs.gov/qio/). The QIO is under contract with CMS in what is called a *scope of work*. The scope of work outlines the expectations of CMS for the QIO. Health records and health information remain a vital part of this process.

Exercise 10-2

History and Evolution of Health Care Quality

1. Which association was the first to recognize a need for quality in health care and was organized for the purpose of promoting it?
2. What was the name of the first program (set of standards) designed to measure quality in a health care setting?
3. Voluntary accreditation attained by successfully undergoing a survey according to the standards set forth in the comprehensive accreditation manual for hospitals is given by which of the following organizations?
   a. MCOP
   b. CMS
   c. Medicare
   d. JCAHO
4. Which of the following groups was the predecessor of JCAHO?
   a. Hospital Standardization
   b. AHIMA
   c. NCQA
   d. ACS
5. The _____ preceded JCAHO in the survey of hospitals against set standards.

Monitoring the Quality of Health Information

In the evolution of quality in health care, several associations and organizations were founded to promote quality. Some of them accredit or certify facilities. Health records are among the primary documents used by health care facilities to evaluate compliance with the standards set by the accreditation or certification agencies. In brief, health information is analyzed for quality as a part of patient care, and during this analysis the facility recognizes opportunities to improve its performance. This analysis of quality should occur concurrently (while the patient is in the facility) and retrospectively (after the patient has been discharged).

The HIM department is responsible for monitoring the quality of health information. Each function in the HIM department exists to enable quality; however, the functions must be monitored to ensure quality. The department, typically led by a credentialed HIM professional, coordinates several functions to ensure the health information is timely, complete, accurate, and valid. Essential HIM functions are collection (assembly/abstracting), analysis, coding, storage, and retrieval. The director of HIM must manage the department functions in a manner that promotes useful and accurate information. The director and other personnel ensure quality by reviewing the functions of the HIM department.

Hit-Bit

Timely, Complete, Accurate, and Valid Health Information

TIMELY HEALTH INFORMATION

Timeliness of health information relates to documentation of an event close to the time it occurred. Health information should be documented as events occur, treatment is performed, or results are noticed. Delaying documentation could cause information to be omitted. Reports must be dictated and typed in a timely manner.

The following are examples of timeliness:
- In the physician's office, the patient documents the history before seeing the physician, and the physical examination is completed during the office visit.
- In an acute care facility, the history and physical (H&P) must be on the record within 24 hours of the patient's admission to the facility, and progress notes must be documented daily. Physician's orders must be dated and timed. A discharge summary should be recorded when the patient is discharged and no later than 30 days after discharge.

COMPLETE HEALTH INFORMATION

Completeness of health information requires that the health care record contain all pertinent documents with all of the appropriate documentation—that is, face sheet, H&P, consent forms, progress notes, anesthesia record, operative report, recovery room record, discharge notes, nursing documentation, and so on (see Chapter 5 for the contents of a complete health record). A complete health record can be used in many more ways than an incomplete one. Review of health records to ensure that each record is complete is called *quantitative analysis*.

ACCURATE HEALTH INFORMATION

Accuracy of health information requires that the documentation reflect the event as it really happened, including all pertinent details and relevant facts. Review of health records for pertinent documentation involves examination of the content of each document. All of the pages in the health record must be for the same patient and also for the same visit.

VALID HEALTH INFORMATION

Validity of health information requires that the data or information documented be of an acceptable or allowable predetermined value or within a specified parameter. This particularly pertains to the documentation of clinical services provided to the patient. For example, there are predetermined accepted values for blood pressure and temperature.

QUALITY ASSURANCE

Several aspects of monitoring quality involve ensuring the employees in the HIM department are performing their functions appropriately and that the functions work correctly to promote the employees' productivity. Assembly, analysis, coding, abstracting, completion of records, filing, release of information, and transcription all must happen within specified time frames to enhance the timeliness, completion, accuracy, and validity of the record. The monitoring of these functions is called quality assessment or **quality assurance (QA).** QA monitoring ensures that HIM functions are working effectively within the department's standards. QA is a retrospective analysis, performed at the end of a patient's visit.

The 1984 JCAHO standards outlined specific instructions requiring each department in the health care facility to develop a monitoring and evaluation program. By requiring the participation of all staff and departments in the facility, JCAHO planned to move health care facilities from retrospective QA to quality improvement. Table 10-2 demonstrates the JCAHO 10-step plan, introduced in 1984, as used by the HIM department. The 10 steps required that the facility recognize and assign responsibility, identify important aspects of care and service, determine indicators of quality for these services, set thresholds that would require action when exceeded, develop an organized method for collecting the data according to the indicators, make an assessment of any actions taken to improve service, and communicate the results of the reviews and process to those affected.

According to the original standards, HIM department managers set the standards for HIM functions. The HIM department had a written plan to monitor the effectiveness of its functions. Taking into consideration all of the regulations governing health records, HIM professionals determined for their facility the appropriate level of quality and productivity for each function. For example, the HIM professional determined that assembly and analysis should occur within 24 hours of the patient's discharge, and the records should be assembled correctly 100% of the time (Table 10-3). This standard required that patient records be checked to ensure that the function was happening according to the standard. If the review revealed that the records were not being assembled correctly 100% of the time or not being assembled within the 24-hour time frame, then action was taken to correct the problem. The same process was applied to the other standards set for HIM functions; reviews were performed, compliance was noted, and any problems were actively addressed to prevent recurrence. QA reviews of coding ensured that the coding staff was accurately coding all records in a timely fashion. In a QA review of the release of information function, the HIM supervisor reviewed several requests to ensure that the release occurred in a timely fashion and that the facility's procedure for release of information was followed.

Today, the evaluation and monitoring of HIM functions remain important. JCAHO continues to require that facilities monitor the quality of their functions. The focus, however, is on quality improvement. The quality improvement process requires that the HIM department monitor its functions by collecting data to identify areas that need to be improved.

PERFORMANCE IMPROVEMENT

Performance improvement (PI), also known as *quality improvement (QI)* or *continuous quality improvement (CQI),* refers to the process by which a facility reviews its services or products to ensure quality. It is no longer acceptable to simply meet a standard; the facility should always seek to improve its performance. PI is a hospital-wide function that occurs interdepartmentally and intradepartmentally. It is multidisciplinary because it involves the facility's entire staff. The employees participate in teams to reach a solution to improve a process. All employees are encouraged to improve their work, surroundings, efforts, processes, and products. The philosophy of PI is that by improving the process, the outcome—patient care—will ultimately be improved.

The PI process begins with a formal policy or statement of how the facility will conduct and document improvement efforts. The organization-wide PI process is directed by a committee, either the medical executive committee (discussed later in this chapter) or another committee established strictly for this purpose. All departments are required to improve processes both internally and in their relationships with other departments. Most facilities choose a model designed by a QI philosopher. The model not only helps the facility document the PI process to

TABLE 10-2	Transcription Example Using the JCAHO 10-Step Process

JCAHO 10 STEPS	HEALTH INFORMATION DEPARTMENT EXAMPLE
1. Assign responsibility.	Someone must be designated to perform the audits of the identified aspects of care—transcription supervisor.
2. Delineate scope of care and service.	The transcription department converts dictated clinical information into reports for the health record.
3. Identify important aspects of care and service.	History and physical (H&P) and operative reports must be typed with 98% accuracy within 12 hours of dictation in order for the reports to be returned to the paper record within 24 hours of dictation.
4. Identify indicators.	H&P is transcribed within 12 hours of dictation, with 98% accuracy. Operative report is transcribed within 12 hours of dictation, with 98% accuracy.
5. Establish thresholds for evaluations.	Error rate 2%.
6. Collect and organize data.	Supervisor reviews random sample of H&P and operative reports for 98% accuracy. Supervisor monitors the transcription system daily to determine compliance with the turnaround time of 12 hours. Reports are generated from the transcription system monthly to determine compliance with the 12-hour turnaround.
7. Initiate evaluation.	The data described in Step 6 are collected and reported to the HIM director monthly. All concerns and problems should be discussed in a timely fashion.
8. Take action to improve care or service.	Review of the data from Step 6 determines whether the transcription department is meeting the quality standard. Failure to meet the standard requires action to improve compliance—that is, increase of transcription staffing, appropriate assignment of transcriptionists to priority work.
9. Assess the effectiveness of actions and maintain the gain.	Continuous collection of the data in Step 6, even after action is taken, will determine whether actions are effective.
10. Communicate results to affected individuals and groups.	Results of the audits should be reported to the employees in the transcription area during the monthly department meeting.

Modified from Mervat Abdelhak, Sara Grostick, Mary Alice Hanken, and Ellen Jacobs. *Health Information Management of a Strategic Resource*. 2nd ed. Philadelphia: Saunders, 2001, p 386.

Hit-Bit

Interdepartmental or Intradepartmental

The prefix *inter-* means "between" (e.g., *inter*state highways, which run from state to state). **Interdepartmental** means "between departments." The prefix *intra-* means "within" (e.g., *intra*venous injections, which are delivered into, or within, the blood vessels). **Intradepartmental** means "within a department."

TABLE 10-3	Quality Monitors for HIM Functions	
HIM FUNCTION	**STANDARD (EXAMPLE)**	**HOW THE FUNCTION IS AUDITED**
Assembly	Health records are assembled within 24 hours of discharge with 100% accuracy.	Supervisor reviews a sample of records monthly to check accuracy.
Analysis	Health records are analyzed (quantitative) within 24 hours of discharge with 100% accuracy.	Supervisor reviews a sample of records monthly to check accuracy.
Coding	All records are coded within 48 hours of discharge with 100% accuracy.	Supervisor reviews a sample of records monthly to check accuracy.
Abstracting	Health information is correctly abstracted on all patient records within 72 hours of discharge.	Supervisor reviews a sample of records monthly to check accuracy.
Filing	Health records are filed in correct filing order 100% of the time.	Supervisor reviews a section of the file area monthly to check accuracy.
Release of information	Requests for information are processed according to law and hospital policy within 48 hours of the request, 100% of the time.	Supervisor reviews a sample of requests monthly to check accuracy.

support accreditation and certification standards but also provides a measure for the facility to monitor its efforts internally. Multidisciplinary teams use the chosen model to accomplish PI.

There are several QI models that provide a structure for a health care facility to follow. Ultimately, one model is chosen, and the entire organization uses this model to facilitate and document PI. A popular method for monitoring and improving performance is the *Plan, Do, Check, and Act method,* also called the *PDCA method,* which was developed by Walter Shewhart.

The PDCA method is easy to understand and use and therefore is one of the most widely used models (Figure 10-3). The Plan phase consists of data collection and analysis to propose a solution for the identified problem. The Do, or implementation, phase tests the proposed solution. The Check phase monitors the effectiveness of the solution over time. The Act phase formalizes the changes that have proved effective in the Do and Check stages (Abdelhak et al. 2001, p 393).

The key point to remember is that a process is being improved. The area of concentration is the process and not the employee performing the job. To improve a process, all persons who are involved in the process must be part of the team. For example, an interdepartmental PI team has employees representing each department involved in a process that affects them. An intradepartmental PI team works to improve a process within a department; for example, the HIM department could organize a team to improve the effectiveness of the chart locator system (discussed in Chapter 8).

Consider another example: A facility is required by state law to inform its patients about advance directives. At this facility, patients must sign a form stating they received information about advance directives when admitted to the facility. This form is called an *acknowledgment form.* To improve the collection of the acknowledgment form for advance directives, all persons involved in the advance directive should be a part of the team.

Because the customer's perspective must be considered to truly evaluate the quality of a process or product, a patient should be on the team for PI of the advance directive's acknowledgment statement. Figure 10-4 describes additional members of a hypothetical advance directive PI team.

A patient is introduced to the advance directive at admission to the health care facility. State laws regarding advance directives vary dramatically. In our example, the state assigns the responsibility of advance directives, patients' rights, and health care options to the hospital (this may or may not be the case in your state). The law does not require the patient to have an advance directive or to make any decisions immediately; it simply states that the patient must be made aware of his or her rights. To prove compliance with this state law, the facility requires the patient

Hit-Bit

Patient Self-Determination Act of 1990

The Patient Self-Determination Act of 1990 promotes public awareness of patients' rights, health care options, and advance directives. An advance directive is a living will or durable medical power of attorney that allows a patient to inform health care professionals of his or her wishes if the patient becomes incapable.

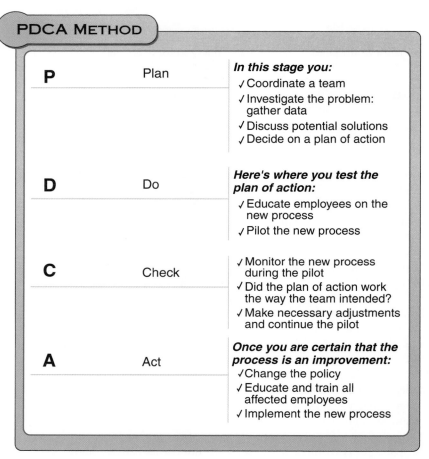

PDCA METHOD

P	Plan	**In this stage you:** ✓ Coordinate a team ✓ Investigate the problem: gather data ✓ Discuss potential solutions ✓ Decide on a plan of action
D	Do	**Here's where you test the plan of action:** ✓ Educate employees on the new process ✓ Pilot the new process
C	Check	✓ Monitor the new process during the pilot ✓ Did the plan of action work the way the team intended? ✓ Make necessary adjustments and continue the pilot
A	Act	**Once you are certain that the process is an improvement:** ✓ Change the policy ✓ Educate and train all affected employees ✓ Implement the new process

◆ **Figure 10-3**
PDCA method.

to sign an advance directive acknowledgment form. This acknowledgment form, signed by the patient and the admitting clerk, serves as proof that the patient was given the advance directive information. A social services employee is called in to assess whether the patient has any questions regarding the advance directive. Therefore the social service representative must be knowledgeable of both the content of the advance directive and the patient's concerns and other related issues. An advance directive is often an end-of-life determination. Pastoral care services assist the patient and family members with spiritual and emotional concerns. Their representation on the team may provide additional insight regarding other concerns affecting the patient or family during consideration of the advance directive statements. The nurse, being very involved in the patient care process and communicating often with the patient, is also an important member of the PI

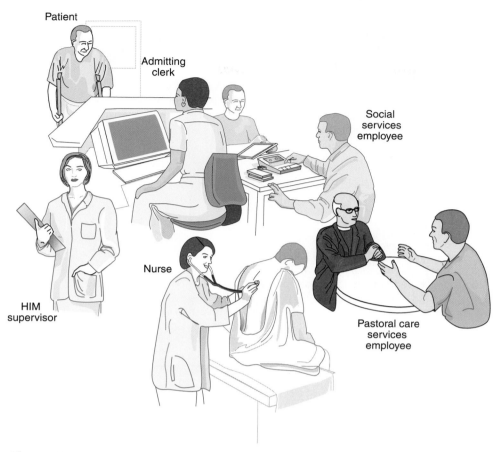

◆ **Figure 10-4**
Advance directive team members.

team. From the HIM department, a quantitative analyst employee should be represented because of his or her knowledge of the record review process. To be effective, all people who are a part of this process must be included on the PI team, and so a patient is also a key member of the team.

BENCHMARKING

Benchmarking is a QI technique used by one facility to compare its process with that of another facility with noted superior performance; sometimes it is used internally to compare current performance with a previous exemplary performance. By reviewing a process that is effective in another facility, the HIM department may discover methods or processes that would improve its own facility. Some processes are better served by throwing out the old model (the way things have always been done) and starting with a clean slate. Sometimes, the benchmarking technique provides the facility with new and better methods for accomplishing the same tasks. Benchmarking internally, against previous performance, allows the facility to compare previous practices to current ones.

 ## HEALTH INFORMATION IN QUALITY ACTIVITIES

Review of health records provides useful information to committees, physicians, administrators, and outside organizations. Quality analysis of health records involves two processes: quantitative analysis and qualitative analysis. Our focus in this chapter is on qualitative analysis. Typically, these two reviews are performed separately, but they can occur simultaneously.

Exercise 10-3

Monitoring the Quality of Health Information

1. What type of quality monitoring does JCAHO require health care facilities to perform?
2. In the popular PDCA quality improvement method, which step of the process involves monitoring the effectiveness of the solution over a period of time?
   a. Plan
   b. Do
   c. Check
   d. Act
3. Which of the following abbreviations is used to describe the continuous improvement of processes within a facility?
   a. QA
   b. QM
   c. QI
   d. UM
4. To improve quality according to a standard, a health care facility may use _____, comparing its performance to that of a similar facility.
5. Retrospective review of the product of a service is _____.
6. A quality improvement effort regarding scanning of loose reports would require a(n) _____.
7. A quality improvement effort regarding completion of the patient advance directive would require a(n) _____.
8. The alternative to quality assurance, _____, is an ongoing effort to improve processes within the health care facility.

QUANTITATIVE ANALYSIS

To evaluate the quality of patient care, the health record must be complete, which means that all of the information must be included in the record. Analysis of the record to ensure that the documentation is complete is called *quantitative analysis* (see Chapter 5). An example of quantitative analysis is the review of an inpatient record for a history and physical (H&P) and discharge summary. Likewise, the operative reports, laboratory reports, radiology reports, and notes must be present and authenticated by the health care professional who authored the notes, reports, or information. Quantitative analysis includes review of the record for the authentication or signatures. This analysis is performed on every health record.

QUALITATIVE ANALYSIS

Qualitative analysis is the review of the health record for accuracy and timeliness of contents. The information must be correct and appropriate as it pertains to the patient's care. In qualitative analysis, the patient's diagnoses, procedures, and treatment are analyzed. Qualitative analysis checks the validity of health information and the timeliness of data entries. A detailed review of the actual documentation in the record is performed to assess whether the clinically pertinent information has been recorded. Figure 10-5 provides an example of a generic (qualitative analysis) record review form that looks for basic information about the timeliness, completeness, accuracy, and validity of the health record.

The reviewer will use this generic form to determine whether the health record meets the minimum requirements set by the JCAHO. Notice that the form captures information about the timeliness of the H&P: whether it was completed within 24 hours of admission. It also captures information about the content of the document: whether it contains the chief complaint, history of present illness, family history, mental status, and so on. This information is required by the JCAHO. When JCAHO representatives survey a health care facility, they review the health records

GENERIC RECORD REVIEW FORM

MR#_____ Attending physician: _____

Admit date: _____ Discharge date: _____

DRG: _____ Procedure:_____ Reviewer: _____ Review date: _____

CRITERIA	Y	N	N/A
Advance directive acknowledgement form signed by patient			
Patients with advance directives have copy on the health record			
H & P documented within 24 hours of admission (and prior to surgery)			
H&P contains: Chief complaint			
Medical history			
Family history			
Psychological status			
Social status			
Review of systems			
Physical examination			
Plan			
Initial nursing assessment documented within 24 hours of admission			
Discharge planning addressed			
All entries dated and authenticated			
Goals and treatment plans documented			
Progress notes documented daily			
Surgery/procedure performed			
Informed consent documented in the health record			
Preanesthesia assessment documented			
Immediately prior to procedure patient is reassesed for anesthesia			
Postoperative monitoring of the patient			
Postoperative monitoring includes: Physiologic status			
Mental status			
IV fluids			
Meds			
Unusual events			
Operative report is documented immediately following the procedure			
Operative report includes: Procedure			
Findings			
Specimen(s) removed			
Postop Dx			
Surgical progress note documented immediately following procedure			
Discharge summary signed and documented within 30 days of discharge			
Discharge summary includes documentation of: Diet			
Meds			
Follow-up			
Activity			
Diagnosis			

◆ **Figure 10-5**

Generic record review form.

to see whether this information is a part of the H&P. The record must be monitored before the survey to ensure that the information is present.

Ideally, a qualitative review should be performed on every health record. However, because it takes a significant amount of time to perform qualitative analysis on paper records, a determination is made about which records to review. Accreditation agencies set the guidelines for this type of record review. Typically, qualitative analysis should be performed at least quarterly. The records chosen for review should represent a sample—usually 30 records or 5% of the monthly average (whichever is greater). Record review may be based on the categories of medical staff in the facility or on specific diagnoses or procedures performed. To prevent a biased result, records must be reviewed for each physician on staff.

Record Review

The quantitative and qualitative review functions performed by HIM professionals to ensure quality of documentation in patient health records are also known as *record review.* The record review is required by JCAHO standards to be performed quarterly by a multidisciplinary team of health care professionals who are involved in patient care. HIM professionals read and understand the JCAHO guidelines and then coordinate the review of the patient records at the facility. The HIM professional typically is responsible for ensuring that the documentation in these records complies with the standards set by the JCAHO. Much of the record review that occurs now is concurrent because of a new methodology that JCAHO uses during the facility survey called **tracer methodology**.

Tracer Methodology

The JCAHO tracer methodology basically traces a current patient's stay in the health care facility. At the beginning of the JCAHO survey, the surveyors request a current patient census for the facility. From that census, the surveyors choose the charts that they are going to review during the survey. These charts are reviewed concurrently during the survey of those patients who are currently in the facility. From the review of these inhouse charts, the surveyors determine which physicians they are going to review, which staff members they are going to interview, and which policies and procedures they will review. In previous JCAHO surveys, the management team sat in a meeting and answered all of the surveyor's questions on policy and procedures, were able to choose (with some restrictions) the charts the surveyors would review, and could sometimes even select the physicians who were involved. With the tracer methodology, the surveyors interview the staff members who are involved in patient care and ask them questions about policies and procedures. This is also how the surveyors determine which physicians are going to be reviewed in the credentialing portion of the survey and which employee files to review in human resources. This process shows whether all of the facility employees know the policies and procedures, rather than just the managers. In essence, the whole survey process revolves around the review of the concurrent health records of the facility during the survey. Therefore the concurrent review of health records is more important today then it was in previous years. The facility should have in place a process for regularly performing this type of record review before the JCAHO survey takes place.

Clinical Pertinence

The qualitative review that analyzes the patient's care specific to a diagnosis or procedure is known as **clinical pertinence.** Clinical pertinence is the review of patient health information to determine whether the care provided was appropriate given the patient's diagnosis. To determine which aspects of each diagnosis or procedure to review, HIM professionals work with physicians within the facility or use a published source to develop indicator screens.

The same rule for the record sample used in qualitative analysis applies to record review: usually 30 records or 5% of the monthly average (whichever is greater). Be aware that both inpatient and outpatient diagnoses and procedures are reviewed. The generic review and the clinical pertinence review can be performed simultaneously so that the reviewer does not duplicate his or her efforts.

An example of clinical pertinence is the review of a health record in which the patient comes to the emergency room (ER) with a productive cough and shortness of breath. The ER physician suspects pneumonia. A sputum culture is requested to identify the organism and confirm the diagnosis of pneumonia. The review of the health record for documentation of the physician's order and test is an example of qualitative analysis. A thorough review of all pneumonia cases in a facility over a given period helps a facility determine whether patients are receiving pertinent care; it also reveals ways to improve the quality of care, if necessary. Figure 10-6 provides an example of the clinical pertinence form for a patient with congestive heart failure (CHF). Note that the indicators on the form are specific to the type of care and treatment a patient with CHF would receive.

Value of Record Review

Qualitative review of health information serves several purposes. The most important reason to perform this review is to evaluate the quality of patient care. Consider the pneumonia scenario again. On review of a sample of patients with a diagnosis of pneumonia, it is found that a sputum culture was ordered in 50% of the cases. Additionally, the culture was obtained immediately after a diagnosis of pneumonia was suspected. The general treatment for pneumonia is to start the

CLINICAL PERTINENCE FORM—CONGESTIVE HEART FAILURE

MR#_____ Attending physician: _____

Admit date: _____ Discharge date: _____

Criteria		Y	N
Assessment			
H & P present within 24 hours of admission			
History contains documentation of:	Shortness of breath		
	Orthopnea		
Physical examination contains documentation of:	Lungs—rales		
	Heart—tachycardia		
	Liver—hepatomegaly		
	Extremities—edema		
Diagnostic workup			
Diagnostic workup includes:	Chest x-ray		
	ECG		
	Electrolyte profile		
	CBC		
	UA		
Orders			
Orders included:	Activities		
	Vital signs q 4 hours		
	Diet		
	Oxygen		
	Intake and output		
	Daily weights		
Complications documented			
Discharge status			
Discharge status includes:	Breathing improved		
	Clear x-ray		
	Potassium (K+) within normal range		
	Weight decrease		
Discharge plan			
Discharge plan includes:	Diet		
	Medications		
	Activities		
	Follow-up plans		

◆ **Figure 10-6**

Clinical pertinence form for patient with congestive heart failure.

patient on some type of antibiotic. However, if the sputum culture reveals a gram-negative specimen, normal antibiotics will not resolve the patient's pneumonia. The patient must be put on a more specific medicine. Early detection of the organism facilitates prompt medication and, ideally, a shorter period of recovery. The facility uses this information to educate the physicians and the clinical staff. The information shows the difference in patient outcome between those who received appropriate care and those who did not. The information can also show the effect of the treatment on cost of health care or reimbursement.

These analyses—qualitative analysis, record review, and clinical pertinence—are also essential to the accreditation of the health care facility. Accreditation bodies expect facilities to analyze their compliance with predetermined standards. The quarterly review of health information to determine this compliance can prevent a facility from failing an accreditation survey. If detected early, noncompliance with standards can be corrected before a survey.

During a JCAHO survey, the record review is performed by a surveyor on *open* patient charts. The results of this review are included in the accreditation decision. Therefore it is important that facilities implement concurrent and open record reviews to ensure compliance with the standards.

Record Review Team

It is important to formalize your record review practices as a policy stating who will perform the record reviews. Multidisciplinary or interdisciplinary teams are organized for this function. Health care professionals who document information in the patient health record meet at least quarterly to review records against the standards. Record review teams include physicians, nurses, physical therapists, occupational therapists, radiologists, laboratory workers, dietitians, case managers, pharmacists, and others. Members of the record review team are challenged to determine whether a record is in compliance with JCAHO standards. Record review requires team members to know where and by whom health information is documented. In the multidisciplinary team record review, health care professionals who document information in the health record are made aware of the importance of the documentation. For example, a nurse reviewing records to measure compliance with patient education standards may realize that the documentation in the records does not support that patient education is actually being accomplished. This may not have been identified and corrected without the record review.

The results of the record reviews must be communicated to the medical staff committee or a quality care review committee that understands the importance of health information and the effect it has on the quality of patient care as well as on facility accreditation.

Electronic Health Record Applications of Qualitative Analysis

The electronic health record (EHR)also requires quantitative and qualitative analysis. The EHR is only as good as the information that is entered. It is important that analysis of the health information remain a key function. However, it is expected that quantitative and qualitative analyses will primarily occur concurrently in the EHR. Concurrent analysis provides information in a timely manner that can have an impact on patient care.

One anticipated aspect of the EHR is the decision support feature. Computers can be programmed to recognize the data as information. This feature allows the computer to determine or prompt the next course of action. In some cases, the computer will analyze each course of action. For example, in the pneumonia scenario, when pneumonia is entered as a suspected diagnosis, the computer searches for a physician's order to obtain a sputum culture. In addition, the computer recognizes the laboratory results of the sputum culture and is able to suggest the next course of action to the attending physician. This automation is discussed in more detail in Chapter 12.

CLINICAL PATHWAYS

A **clinical pathway** is the "multidisciplinary plan of best clinical practice" for a specific diagnosis (http://www.openclinical.org/clinicalpathways.html). The plan can come from industry leaders or the organization can, after studying or reviewing a significant number of health records for patients with a particular diagnosis, develop a guide or plan for patients with that diagnosis. By doing so, a facility can streamline the patient's stay in the hospital, coordinate multidisciplinary care, and ideally eliminate any unnecessary time spent in the facility or in a particular level of care. The goal is to provide high-quality patient care in an efficient and effective manner. It is

Hit-Bit

Decision Support

The programming of decision support information involves the HIM professional. Criteria must be established, decision support information entered, and scenarios analyzed to ensure that these functions work as expected in the health care environment.

important to note that this does not mean that all patients will be treated the same. If the patient's condition warrants a change from the clinical pathway, appropriate treatment is rendered, and, ideally, the patient's condition improves.

UTILIZATION MANAGEMENT

Utilization management (UM), also known as *utilization review (UR),* is the function or department that ensures appropriate, efficient, and effective health care for patients. It also monitors patient outcomes and compares physician activities. *Appropriate* may also refer to what is covered by the patient's insurance plan. A health insurance plan may require a specific test before approving a specific treatment or procedure. The expectation is that the test will provide definitive information regarding the necessity of the treatment or procedure. For example, before approving arthroscopy of the knee, an insurance company may require magnetic resonance imaging (MRI). In the past, the physician had sole responsibility for determining the procedures and treatments that a patient would or would not receive. Today, such decisions may be heavily influenced by the third party paying the bill.

Payers study historical patient treatment by analyzing patient health records to identify "best practices," or a specific plan of treatment that is most likely the best standard. This is not to say that physicians do not order tests that payers do not approve. Nor does it imply that payers over-rule physician orders. However, there is significant controversy over the influence of payers in medical decision making.

CASE MANAGEMENT

Case management is the coordination of the patient's care within the facility. Case management is performed by health care professionals within the facility as well as by the payers who send their employees into the facility to oversee or coordinate care. The health care professional coordinating the care is called a *case manager*. Case management in practice is multidisciplinary. The coordinator interacts with all of the health care professionals involved in the patient's care. With such a team, the expectation is that the communication among the disciplines (e.g., physical therapy, occupational therapy, nursing, medical) will facilitate appropriate, effective, and efficient health care for the patient.

Typically, the case manager is the employee assigned to review the patient's care, interact with the health care team, and ensure that the services provided are covered by the patient's insurance. The case manager is assigned to the patient when the patient is admitted to the facility. Review of the patient's health information to determine the plan of care happens concurrently. Case management also includes multidisciplinary meetings of health care professionals to coordinate the patient's plan of care and continually update each discipline on the patient's progress.

The team members in this multidisciplinary effort may include, but are not limited to, physicians, nurses, physical therapists, occupational therapists, respiratory therapists, speech therapists, HIM coders, and patients (in some settings). Each person on the team attends the case management meeting to discuss the development or progress of the patient's care. Each team meeting is documented and becomes a part of the patient's health record. When necessary, the plan of care is also updated.

RISK MANAGEMENT

Risk management is the coordination of efforts within a facility to prevent and control **potentially compensable events (PCEs).** A PCE is any event that could cause a financial loss or lead to litigation. The health record serves as evidence of patient-related events that occur within the facility. The patient health record includes documentation of the facts of an incident as they are related to the care of the patient. For example, if a patient falls out of the bed during his or her stay in the health care facility, the documentation in the patient's record would indicate the time and date of the occurrence. It would also document the position of the patient's bed, use of side rails, and other pertinent information, such as the patient's diagnosis, medications administered, and instructions given to the patient before the incident.

This type of documentation in the health record is different from the *occurrence,* or *incident, report* completed when there is an inadvertent occurrence (Figure 10-7). An incident report is an administrative discovery tool used by the facility to obtain information about the incident. The incident report is *not* a part of the patient's health record, nor is it mentioned in any documentation.

Incident reports should be completed immediately by the employee or employees most closely associated with the incident. The incident report is used to perform a mini-investigation into the facts surrounding the incident. Facts discovered immediately after the incident can significantly affect the facility's ability to defend, comprehend, or determine the cause of the incident or the liability of the parties in an incident. Examples of inadvertent occurrences are listed in Figure 10-8.

Occasionally, events are not recognized as incidents during the patient's stay. Review of documentation by HIM staff members may identify a PCE. As a result, health information is used in risk management to gather facts surrounding an occurrence; support the claim, should it require litigation; or provide information to prevent a future occurrence.

Hit-Bit

Sequestered File

The HIM department maintains a sequestered file for all cases that are identified as PCEs or that are currently involved in litigation against the facility. This file is kept in a locked cabinet that contains the health records. Access to the file is generally limited to the department director. Records released from the file must not leave the department and can be reviewed only under direct supervision.

Exercise 10-4

Health Information in Quality Activities

1. Specify the number of records that would be reviewed at the following facilities using the rule of 5% or 30 discharges (whichever is greater).
   Hospital A has 1200 discharges each month.
   Hospital B has 400 discharges each month.
   Hospital C has 150 discharges each month.
2. Health records contain demographic, socioeconomic, financial, and clinical data. If one of the JCAHO standards requires that the health record contain personal identification information for each patient, where could this information be found in the health record?
3. What would you need to do if an employee reports that he or she fell while on a nursing unit, injuring his or her left knee?
4. A predetermined course of treatment for a patient with a particular diagnosis is known as a(n) _____.
5. A method used to effectively manage patients during their hospitalization is known as _____.
6. _____ is the qualitative review of health care records to determine the appropriateness of care according to the patient's diagnosis.
7. Thorough review of the patient's health information to determine pertinence, appropriateness, or compliance with standards is _____.
8. The _____ process would be initiated after a patient fall from the bed to gather information and coordinate the claim.
9. Ensuring appropriate, efficient, and effective patient care is a process of _____.
10. Which of the following is an important process in the determination of the facility's compliance with documentation standards?
    a. Physician profile review
    b. Record review
    c. Mediation review
    d. PDCA

Incident Report
Do Not File in Medical Records

Confidential and privileged health care quality improvement information prepared in anticipation of litigation

Name: _____ Employee ☐ Patient ☐ Visitor ☐

Attending physician: _____
MR # _____ SS # _____
D.O.B. ___/___/___ Sex: M[ ] F[ ]
Admission date: ___/___/___
Primary diagnosis: _____

Facility name: _____
_____
Site (if applicable) _____
City _____
Facility ID# _____
State _____
Phone # _____

SECTION I: General Information

General Identification (circle one)
001 Inpatient
002 Outpatient
003 Nonpatient
004 Equipment only

Location (circle one):
005 Bathroom/toilet
006 Beauty shop
007 Cafeteria/dining room
008 Corridor/hall
009 During transport
010 Emergency department
011 Exterior grounds
012 ICU/SCU/CCU
013 Labor/delivery/birthing
014 Nursery
015 Outpatient clinic
016 Patient room
017 Radiology
018 Recovery room
019 Recreation area
020 Rehab
021 Shower room
022 Surgical suite
023 Treatment/exam room

Treatment Rendered (circle one):
024 Emergency room
025 First aid
026 None
026 Transfer to other facility
027 X-ray

SECTION II: Nature of Incident (Circle all that apply):

001 Adverse outcome after surgery or anesthetic
002 Anaphylactic shock
003 Anoxic event
004 Apgar score of 5 or less
005 Aspiration
006 Assault or altercation/combative event
007 Blood or IV variance
008 Blood/body fluid exposure
009 Code/arrest
010 Damage/loss of organ
011 Death
012 Dental-related complication
013 Dissatisfaction/noncompliance*
014 Equipment operation*
015 Fall with injury*
016 Fall without injury*
017 Handling of and/or exposure to hazardous waste
018 Informed consent issue
019 Injury to other
020 Injury to self
021 Loss of limb
022 Loss of vision
023 Medication variance*
024 Needle puncture/sharp injury
025 Paralysis
026 Patient-to-patient altercation
027 Perinatal complication*
028 Poisoning
029 Suspected nonstaff-to-patient abuse
030 Suspected staff-to-patient abuse
031 Thermal burn
032 Treatment/procedure issue
033 Ulcer: nosocomial stage III/IV

* Complete appropriate area in Section III

SECTION III: Type of Incident

If death, circle all that apply:
001 After medical equipment failure
002 After power equipment failure or damage
003 During surgery or postanesthesia
004 Within 24 hours of admission to facility
005 Within 1 week of fall in facility
006 Within 24 hours of medication error

Blood/IV Variance Issues (circle all that apply):
007 Additive
008 Administration consent
009 Contraindications/allergies
010 Equipment malfunction
011 Infusion rate
012 Labeling issue
013 Reaction
014 Solution/blood type
015 Transcription
016 Patient identification
017 Allergic/adverse reaction
018 Infiltration
019 Phlebitis

Dissatisfaction/Noncompliance (circle all that apply):
020 AMA
021 Elopement
022 Irate or angry (either family or patient)
023 Left without service
024 Noncompliant patient
025 Refused prescribed treatment

Falls (circle all that apply):*
001 Assisted fall
002 Found on floor
003 From bed
004 From chair
005 From commode/toilet
006 From exam table
007 From stretcher
008 From wheelchair
009 Patient states—unwitnessed
010 Unassisted fall
011 While ambulating
012 Witnessed fall

* For any marks in this field, Section V must be completed

Medication Variance Issues (circle all that apply):
013 Contraindication/allergies
014 Delay in dispensing
015 Incorrect dose
016 Expired drug
017 Medication identification
018 Narcotic log variance
019 Not ordered
020 Ordered, not given
021 Patient identification
022 Reaction
023 Route
024 Rx incorrectly dispensed
025 Time of dose
026 Transcription

◆ **Figure 10-7**
Incident report.

ORGANIZATION AND PRESENTATION OF DATA

To effectively communicate the information that you have learned in the previously discussed QI activities and record reviews, you need to know how to organize and present the data in a brief but effective format. The information is commonly presented in a meeting.

EXAMPLES OF INADVERTENT OCCURRENCES

- An employee falls in the hallway on a slippery floor, injuring his knee.
- A visitor entering the elevator is struck by the door as it closes.
- A missing patient is found on the roof of the health care facility.
- A patient falls out of bed; assessment of the patient found on the floor in the room reveals a broken arm.
- A nurse injures her back during transport of a large, uncooperative patient.

◆ **Figure 10-8**
Examples of inadvertent occurrences.

MEETINGS

Meetings are an important method for bringing people together to improve performance. Meetings can be used to gather information or impart information. At a meeting, you can inform everyone of the purpose of your presentation: Everyone gets the same message at the same time. During a meeting, you can gather information about the process from the people who are involved, educate other members of the team, and keep the team focused on the goal of improving the process.

The *facilitator* plays an important role in the PI team meeting. The facilitator is the person who keeps the team focused on the goal (e.g., improvement in the collection of patient advance directives). During improvement efforts, it is common for a team to get sidetracked by equally pressing issues that need to be corrected. A facilitator makes sure that the team does not deviate too far off course. Such deviation could impair the team's ability to accomplish its goal.

QUALITY IMPROVEMENT TOOLS

Many tools facilitate the use of data in the QI process. There are tools to gather information and to organize or present the information in a useful manner. Data-gathering tools assist the team in exploring or at least acknowledging issues surrounding the process of concern. Organization and presentation tools make a statement about the information that is gathered. Two data-gathering tools, brainstorming and surveys, are discussed below, as well as several organization and presentation tools: bar graphs, line graphs, pie charts, decision matrices, and flowcharts.

Data-Gathering Tools

Brainstorming is a method in which a group of people discuss ideas, solutions, or related issues on a topic or situation. It is a data-gathering tool used to identify as many aspects, events, or issues surrounding a topic as possible. This process encourages the involvement of everyone in the group. All ideas are accepted, no matter how insignificant they may appear. To brainstorm, you need only to have a topic and a place to write down the ideas mentioned by the group. To begin the process, the team's facilitator explains that this tool is used to gather all ideas related to the issue—regardless of how unusual they may seem.

For example, a QI team is organized to reduce the length of time that a patient waits to receive treatment in the ER. At the team's first meeting, the members brainstorm all of the possible factors that could have an impact on the patient's wait in the ER. The team members are encouraged

Hit-Bit

Meeting Roles

A few people in the meeting play key roles to ensure that the meeting is organized and orderly:

Leader: The leader is responsible for organizing the meeting and motivating the participants toward the goal.

Facilitator: The facilitator keeps the meeting on track, making sure that it is proceeding as necessary to accomplish the goal. The facilitator is not necessarily a member of the meeting or team but is there to ensure that the meeting progresses.

Recorder: The recorder acts as a secretary, taking minutes of the meeting and documenting the necessary proceedings of the meeting. The events of a meeting should be recorded and documented in the minutes of the meeting, which help the team track its progress and stay focused on the goal. The recorder's responsibilities should also include taking attendance, noting each member who is present and absent. Minutes keep the team aware of any unresolved issues. Meeting agendas and minutes are discussed in more detail in Chapter 13.

Time-keeper: The time-keeper is responsible for keeping the team on schedule, making sure that the meeting starts and ends on time, and so on.

Hit-Bit

Brainstorming Rules

1. Collect as many ideas as possible from all participants, with no criticisms or judgments made while ideas are being generated.
2. All ideas are welcome no matter how silly or far out they seem. Be creative. The more ideas, the better because at this point no one knows what might work.
3. Absolutely no discussion takes place during the brainstorming activity. Talking about the ideas will take place after brainstorming session is complete.
4. Do not criticize or judge. Don't even groan, frown, or laugh. All ideas are equally valid at this point.
5. Do build on others' ideas.
6. Do write all ideas on a flip chart or board so the whole group can easily see them.
7. Set a time limit (e.g., 30 minutes) for the brainstorming session.

From Maricopa Community College: http://www.mcli.dist.maricopa.edu/authoring/studio/guidebook/ brain.html

to mention anything that could affect the patient's wait time. Note that at this stage the members do not need to prove that the factors they mention actually affect the patient's wait time. Brainstorming is simply a data-gathering tool. Later, you will learn the use of an organization tool to narrow your improvement effort.

A **survey** is set of questions designed to gather information about a specific topic or issue. A survey can be used routinely to gather information from a group, or it can be designed as part of a QI team's efforts. For example, many facilities conduct a survey of patients after a visit to the facility. The data collectors want to find out how the patient perceived the service. This type of survey can be used to measure patient satisfaction. When significant dissatisfaction is observed, the facility may organize a PI team to address the issue. In the previously mentioned emergency room example, the PI team could develop a survey to ask patients why they think it took so long to receive treatment. The questions on a survey can be open ended, which means that the response area is blank. With open-ended questions, patients are free to answer the question in their own words. However, this method of questioning may not provide enough information to determine how much improvement is necessary. Table 10-4 provides an example of the same survey question asked in two different ways.

Data Organization and Presentation Tools

Data organization and presentation tools are used to communicate information quickly to another person or group. Because QI is a team effort, you will routinely need to organize information and display it so that the group can interpret or understand it. Such tools include graphs, tables, and charts. A **graph** is an illustration of data. A **table** organizes data in rows and columns. These visual tools can be quite persuasive, and positive information can be emphasized just as easily as negative information. Consider the following example: The number of cigarette-smoking freshmen on a college campus declined 40% between 1996 and 2000. However, overall smoking prevalence on the campus was virtually unchanged during that time. We can take the positive data—the decrease in the number of freshmen who smoked from 1996 to 2000—and plot it on a graph to show a positive trend in smoking cessation (Figure 10-9).

However, the same statement can also provide a negative picture because the overall number of people smoking on the campus remains about the same. The same statement could be graphed in two different ways: The positive graph shows that the number of freshmen who smoke has decreased, and the negative graph shows that the total percentage of people who smoke remains unchanged.

Bar and Line Graphs

Bar and *line graphs,* also known as *charts,* relate information along the horizontal (*x* axis) and the vertical (*y* axis). In a bar graph, one axis is used to represent the group or indicator, and the other axis is used to plot the data for the group. For example, Figure 10-9 is a bar graph showing the categories (2001, 2002, 2003, 2004, 2005) along the *x* axis that represents the years in which freshmen smoking was measured. The data plotted along the *y* axis indicate the percentage of freshmen who smoke for each year. If you change the bar graph to a line graph, you could follow the percentage of people smoking over the course of the 5-year period. In Figure 10-10, the bars have been replaced with points that are connected by lines. Line graphs are used to plot data over time. This graph is an easy way to depict the trend of the same data as they are measured continuously, month to month or year to year.

Note the labels and headings used in Figures 10-9 to 10-11. The headings describe the graph or chart, giving the reader an idea of what information is included. On bar and line graphs, the labels on the axes identify what is being measured and how it is being measured. On the pie chart, a key might be used to indicate which color is associated with each group. The following is a list of reminders for creating graphs:

TABLE 10-4	**Survey Questions**
OPEN QUESTION	**LIMITED ANSWER QUESTION**
How would you describe your visit to our emergency room?	Choose one of the following to describe the emergency room during your recent visit: a. Very clean b. Adequately clean c. Unclean d. Very dirty
How long did you wait in the emergency room before being seen by a physician?	How long did you wait in the emergency room before being seen by a physician? a. Less than 1 hour b. 1 to 2 hours c. 2 to 3 hours d. Longer than 3 hours

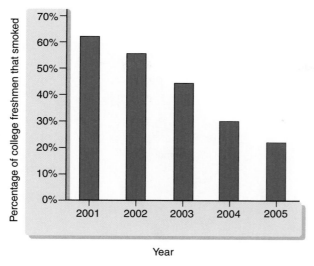

◆ **Figure 10-9**

Bar graph of college freshmen who smoked cigarettes, 2001 to 2005.

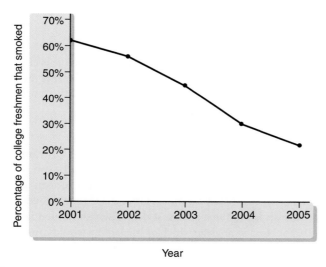

◆ **Figure 10-10**

Line graph of same data as in Figure 10-9.

- Include information about the time frame of the data or the date on which the data were collected.
- Make sure that your graph is legible, especially if you plan to present the information on an overhead projector to a large group.
- Choose the best graph for the data that you are presenting—for example, percentages relate well on a pie chart, but the total of the percentages must equal 100% for the pie chart to be accurate.
- Be prepared to explain your graph if you are questioned by the audience.

    Software programs such as Microsoft Excel can simplify the creation of the aforementioned graphs, tables, and charts. These software products make it very easy to turn your data into an easy-to-read presentation tool.

Pie Chart

A *pie chart* is a graphical illustration of information as it relates to a whole. For example, you can use a pie chart to illustrate the percentage of people on campus who smoke. When you think

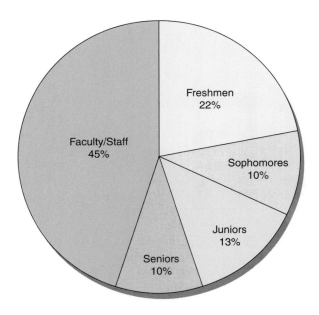

◆ **Figure 10-11**
Pie chart of the percentage of people on campus who smoke.

about this type of chart, imagine a pie. The pieces of the pie represent percentages. If the pie is cut into even slices, all of the pieces will be equal. However, when the size of each piece represents the various smoking populations on campus, we can easily determine which group smokes the most because the sizes vary (Figure 10-11).

Decision Matrix

A **decision matrix** can help a group organize information. This tool is used when the QI team must narrow its focus or choose among several categories or issues. For example, if a PI team is organized to decrease smoking on the college campus, the members may begin by brainstorming to determine all of the issues that influence a person's decision to smoke. Once the team has identified the factors on campus that influence this decision, the team must decide which influential factors they can change. A decision matrix can be used to analyze which of the factors would cause a decrease in the number of smokers if removed. Table 10-5 shows a decision matrix in which each group of smokers is analyzed to determine which issue has the greatest influence on that group's decision to smoke.

First, note that we have set up a table, with the first row identifying the groups of smokers and the first column identifying the issues that may influence a person's decision to smoke. To complete the decision matrix, the PI team analyzes each group according to the influences that the team identified. Team members can write their comments in the squares, or they can assign a value—in this case, *1* for least likely to influence the person to smoke, *2* for moderate influence, and *3* for most likely to influence the person to smoke. The final column on the right is a total, or decision, column. The influence with the highest rating or the influence that occurred in each of

TABLE 10-5	**Decision Matrix**					
	FRESHMAN	**SOPHOMORES**	**JUNIORS**	**SENIORS**	**FACULTY-STAFF**	**TOTAL**
Commercials	2	2	2	2	1	9
Smoking areas	3	3	3	3	3	15
Peer pressure	3	3	2	2	1	11

the categories would be the team's target. In this case, the first, and by far easiest, way to decrease smoking on campus would be to eliminate some of the smoking areas.

Flowchart

A *flowchart* is a tool used to organize the steps involved in a process. Because the PI team is inter-disciplinary, some of the team members may not understand the process they are intended to improve. The flowchart provides an illustration of how the process works within the facility. For an example, refer to the advance directive process shown in Figure 10-4. Figure 10-12 is a flowchart of the advance directive process showing how the facility informs the patient about the advance directive and how the health care professional obtains the patient's signature on the acknowledgment form. Flowcharts help the team streamline a process and eliminate unnecessary steps.

Exercise 10 - 5

Organization and Presentation of Data

1. Which graph would you use to show that the overall percentage of people smoking on campus has remained unchanged?
2. _____ is a quality improvement technique used to solicit participation and information from an entire group.
3. A supervisor and her team of employees are confronted with two solutions to a problem. Each solution involves time, money, and space. Which quality management tool might the supervisor use to choose a solution?

HEALTH CARE FACILITY COMMITTEES

Committees are formal organizational tools that facilities use to conduct business. The committee structure of the health care facility is outlined in the medical staff bylaws, rules, and regulations. Some committees are required by accreditation agencies. Although all health care facilities have committees, the roles and functions of committees in each facility vary. Examples of committees within a health care facility are medical staff departments, infection control, safety, surgical case review, pharmacy and therapeutics, and HIM. The following discussion briefly explains how these committees use health information.

MEDICAL STAFF COMMITTEES

The medical staff of a health care facility is a self-governed group of physicians divided into departments based on their practice, such as the department of medicine, department of surgery, department of obstetrics, and department of pediatrics. The medical staff structure is directed by an elected group of physicians; such positions include chief or president of the medical staff, president-elect (incoming chief of staff), and chairperson of each department. Each medical staff department has a committee meeting in which business directly related to that field of medicine is discussed. The committee reviews patient cases, determines appropriate documentation, and discusses standards of care, as necessary. The medical staff departments also use statistics acquired from health information to make decisions regarding physician membership, privileges, and compliance with accreditation standards.

Accreditation by JCAHO requires that a facility review specific cases of patient care in the areas of surgery, medication usage, and blood and tissue usage. For example, the department of surgery will perform *surgical case review* as an accreditation requirement. The facility reviews statistics related to surgeries and the health records of surgical cases with unexpected outcomes (e.g., a patient who goes into cardiac arrest during an appendectomy or a case in which the wrong operation was performed). *Medication usage* is typically reviewed by the pharmacy and thera-peutics (P&T) committee. The P&T committee is composed of members of the medical staff, with

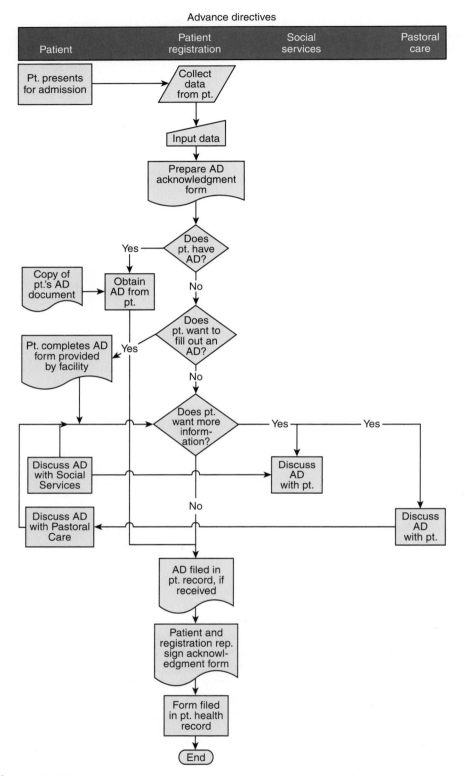

◆ **Figure 10-12**

Flow chart of the advance directive process showing how the facility informs the patient about the advance directive and how the health care professional obtains the patient's signature on the acknowledgment form.

representatives from nursing, administration, and the pharmacy also represented. The committee reviews medications administered to patients, specifically targeting any adverse reactions that a patient has had as a result of medication. The P&T committee also oversees the hospital formulary, which is a listing of the drugs used and approved within the facility. *Blood usage* is also a review that requires participation from the medical staff. This review analyzes the appropriate protocol, method, and effects for patients receiving blood transfusions (or blood products).

The business and decisions of the departments of the medical staff are reported to the medical executive committee for action, recommendation, or correspondence to the governing board. The "med exec committee," as it is commonly called, acts as a liaison to the governing board of the facility. This committee is composed of the chief of staff and elected positions, with a representative from each of the medical staff departments.

HEALTH INFORMATION MANAGEMENT COMMITTEE

The HIM committee, commonly referred to as the *medical record committee,* serves as a consultant to the director of the HIM department. At a minimum, the HIM committee acts as the forms committee, as discussed in Chapter 3. However, in some facilities, the HIM committee is also responsible for reviewing the documentation in patient health records and assisting in compliance with accreditation standards. There are many important health information issues that can be addressed by this committee. Figure 10-13 is a sample agenda for the HIM committee; the committee can review the findings of the record review teams, the percentage of delinquent medical records, and QA and QI activities. Members of the HIM committee include the director of HIM, physicians from each department of the medical staff, nursing staff, and quality management personnel.

INFECTION CONTROL COMMITTEE

The infection control committee is organized to analyze the rate of infection of the patients within a facility. This committee meets regularly to determine whether patients are entering the facility with infections that can harm the staff or other patients or whether patients are acquiring infections within the facility that affect their care, treatment, and length of stay.

The infection control committee is also involved in preventing and investigating infections. Members of the infection control committee include physicians, nurses, quality management personnel, and HIM personnel. To evaluate infection control rates within a facility, the committee must analyze information from patient health records.

SAFETY COMMITTEE

The safety committee is organized to assist the safety officer, who is responsible for providing a program to create a safe environment for patients, visitors, the community, and staff. Health care facilities must adhere to numerous requirements from the Occupational Safety and Health Administration (OSHA), JCAHO, state licensing boards, and federal agencies. The safety committee evaluates the information presented by the safety officer, ensures safety of the environment, and performs disaster planning. Occasionally, the safety committee also reviews the incident reports of cases related to the facility's environment. Members of the safety committee are appointed and may include clinical and nonclinical employees.

Hit-Bit

Nosocomial Infections

Nosocomial infections are infections acquired by patients while they are in a health care facility.

AGENDA FOR HIM COMMITTEE

Health Information Management Committee
Meeting: October 19, 2006

Agenda
　　I. Call to order
　　II. Review of minutes
　　III. Old business
　　IV. Record review
　　V. New business
　　VI. Reports
　　　　Delinquent record count
　　　　Quality audit of HIM functions
　　VII. Adjourn

Next Meeting: November 16, 2006

◆ **Figure 10-13**
Agenda for HIM committee.

Exercise 10-6

Health Care Facility Committees

1. Which of the following is the committee often responsible for reviewing health care records according to accreditation standards, checking physician record completion statistics, and acting as the consultant to the director of health information management?
   a. HIM committee
   b. Safety committee
   c. Infection control committee
   d. P&T committee
2. Infections acquired by patients while they are in the hospital are known as
   a. nosocomial infections
   b. comorbidities
   c. secondary infections
   d. opportunistic infections
3. Which of the following committees acts a liaison to the governing board of the facility?
   a. Surgical case review
   b. P&T committee
   c. Medical executive committee
   d. Credentials committee
4. Which of the following medical staff committees reviews medication usage?
   a. Surgical case review
   b. P&T committee
   c. Medical executive committee
   d. Credentials committee

USES OF HEALTH INFORMATION

Now that you have learned about the use of health information to ensure quality within the health care facility, it is time to move on to some of its other uses. Within the health care facility, health information is used for the following reasons:

- To improve patient care
- To support and collect reimbursement
- To support and prove compliance for licensing, accreditation, and certification
- To support the administration of the facility
- To provide evidence in litigation
- To educate future health care professionals

Agencies outside of the health care facility use health information for the following reasons:

- To study the prevalence and incidence of mortality and morbidity
- To support litigation
- To develop community awareness of health care issues
- To influence national policy on health care issues through legislation
- To educate patients and health care professionals
- To develop health care products

The aforementioned uses are the most obvious, but they may not include every possible use of health information.

IMPROVING PATIENT CARE

Health information is used to improve the quality of care provided to patients. Have you ever been treated by a physician or in a health care facility and thought that a few things could have been improved? For instance, did you have to wait too long to see the physician? Was communication among the health care professionals inadequate? Maybe you were given the impression that no one knew exactly what was going on with your care.

Historically, HIM professionals have reviewed the documentation of patient health care after the patient is discharged to determine whether patients received appropriate care. Review of the patient's record after discharge is called **retrospective review;** this method of review analyzes how, when, and where the patient received care. Retrospective reviews provide statistical information to support decisions that will improve care for future patients. Although retrospective reviews can be effective in improving future care, they cannot change or improve the outcome for patients who have already been discharged. The alternative to retrospective review is **concurrent review.** Concurrent reviews of patient health information provide timely information that is used to support decisions made while the patient is still in the hospital. Concurrent information provides an opportunity that *can* change or improve the patient's outcome. This process is discussed in greater detail later in this chapter, in the section about health information in quality activities.

SUPPORT AND COLLECTION OF REIMBURSEMENT

Reimbursement is the amount of money that the health care facility receives from the party responsible for paying the bill. Health care, although personal in service, has evolved into a large and sometimes very impersonal industry. All health care facilities have a vested interest in their financial operations. As with any other business, a health care facility provides a service or product and then charges a fee for that service or product. The facility may obtain reimbursement from several different parties—the patient, an insurance company, a managed care organization, or the state or federal government.

The patient's health record, with documentation of all of the patient's care, enables the facility to charge for services and supplies. The health record contains documentation of the type of product or service, the date and time at which the service was provided, and the employee who provided the service to the patient.

HIM coding personnel review the patient's health record to identify the correct diagnoses and procedures and then assign the appropriate codes, found in the International Classification of Diseases, Ninth Revision—Clinical Modification (ICD-9-CM) and the Current Procedural Terminology (CPT). These codes are documented on the UB-92 or the CMS-1500 form (see Chapter 6); they tell the payer why the patient received health care (the diagnosis) and whether any procedures were performed that affect reimbursement. Accurate coding requires a thorough analysis of the complete health record. Inaccurate coding causes the facility to submit false claims for reimbursement. Submission of false claims is a crime punishable by law; therefore HIM coders are educated in the review of records and the appropriate assignment of codes for reimbursement.

Hit-Bit

Reimbursement for Health Care

Several people may be involved in reimbursement for health care. The patient can pay for health care services out of pocket or through an insurance plan. Paying out of pocket involves two people, or parties, making the transaction. If the patient chooses to pay with insurance, a third party is introduced. The insurance company becomes a third party payer. In health care, a payer is the person or party responsible for the bill.

Hit-Bit

Fraud

Fraud is the term most often used to describe a false claim. The facility should have a compliance officer to ensure that the coding of health information and the billing comply with federal, state, and coding guideline requirements.

LICENSURE, ACCREDITATION, AND CERTIFICATION

Health care facilities must have a license to operate. *Licensure* of health care facilities is performed by the state in which the facility is located. Among the many requirements necessary to receive a license, the facility must maintain documentation (a health record) on all patients.

As discussed in Chapter 1, health care facilities that provide care to Medicare and Medicaid patients receive reimbursement from the federal government. The Centers for Medicare and Medicaid Services (CMS) oversee the federal responsibilities of the Medicare and Medicaid programs. For a facility to receive reimbursement from the federal government, it must be certified under Medicare's Conditions of Participation (COP). The COP are the CMS rules and regulations (standards) that govern the Medicare program. **Certification** under the COP, performed by the states, attests that the health care facility has met the CMS standards.

Accreditation is another means by which some health care facilities may be approved to serve state and federally funded patients. Accreditation, like certification, recognizes that a facility has met a predetermined set of standards. However, accreditation is voluntary. Facilities are not mandated to attain accreditation, but they may be motivated by third party payer requirements for reimbursement and the perception that accreditation indicates a certain quality of care necessary to compete in the marketplace. Accreditation is performed by organizations such as JCAHO, CARF, and the AOA. In some health care settings, a successful survey by JCAHO and some other accreditation agencies results in *deemed status* assignment by CMS in which JCAHO accreditation is accepted in lieu of the Medicare COP certification.

What does any of this have to do with health information? Licensure, certification, and accreditation require that a facility prove compliance with regulations or standards. Much of the proof necessary to validate certification and accreditation standards is found in a review of the facility's patient records. The certification or accreditation survey of the facility records reveals the quality of care delivered to patients within a facility. The survey record review is coordinated to determine whether the facility is providing care within the established guidelines. For example, JCAHO requires that an operative report be completed immediately after surgery. In cases in which the physician chooses to dictate the operative report, an operative note should be made part of the patient's chart and should include information pertinent to the operation that a health care professional might need to know in the absence of the detailed operative report. To

Hit-Bit

Transcription Report Data

A transcriptionist records on each operative report the date on which the report was dictated by the physician and the date on which it was transcribed, along with the transcriptionist's initials. This information is found at the end of each transcribed report.

check compliance with this standard, a sample of surgery records would be pulled for review. The surveyor, HIM personnel, or others would review the record to determine the date and time of surgery. The date and time of the surgery are used for comparison with the dates on which the operative report was dictated and transcribed, both of which are indicated on the operative report in Figure 10-14.

At the end of the report, the transcriptionist's initials, the date dictated (DD), and date transcribed (DT) are indicated as follows: mm/dd/yy and mm/dt/yy, respectively. This information identifies when the report was dictated, who the transcriptionist was, and when it was transcribed. During record review, this information is very helpful in determining whether the facility has met the predetermined standards.

ADMINISTRATION

Administration is the common term used to describe the management of the health care facility. To manage health care, the services that are provided must be evaluated. Managers want to be certain that they are providing health care services in an efficient and effective manner. The administrators responsible for a facility are concerned with personnel and financial and clinical operations of the health care facility. Health information is used in administrative aspects to support reimbursement, make decisions regarding services, and analyze the quality of patient care.

The administrators of the facility rely on the review of health information to make decisions regarding the management of the facility. For example, review of health information may indicate that improper coding, which affects reimbursement, caused a significant decrease in revenue or that patients who receive physical therapy soon after heart surgery recover in a shorter period of time. Health information is also used to make decisions regarding the health care services offered, to formulate policies, and to design an organizational structure.

Administrators also use health information to negotiate and evaluate contracts with managed care companies or other vendors, such as surgical supply companies and laundry companies. For surgical supply companies and laundry companies, the facility uses statistics from its database to negotiate terms of a contract. The statistics help the facility determine the proper quantities of supplies to purchase.

PREVALENCE AND INCIDENCE OF MORTALITY AND MORBIDITY

Health care facilities are required to report statistics on communicable and infectious diseases to agencies of the federal government, as discussed in Chapter 9. The agencies use this information to aid in the prevention and treatment of these diseases. In this use of health information, you need to understand some new statistical terms. **Prevalence** is the extent to which something occurs (Random House Webster's College Dictionary, 1991)—that is, the number of existing cases. **Incidence** is the rate of occurrence (Webster's Tenth New Collegiate Dictionary, 1993)—that is, the number of new cases (Abdelhak et al., 2001, p 317). *Prevalence* and *incidence* are very similar terms, but they differ in that *incidence* captures only new cases of a disease, and *prevalence* captures all existing cases of the disease. By studying the number of cases and the speed at which a disease is spreading in a given population, the government can target areas for prevention and treatment.

OPERATIVE REPORT

Patient's name: Mary Davidson

Hospital no.: 400130

Date of surgery: 01/07/2006

Admitting Physician: Mark Ellis, MD

Surgeon: Fred Cotter, MD

Preoperative diagnosis: Nodular lymphoma
Postoperative diagnosis: Nodular lymphoma
Operative procedure: Regional lymph node excision

PROCEDURE AND GROSS FINDINGS: Under general anesthesia, after usual sterile preparation and draping, the patient was...

The patient tolerated the procedure well. Approximate blood loss 200 mL.

Fred Cotter, MD

FC/mt
DD: 01/07/2006
DT: 01/07/2006

◆ **Figure 10-14**
Operative report with date dictated (DD) and date transcribed (DT).

The other statistics that are reported as a result of the review of health information are mortality and morbidity. **Mortality** refers to death. **Morbidity** refers to disease or sickness. As a society, we are very concerned with death and disease. As a population, we are living longer, but some diseases remain fatal for many people. Federal agencies monitor, study, and determine the impact of diseases on the American public.

Within our national government the Department of Health and Human Services (DHHS) is responsible for overseeing many agencies that have an impact on health care. DHHS was reviewed in Chapter 1, so you are familiar with the role of the CMS. The mission of the Centers for Disease Control and Prevention (CDC) is "to promote health and quality of life by preventing and controlling disease, injury, and disability" (CDC, 2000). The agencies of the CDC use health information to study diseases and support their mission. The centers, institutes, and offices in the CDC are responsible for a wide variety of health issues including minority health, human immuno-deficiency virus, sexually transmitted diseases, tuberculosis prevention, occupational safety and health, chronic disease prevention and health promotion, infectious diseases, and genetics.

NATIONAL POLICY AND LEGISLATION

Federal and state governments use health information when making decisions related to health care. Sometimes their decisions have an impact only on Medicare and Medicaid beneficiaries; at other times, their decisions influence the legislation that governs other areas of health care. For example, the Health Insurance Portability and Accountability Act (HIPAA) of 1996 affects health plans, health care clearinghouses, and providers. This legislation affects many aspects of health care including the portability of health insurance and standardization of electronic transfer of health information. Another type of legislation has an impact on health maintenance organizations (HMOs), which administer health insurance. In some states, a patient has the right to sue an HMO; in other states, such lawsuits are illegal. Many insurance carriers reduced the length of stay (LOS) for obstetrical deliveries: 48-hour LOS for a cesarean section and a 24-hour LOS for a vaginal delivery. State legislation has an impact on the insurance carriers' decision requiring assessment and prevention of premature discharge for these maternity cases.

Health information is used to determine the type of coverage that Medicare or Medicaid patients receive. In other words, the government looks at the history of care provided to its beneficiaries and determines the cost and quality of that care to make decisions and enact legislation. These decisions and the legislation affect future coverage, reimbursement, and availability of services for Medicare and Medicaid beneficiaries.

Health care policy is another method the federal government uses to influence health care. The Surgeon General is an advisor, spokesperson, and leader concerning many health issues that affect the U.S. public. For example, a familiar influence of the Surgeon General is the warning on tobacco and alcohol products manufactured in the United States (Figure 10-15).

How did the Surgeon General's office decide that this warning was necessary? The incidence and prevalence of certain diseases, combined with research requiring review of health information, indicate that tobacco and alcohol products can cause harm to society. The warning statement is one way the government has tried to affect how and when people use these products. The Surgeon General also works to educate the public and advise the President about disease prevention and health promotion in the United States.

DEVELOPMENT OF COMMUNITY AWARENESS OF HEALTH CARE ISSUES

Many diseases in our society have caused people to organize into groups to promote awareness, raise money for research, and increase prevention. Have you seen a person wearing a pink or red ribbon on a lapel to promote awareness of a particular disease? Breast cancer and acquired immunodeficiency syndrome (AIDS) awareness groups are quite common. These groups use widely known symbols (i.e., the pink and red ribbons) to promote public education. Since these groups became involved in health care, more people are educated about the prevention, detection, and treatment of various diseases. These groups use health information, research, and statistics to inform the public. Health information in this case may relate to different populations' exposure to the disease. Health information about the prevention, cause, and treatment of a particular disease can improve the recognition of the disease in a population. Typically, a disease diagnosed at an early stage is easier to treat, and the patient's prognosis is better.

LITIGATION

Litigation is the process by which a disputed matter is settled in court. During litigation, health information is used to support a plaintiff's or a defendant's case. Health records can support or

---

SURGEON GENERAL'S WARNING:

Quitting smoking now greatly
reduces serious risks to your health.

◆ **Figure 10-15**
Surgeon General's warning on tobacco and alcohol products.

validate a claim of physician malpractice. However, the opposite can be proved if there is complete and accurate documentation showing that the physician was not at fault. The health record, when admissible in court, provides evidence of the events that are alleged in a lawsuit. Chapter 11 includes more information about the use of health information in litigation.

Standards of care, expert testimony, and research are other sources of health information that may be used as evidence in a trial. Standards of care provide information regarding the typical method of providing services to a patient with a particular diagnosis. Expert testimony in health care provides the jury with information or an explanation that helps them understand the highly technical language used in the health care profession. Research information provides information that the judge or jury can use to make decisions as well. Health information, whether specific to a patient or a disease, is helpful in litigation that involves a person's health or injury.

EDUCATION

Health information is used in the education of health care professionals and patients. For example, physicians, nurses, physical therapists, and pharmacists need health information for instruction and examples as they learn how to perform their duties. The documentation of past occurrences provides an excellent opportunity to show others how to handle patient care in the future. Medical institutions use case studies of patients to teach new students about a disease process. Some health care professionals are required to earn continuing education credits in their field to keep their credentials current and comply with professional standards. These professionals perform case studies on new and intriguing cases or present new technology for the education of their peers.

Likewise, health information is presented to patients and the community to inform them of the prevention, causes, incidence, and treatment for many diseases. This use of health information involves research, statistics, and information on new technology for treatment or prevention of disease.

RESEARCH

Research is the systematic investigation into a matter to obtain or increase knowledge. Health-related research requires a tremendous amount of investigation of health information. In the health care profession, documentation from previous patient care, combined with the scientific process, allows physicians and other researchers to improve, invent, or change patient care and technology. The intention, of course, is to affect health care by giving patients the technology, medication, or opportunity to live longer, healthier, happier lives.

Researchers review the health information from past or present patient health care. They retrieve data specific to their topic and analyze it to look for trends or suggested ways to enhance a treatment, disease, or diagnosis. They can analyze a patient's response to medication or treatment, prognosis, and the stages of a disease process—that is, the way in which the disease develops. Health information is documented during the course of the research. Although the health information may not be reported in the traditional form of a health record, it must be organized and stored in a manner that facilitates its retrieval and reference at a later date.

MANAGED CARE

Managed care is the coordination of health care benefits by the insurance company to control access and emphasize preventive care. Managed care organizations use health information internally and in their relationship with health care providers. A managed care organization chooses to use a health care provider's services on the basis of an analysis of the provider's performance. The managed care organization requires the health care facility to provide information about its services, performance, patient LOS, outcomes, and so on. The managed care organization uses this information to determine whether to include the facility as a provider for the organization's beneficiaries.

This data gathering is part of the contract negotiation and evaluation. Before entering into a managed care contract, a great deal of health information is exchanged between the managed

Hit-Bit

Research

Pharmaceutical companies perform a great deal of research on medications before receiving approval to market them to the consumer. This research involves clinical trials in which patients with a known diagnosis or predisposition are given the medication or a **placebo** or routine treatment. While receiving the medication, the patients are monitored to determine the impact of the medication on their condition. In later clinical trials, the new medication is administered to a wider group for more extensive study. Results of this monitoring are reported in the patients' health records.

Hit-Bit

The National Committee for Quality Assurance

The National Committee for Quality Assurance (NCQA) was founded in 1979.

care organization and the health care provider. While the facility is providing this information to the managed care organization, it also begins evaluating its own data to determine its ability to provide health care to this group of beneficiaries. With this information, the facility can determine whether the contract is viable.

Managed care organizations can also be accredited by the National Committee for Quality Assurance (NCQA). The NCQA requires that managed care organizations comply with clinical and administrative performance standards, including a requirement for health records. Therefore the use of health information within a managed care organization has an impact not only on the benefits of the group members but also on the accreditation of the organization.

MARKETING

Marketing is the promotion of products and services in the hope that the consumer chooses them over the products and services of a competitor. Health information can be used for marketing. Health care facilities are in business to make a profit. Regardless of their status, for profit or non-profit, they must raise enough funds to sustain their business. Facilities routinely involve themselves in situations that allow them to compare their business with that of the competition. They analyze market share and compare usage and cost of particular services and information about patient LOS. In other words, they analyze statistical information obtained from health care information databases (see Chapter 9) to determine whether there is a need for new treatment or technology in the community. Perhaps the study reveals that the facility has a significant share of the maternity market. There are methods that the facility can use to promote other services to that group of patients. They also analyze trends that show a need for a specific type of health care, such as dialysis care, midwifery, sports medicine, or laser surgery.

The marketing department also uses a successful survey by an accreditation agency as a way to promote the facility in the community. Because the accreditation recognizes compliance with set standards, an accredited facility is perceived as better than one that is not accredited.

Table 10-6 reviews all of the uses of health information mentioned in the previous sections.

TABLE 10-6	Uses of Health Information

USE	EXAMPLE/EXPLANATION
Improvement in patient care	The health care facility uses the documentation in the health record to determine patient care.
Support and collection of reimbursement	Documentation of health care is used to support and collect reimbursement for services rendered to patients.
Licensing, accreditation, and certifications	Health information must be maintained as a requirement of licensure. Likewise, it supports compliance with certification requirements and accreditation standards.
Administration	Health information is used to make decision regarding the delivery of health care services.
Prevalence and incidence of morbidity and mortality	Statistics are reports to aid in the prevention and treatment of certain diseases.
National policy and legislation	Research and statistics are references to establish policy and legislation related to health care (i.e., Medicare and Medicaid).
Development of community awareness of health care issues	Research and literature are used to educate the public regarding health care issues (e.g., cancer awareness programs).
Litigation	Health information is used to support or prove a fact in a lawsuit.
Education	Health information is used to educate patients, clinicians, allied health professionals, and the public.
Research	Health information is used to support and document health care research.
Managed care	Managed care organizations evaluate health information (statistics) to determine whether to include a facility in their plan. Also, managed care organizations use health information to analyze services provided to their beneficiaries.
Marketing	Analysis of health information provides statistical information that the marketing department can use to promote the facility within a community.

Exercise 10-7

Uses of Health Information

1. Can you think of another use for health information besides those listed in this chapter?
2. Each month the tumor registry personnel are required to report the _____ of breast cancer for the facility. They report this statistic by determining the number of new cases of breast cancer for the month.
3. The method of reviewing patient information during hospitalization is known as _____.
4. Successful completion of a Medicare Conditions of Participation survey results in _____ for the health care facility.
5. Health information may be used in _____ to support the plaintiff's claim.
6. _____ refers to death within a population.
7. Health information may be analyzed to support a _____ campaign to promote the facility within its community.
8. The number of existing cancer cases reported by the tumor registry is known as _____.
9. _____ refers to disease within a population.
10. The monies collected by the health care facility from the payer is known as _____.
11. Physicians may perform _____ to determine the cause or best treatment for a particular disease.
12. The postdischarge review of the record is known as _____.
13. Certification may be obtained by complying with which one of the following:
    a. MCOP
    b. MPI
    c. Medicaid billing regulations
    d. JCAHO

■ WORKS CITED

Abdelhak Mervat, Sara Grostick, Mary Alice Hanken, and Ellen Jacobs. *Health Information: Management of a Strategic Resource.* 2nd ed. Philadelphia: Saunders, 2001.

Rudman, William J. *Performance Improvement in Health Information Sciences.* Philadelphia: Saunders, 1997.

■ SUGGESTED READING

Merriam-Webster's Collegiate Dictionary. 10th ed. Springfield, MA: Merriam-Webster, Inc., 1993.

Random House Webster's College Dictionary. New York: Random House, 1991.

WEB SITES

American College of Surgeons: http://www.facs.org.

American Hospital Association: http://www.aha.org/about/history.html

Centers for Disease Control: http://www.cdc.gov/aboutcdc.htm

OpenClinical: http://www.openclinical.org/clinicalpathways.html

NCQA: http://www.ncqa.org

CHAPTER ACTIVITIES

CHAPTER SUMMARY

Health information is widely accepted as an important part of the health care industry, and people take for granted that it will be timely, complete, accurate, and valid. This chapter reflects the importance of continued efforts to ensure high-quality health information so that it may be used effectively to make decisions about patient care. Having standardized information for all patients, as first required by ACS minimum standards, is important. With standardized information, health care professionals are able to compare one patient's care with another's and determine the quality of each. Standardized information allows for similar information to be shared as well as compared.

Perhaps the most eye-opening issue surrounding data quality is that outsiders do not recognize its importance until an HIM professional points it out or, more pointedly, until what is needed is not available, as ACS recognized in 1917.

High-quality health information allows others to use this vital information for the benefit of patients, communities, payers, and providers.

Review Questions

1. List and describe 10 uses of health information.
2. How is health information used to measure quality of patient care?
3. Explain the PDCA method for quality improvement.
4. Identify three committees and how they use health information.
5. Briefly explain the philosophy of Deming, Juran, and Crosby.
6. Explain the medical staff committee structure.
7. List the tools used for data gathering.
8. List the tools used for data organization and presentation.
9. Explain the purpose and composition of the HIM committee.
10. Explain the difference and similarity among risk management, utilization management ,and case management.

Assistant Director, HIM

My name is Kim, and I am the assistant director of the health information management (HIM) department. I am responsible for coordinating review of health records to ensure compliance with Joint Commission on Accreditation of Healthcare Organizations (JCAHO) standards. Record review is performed on a monthly basis at Parker Hospital, a 500-bed acute care facility. According to standards, my staff and I review 50 records each month. I make sure that all of the records are pulled before the meeting and prepare enough forms for review of the 50 records. During the multidisciplinary review meeting, I help the team members when they have a problem interpreting a standard or locating information in the health record. When all 50 records are reviewed, I collect the forms and tabulate the scores to determine the compliance with each standard. I then present the results of this review to the HIM committee for recommendation and action, as necessary. If the committee suggests a corrective action to improve compliance with a standard, I coordinate that effort. After the implementation of the corrective action, I report back to the HIM committee to show whether compliance has been achieved.

APPLICATION

Record Review

As a member of the record review team, you will perform a mock record review. Use the health record forms provided on the Introduction to Health Information Technology Companion Web site, discussed in Chapter 4, and the generic record review form (see Figure 10-5) to identify where the information on the record review form should be located in the patient's record.

LEGAL AND SUPERVISORY ISSUES IN HEALTH INFORMATION

Chapter 11

CONFIDENTIALITY AND COMPLIANCE

CHAPTER OUTLINE

By the end of this chapter, the student should be able to

- Distinguish between privacy and confidentiality.
- Explain the foundation for privacy regulation.
- List and describe the federal laws and regulations governing patient privacy and confidentiality.
- Explain the components of the HIPAA privacy regulations.
- List and describe the types of subpoenas.
- Define *jurisdiction*.
- Prepare information for copying, photocopy it, and send it out.

- Differentiate between release of patient information with and without consent.
- Develop and implement departmental policies and procedures regarding release of information to patients.
- Develop and implement departmental policies and procedures regarding release of information to care providers.

VOCABULARY

access

accounting of disclosures

amendment

business record rule

certification

competency

compliance

Conditions of Admission

confidential communications

confidentiality

consent

correspondence

court order

custodian

defendant

designated record set

disclosure

discovery

emancipation

exceptions

Federal Drug and Alcohol Abuse Regulations

hearsay rule

Health Insurance Portability & Accountability Act (HIPAA)

informed consent

Joint Commission on Accreditation of Healthcare Organizations

jurisdiction

litigation

minimum necessary

Notice of Privacy Practices

outsourced

permitted disclosure

personal health record

physician-patient privilege

plaintiff

power of attorney

privacy

privacy officer

prospective consent

protected health information (PHI)

public priority exception

release of information

required disclosure

restriction

retention

retrospective consent

right to complain

right to revoke

subpoena

subpoena ad testificandum

subpoena duces tecum

use

verification

he topic of confidentiality was touched on briefly in Chapter 4 with regard to the function of release of information. In this chapter, you will learn about the release of information and confidentiality as it relates to the actions of health care workers and outside parties. There is also an overview of the federal **Health Insurance Portability and Accountability Act (HIPAA)** Privacy Regulations, including patient rights as well as uses and disclosures of health information. The function of release of information is generally the responsibility of the health information management (HIM) department, but a number of other individuals are also involved at various junctures. You will also learn about the importance of confidentiality, the rules that are critical to ensuring the confidentiality of a health record, and problems that can occur when requests for release of health information are received.

CONFIDENTIALITY

DEFINITION

Although the terms *privacy* and *confidentiality* are often used synonymously, they do have slightly different meanings. **Confidentiality** implies the use of discretion in the disclosure of information. In very simple terms, it's like keeping a secret. When a patient is receiving medical care, no matter what the facility, no matter whom the provider, that information is confidential—it is secret. It may not be released to a person who is not authorized to receive it. **Privacy** is the right of the individual to control access to that information.

LEGAL FOUNDATION

The foundation for confidentiality is **physician-patient privilege.** This concept refers to communication between the patient and his or her physician. To promote complete and honest communication between the physician and patient, such communication cannot be disclosed to other parties without authorization. Although the facility owns the physical or electronic record, the patient owns the information in the record. Only the patient can waive the right to keep that communication confidential. The concept of physician-patient privilege has been upheld in court.

SCOPE

The scope of confidentiality is very broad. It includes not only the confidentiality of the written or electronic record but also spoken information. There are some basic guidelines that a health care professional can follow when working in a health care facility. First, health care professionals should never discuss patients in a public place, such as the cafeteria, elevators, or hallways, because others may be able to hear their conversations.

If it becomes necessary to discuss a patient in a public place, the patient should be discussed only by diagnosis or in some manner that prevents eavesdroppers from being able to identify the patient. However, care should be taken even in this regard. For example, discussing a patient by room number can violate the patient's privacy if the conversation is overheard by someone who knows what room the patient is in (e.g., a family member). This may seem like common sense to you, but it is one of the most frequently committed violations of a patient's right to confidentiality.

All employees should sign a confidentiality agreement when they are hired. Annual re-signing of that document, along with in-service training in the necessity for understanding and complying with the facility's confidentiality policies and procedures, is recommended. Figure 11-1 is a sample confidentiality agreement.

A second issue in confidentiality is the physical maintenance of the patient's health record. Physical documents should be kept in a binder or folder at all times. Binders or folders containing a specific patient's documents should be identified only with the patient's name, health record number, and room number (if applicable). No matter how the record is maintained, the outside of the folder or binder should not contain any diagnostic information or anything of significance that could be read by a casual passerby. On the nursing unit, only the bed number should be visible on the patient's binder. An important exception to this rule is a warning about allergies.

DIAMONTE HOSPITAL

Diamonte, Arizona 89104 • TEL. 602-484-9991

CONFIDENTIALITY AGREEMENT

I, _____ , understand that I have a legal and ethical duty to maintain the confidentiality of the private health information of all patients treated at this facility. During the course of my employment or assignment at Diamonte Hospital, I will have access to confidential patient information.

I understand that I am obligated by state law, federal law, and Diamonte Hospital to protect and safeguard the privacy of all patient data and/or health information. I agree that I will not disclose any patient information to any person, even after my term of employment or assignment ends. In addition, I will not allow any person to examine or make copies of any patient information except that which is necessary in the course of my employment or assignment.

I understand that violation of this agreement may result in punitive legal action and disciplinary action, possibly including termination of my employment or assignment.

_____   _____
Signature of Employee/Student/Volunteer   Date

_____   _____
Signature of Witness   Date

◆ **Figure 11-1**
Confidentiality agreement.

Patient allergies should be clearly noted on the front of the binder. Employees are often tempted to mark the binder with clinically significant information, such as "HIV Positive." Such sensitive information should not be visible. Some facilities place color-coded stickers or other symbols on the outside of the binder to circumvent this rule; however, these symbols should not be easily recognizable by the casual observer.

Confidentiality procedures extend to the hallways and to the patient's room itself. The patient's actual diagnoses, procedures, and appointments should not be displayed where the casual observer can see them. This is a common failing in facilities where multiple individuals need to know the activities of a patient. For example, in an inpatient rehabilitation facility, patients do not generally remain in their rooms. They are transported to other parts of the facility for various therapies, or they may be taken out of the facility for a procedure. The temptation is to write this information in a common area where all health care providers can see it. To protect the patient's privacy, however, such postings should be confined to restricted areas.

In a computer-based environment, certain special considerations apply. Computer screens should be placed so that they are not in public view. A health care professional accessing a patient's record at a computer terminal may be called away temporarily. It is very important for the person to log off the computer before leaving so that patient information is not visible to anyone who is not authorized to view it.

Even health care professionals do not have a right to access a patient's record unless they are actually working with the patient. Computer-based systems should always provide an automatic log-off after a certain period of idle time. A typical computer screen saver is not sufficient unless it is password protected. The entire record should be logged off and made inaccessible without a specific user name and password. Passwords should not be shared among caregivers, even for reasons of efficiency. Passwords should not be written near computers or anywhere that unauthorized users could obtain them.

LEGISLATION

A statute is a law that has been passed by the legislative branch of government. Legislation dealing with confidentiality and health information varies at the state level. Federal regulations, as discussed in the following section, must also be followed.

Each state has licensure requirements for health care facilities. Generally, states also have regulations regarding medical records. Health care facilities must comply with these regulations to maintain their facility license. A facility often has to follow federal laws, federal regulations, state laws, and state regulations. HIPAA clarifies that when the privacy regulations conflict with state law, the regulation or law that gives the patient more rights or is more restrictive should prevail. Therefore practices vary from state to state, and HIM professionals must become familiar with applicable state laws and licensure rules and regulations as well as federal laws and regulations.

Exercise 11-1

Confidentiality

1. What is the difference between privacy and confidentiality?
2. What is the legal foundation for confidentiality?

HEALTH INSURANCE PORTABILITY AND ACCOUNTABILITY ACT

Public Law 104-191 is the legal reference for the Health Insurance Portability and Accountability Act of 1996, commonly known as HIPAA. Title II contains the Administrative Simplification Section. Within Title II are major categories dealing with health information: Electronic Transactions and Code Sets, Unique Identifiers, the Privacy Rule, and the Security Rule. The purpose of Title II is to improve the Medicare and Medicaid programs and to improve the efficiency and effectiveness of health information systems by establishing a common set of standards and requirements for handling electronic information.

The HIPAA Privacy Regulations address the use and disclosure of protected health information. The HIPAA Security Regulations address administrative, physical, and technical safeguards to protect health information that is collected, maintained, used, or transmitted electronically.

Health care providers, health care plans, and health care clearinghouses must comply with the HIPAA privacy and security regulations. They are known as *covered entities*. Business associates must also comply. Business associates are those contracted vendors that use confidential health information to perform a service on behalf of the covered entity. They must comply indirectly with certain HIPAA provisions. Figure 11-2 illustrates the major sections of HIPAA.

PRIVACY REGULATIONS

This chapter focuses on the Privacy Rule because health information professionals play key roles in assisting health care facilities with HIPAA privacy compliance. The rule introduces the role of **privacy officer**. Facilities must appoint a privacy officer to handle privacy compliance and must also designate a person to handle any complaints. The privacy officer usually handles this role as well. Health care facilities were required to be in compliance with HIPAA's Privacy Rule on April 14, 2003.

TITLE I	TITLE II	TITLE III STANDARDS	TITLE IV	TITLE V
Health care access, portability, and renewability	**Preventing fraud and abuse**	Tax-related health provisions	Application and enforcement of group health plan requirements	Revenue offsets

Administrative Simplification (Title II)

Electronic data interchange (transactions, code sets)   Unique identifiers   Privacy   Security

◆ **Figure 11-2**
The major sections of HIPAA.

Hit-Bit

Examples of Business Associates

Typical business associates of the health information department are an outsourced medical transcription company, the release of information vendor, legal counsel representing the health care facility, reimbursement consultants, and the microfilm/imaging/storage vendor. They are not members of the facility's workforce, but they use or disclose health information to perform a function or activity on behalf of the health care facility.

Hit-Bit

Privacy and Security Credentials

Many health information professionals serve as privacy officers for their facilities. AHIMA offers a special credential: CHPS (Certified in Healthcare Privacy and Security). Exams no longer administered after March 2007 are the CHP (Certified in Healthcare Privacy) and the CHS (Certified in Healthcare Security).

PROTECTED HEALTH INFORMATION

The Privacy Rule addresses the uses and disclosures of **protected health information** (**PHI**). PHI is individually identifiable health information that is transmitted or maintained in any form or medium by covered entities or their business associates. This includes oral, written, and electronic information. Some examples of PHI are name, address, telephone number, fax number, e-mail address, social security number, medical record number, health plan number, account number, driver's license number, license plate number, URL, Internet service provider address, biometric identifiers (e.g., finger prints), photos, and all relevant dates (e.g., date of birth, admission, and discharge). These data items could identify a person, thereby violating his or her right to privacy.

USES AND DISCLOSURES

Health information is used to treat patients. When a physician reviews a test result, it is a **use** of PHI. A **disclosure** occurs when PHI is given to someone. For example, an insurance company is given a copy of an emergency room record to verify that the patient's condition was indeed an emergency, as defined in the patient's health insurance policy. This disclosure may be necessary to obtain reimbursement from the insurer.

PHI cannot be used or disclosed unless the Privacy Rule requires or permits it to be used or disclosed. There are two types of **required disclosures**: disclosures to the patient and disclosures to the Secretary of the Department of Health and Human Services for compliance auditing purposes. There are several **permitted disclosures** outlined in the Privacy Rule. All disclosures that are specifically authorized by the patient are permitted. Disclosures for treatment purposes, payment of the patient's bill, or health care operations such as risk management are all permitted and do not need to be authorized by the patient. Disclosures for research purposes are permitted under specific conditions.

Uses and disclosures of PHI without patient authorization are also permitted for certain public priorities. These are considered **exceptions**. Covered entities must comply with the conditions in the exceptions. The following are some exceptions:

- As required by law
- For public health activities
- About victims of abuse, neglect, or domestic violence
- For health oversight activities
- For judicial and administrative proceedings
- For law enforcement
- About decedents (to coroners, medical examiners, funeral directors)
- To facilitate cadaver organ donation and transplants
- For certain research
- To avert a serious threat to health or safety
- For specialized government functions (e.g., military, veterans' groups, national security, protective services, State Department, correctional facilities)
- For workers' compensation (as authorized by law)

Hit-Bit

Uses for Health Care Operations

Some examples of health care operations are risk management, infection control, quality improvement, legal counsel, and case management. For example, an infection control nurse is allowed to review the medical records of a patient with an infectious disease without authorization to investigate the outbreak, keep statistics, and prevent the spread of a disease to other patients.

NOTICE OF PRIVACY PRACTICES

Covered entities are required to establish policies and procedures addressing HIPAA privacy issues. One of the most important policies is the **Notice of Privacy Practices**. This document summarizes the facility's privacy policies and explains how the facility may use or disclose patient health information. The notice must be written in clear and simple language and provide examples. Contact information, such as telephone number, for the privacy officer/complaint designee must be included in the notice. Facilities must also obtain a signed acknowledgment from the patient that the notice was received.

PATIENT RIGHTS

The Privacy Rule gives patients certain rights, including the right to receive a notice of the privacy practices. In some situations, patients may request a higher level of privacy. In this case, they have the right to ask for additional **restrictions** on the use of their PHI or additional limitations on the amount of PHI disclosed. For example, a patient may ask that the facility not allow her next-door neighbor, a nurse who would normally have access to the record for patient care, to have access to her PHI. Facility administrators must decide whether they can comply with the patient's request. They do not have to honor such a request. For example, the facility may be small, with a limited nursing staff, and the next-door neighbor may need to be involved in the patient's care on account of a staffing shortage. A common restriction (called an *opt-out* in HIPAA) is a patient's request to be removed from the patient directory. In other words, individuals calling the facility would not be told that the patient is there, and calls would not be forwarded to the patient. The patient may also ask for **confidential communications**. For example, the patient may ask that the bill be mailed to another address instead of the home address.

Patients have the right of access to their health information. **Access** refers to the ability to learn the contents of a health record by reading it or obtaining a copy. There are many reasons that patients would want access to their record. Many patients are now keeping their own **personal health record**. The purpose of a personal health record is to document their history and provide information for continuing patient care. The American Health Information Management Association (AHIMA) and the American Medical Association (AMA) are both encouraging patients to track their own health information.

The patient is generally required to sign an authorization form or a request-for-access form to obtain or read copies of his or her health information. State laws and regulations vary regarding **retention**, but many facilities do destroy old records after the required retention period has passed. If a patient's appendectomy took place 30 years ago, the paper record may no longer exist. Therefore it is in the patient's best interest to maintain a personal file of health information.

The only legitimate reason to deny access to a patient is if the patient's health care provider decides that the information in the record would be harmful to the patient. This is an unusual circumstance that pertains primarily to behavioral health cases. If knowledge of the information in the record would be harmful to the patient, the provider must document reasons for the refusal of access. Health care providers must also follow a formal appeals process if access is denied. Figure 11-3 illustrates the flow of the decision-making process with regard to access requests.

Hit-Bit

Record Retention

HIPAA requires that any documentation associated with the Privacy Regulations must be kept for 6 years. For example, documentation regarding release of information, such as subpoenas, requests, authorizations, and correspondence logs, must be kept for 6 years. Other examples are policies and procedures, acknowledgments of notice of privacy practices, and amendment documentation—basically any documentation that the Privacy Rule discusses.

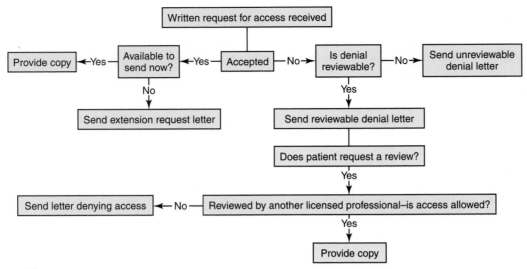

◆ **Figure 11-3**
The flow of the decision-making process with regard to access requests.

The HIPAA Privacy Regulations require health care providers to define their **designated record set** to respond to an individual's right to request access, request amendment, and request restriction to his or her PHI. The designated record set must include the legal medical records, the billing records of the patient, and any other information with which a decision was made that affects the patient. Patients have full access to the designated record set. Access by others will be discussed later in this chapter.

Patients may not always agree with the information in their designated record set. The HIPAA privacy regulations give patients the right to request an **amendment** of their health information. When patients ask to amend their health information, they should be given an amendment/correction request form to complete. It is generally given to the privacy officer for review and response to the patient within 60 days. If the facility cannot respond within 60 days, one 30-day extension is allowed. However, the patient must be informed in writing that there is a delay and given an expected date of response. The amendment can be denied if any of the following applies:

- The information was not created by the facility.
- The information is not part of the designated record set.
- The information is not available for access.
- The information is accurate and complete.

Patients are also given the **right to revoke** authorization to disclose their PHI. For example, a patient may authorize his or her attorney to receive a copy of his or her medical record and later

Hit-Bit

Request for Amendment

Usually, the privacy officer will contact the physician or health care professional whose documentation the patient is contesting. This professional will review the request and decide whether to correct the information. If the professional stands by the information as being correct, the patient is notified that his or her request is denied because the information is accurate and complete. If the patient disagrees with the denial, they must be given the opportunity to provide a statement of disagreement. The patient may request that all future releases include a copy of his or her request for amendment, the facility's denial letter, and his or her disagreement statement.

change attorneys. The patient would be allowed to revoke the original authorization to Attorney A and authorize a new disclosure to Attorney B.

Facilities are also required to give patients an **accounting of disclosures** upon request. This accounting is basically a list indicating who received information about the patient as well as when, why, and how the disclosure was made. Some disclosures do not require this accounting. Disclosures for treatment, payment, some health care operations, and patient authorized disclosures do not require accounting. Most facilities track all disclosures, even those for which accounting is not required, because thorough documentation is a good practice. HIPAA requires health care facilities to keep all documentation with regard to an accounting of disclosures for 6 years.

Finally, patients have a **right to complain**. They must be given the ability to discuss their concerns about privacy violations with a staff member and ultimately with the Department of Health and Human Services (DHHS). The Office of Civil Rights has been given DHHS authority to investigate complaints, enforce the privacy rule, and impose penalties for HIPAA violations. Penalties may be civil or criminal and may involve fines and imprisonment depending on the circumstances.

Exercise 11-2

HIPAA

1. Describe HIPAA. Why is it important?
2. What is PHI?
3. What is a covered entity?
4. What is a business associate?

ACCESS

Despite the need for privacy, there are legitimate reasons for various parties to have access to a patient's PHI. These reasons include the following: treatment (continuing patient care), payment (reimbursement), and health care operations. In addition, the patient may wish to provide access to third parties, such as lawyers.

CONTINUING PATIENT CARE

Confidentiality presents some interesting issues for continuing patient care. The attending physician and direct care providers involved with the patient should have full access to the patient's health information in order to treat the patient. However, what if a physician wishes to review his neighbor's medical record? Should he be given access simply because he is a physician? No. The health care professional must have direct patient involvement or a specific "need to know" in order to obtain the patient's information. Any other access to a patient's record requires specific patient authorization. An example of inappropriate access is a facility employee who looks at a family member's medical record without the patient's permission. This misuse of access would be a confidentiality violation. Electronic records systems should provide audit trails indicating who accessed what patient information so that compliance with confidentiality can be documented and violations identified.

It is important to convey to employees of the HIM department and the facility in general that inappropriate access to a record is illegal and will lead to punishment. The HIPAA Security Regulations discussed earlier in this chapter have a section dealing with workforce security and termination procedures if someone violates the rules. Dismissal of employees who inappropriately access health records is not excessively harsh; it is common.

Health care professionals outside of the facility in which the patient was originally treated may also need certain health information. HIPAA's Privacy Regulations allow the use and disclosure of health information for continuing patient care, without specific patient authorization. However, it is common practice to ask for authorizations or at least written requests from outside health care providers because thorough documentation is good practice.

REIMBURSEMENT

Another reason to disclose health information is for reimbursement purposes. In the current health care environment, various payers may need to review the record. HIPAA's Privacy Regulations allow the use and disclosure of health information for payment purposes without authorization. However, it is common practice to have patients sign a **Conditions of Admission** form upon admission to a hospital; this form includes authorization for the release of health information to the party who is financially responsible. This type of authorization constitutes **prospective consent**. In other words, the patient is authorizing the release of information before that information has been generated.

Although this authorization is not required because HIPAA allows release of health information for payment purposes without authorization, it is a common practice because it informs patients that their health information may be disclosed in order for the bill to be paid. In addition, the Notice of Privacy Practices informs the patient that his or her health information may be disclosed for reimbursement purposes.

In most other cases, such as third-party release of information for legal purposes, **retrospective consent** is necessary. Retrospective consent means that the patient authorizes the use or disclosure of health information after care has been rendered.

HEALTH CARE OPERATIONS

HIPAA's Privacy Regulations also allow the use and disclosure of health information for health care operations purposes without authorization. Health care operations include functions such as risk management, infection control, case management, and quality improvement. Disclosures for health care operations must comply with the **minimum necessary** rule. Health care providers must disclose only the minimum amount of information necessary to accomplish a task. For example, a nurse manager auditing the record for compliance with restraint rules would not require access to billing records.

LITIGATION

Litigation is an area of disclosure in which authorization to release information is required (unless it is to the health care provider's attorney for defense—an operations purpose). **Litigation** is the process by which one party sues another in a court of law. Litigation often results when a patient has been injured, either accidentally or intentionally. The party who is suing is the **plaintiff**. The party who is being sued is the **defendant**.

The legal aspects of health information and health care in general are too broad to discuss in this book. However, a general understanding of how a trial works is helpful knowledge for the HIM professional. Most lawsuits that require disclosure of medical records are based on some injury to the patient. A shopper slips and falls in the grocery store, spraining her back, and sues the store. A physician amputates the wrong foot, and the patient sues the physician and the hospital. A pedestrian is hit by a car, breaks a leg, and sues the driver of the car.

The plaintiffs in these cases file a complaint with the court that states the issues, the reason they chose that particular court, and what outcome they desire. In the grocery store example, the plaintiff may file a complaint in a state court stating that the grocery store's floor was wet and posed a hazard, which was the cause of the accident. The complaint is filed in that court because the store is located in that state and the plaintiff lives in that state. The plaintiff wants the court to agree that the store was at fault and to order the store to pay for the plaintiff's medical care and loss of income. The steps in this type of litigation are listed and defined in Table 11-1.

There are two steps in the aforementioned lawsuit in which health records may be required. The first step is during the **discovery** process. During discovery, the lawyers may want a copy of the documentation of the plaintiff's treatment to verify the extent and timing of the injuries as

TABLE 11-1	**Steps in Personal Injury Litigation**
Complaint	This is the plaintiff's written claim, including a description of compensation or other relief and an expression of the court's jurisdiction in the matter. Complaint may be followed by a counterclaim and other communications establishing the position of both parties on the issue.
Discovery	This is an investigation of the facts of the case, including taking statements, interviewing witnesses, and obtaining and reviewing documentation.
Pretrial conference	This is a meeting of the parties with the trial judge to resolve or clarify outstanding issues and explore potential settlement.
Trial*	The trial is the presentation of both sides of the case in court. Judgment may be rendered by a judge or jury. In some cases, a judge may override the verdict of a jury.
Appeal	The loser of the trial may request a review of the trial proceedings by a higher court. Appeals must be based on perceived errors or problems with the original trial, not purely on dissatisfaction with the outcome.
Satisfying the judgment	This is the final disposition of the case, such as the collection of damages.

Data from Dana McWay. *Legal Aspects of Health Information Management.* Albany, NY: Delmar, 1996.
*Trials vary, depending on the type of case, the jurisdiction, and the type of court. Local court rules vary from state to state. HIM professionals are frequently asked to provide documentation at the discovery and trial steps. New York: Delmar.

well as the nature, extent, and cost of care. The record may be needed again in court during the trial if it is used as evidence. During both of these steps, a certified or notarized copy of the original record is usually required. **Certification** is the process whereby the official custodian of the medical records certifies that the copies are true and complete copies of the original records. The **custodian,** usually the HIM director, is the official keeper of the medical records.

The certification and use of health records as evidence in court is based on the **business record rule.** The business record rule states that health records may be accepted as evidence in the following instances:

■ They are kept in the normal course of business.
■ They are recorded by individuals who are in a position to be knowledgeable of the events that are being recorded.
■ They are documented contemporaneously with those events.

The business record rule is an exception to the **hearsay rule,** which prohibits secondhand accounts of events. If the hearsay rule applied to health records, then a nurse's documentation of a patient's statements or a physician's subjective notes would not be admissible evidence (i.e., it would not be allowed to be presented in court).

The choice of a court in which to file the complaint is primarily a matter of **jurisdiction.** *Jurisdiction* means that the court has authority over the issue, the person, or both. There are courts of limited jurisdiction, such as traffic court, which may decide only certain types of cases. Other courts have general jurisdiction, such as state courts, and they may decide a wide variety of cases. In general, these courts have jurisdiction over citizens of the states in which they operate. There are also federal courts, whose jurisdiction extends to issues regarding federal statutes, regulations, and treaties; events that occur on federal land; and citizens of different states.

There are several different avenues through which access to the record can be obtained during litigation. First, the patient can sign an authorization to release the information to either the patient's lawyer or the defendant's lawyer. It is presumed that when a patient institutes litigation and uses the medical condition as a foundation for the litigation, he or she is waiving the right to confidentiality.

Another avenue of approach is through the **subpoena** process. A subpoena is a direction from an officer of the court. The direction may be to testify (**subpoena ad testificandum**) or to provide documentation (**subpoena duces tecum**; Figure 11-4). The HIM department may receive a

AO 88 (Rev.1/94) Subpoena in a Civil Case

Issued by the
UNITED STATES DISTRICT COURT
DISTRICT OF

SUBPOENA IN A CIVIL CASE

V.

CASE NUMBER: [1]

To:

☐YOU ARE COMMANDED to appear in the United States District Court at the place, date, and time specified below to testify in the above case.

PLACE OF TESTIMONY	COURTROOM
	DATE AND TIME

☐YOU ARE COMMANDED to appear in the United States District Court at the place, date, and time specified below to testify at the taking of a deposition in the above case.

PLACE OF TESTIMONY	COURTROOM
	DATE AND TIME

☐YOU ARE COMMANDED to produce and permit inspection and copying of the following documents or objects at the place, date, and time specified below (list documents or objects):

PLACE	DATE AND TIME

☐YOU ARE COMMANDED to permit inspection of the following premises at the date and time specified below.

PREMISES	DATE AND TIME

Any organization not a party to this suit that is subpoenaed for the taking of a deposition shall designate one or more officers, directors, or managing agents, or other persons who consent to testify on its behalf, and may set forth, for each person designated, the matters on which the person will testify. Federal rules of Civil Procedure, 30(b) (6).

ISSUING OFFICER SIGNATURE AND TITLE (INDICATE IF ATTORNEY FOR PLAINTIFF OR DEFENDANT)	DATE
ISSUING OFFICERS NAME, ADDRESS AND PHONE NUMBER	

(See Rule 45, Federal Rules of Civil Procedure, Parts C & D on Reverse)
[1]If action is pending in district other than district of issuance, state district under case number.

◆ **Figure 11-4**
Sample subpoena to testify in a civil case. (From Dana McWay. *Legal Aspects of Health Information Management*. New York: Delmar, 1996.)

subpoena from the patient's lawyer or from the defendant's lawyer. A subpoena is valid for access to health records only if the subpoena itself is valid and the court through which the subpoena is issued has jurisdiction over the party to whom the subpoena is addressed. Figure 11-5 lists the common elements of a valid subpoena.

The HIPAA Privacy Regulations state that a covered entity may disclose protected health information in the course of any judicial or administrative proceeding in response to the following:

AO 88 (Rev.1/94) Subpoena in a Civil Case

PROOF OF SERVICE

	DATE	PLACE
SERVED		

SERVED ON (PRINT NAME)		MANNER OF SERVICE

SERVED BY (PRINT NAME)		TITLE

DECLARATION OF SERVER

I declare under penalty of perjury under the laws of the United States of America that the foregoing information contained in the Proof of Service is true and correct.

Executed on (date)	SIGNATURE OF SERVER
	ADDRESS OF SERVER

Rule 45, Federal Rules of Civil Procedure, Parts C & D:

(c) PROTECTION OF PERSONS SUBJECT TO SUBPOENAS.

(1) A party or an attorney responsible for the issuance and service of a subpoena shall take reasonable steps to avoid imposing undue burden or expense on a person subject to that subpoena. The court on behalf of which the subpoena was issued shall enforce this duty and impose upon the party or attorney in breach of this duty an appropriate sanction which may include, but is not limited to, lost earnings and reasonable attorney's fee.

(2) (A) A person commanded to produce and permit inspection and copying of designated books, papers, documents or tangible things, or inspection of premises need not appear in person at the place of production or inspection unless commanded to appear for deposition, hearing or trial.

(B) Subject to paragraph (d) (2) of this rule, a person commanded to produce and permit inspection and copying may, within 14 days after service of subpoena or before the time specified for compliance if such time is less than 14 days after service, serve upon the party or attorney designated in the subpoena written objection to inspection or copying of any or all of the designated materials or of the premises. If objection is made, the party serving the subpoena shall not be entitled to inspect and copy materials or inspect the premises except pursuant to an order of the court by which the subpoena was issued. If objection has been made the party may, upon notice to the person commanded to produce, move at any time for an order to compel the production. Such an order to compel production shall protect any person who is not a party or an officer of a party from significant expense resulting from the inspection and copying commanded.

(3) (A) On timely motion, the court by which a subpoena was issued shall quash or modify the subpoena if it

(i) fails to allow reasonable time for compliance:

(ii) requires a person who is not a party or an officer of a party to travel to a place more than 100 miles from the place were that person resides, is employed or regularly transacts business in person, except that, subject to the provisions of clause (c) (3) (3) (iii) of this rule, such a person may, in order to attend trial be comman-

ded to travel from any such place within the state in which the trial is held, or

(iii) requires disclosure of privileged or other protected matter and no exception or waiver applies, or

(iv) subjects a person to undue burden.

(B) If a subpoena

(i) requires disclosure of a trade secret or other confidential research development, or commercial information, or

(ii) requires disclosure of an unretained expert's opinion or information not describing specific events or occurrences in dispute and resulting from the expert's study made not at the request of any party, or

(iii) requires a person who is not a party or an officer of a party to incur substantial expense to travel more than 100 miles to attend trial, the court may, to protect a person subject to or affected by the subpoena, quash or modify the subpoena, or, if the party in whose behalf the subpoena is issued shows a substantial need for the testimony or material that cannot be otherwise met without undue hardship and assures that the person to whom the subpoena is addressed will be reasonably compensated, the court may order appearance or production only upon specified conditions.

(d) DUTIES IN RESPONDING TO A SUBPOENA

(1) A person responding to a subpoena to produce documents shall produce them as they are kept in the usual course of business or shall organize and label them to correspond with the categories in the demand.

(2) When information subject to a subpoena is withheld on a claim that it is privileged or subject to protection as trial preparation materials, the claim shall be made expressly and shall be supported by a description of the nature of the documents, communications, or things not produced that is sufficient to enable the demanding party to contest the claim.

◆ **Figure 11-4 (*cont'd*)**

- A court order, but only the protected health information expressly authorized for release by the order
- Subpoena duces tecum, provided that the covered entity
  - receives a written statement and accompanying documents from the party seeking the information that reasonable efforts have been made to ensure that the individual who is the subject of the information has been notified of the request or that reasonable efforts have been made to secure a qualified protective order for the information.

COMMON ELEMENTS OF A VALID SUBPOENA

1. Name of the court where the lawsuit is brought

2. Names of the parties to the lawsuit

3. Docket number of the case

4. Date, time, and place of the requested appearance

5. Specific documents to be produced, if a subpoena duces tecum is involved

6. Name and telephone number of the attorney who requested the subpoena

7. Signature, stamp, or seal of the official empowered to issue the subpoena

8. Witness fees, where provided by law

◆ **Figure 11-5**
Common elements of a valid subpoena. (From Dana McWay. *Legal Aspects of Health Information Management.* New York: Delmar, 1996.)

■ makes reasonable efforts to limit the protected health information used or disclosed to the minimum necessary to respond to the request.

The requirement to provide sufficient notice to the individual is when a party provides a written statement and accompanying documentation that demonstrates the following:

■ A good faith attempt was made to notify the individual.

■ The notice included sufficient information to permit the individual to raise an objection with the court.

■ The time for the individual to raise objections has lapsed, no objection was filed or objections have been resolved by the court, and the disclosure is consistent with the resolution.

A qualified protective order is an order of a court that prohibits the parties from using or disclosing the PHI for any purpose other than the litigation or proceeding for which such information was requested and requires the return to the covered entity or destruction of the PHI (including any copies) at the end of the litigation or proceeding.

Exercise 11-3

Access

1. What is jurisdiction?
2. What is the hearsay rule? How does it affect cases involving health records?
3. What are the components of the business record rule?
4. Explain the difference between retrospective and prospective consent. Why is the difference important?
5. Over what events or circumstances does a federal court have jurisdiction?
6. Number the steps in a civil lawsuit in their correct order:

_____ Appeal

_____ Complaint

_____ Discovery

_____ Pretrial conference

_____ Satisfying the judgment

_____ Trial

COMPONENTS OF A VALID COURT ORDER AUTHORIZING DISCLOSURE

1. Name of the court issuing the order authorizing disclosure

2. Names of the parties to the lawsuit

3. Docket number of the case

4. Limitations for disclosure of only those components of the patient's records that are essential to fulfill the objective of the order

5. Limitations for disclosure to those persons whose need for information is the basis for the order

6. Any other limitations on disclosure that serve to protect the patient, the physician-patient relationship, and/or the treatment given, such as sealing the court proceeding from public scrutiny

◆ **Figure 11-6**

Court order components of a valid court order authorizing disclosure. (From Dana McWay. *Legal Aspects of Health Information Management.* New York: Delmar, 1996.)

A **court order** is the direction of a judge who has made a decision that an order to produce the records is necessary. Again, the issue of jurisdiction arises. For example, if an elderly patient's children seek to declare the patient legally incompetent (unable to make decisions about his or her affairs), the judge may issue a court order to obtain the patient's health records. Figure 11-6 gives the components of a valid court order authorizing disclosure.

 CONSENT

In health care, **consent** refers to the patient's agreement to allow something to occur. Consents underlie virtually all of a patient's contacts with health care professionals. Consents may be either implied or expressed. When a patient makes an appointment with a physician to get a flu shot, consent to have the shot is implied because they showed up for the appointment. Express consent, however, would involve signing a consent form to take the shot.

INFORMED CONSENT

For a patient to give consent, the patient must be of legal age, competent, and provided with sufficient information to make a reasonable decision about the issue to which he or she is consenting.

Legal age generally refers to having achieved the statutory age, which is determined by state law. Statutory age is generally 18 or 21 years old. There are some exceptions, such as emancipated minors and minors receiving psychiatric treatment, chemical dependency counseling, or prenatal care. State laws outline the conditions in which minors are given **emancipation** (i.e., consideration as an adult even though they are younger than the statutory age). A common reason for emancipation is marriage.

Competency is the patient's ability to make reasonable decisions. A patient who has been declared incompetent by a court has a guardian who can consent on behalf of the patient. This guardian is given a health care **power of attorney**. In general, a patient is assumed to be competent unless there is evidence to the contrary. When the patient's competence is in doubt, the patient's physician and hospital attorney should be contacted for guidance.

Informed consent requires an explanation of the process, procedure, risks, or other activity to which the patient is consenting. Sufficient information must be provided to the patient so that he or she can make an informed decision about the matter. Documentation of this informed consent is required before health care can be rendered.

ADMISSION

For admission to a health care facility or a visit to a physician's office, the patient is asked to sign a document consenting to medical treatment. This type of consent is very general and covers routine procedures, such as physical examinations and medical therapies, nutrition counseling, and prescribing medications. In an inpatient facility, this consent is usually called the **Conditions of Admission** (Figure 11-7). The Conditions of Admission form generally also includes permission for the facility to use patient information for education, research, and reimbursement.

Community Hospital
555 Street Drive
Town, NJ 07999
(973) 555-5555

| 554879 |
| Green, John |
| 44 Avenue Street |
| Town, NJ 07999 |
| |
| Dr. Ramundo |

Admission Consent

1. I understand that I am suffering from a condition requiring diagnosis and medical and/or surgical treatment. I voluntarily consent to such medical treatment deemed necessary or advisable by my treating physician, his associates, or assistants, in the treatment and care rendered to me, while a patient in Community Hospital. I also give permission for the services of any consulting physician that my attending physician deems necessary in his/her treatment of me.

2. I authorize Community Hospital, its medical and surgical staff, and its medical and other employees to furnish the appropriate hospital service and care deemed necessary by my condition.

3. I am aware that the practice of medicine and surgery is not an exact science and I acknowledge that no guarantees have been made to me as to the results of any diagnosis, treatment, or hospital care that I may receive at Community Hospital.

4. I authorize the transfer of medical information to any federal, state, or local government institution, or any agency, nursing home, or extended care facility to which I may be transferred or from which I may require assistance.

5. I certify that the information given by me regarding my health insurance is current and accurate, to the best of my knowledge. I authorize the release of any information needed to act on obtaining reimbursement from the parties so named. I understand that I am responsible for any health insurance deductibles or copayments and I do hereby agree to pay all bills rendered by Community Hospital for my hospital, medical, and nursing care that are not covered by these parties.

6. I authorize Community Hospital to retain, preserve, and use for scientific or teaching purposes, or dispose of at their convenience, any specimens or tissues taken from my body and any x-rays, photographs, or similar data taken during my hospitalization.

7. This form has been fully explained to me and I certify that I understand its contents.

_____   _____   _____
Witness   Signature of patient, agent,   Date
                                                     or legal guardian

---

◆ **Figure 11-7**
Conditions of admission.

MEDICAL PROCEDURES

The Conditions of Admission form includes only routine procedures and administrative issues. For invasive procedures, such as surgery, a specific consent is required. Anesthesia delivery and human immunodeficiency virus (HIV) testing are examples of other procedures that require specific consent. These consents are intended, in part, to document the extent to which procedures have been explained to patients, including the known risks of the procedures. Figure 11-8 shows a consent for surgery form.

Community Hospital
555 Street Drive
Town, NJ 07999
(973) 555-5555

```
554879
Green, John
44 Avenue Street
Town, NJ 07999

Dr. Ramundo
```

Consent to Operation
or Other Procedure(s)

1. I understand that _____ is proposed to be performed by_____ and/or his/her associates and whomever may be designated as assistants.

2. I understand that the nature and purpose of the operation or procedure is to _____ _____ _____

3. I understand that possible alternative methods of treatment are _____ _____ _____

4. I understand that the risks and possible complications of this operation or procedure are _____ _____

5. I am aware that the practice of medicine and surgery is not an exact science and I acknowledge that no guarantees have been made to me as to the result of this procedure.

6. I consent to the examination and disposition by hospital authorities of any tissue or parts which may be removed during the course of this operation or procedure.

7. I understand the nature of the proposed operation or procedure(s), the risks and possible complications involved, and the expected results, as described above, and hereby request that such operation or procedure(s) be performed.

_____ _____ _____
Witness (may not be a   Signature of patient, agent,   Date
member of operating team)   or legal guardian

I have discussed with the above patient the nature of the proposed operation or procedure(s), the risks and possible complications involved, and the expected results, as described above.

_____
Signature of
counseling physician

◆ **Figure 11-8**
Consent for surgery.

Exercise 11-4

Consent

1. Permission to perform a medical procedure generally requires the patient's _____.
2. A 16-year-old patient presents in the emergency room for treatment of stomach pain. She is conscious, alert, and oriented. Who is the appropriate individual to sign the consent for treatment?
3. What are the elements of a valid authorization for release of information?
4. A permission that is given after the event to which the permission applies is _____.

▋ RELEASE OF INFORMATION

In both paper-based and electronic environments, portions of the record must sometimes be disclosed. Duplication may be accomplished by photocopying the paper record, printing a copy from a computer or microfilm printer, or transmitting the information electronically, such as by faxing it from an electronic system. In practice, the duplicate is generally provided in paper format, regardless of how it is stored or maintained. The function of disclosing health information in the HIM department is often called **release of information** or **correspondence.** This function is often **outsourced** (i.e., performed by outside contractors instead of facility personnel).

REQUIRED DISCLOSURES

HIPAA's Privacy Rule discusses two types of required disclosures:
- To the individual who is the subject of the information
- To the secretary of the DHHS for purposes of determining compliance

PERMITTED DISCLOSURES

All other disclosures are permitted. The following are permitted disclosures:
- To the individual or his personal representative
- For treatment, payment or health care operations
- For public priority purposes (exceptions)
- As authorized by the patient

AUTHORIZED DISCLOSURES

The patient may authorize the release of his or her information to anyone. Remember that only the patient (or his or her personal representative) can waive the physician-patient privilege. Documentation of the patient's consent to release information is accomplished by completion of an authorization form. As with consents for medical procedures, the concept of informed consent applies. The patient must know in advance the nature and purpose of the consent for disclosure. Therefore consents for release of information should be retrospective. In other words, the patient cannot be fully informed about what is being released until after the information has been generated.

Technically, it is not necessary for a patient to complete a specific form in order to authorize the release of information. Each health care facility should have an access policy. A letter addressed to the facility should suffice if it contains all of the elements of a valid authorization, but many facilities still require the use of a specific authorization form. HIPAA compliant authorizations require these core elements:
- *Identification of the party being asked to release the information.* The owner of the actual documents (i.e., the facility or health care provider who has custody of the documents) is named.

Hit-Bit

Personal Representative

A personal representative is an individual who is authorized to act on behalf of the patient. For example, a parent is generally a personal representative of his or her minor child. This title would also apply to a legal guardian or person acting "in loco parentis" of a minor child. In addition, if state law gives a person authority to act on behalf of a deceased individual (usually the executor, administrator, spouse, or next of kin), then that person would be considered a personal representative.

■ *Patient name/identification.* The patient's name is the primary identifier. However, because many individuals have the same or similar names, additional identifiers such as date of birth or social security number should be documented. The medical record number or account number is also very useful, if known.

■ *Identification of the party to whom the information is to be released.* The person or class of persons to whom information is being released must be listed. This may be the name of a facility, a health care provider, or any other party. In other words, to whom does the patient want the information to be sent? It is also important to include the accurate address of this party.

■ *Specific information to be released.* The authorization must include description of the information to be used or disclosed that identifies the information in a specific and meaningful way.

■ *Description of the purpose of the use or disclosure.* Common purposes for disclosure are for treatment purposes, legal reasons, application for disability benefits, application for life insurance, or simply "at the request of the individual."

■ *Expiration date.* The authorization form must list an expiration date or expiration "event." For example, the patient may document an expiration event of "upon my death" or "upon the event of my favorite National Football League team (must be named) winning the Super Bowl."

■ *Signature of the patient or personal representative authorizing the disclosure.* If the personal representative of the patient signs the authorization, a description of such representative's authority to act for the individual must also be provided. For example, if a mother authorizes a disclosure on behalf of her minor child, she must sign and document the disclosure "as mother or parent." If a patient is deceased, the executor of the will provides such documentation as the patient's representative.

■ *Date.* This is the date on which the patient makes the consent and signs the authorization documenting his consent.

In addition to the core elements, there are some required statements:

■ *Patient's right to revoke the authorization.* The patient or authorized agent has the right to revoke the consent for release of information in writing at any time before the actual distribution of the information. This should be explicitly stated on the authorization form.

Hit-Bit

Assisting Patients with Authorization Forms

It is often necessary to assist a patient with completion of the authorization form to ensure that it is properly completed when a patient visits the HIM department to obtain copies. Patients must always understand what they are signing.

- *Redisclosure statement.* The information used or disclosed may be subject to redisclosure by the recipient and may no longer be protected.
- *Conditions of authorization.* Whether the covered entity is permitted to condition treatment, payment, enrollment, or eligibility for benefits on the authorization.

DEFECTIVE AUTHORIZATIONS

An authorization is considered invalid in the following instances:

- If any of the core elements are missing
- If the expiration date or event has passed
- If it is filled out incorrectly
- If it is known that it was revoked
- If any information in the authorization is known to be false
- If the authorization is not in plain language (i.e., in simple language that a person with a sixth-grade education would be able to understand)

Figure 11-9 provides a checklist to ensure authorization validity.

AUTHORIZATION VALIDITY CHECKLIST:

_____ Discloser (facility) name listed (ex: Hospital Medical Center)

_____ Requestor name listed (ex: attorney John Doe)

_____ Specific description of information to be disclosed (ex: mammogram 3/01/06)

_____ Is the disclosure purpose listed or does it state something to the effect "at the request of the individual"? (ex: to take to new physician)

_____ Is there an expiration date or event that has not passed? (ex: an actual date or an event like "upon completion of this request" or "upon my death")

_____ Is it signed by the patient or by a personal representative with his or her authority documented? (ex: parent of a minor)

_____ Is it dated? (ex: must include the date the patient signed it)

_____ Is there a statement of the individual's right to revoke the authorization?

_____ Is this authorization still valid, i.e., has not been revoked? (Check for revocation.)

_____ All of the information in the authorization appears to be true. (If you know that any information in the authorization is false, it will not be valid.)

_____ Is the authorization written in plain language? (ex: a non-lawyer can understand it.)

DECISION: _____ VALID or _____ INVALID

Employee _____   Date _____

◆ **Figure 11-9**

A sample checklist to help ensure that an authorization is valid. *Individual states may require additional elements for valid authorization.*

EXCEPTIONS

Another aspect of release of information is **public priority exceptions**. These are permitted disclosures in which authorization is not required as long as state law allows these exceptions. For example, many states require reporting of conditions of public health interest. Some of these conditions include cancers, birth defects, and infectious diseases. In these cases, patient consent is not required to file reports with the appropriate governmental agency. Suspected child abuse is another instance in which reporting may occur without patient consent. Other examples are disclosures to coroners, law enforcement officials, and health licensing agencies and for organ transplant activities, for certain research, for prevention of a bio-terrorism event, and other specific government functions and workers' compensation activities.

SPECIAL CONSENTS

In terms of special consents, we must consider federal law, state law, and federal and state rules and regulations. In general, health records containing chemical dependency information, HIV and acquired immunodeficiency virus (AIDS) information, mental health information, and adoption information are often addressed in state laws and regulations. As previously mentioned, whatever gives the patient the highest level of protection should be followed. Most health care facilities have designed their authorization forms to be compliant with HIPAA and any state laws or regulations, but some facilities have a separate authorization form for special consents. In general, the authorization must specifically list the special nature of the health information that is to be disclosed.

The Code of Federal Regulations (42 CFR Part 2), commonly referred to as the **Federal Drug and Alcohol Abuse Regulations,** outlines the requirements for disclosing chemical dependency information. A subpoena for disclosure of chemical dependency information is not good enough—a court order is required.

Exercise 11-5

Release of Information

1. A patient presents in the HIM Department requesting a copy of the record for his recent appendectomy. Upon inquiry, the patient reveals that, in addition to wanting a record of the operation, he had an allergic reaction to the anesthesia and wants to keep a record of this event in order to prevent a similar problem in the future. What else should the patient be advised to request?

PREPARING A RECORD FOR RELEASE

There are several steps to take to properly release health care information. Each facility should have formal written policies and procedures regarding these steps. The specific policies and procedures vary among facilities; however, the issues can be discussed in general. Care should be taken to train and continually remind personnel of the confidential nature of health information.

VALIDATION AND TRACKING

After a request for information is received, the request should be recorded either in a manual log or in a computer database. The purpose of recording the request is so that its status and disposition may be tracked. Many state regulations require that facilities fulfill such requests within a specific time frame. A correspondence-tracking log serves to document compliance and fulfill HIPAA's requirements regarding accounting of disclosures.

Every request should be fully read, and every accompanying authorization form should be analyzed to determine whether there is valid authorization. In addition, there should be **verification** that the patient indeed has consented. The signature of the patient should be validated in an appropriate manner. This may be as simple as comparing the signature on the authorization form with the signature on file in the health record. If such validation cannot be accomplished or is not clear, notarization of the signature or additional proof of identity may be required. It is also important to verify identity when a patient comes to the facility to obtain copies of records. Proof of identity should always be requested to verify that the person to whom records are disclosed is indeed the person who is authorized to receive them.

Figure 11-10 lists sample data elements contained in a typical correspondence-tracking log. Most logs today involve an electronic database.

RETRIEVAL

Retrieval of the patient's information is based on the specific information requested. It is very important to release only those portions of the record that are authorized for disclosure. Care should be taken to ensure that the information retrieved is complete. This verification may be complicated by the decentralization of paper-based records among facility clinics or by incomplete processing of the record. Incomplete records should not, as a general rule, be released unless it is for treatment purposes and the facility is sending whatever is available. If an incomplete record is disclosed in response to a subpoena, the status of the record as incomplete should be clearly stated in the certification statement, affidavit, or cover sheet.

CORRESPONDENCE TRACKING LOG DATA ELEMENTS

- Request ID number
- Date request received
- Patient name
- Medical record number/account number
- Admission date/discharge date
- Request type
- Requestor name (including address or fax number)
- Information requested
- Purpose
- Information sent
- Date request cancelled or returned (if applicable)
- Date information sent
- Basis for allowing disclosure (authorization, permitted use, etc.)
- Notes or comments
- Invoice number
- Invoice amount
- Employee name/initials of person who processed request

◆ **Figure 11-10**
Correspondence tracking log data elements. (From Alice A. Andress. *Saunders' Manual of Medical Office Management.* Philadelphia: Saunders, 1996, p 150.)

REPRODUCTION

Photocopies or printed reproductions are made of the specific information requested. Every effort should be made to ensure the quality of the reproductions. When photocopying, personnel should compare the reproduction with the original to ensure completeness and clarity.

CERTIFICATION

When a copy of a record is required as evidence in a trial, a certified or notarized copy is usually acceptable in court. However, sometimes the original record is subpoenaed, and the custodian of the medical record accompanies the record to court. The custodian may be required to testify on the facility's procedures regarding development and retention of the record. When appearance by the custodian is required, a witness subpoena is usually issued in addition to the subpoena duces tecum for production of the record.

A certified copy contains a certification cover sheet signed by the custodian of the medical records, which states that the copy is a true and complete reproduction of the original record that is on file at the facility. The facility's policies and procedures should include the process by which verification of completeness can be obtained. With a paper record, this can be verified by numbering all of the pages in the original record before copying it. The copies will then contain a sequential numbering of the pages.

COMPENSATION

Most states permit facilities to charge a fee for providing copies of health records. Some states place a cap, or maximum, on the fees that may be charged. The fee covers the actual services performed: retrieval of the record (search fee), reproduction of the record, and delivery charges (postage). Therefore an important component of the release of information process is the preparation of the invoice. Some facilities may require that requesters pay the fee in advance, particularly for large records. As a professional courtesy, health care providers do not generally charge other health care providers for copies of records. In many cases, insurance companies and other payers have established set amounts that they will pay for copies of records. These fees may differ from the fees charged by the facility to other parties. HIPAA does not allow facilities to charge a retrieval or search fee to patients. Generally, the rate should be based on the actual cost to the facility of providing copies to the patient.

DISTRIBUTION

When a record is released, inclusion of a confidentiality notice is common practice. A typical notice might say, "This information is confidential and may not be used for other than the intended purpose and may not be re-released." This is to remind the recipient that the information belongs to the patient—not the recipient. Table 11-2 lists the general steps in release of information.

The patient or the individual to whom the record is being released may arrive in person to pick up the record. Policies and procedures should define how the patient or individual's identity should be verified, and the individual picking up the record should sign a receipt. Usually, the copies are mailed. Care must be taken to ensure that the address is correct and legible on the envelope so that the record is not misdirected. Records may also be sent electronically, by fax machine or e-mail. Extra care should be taken when electronically transmitting health information, as specifically addressed in the HIPAA Security Rule, which is covered in Chapter 12.

A cover sheet should accompany records sent by fax machine. The cover sheet should contain a confidentiality statement (Figure 11-11). Internet transmission of confidential information is becoming more common, particularly in the physician's office setting. Consideration should be given to the transmission security and whether the recipient is able to handle the information confidentially. For example, many employers automatically monitor their employees' e-mails. Therefore sending medical information to a patient at his or her place of business may jeopardize confidentiality. The patient must be made aware of the issues before authorizing transmittal in this manner.

TABLE 11-2	Steps in Release of Information
PROCEDURE	**COMMENTS**
Log in request.	Log request into a computer tracking system or onto a paper form.
Validate request.	Check signature, review the request for completeness. Obtain missing information if possible. Verify the validity of the subpoena or court order.
Obtain record.	Retrieve the record from storage. Incomplete records should be completed before release.
Copy record.	Photocopy or print from computer system. Copy only the required sections, as specified in the request.
Prepare invoice.	Calculate charges, and prepare an invoice.
Distribute copy.	Obtain signed receipt if picked up in person.

This facsimile message and the document(s) accompanying this telefax transmission may contain confidential information which is legally privileged and intended only for the use of the addressee named above. If the reader is not the intended recipient or the employee of the intended recipient, you are hereby notified that any dissemination, copying, or distribution of this communication is strictly prohibited. If you received this communication in error, please notify us immediately by telefax or telephone and return the original documents to us via the U.S. Postal Service at the above address. Thank you for your help.

◆ **Figure 11-11**

Sample confidentiality notice for faxed information. (From Alice A. Andress: *Saunders Manual of Medical Office Management*. Philadelphia: Saunders, 1996, p. 150.)

Exercise 11-6

Preparing a Record for Release

1. Your facility charges a $10 search fee plus $1.00 per page to copy records up to 100 pages. All pages in excess of 100 incur a charge of $.50 per page. Based on these rates, what is the fee for a 125-page record?

INTERNAL REQUESTS FOR INFORMATION

Now that you understand the nature of consent and confidentiality, we are ready to learn about the issues that arise in everyday practice within a health care facility. There are numerous instances in which facility personnel routinely request health information. Some of these requests include utilization review, performance improvement, and a variety of ongoing clinical reviews (e.g., surgical case review and infection control). These requests should be documented in writing both for internal control purposes (chart tracking) and to ensure that the request is valid.

The routine release of information for patient care should be handled with some caution. Even within a facility, many attempts are made to obtain information inappropriately. The culprits range from overly curious friends and family members who inquire about a patient's condition to unethical health care professionals who spy on one another. In the case of a physician's request, authorization is easily determined by checking the record to ensure that the physician requesting the chart is listed as an attending or consulting physician for that particular case. HIM departmental policies and procedures should be clear and specific regarding the release of information internally and should also include the steps to be taken when the legitimacy of the request is in question. Staff members should be allowed access to health information only on a "need to know" basis. In other words, what is the minimum amount of information necessary for the staff members to do their jobs?

Exercise 11-7

Internal Requests for Information

1. What special procedures, if any, should be in place to handle the records of employees who are patients in the facility?

SENSITIVE RECORDS

There are two major types of sensitive records: employee patients and legal files. Although there may be no statutory or regulatory requirement to handle these records differently from others, certain practical considerations apply. In the electronic environment, knowledge that an audit trail of access to the record will be monitored may serve as a deterrent to inappropriate access.

EMPLOYEE PATIENTS

Maintaining the confidentiality of employee records is particularly difficult. In a small facility, a paper record can be maintained in a secure file. In a large facility, this may be impractical. Therefore facility policies and procedures should include specific language regarding the sensitivity of health information pertaining to fellow employees. The confidentiality statement shown in Figure 11-1 includes such language.

LEGAL FILES

Special attention should be paid to records that have been requested for litigation involving the facility, health care personnel, or a physician. Every effort should be made to obtain control of those records immediately on receipt of the notification, and special care should be taken to safeguard these records in a special area inaccessible to all but authorized personnel. If possible, the records should be locked in a file used exclusively for that purpose.

Although photocopies of the records can be circulated for review and discussion, HIM personnel should safeguard the original records. Staff members may be tempted to alter or remove incriminating records when a health care practitioner is being sued. Safeguarding the records in the aforementioned manner removes that temptation and ensures the safety and availability of the records for legal proceedings.

FEDERAL, CORPORATE, AND FACILITY COMPLIANCE

An increasingly important responsibility of the HIM professional is that of ensuring **compliance** with the many statutes, regulations, and other rules imposed on the facility and the professionals who work there. Part of the compliance function is monitoring data quality. Another function is ensuring the completeness and timeliness of records. The following sections discuss the most common areas of concern to HIM professionals.

LICENSURE

As discussed in Chapter 1, individual states license facilities for operation within that state. A state's licensure requirements, which can be found in the state's administrative code, may contain very specific provisions for the content and retention of specific clinical documentation. These provisions may take the form of a listing of elements to be maintained in a health record. They may also be included in statements about a facility's medical staff. The provisions for health records may be as detailed as specifying which documents should be included or which types of data should be collected. Whatever provisions are listed for a specific type of facility, HIM personnel must be aware of these rules and ensure that any activities under their span of control are in compliance with those rules.

The first step in ensuring compliance with any rule is to review the rule and understand what it really means. Therefore every HIM professional should have access to a copy of the specific portions of the licensure regulations that apply to his or her activities. Although it is not necessary in terms of everyday practice for each person to have a copy of the document, it is certainly appropriate for such a document to be available to personnel in the facility.

In practice, each employee in the facility is responsible for a small portion of the compliance with the specific regulations. The responsibility for overall compliance with the particular regulations rests with the director of the particular department. In the case of the HIM department, the director typically is responsible for compliance.

One of the best ways to teach HIM employees how to comply with various regulations is to ensure that there are written policies and procedures in the department that address these particular issues. Employees should be trained with these issues in mind. It is also important to cross-reference the policies and procedures to the specific regulations for compliance.

HIM professionals often become involved in researching and interpreting regulations and assisting in the development of policies and procedures to comply with those regulations. Frequently, HIM professionals become involved in facility-wide compliance issues. This occurs because of the pervasive nature of the documentation that is handled after a patient's discharge. For example, if a regulation dictates that physician telephone orders be signed within a certain time frame after being ordered, HIM personnel are frequently involved in the development of the procedures and controls to ensure the monitoring of that activity because by analyzing the chart after the patient's discharge, they are in a position to note noncompliance with this regulation.

ACCREDITATION

State licensure of a facility is mandatory. Accreditation is optional. Remember that accreditation is the process by which independent organizations verify that a facility complies with standards of practice developed by that organization. There are accrediting bodies that deal with a specific type of health care facility, and there are accrediting bodies that deal with many different types of health care facilities. The **Joint Commission on Accreditation of Healthcare Organizations (JCAHO),** known primarily for accrediting acute care facilities, also accredits other facilities such as rehabilitation, long-term care, and ambulatory care facilities. Because JCAHO is so important, it is used in this chapter to exemplify how accreditation works. The accreditation process is very similar, regardless of the accrediting body.

JCAHO publishes its standards annually in several formats, including a *Comprehensive Guide* that pertains to each setting. The standards are updated annually to reflect changes in health care delivery, organizational philosophy, and environment. To become accredited, a facility applies to the JCAHO, completes a detailed questionnaire, and undergoes an intensive site visit called a *survey.* JCAHO surveys facilities approximately every 3 years. Unannounced surveys or surveys focusing on previously identified problems may take place between formal surveys. Because JCAHO standards are modified frequently, reference to the most recent publications is essential to ensure compliance. See the JCAHO Web site for current publications and other information: http://www.jcaho.org.

Routine JCAHO surveys are planned well in advance. Ideally, a facility should be in continuous compliance with the standards; however, because the standards change annually, it may take facilities a little time each year to adjust their operations accordingly. Many facilities spend a great deal of time preparing for a survey, ensuring that documentation and various procedures are in compliance. Although it is important to discuss the preparation for a JCAHO survey, it should go without saying that if a facility is in continuous compliance with JCAHO standards, continually updates its procedures to ensure compliance, and structures its reporting to document that compliance, then very little preparation is needed before a JCAHO survey. Nevertheless, in reality, verifying JCAHO compliance is a time-consuming process, and facilities should scrutinize their compliance documentation and procedures on a periodic basis rather than a continuous basis.

The preparation for a routine JCAHO survey frequently begins with the appointment of a JCAHO steering committee or task force. It is very important that the HIM department be represented on the steering committee. In some cases, the director of the HIM department chairs or co-chairs that committee. Other members of the committee may include a variety of department directors and managers. The director of nursing or his or her designee and a physician's representative are critical participants. There are a number of management-level staff members on the committee, and they divide the responsibilities for reviewing compliance among themselves.

Some of the activities of the JCAHO steering committee are to review current JCAHO standards and compare them to current policies and procedures, to ensure that the policies and procedures are updated, to conduct mock surveys, to prepare staff for the JCAHO visit, to review reports that will be required, and to assemble large quantities of documentation that are required by the JCAHO surveyors. These activities are largely delegated to the appropriate department manager, but many employees become involved in preparing for the JCAHO survey. In corporate environments, a team from the home office usually conducts mock surveys before the actual JCAHO survey.

COMPLIANCE

As a result of increasing pressure from the federal government, health care organizations have spent a great deal of time and effort in recent years to demonstrate their commitment to data quality, particularly in terms of accurate billing. Some of this pressure comes from the federal DHHS Office of the Inspector General (OIG), which has received increased funding in recent years for enforcing accurate billing through audits and penalties. In addition, the HIPAA legislation of 1996 and the Balanced Budget Act of 1997 increased the penalties for failure to comply with regulations.

A compliance program is a facility-wide system of policies, procedures, and guidelines that help to ensure ethical business practices. These policies, procedures, and guidelines should include, for example, ethics statements, strong leadership policy, commitment to compliance with regulations, and ways for employees to report unethical or noncompliant activities and behaviors. Part of a compliance effort is a coding compliance program. A coding compliance program ensures accurate coding and billing through training, continuing education, quality assurance, and performance improvement activities. An excellent beginning reference source for learning about corporate compliance is the American Health Information Management Association's practice brief, *Seven Steps to Corporate Compliance: The HIM Role.*

PROFESSIONAL STANDARDS

Finally, there are professional standards with which health care professionals must comply. As mentioned in Chapter 1, each profession has a code of ethics and a set of standards that are imposed by the credentialing body or the licensing agency for that profession (or both). HIM professionals comply with the code of ethics of the American Health Information Management Association (AHIMA). In addition, AHIMA supports the profession by issuing a variety of publications designed to guide and promote excellence in professional practice. AHIMA regularly issues practice briefs, documenting best practices in areas of interest to HIM professionals.

Exercise 11-8

Compliance

1. What is the purpose of the JCAHO Steering Committee?
2. What is compliance? Why is it important?

■ SUGGESTED READING

Privacy Forms Toolkit- AHIMA HIM Body of Knowledge.

Abdelhak, Mervat, Sara Grostick, Mary Alice Hanken, and Ellen Jacobs. *Health Information: Management of a Strategic Resource.* Philadelphia: Saunders, 2001.

Hjort, Beth. "Practice Brief: Release of Information Reimbursement Laws and Regulations" (updated March 2004) <http://library.ahima.org/xpedio/groups/public/documents/ahima/pub_bok1_023132.html>.

Hjort, Beth. "Practice Brief: Understanding the Minimum Necessary Standard" (updated March 2003) <http://library.ahima.org/xpedio/groups/public/documents/ahima/pub_bok1_022114.hcsp?>.

Hughes, Gwen. "Practice Brief: Defining the Designated Record Set." *Journal of AHIMA* 74.1(2003): 64A-D.

Hughes, Gwen. "Practice Brief: Notice of Information Practices" (updated November 2002) <ahima.org/xpedio/groups/public/documents/ahima/bok2_000116.hcsp?>.

McWay, Dana. *Legal Aspects of Health Information Management.* Albany, NY: Delmar, 1996.

"Practice Brief: E-mail Security" (Updated). AHIMA Practice Brief. *Journal of AHIMA,* 71.2(2000): 72A-72D.

"Practice Brief: Facsimile Transmission of Health Information." *Journal of AHIMA,* 72.6(2001):64E-64F.

"Practice Brief: Seven Steps to Corporate Compliance: the HIM Role." *Journal of AHIMA,* 70.9(1999): 84A-84F.

Standards for Privacy of Individually Identifiable Health Information; Final Rule. 45 CFR Parts 160 and 164. Federal Register 67, no. 157 (August 14, 2002) <http://aspe.hhs.gov/admnsimp/>.

WEB SITES

Centers for Medicare and Medicaid Services: http://www.cms.hhs.gov/hipaa/hipaa2

United States Department of Health and Human Services: http://www.os.dhhs.gov/ocr/hipaa

Substance Abuse and Mental Health Services Administration, an Agency of the United States Department of Health and Human Services: http://www.hipaa.samhsa.gov

CHAPTER ACTIVITIES

CHAPTER SUMMARY

This chapter covered the legal and regulatory issues governing the development and retention of health information. Informed consent underlies patient admission, treatment, and release of information. Health information is confidential. Patient-physician privilege dictates confidentiality and release of records only with the consent of the patient. A valid consent for release of information comprises eight elements: identification of the party being asked to release the information, patient name/identification, identification of the party to whom the information is to be released, specific information to be released, description of the purpose of the use or disclosure, expiration date, signature of the patient or personal representative authorizing the disclosure, and date. However, in an emergency, records may be released without patient consent. Other important issues include compliance with regulatory, accrediting, and professional standards. Health care facilities should make every effort to ensure continuous compliance with the standards imposed by authoritative bodies.

Review Questions

1. Discuss the steps to release patient information.

2. List and describe the elements of a valid authorization for release of information.

3. Describe situations in which authorization is not necessary to release information.

4. Compare and contrast the procedures for preparing a record for release to the patient versus a certified copy for court.

5. Locate the licensure regulations for your state.
   a) What are the provisions for the content of a health record?
   b) What are the rules regarding the timeliness of completion of a record?

6. Locate any state laws regarding health information or medical records for your state.
   a) Are there retention statutes for medical records?
   b) Are there references to the costs of providing copies of medical records?

7. Describe the accreditation process.

APPLICATION

Is It Confidential?

You are the director of health information management (HIM) in a small community hospital. One day, an employee in the incomplete file area comes to you with a coat. One of the physicians left it in the dictation room, but the employee does not know to whom it belongs. You decide to look in the pockets of the coat to see if any identification is present. You find in one of the pockets a prescription bottle of Antabuse, a medication given to alcoholics to help them stop drinking. The patient named on the bottle is a physician at your facility. What should you do with this information? What are the confidentiality issues? Should you have handled this situation differently?

Chapter 12

∿

ELECTRONIC HEALTH RECORDS

CHAPTER OUTLINE

By the end of this chapter, the student should be able to

- Define *electronic health record*.

- Compare and contrast an electronic health record with a hybrid electronic health record.

- Explain the history and future of the electronic health record.

- Explain the difference between the interoperable use and the longitudinal use of an electronic health record.

- Identify the advantages and disadvantages of the electronic health record.

- Discuss government and private sector intervention in the development of an electronic health record.

- Define *electronic health records management*.

- Compare and contrast health information management functions associated with the use of a paper record versus an electronic record.

- Discuss health information management career opportunities with reference to the electronic health record.

VOCABULARY

algorithm

computer output to laser disk (COLD)

computerized physician order entry (CPOE)

data repository

data warehouse

digital signature

digitized signature

document imaging

electronic health record (EHR)

electronic health record management

electronic signature

encryption

evidence-based decision support

Health Level Seven (HL7)

hybrid record

indexing

infrastructure

integrity

interfaced

interoperable

longitudinal

nonrepudiation

personal identification number (PIN)

queue

workflow

he **electronic health record** (**EHR**) is discussed in conjunction with the paper record throughout the chapters of this book. At the present time, both are in use in various health care settings. Some facilities use only a paper record, a few have made the transition to a completely electronic record, whereas the majority maintain records containing both electronic and paper reports. The need for an EHR is no longer being advocated only by health information management (HIM) professionals; it is being forcefully advocated by the government, several of its agencies, and private consumer groups. This chapter is an introduction to the EHR, including the EHR as we know it now and the vision for the EHR in 2014. This chapter also covers the changes that the EHR will bring to the HIM profession, both in practice and in professional career opportunities. It does not address every aspect of the EHR because new information emerges daily. The Internet is the most useful tool to keep abreast of the evolution of the EHR.

THE EVOLUTION OF THE ELECTRONIC HEALTH RECORD

THE PAPER RECORD

As discussed throughout this book, the medical record has been traditionally maintained in a paper format. Each department within a facility may develop a form to document treatment, tests, and other results pertinent to that department's functions. For example, the paper record is generated at the time of the patient's admission or encounter and moves with the patient as he or she receives treatment throughout the health care facility. The paper record is manually processed after discharge and filed in the HIM department. When the patient is readmitted or the paper chart is needed for other purposes, it is obtained from the HIM department file area, as discussed in Chapter 8. Many facilities still use a paper record.

THE HYBRID RECORD

Many hospitals are currently using a **hybrid record**. In this type of record, part of the data collection into the record is paper based and part of it is computer based. There are various degrees of computerization in the hybrid record, ranging from only one department generating electronic reports to many departments generating electronic reports with limited data being captured electronically. One of the first hybrid records seen in health care facilities was created when the financial departments **interfaced** (two independent systems configured to communicate with each other) with the Master Patient Index. The financial system shared information with the HIM system, enabling the facility to generate a computerized face sheet or admission record.

Eventually, other ancillary departments, such as laboratory, radiology, and pharmacy, began using computers to collect data and generate their reports. Their data were either held in a separate database or interfaced with the HIM and/or financial systems.

Some transcribed reports, such as the history and physical and the operative report, are interfaced with the HIM system, allowing caregivers remote access to the computerized reports.

Some facilities use a **computerized physician order entry** (**CPOE**) system. In a paper-based system, the physician writes an order, the nurse communicates the order to the pharmacy, the

Exercise 12-1

Introduction

Use the Internet, to find three other definitions of an EHR by other organizations. Make a table comparing the similarities and the differences among the components of the definition of an EHR.

1. The EHR does not provide patient-centric information. True or False
2. The EHR can be used for public health disease surveillance. True or False
3. Evidence-based decision support is not a part of the EHR. True or False

pharmacy dispenses the medication, and the nurse administers the medication. If the physician has questions about a medication (e.g., dosage, drug interactions, contra-indications), looking up the answers is time consuming. A CPOE provides the physician with a list of medications that can be used for the specific treatment of the patient's diagnosis. It offers decision support (i.e., information to help the physician select the appropriate drug) such as generic drug ordering, drug interaction information, and lab information that may be needed before prescribing the medication. CPOEs are an important part of a fully electronic health record because they help to reduce medication errors.

Facilities with hybrid records may choose to retain part of the record electronically or to print out a paper copy of the computer-based portions. In other facilities, the paper-based portion is copied to a computer-based format using a **document imaging** system. In document imaging, a scanner or a fax machine may be used to store the paper document electronically into a computer program or onto an optical disc. Document imaging can be performed after discharge or at the point of care. An example of this is illustrated in Figure 12-1. In this example, the admit clerk scans the consent forms and identification information into the electronic file from the admit office for Patient A. At the same time, Patient B is seen by a physician in a clinic across town. The clinic staff faxes the physician's progress note to the electronic file. Patient C is being discharged from the hospital, where he was admitted several days ago for surgery. After discharge, the inhouse documents are sent to the HIM department, where they are processed and scanned using a large scanner suitable for high-volume scanning into the electronic file.

As the documents are scanned or faxed into the system, the different types of reports are then indexed (discussed in Chapter 8). **Indexing** sorts the records by the different report types, making the viewing of the record uniform. It is similar to the plastic tab separators used in the paper records. Bar coding is sometimes used to decrease errors and improve productivity in the indexing process. Document imaging makes the record available for viewing from various areas networked to the computer system. It also allows various functions to be performed electronically, such as coding, analysis, and physician chart completion. In this hybrid record, each sheet of paper contained in the record can be viewed from the computer, but this method does not allow for data capture and later retrieval of the data for reporting and decision making. When a patient returns for treatment, the caregivers must retrieve the computerized copy of the record.

Some facilities, however, are venturing into the use of an electronic record in which limited data is captured. This type of hybrid record has both paper and electronic components and is similar to the hybrid records described previously. The difference in this record is that the electronic

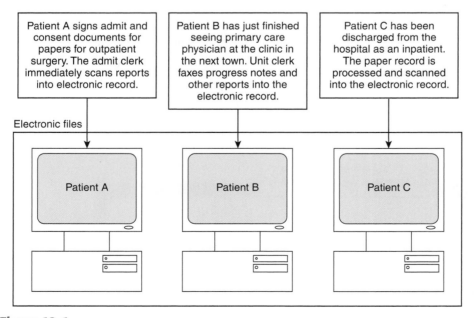

◆ **Figure 12-1**
Example of paper documents being scanned or faxed from various hospital departments.

components capture data elements used to generate reports. For example, consider the sequence of events that take place when a physician or dietitian orders nutrition management for a patient with amyotrophic lateral sclerosis (ALS), or Lou Gehrig's disease (Miller et al 1999). When ordering nutrition, the physician or dietitian may use an **algorithm,** which is a formula or set of steps for solving a particular problem, to determine the correct management of the patient based on the patient's condition. Using the ALS algorithm, the patient's forced vital capacity (FVC) score is going to determine the course of treatment. The FVC test shows the total amount of exhaled air during a forced breath and checks how well the lungs are working. The nutritional program interfaces with the electronic record abstracting program, allowing the retrieval of specific data electronically to generate reports on the basis of the data collected. For example, a quality improvement team may want to generate statistics on the number of patients with FVC >50% who had a PEG (percutaneous endoscopic gastrotomy) inserted. Although this hybrid record collects some data, it does not share data with other computer software programs; therefore it does not meet the definition of an electronic record. Figure 12-2 shows an algorithm used for nutrition management in patients with ALS.

THE ELECTRONIC HEALTH RECORD

The Health Information Management Systems Society (HIMSS) Electronic Health Record Committee defines the EHR as follows (http://www.himss.org/content/files/EHRAttributes.pdf):

> The Electronic Health Record (EHR) is a secure, real-time, point-of-care, patient-centric information resource for clinicians. The EHR aids clinicians' decision making by providing access to patient health record information where and when they need it and by incorporating **evidence-based decision support** (the best care results from the conscientious, explicit, and judicious use of current best evidence). The EHR automates and streamlines the clinician's workflow, closing loops in communication and response that result in delays or gaps in care. The EHR also supports the collection of data for uses other than direct clinical care, such as billing, quality management, outcomes reporting, resource planning, and public health disease surveillance and reporting.

An EHR results from computer-based data collection. Physicians and other clinicians capture data at the point of care, with the ability to retrieve the data later for reporting and use in research or administrative decision making. Health care workers document via computers on the various clinical units, using lap tops, handheld computers, and bedside terminals. Very few, if any, paper reports are generated. The EHR allows the nursing department to document care on the computer. The electronic record should provide a CPOE. Optimally, it will also include decision-making algorithms, as described previously. An EHR can provide certain prompts or alerts specific to the physician's orders.

The EHR can provide clinical decision-making algorithms for nonphysician caregivers. Care paths, or clinical pathways, are electronic aids that help caregivers make decisions about treatment. Reference material may be available for electronic use when specific diagnoses are documented.

In many systems, a **data repository** is used. The data repository stores data from unrelated software programs. These software programs can be created by different vendors and have different applications. Health care organizations should be able to integrate the data and provide a multidisciplinary view of their elements. A data repository can store the data from these different systems and make them usable without the need to run reports from each system. For example, data may be collected from three separate software programs and stored in the data repository. Consider a patient who has diabetes: the data repository would store data from the pharmacy software program (e.g., the amount of insulin that the patient receives, from the medication administration report), the laboratory software program (e.g., the patient's glucose levels, from the laboratory findings), and the nursing notes (the glucose monitoring results, from the nursing flow sheets). The repository data are then collected and reorganized in a **data warehouse**. The data warehouse collects information from different databases and organizes it for use in ad hoc reports and analytical research. The data warehouse may not include patient identifying information. Data warehousing is used for analyzing revenue (e.g., to calculate the cost of treating a patient with diabetes) and for clinical (e.g., to determine the average amount of insulin needed by a patient

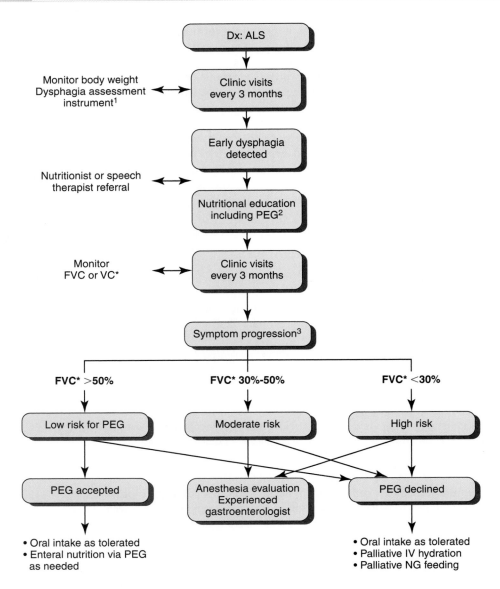

Monitor body weight
Dysphagia assessment
instrument[1]

Nutritionist or speech
therapist referral

Monitor
FVC or VC*

Dx: ALS

Clinic visits
every 3 months

Early dysphagia
detected

Nutritional education
including PEG[2]

Clinic visits
every 3 months

Symptom progression[3]

FVC* >50%   **FVC* 30%-50%**   **FVC* <30%**

Low risk for PEG   Moderate risk   High risk

PEG accepted   Anesthesia evaluation Experienced gastroenterologist   PEG declined

- Oral intake as tolerated
- Enteral nutrition via PEG as needed

- Oral intake as tolerated
- Palliative IV hydration
- Palliative NG feeding

[1] Rule out contraindications

[2] Prolonged mealtime, ending meal prematurely because of fatigue, accelerated weight loss due to poor caloric intake, family concern about feeding difficulties

* Forced vital capacity (FVC) or vital capacity (VC) can be used. VC may be more accurate in patients with bulbar dysfunction

[3] For example, Colorado Dysphagia Disability Inventory, bulbar questions in the ALS Functional Rating Scale, or other instrument

◆ **Figure 12-2**

An algorithm for nutrition management for ALS patients. (From American Academy of Neurology. *Guideline Summary for Physicians:* http://www.aan.com/ professionals/practice/pdfs/manageals.pdf)

with diabetes in a specific age group), operational (e.g., to assess the staffing pattern for patients on a diabetic nursing unit), and outcome management (e.g., to estimate the percentage of patients who showed improvement after treatment). In a true EHR, data are collected, used, and shared with other third parties as authorized and shown in Figure 12-3. The HIM functions can be performed electronically, either concurrently or after discharge (Clinical Research Information System 2006).

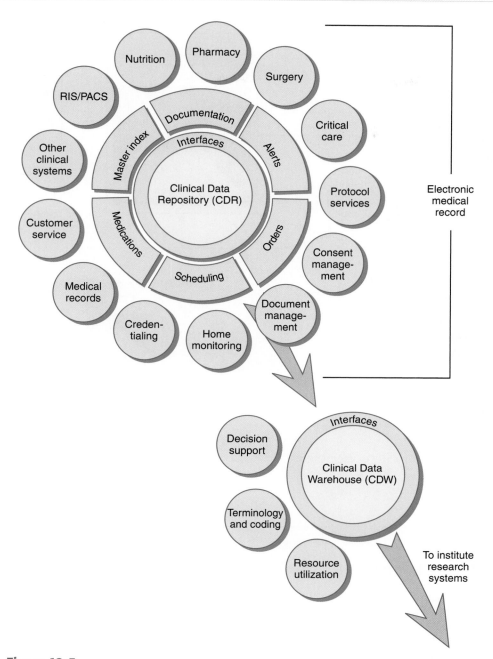

◆ **Figure 12-3**

Data repository and data warehouse. (From National Institute of Health Clinical Research Information System: http://cris.cc.nih.gov/public/project.html.)

THE FUTURE OF THE ELECTRONIC HEALTH RECORD

As useful as an EHR is to the facility that uses it, the system stands alone. It is still necessary to print out reports in hard copy or convert data to other formats to share information with other facilities. As the EHR continues to be developed, the goal is to make it **interoperable.** *Interoperable* means that the software and hardware can be used on different machines from different vendors to share data. Interoperability allows the data to be exchanged among health care facilities, physicians, and public health organizations, facilitating the **longitudinal** use of the health care data. *Longitudinal use* means that the information can flow electronically from one type of provider to another along the continuum of care and over time. Figure 12-4 demonstrates the

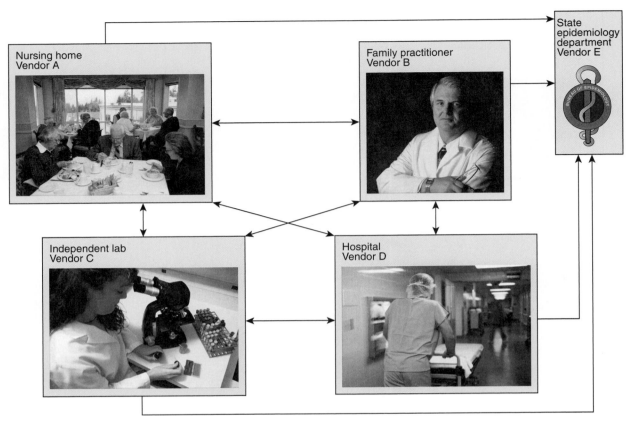

◆ **Figure 12-4**
Example of interoperatibility and longitudinal use of information.

Hit-Bit

Regional Health Care Information Organizations

Regional health care information organizations (RHIOs) or Health Information Exchanges (HIEs) are being formed both regionally and locally by entities such as health care providers and health care businesses in an effort to share health information electronically. These providers and businesses may have been competitors in the past, but they are forming alliances in an effort to improve the quality and safety of health care in their city, state, or region (Gater 18 July 2005).

way in which information is shared interoperably and longitudinally. An example of interoperatibility and longitudinal use is given in the following paragraph:

Mrs. Gift is an 85-year-old nursing home resident with chronic obstructive pulmonary disease, diabetes, and hypertension. The nursing home has an EHR that was purchased from Vendor A. Mrs. Gift visits her family practitioner every 6 months to monitor her illnesses. The family practitioner has an EHR that was purchased from Vendor B. Mrs. Gift usually has her testing performed at an independent laboratory that uses a computer laboratory program from Vendor C. On occasion, Mrs. Gift must go into an acute care hospital near the nursing home because of an exacerbation of her COPD. The acute care hospital has an EHR from Vendor D. Sometimes information regarding Mrs. Gift's diagnosis must be forwarded to the State Epidemiology Department, which uses yet another vendor. Interoperability refers to the ability for each of these different computer systems to use and read the same data. Longitudinal use refers to the ability of the different types of providers to access and share the same patient's information.

Exercise 12-2

The Evolution of the Electronic Health Record

1. Explain the difference between *interoperable* and *longitudinal*. Give an example of each.
2. Describe the two different types of hybrid medical records.
3. Explain why indexing of an EHR is important.
4. Explain how an algorithm can improve quality of care.
5. A medical record that is contains computer-generated reports, collects data, and shares data with outside agencies is a(n) _____.
6. Sorting medical reports by type is _____.
7. _____ describes two independent systems configured to communicate with each other.
8. _____ collects information from different databases and organizes it to be used for ad hoc reports and analytical research.
9. _____ uses scanners or fax machines to store records electronically.

GOVERNMENT AND PRIVATE SECTOR INTERVENTION

HIM professionals are not the only people interested in developing standards for the EHR. Both private consumer groups and government agencies have been working toward this goal.

PRIVATE SECTOR

Several private groups encourage and monitor the use of EHRs. Two notable private groups are the Institute of Medicine and the Markle Foundation. These groups advocate the use of the EHR in an effort to improve patient care and safety. The Institute of Medicine (IOM) is a nonprofit organization chartered in 1970 as a component of the National Academy of Sciences. According to the IOM Web site, the Institute provides unbiased, evidence-based, and authoritative information and advice about health and science policy to policy makers, professionals, leaders in every sector of society, and the public at large. One of its projects is quality of health. The IOM has identified eight functions that any EHR should be able to perform in an effort to promote safety, quality, and efficiency in health care facilities (Committee on Data Standards for Patient Safety 2003). These eight functions are listed in Table 12-1. More information on the IOM can be found on their Web site: http://www.iom.org.

The Markle Foundation initially was founded in 1927 by a husband and wife to encourage the progression of knowledge and the general good of mankind. One of its current goals is to eliminate barriers in the implementation of the EHR. Two of these barriers include lack of interoperability among computer systems and privacy issues. The Markle Foundation fosters collaboration in both private and public sectors through an initiative called Connecting to Health, which seeks to improve patient care by promoting standards for electronic medical information. More information on Connecting to Health can be found on the Markle Foundation Web site: http://www.markle.org.

A nonprofit group composed of providers, vendors, payers, consultants, government groups, and others is working to develop standards that will aid the interoperability of the exchange of electronic data in and across health care organizations. This group, **Health Level Seven (HL7)**, is one of many standards developing organizations (SDOs) producing standards for particular health care domains, such as pharmacy and radiology. HL7 works to provide standards for clinical and administrative domains, specifically the exchange, management, and integration of data supporting clinical patient care and the evaluation of health services. HL7 develops specifications that allow

TABLE 12-1	Functions of the Electronic Health Record
TOPIC	**FUNCTION**
Health Information and Data	Allows caregivers to have immediate access to key information such as allergies, medications, and lab test results
Result Management	Allows caregivers to quickly access new and past test results, increasing patient safety and effectiveness of care
Order Management	Allows caregivers to enter and store orders for prescriptions, tests, or services in a computer-based system that improves legibility, reduces duplication, and increases speed of executing the orders
Decision Support	Allows the use of reminders, alerts, and prompts that will improve compliance with best clinical practices, ensure regular screening, and identify possible drug interactions
Electronic Communication and Connectivity	Allows for efficient, secure, and readily accessible communication among caregivers and patients that will improve the continuity of care, enhance timeliness of diagnoses and treatments, and reduce the frequency of adverse occurrences
Patient Support	Provides tools that give patients access to their own health records, provides Internet education, and assists them carrying out home monitoring and self-teaching, which can help improve chronic conditions
Administrative Processes	Allows for administrative tools such as scheduling, which would improve efficiency and provide more timely service
Reporting	Allows electronic data storage using uniform data standards that will enable organizations to respond to third-party regulatory agencies

From Committee on Data Standards for Patient Safety. 31 July 2003. *The National Academic News*: http://www4.nas.edu/new/nsf.

for transfer of data. An easy example is the use of birthdates. Birthdates can be displayed in several ways, such as

- May 1, 1986
- 5/1/86
- 05/01/86
- 05/01/1986
- 19860501

GOVERNMENT SECTOR

Government agencies such as the National Committee on Vital and Health Statistics (NCVHS) are stressing the need for a national health information **infrastructure** (NHIIS). *Infrastructure* refers to the underlying system of standards and rules that would enable effective data exchange throughout the health care industry. Just as the system of roads, bridges, and highways facilitated the popularization of the automobile, an NHIIS would facilitate the improvement of data exchange. This infrastructure would enable interoperability by using standard operating nomenclature, specifications, or protocols. One of the key issues in developing and implementing an NHIIS is the importance of providing access to data while maintaining confidentiality.

Another government-related entity, Consolidated Health Informatics, is composed of approximately 20 department or agencies, including the Department of Health and Human Services (DHHS), the Department of Defense, and the Department of Veterans' Affairs. This group is working to establish uniform standards for the electronic exchange of clinical health information across federal health care agencies.

The most notable government intervention took place in April of 2004, when President George W. Bush issued Executive Order 13335. This executive order required the widespread adoption of interoperable EHRs within 10 years. It also established the position of a National Coordinator for Health Information Technology within DHHS. In addition, it directed the national coordinator to produce a report on the development and implementation of a strategic plan to guide the nationwide implementation of an interoperable EHR in both public and private sectors.

OFFICE OF THE NATIONAL COORDINATOR FOR HEALTH INFORMATION TECHNOLOGY

Dr. David Brailer was appointed as the National Coordinator for Health Information Technology in May of 2004. His office with the DHHS, the Office of the National Coordinator for Health Information Technology (ONCHIT), submitted the report "The Decade of Health Information Technology: Delivering Consumer-Centric and Information-Rich Health Care." This report discussed the promise of health information technology, reasons that it is not currently being used, the goals and strategies of ONCHIT, incentives to providers to use the EHR, and the key actions necessary to accomplish the goals and strategies of ONCHIT. These goals and strategies are listed in Table 12-2.

Accomplishment of these goals requires communication and coordination among several groups, including vendors, health care providers, government agencies, and SDOs. ONCHIT has been assigned the responsibility for coordinating federal activities relating to health information technology with the various groups.

Exercise 12-3

Government and Private Sector Intervention

1. Explain the function of decision support as stated in the Institute of Medicine's eight functions.
2. Define HL7.
3. Explain Executive Order 13335.
4. Which group is stressing the need for a national information infrastructure?
5. List the four goals of ONCHIT.

TABLE 12-2	**Goals of ONCHIT**		
GOAL 1: INFORM CLINICAL PRACTICE	**GOAL 2: INTERCONNECT PHYSICIANS**	**GOAL 3: PERSONALIZE CARE**	**GOAL 4: IMPROVE POPULATION HEALTH**
Provide incentives for electronic health record (EHR) adoption	Regional collaborations	Encourage use of personal health records	Unify public health surveillance architectures
Reduce risk of EHR investment	Develop a national health information network	Enhance informed consumer choice	Streamline quality and health status monitoring
Promote EHR diffusion in rural and underserved areas	Coordinate federal health information systems	Promote use of telehealth systems	Accelerate research and dissemination of evidence

From Office of the National Coordinator for Health Information Technology. 2006. Directory of Federal HIT programs: http://www.os.dhhs.gov/healthit/federalprojectlist.html#initiativestable

ADVANTAGES OF AND BARRIERS TO IMPLEMENTING AN ELECTRONIC HEALTH RECORD

As discussed earlier in the chapter, many hospitals are already using some form of EHR. There are many advantages to implementing an EHR and NHIIS, including accessibility, standardization, and improved quality of care.

ACCESSIBILITY

One of the most obvious advantages of an NHIIS is the accessibility of the patient's information by the caregivers regardless of the location of the patient. For example, consider a patient who enters a health care facility through the emergency department because of shortness of breath. The physician is able to retrieve the patient's old records through the computer and review any admissions, test results, and treatments that the patient received at that facility or any other facility. A surgery consultation is ordered for the patient. The surgeon is just finishing another patient's procedure and receives the notice of the consultation. While in the surgery unit, he can access the patient's old and current records and have some prior knowledge of the patient's health status before assessing the patient during this treatment episode. The patient undergoes surgery and has an organ removed. The organ is sent to the pathology laboratory for review. The pathologist may access the patient's record to review the clinical history and surgical findings before performing the pathological examination of the organ. The patient is discharged and has a follow-up appointment with the surgeon. The surgeon wants to review the pathology report again before discussing the findings with the patient. He can access the pathology report from his office rather than going to the HIM department and viewing the paper record.

When a paper record is used, the record is accessible wherever the patient is being treated because it goes where the patient goes; therefore only one person at a time is usually able to see the record. The EHR allows the record to be viewed by several caregivers at the same time regardless of the location of the patient or caregivers. In the HIM department, the EHR allows several staff members to use the record at the same time for postdischarge processing. One goal of ONCHIT is to allow authorized users to have access to medical information wherever and whenever it is needed, whether in a physician office, acute care facility, or home health agency. Rural facilities will be able to access the records of urban facilities where the specialists practice. Consumers may have personal health records (PHRs) that they can share with the caregivers at any facility.

IMPROVEMENT IN QUALITY OF HEALTH CARE

The quality of health care will improve because the EHR will assist in reducing medical errors. One of the goals is to prescribe medication electronically. Health care providers will have access to timely and appropriate treatment information to aid in the diagnosis and treatment of diseases. This will include best practice protocols. A reduction of health care costs may be realized because of a reduction in duplicative care, low health administrative costs, and prevention of medical errors. Dr. A at Hospital B will now be able to see that the patient had a similar test performed

---

Hit-Bit

Personal Health Records (PHRs)

According to AHIMA, the personal health record (PHR) is an individual's record of his or her own health information, which may be needed in making health decisions. The individual owns and manages the health information and decides who has access to it. It can be paper based, computer-based, Web-based, or some kind of hybrid thereof. The PHR is maintained separately from any legal record kept by health care providers (AHIMA e-HIM Personal Health Record Work Group 2005).

recently as an outpatient at Lab C. The public health sectors will be able to link information networks to better observe disease outbreaks. Access to public health statistics may hasten biomedical research and bring research findings to the caregivers in a more timely manner.

STANDARDIZATION

Electronic health systems that share data will have to standardize the health record formats used within the various computer systems. The various diagnostic reports will look similar, allowing the caregivers to find the necessary information in less time. HL7 has signed an agreement with SNOMED International, a division of the College of American Pathologists (CAP). The agreement formalizes the organizations' long-standing relationship and enables HL7 to work with SNOMED to help drive coordination between SNOMED Clinical Terms (SNOMED-CT) and the HL7 Reference Information Model (RIM). SNOMED-CT is considered to be the most comprehensive multilingual clinical healthcare terminology available in the world. "The RIM is the cornerstone of the HL7 standard for exchanging messages among information systems that implement healthcare applications," said Franklin R. Elevitch, M.D., Chair, SNOMED International Authority. "Binding SNOMED-CT to the RIM will further improve interoperability for all data exchange in healthcare and ultimately improve quality of care and enhance patient safety" ("HL7, SNOMED" 2005).

A review of all the advantages of the EHR might suggest that no disadvantages exist; however, there are a few barriers, such as costs, training, privacy, and reliability.

COST OF CONVERSION

The biggest disadvantage of the EHR at this time is the cost of converting from a paper record to an electronic record. These costs include the acquisition of both hardware and software. Many facilities use various computer software programs in the different clinical units. These must be reconfigured to interface with the national standard EHR. Those facilities that currently use an EHR must determine whether their system will meet the national EHR standards under development.

TRAINING

Training is a massive undertaking involving all employees and physicians. Even though computers are becoming a part of our daily lives, many individuals are not competent or comfortable using them. Initially, productivity falters as the employees learn the new system. Some employees will be reluctant to convert to a completely electronic environment. Some physicians might consider electronic ordering and documentation to be more time consuming than their previous method. Space must be allocated for training both employees and physicians during the implementation phase and throughout the transition. As updates are added to the EHR, training must follow.

PRIVACY ISSUES

An important barrier under discussion by a number of consumer agencies is the privacy issue. When multiple users have access to the record, the ability to maintain the security of the record becomes a risk. As more people have access to health information in more places, security of the information becomes paramount. Policies, procedures, and sanctions (if there is a breach in security) must be developed.

RELIABILITY

Reliability is another issue that must be considered. The paper record is reliable in the sense that it will be available during a power outage and it is not vulnerable to programming problems. Several HIM clerks ensure that there is a record for each patient, and all the reports are in the record. In the EHR, it is assumed that there is a record and that all the components have properly interfaced with the EHR. It is also assumed that no power outages, no programming errors, and no electromagnet pulses have occurred that would prevent a functioning interface.

Exercise 12-4

Advantages and Barriers to Implementing an Electronic Health Record

1. How will SNOMED be used in the EHR?
2. Explain why the HL7 RIM is important.
3. List the barriers to implementing an EHR.
4. Explain how using electronic medication prescribing will improve quality of care.

ELECTRONIC HEALTH RECORD MANAGEMENT

The October 2004 *Journal of the American Health Information Management Association* (AHIMA) states that the EHR includes information that is

- recorded on any electronic medium (e.g., magnetic medium).
- intended to provide documentation for long-term retention with legal or business evidentiary value.
- potentially produced in response to a subpoena duces tecum.

AHIMA defines **EHR management** as the process by which electronic (e.g., digital) health records are created or received and preserved for evidentiary (e.g., legal or business) purposes (AHIMA Workgroup on Electronic Health Records Management 2004).

HEALTH INFORMATION MANAGEMENT PROCESSING ISSUES

Several issues and decisions must be made when converting from a paper record to an electronic record. If you ever have the opportunity to talk to an HIM director who has experienced this transition, you will hear the same response over and over: "You think you planned for everything, but something you did not expect will always surface and have to be addressed." This chapter covers the more important HIM processing issues and changes that may occur with the transition.

RECORD ASSEMBLY

An important consideration in the transition to the EHR is how the health information is going to get into the EHR. Will a paper record be generated first and then scanned in after discharge by the HIM department? Will all information be either computer generated or scanned in at the point of service? Will the record be a hybrid, with some reports scanned and others computer generated? Will it be a total electronic record in which each caregiver enters documents and orders directly into a computer system? Will clerks be needed to input data in the HIM Department or at the points of service? Whatever the scenario, form control (see Chapter 3) must be closely monitored and becomes more important with a document imaging system and the use of the EHR.

The use of bar codes for both the type of form and patient demographics is advantageous in the hybrid health record. The demographic bar code can be generated on labels and attached to each form. In some systems, the demographic bar code is automatically printed out on each report. The bar code indicating the form name is usually preprinted on the form. The bar codes allow for automatic indexing by patient record and report type. Indexing is discussed in more detail later in this chapter.

Chart order in the EHR is just as important as in the paper record. In the paper record, the order of the reports in the chart are standardized, and the same consideration must be given to the EHR. Users of the EHR will rely on the indexes to find the reports that they need to read; if the format is standardized, they will become familiar with it more quickly.

Computer output to laser disk (COLD) involves the capture of large (typically mainframe-generated) reports on optical media such that sections are accessible as individual documents. COLD technology succeeded computer output on microfilm (COM). COLD software allows the transfer of documents from expensive mainframe storage onto an inexpensive, long-term optical disk storage system.

Another consideration in the assembly of hybrid records is the handling of the paper documents in the in house paper chart, as well as COLD feed documents that are generated from other departments. These could include laboratory reports, clinic reports, and transcribed reports. COLD allows transfer of documents from a computer software program to an optical disk storage system. The feed is the actual transmission of the documents. For example, Hospital A uses a hybrid record in which a paper record is maintained on the nursing unit and then scanned as part of the EHR postdischarge. The radiology reports are typed into a separate transcription system. The transcription system interfaces with the HIM EHR. Once the radiology report is typed, it automatically COLD feeds into the electronic chart. However, the hospital still uses a paper record on the nursing unit, so the radiology report is printed out and becomes part of the paper record. After discharge, the paper record is processed for scanning and indexing. While checking the record, the HIM clerk will pull all COLD-fed reports into the electronic record and secure them to the back of the record labeled "Do not scan." The person scanning the records then knows which reports in the back of the record are not to be scanned.

Whether a paper record or an electronic record is used, the assembly process usually takes place when the HIM personnel verify that all the discharged records were received. This process must also be continued with the EHR. The last step in processing the discharged record is to verify that the EHR is active and available to the appropriate users. This can be accomplished by having the indexer confirm that the chart can be viewed in workflow or by having the analysis clerk confirm that all records being analyzed for a particular discharge day are available.

SCANNING AND INDEXING

Scanning and indexing are necessary functions with both the hybrid record and the EHR. With the hybrid record, the HIM department may be scanning (as discussed in document imaging) the whole record or parts of a record. With the EHR, the HIM department may have only a few reports to scan because most reports are electronically generated. Scanning equipment must be purchased on the basis of the volume of reports (number of pages) to be scanned.

As stated previously, indexing is sorting the records by the different report types, making the viewing of the record uniform. Use of bar codes will automate the indexing process. Indexing is important because users must be able to find the information that they need quickly in the EHR. The creation of an accurate index facilitates future retrieval of the images. By correctly identifying (i.e., indexing and naming) the document for each patient, the computer system is able to locate the correct image when a search is performed. For example, when you scan a document into a computer using a standard flatbed scanner, you must name the file to identify the information stored. Because you name the file when you save it, the next time you access the file index, you are able to identify the contents without opening each file. Therefore indexing in the computer environment facilitates future retrieval.

What happens if the image is indexed by the wrong patient's name? How do you find the missing images of a record in the computer? All computer systems use various search methods to aid in the retrieval of the images. Additional methods to locate missing files require searching the discharge list to identify other patient records indexed on the same day. When records are scanned into a computer system, they are typically scanned in groups or batches. A typical group or batch of records would consist of 1 day of discharges. Therefore looking through the images of all the patients' records scanned on the same day may produce the missing image. Once the missing image is identified, it is renamed or indexed appropriately. Figure 12-5 is an example of an indexed EHR.

RECORD ANALYSIS

As discussed in previous chapters, analysis using a paper record is performed by HIM personnel, who review each page of the record to determine if all the reports are present and any authentication is missing. A tally of what needs to be completed on the record can be maintained using a paper notification system or a computer-generated notification. In a hybrid or electronic record, it must be decided how and when the record will be analyzed. When using a hybrid record, an

Face Sheet
Discharge Summary
History and Physical
Emergency Room Record
Consultation
  Dr. Sign
  Dr. Sick
  Dr. Ill
Operative Report
Progress Notes
Physician Orders
Laboratory
  Chemistry
  Blood
  Urinalysis
Radiology
  Chest
  CT Scan
  MRI
Cardiology
  EKG
  Stress Test
Respiratory
  Notes
  Blood Gas
Dietary
Physical Therapy
Nursing Admit Note
Nursing Flow Sheets
Nursing Narrative Notes
Intake and Output Notes
Graphic Sheet
Nursing Discharge Form
Consents
Admit Forms
	DISCHARGE SUMMARY
	DIAGNOSES:
	1. Cerebrovascular accident
	2. Schizophrenia
	3. Recurrent transient ischemic attacks
	
	PROCEDURES:
	1. Echocardiogram
	2. Holter monitor
	
	HISTORY OF PRESENT ILLNESS:
	This is a 59-year-old, right-handed woman with a history of hypertension, schizophrenia, and a fallopian ovarian tumor resected surgically and with radiotherapy treatment, who presented to the emergency room with a four-hour history of difficulty talking and numbness and weakness on the right side. She was in her usual state of health until early the morning of admission when she woke up and noted numbness on her right side. Her numbness was associated with weakness as well as difficulty speaking, with no associated headache, chest pain, fever, chills, double vision, difficulty swallowing, or palpitations. She reported having a similar incident about 1 month prior to admission when she was seen in the emergency room, but at that time, her symptoms resolved while in the emergency room. CT scan at that time showed bilateral basal ganglion infarcts. Carotid duplex then showed minimal plaque, right greater than left, with no hemodynamic stenosis. At that time, she was sent home on aspirin 1 q.d. which she has been taking except for the day prior to admission, when she missed her dose.
	
	HOSPITAL COURSE: The patient was admitted to the neurology service with concern for an embolic versus ischemic event in the face of aspirin therapy. As an inpatient, she had an echocardiogram which was reported to show mild, concentric, left ventricular hypertrophy with normal left ventricular function, no segmental wall abnormalities, no mitral regurgitation, no aortic regurgitation, and no tricuspid regurgitation. No evidence of coral thrombus. Carotids were not repeated, since she had a carotid study one month prior to admission that showed an occlusion of her carotids. RPR was nonreactive. Blood pressure remained under control during hospitalization. Her psychiatric symptoms were stable during this time. She was seen by physical therapy and occupational therapy, who helped her with ambulation, and by discharge she was making good progress, ambulating, and using her arms, although she remained with weakness on the right more marked than the left. She was discharged in good health.
	
	DISCHARGE MEDICATIONS:
	1. Nortriptyline 25 mg p.o. q.h.s.
	2. Benadryl 50 mg p.o. q.h.s.
	3. Navane 5 mg p.o. q.h.s.
	4. Aspirin 2 p.o. b.i.d.
	
	DISCHARGE INSTRUCTIONS:
	1. Diet: Low-cholesterol, low-fat diet.
	2. Activity: As tolerated.
	
	FOLLOW-UP CARE:
	1. Return to the neurology clinic about 1 month after discharge.

◆ **Figure 12-5**

Indexed electronic health record. The left side of the table is the indexed record. The right side is a report being viewed in the EHR.

analysis clerk may still need to review the record and provide the physician with the chart deficiencies electronically. In the EHR, an automated deficiency analysis program may be included with the electronic record system; this allows the record to be completed at the time of ordering or documenting. Polices and procedures must be established to define what constitutes a deficiency and what constitutes a complete record.

The physicians can complete the records electronically using their passwords and can, in some cases, actually correct their own transcribed documents before signing them. These systems can notify the physician that dictation, signatures, and even text are missing. In some facilities, the physician can complete the record from his office or other areas of the hospital. In a paper context, the physician may complete the records in the HIM department, where procedures were set up to notify the physician of any coding discrepancies or questions that HIM personnel may have about record completion. Because the physician can complete the EHR from areas other than the HIM department, procedures must be established to notify the physician about such matters.

Authentication in a hybrid or electronic record must be carefully considered. A **digitized signature** is an original signature on a report that is then scanned into an electronic document. An **electronic signature** occurs when the authenticator uses a password or **personal identification number** (**PIN**) to electronically sign a document. In some facilities, the authenticator must use both a password and a PIN to sign. HIPAA is in the process of establishing specific guidelines for electronic signatures. A **digital signature** has a means to identify the user, provides **nonrepudiation** (a process that provides a positive identification of the user), and it ensures the **integrity** of the signature (i.e., the document cannot be altered after the signature has been applied).

CODING

In most facilities, the coding function is being assisted with encoders to help assign codes more accurately. During conversion to a hybrid electronic record, staff members must decide whether to use the paper record or the electronic record to assign codes. Some facilities still use the paper record for coding inpatient stays but use the electronic record to code the ambulatory surgery and emergency room records. An example of when the paper record might be used is when there is a backlog of scanning and indexing. The coding function may have to be completed within a specific time period, as outlined by the facility policies. When the electronic record is used for coding, the facility may opt to provide large monitors to the coders that allow them better visualization of the record and the ability to use two windows at once. Some hospitals have elected to assign two monitors to coding personnel for this purpose. In some cases, the coding process may migrate offsite as is common with transcription. If computer-assisted coding becomes a reality, automated coding algorithms will be developed to perform the coding task electronically. The coding function will become more of an audit function to verify the accuracy of the automated coding.

ABSTRACTING

Most HIM departments use a computer program to store the abstracted data and generate reports. When converting to a hybrid electronic record, HIM staff must address how abstracting will occur—in a freestanding program, with an interface, or through a vendor's product that includes report-writing capabilities. It must be determined if data will be captured at the point of care or abstracted retrospectively. In the EHR, the abstracting function could be automated, with data captured at the time of documentation (Figure 12-6). As with coding, abstracting may someday become an auditing function to verify the accuracy of the information.

FILING

During conversion to a hybrid or an electronic record, policies and procedures must be established to define what constitutes a legal document. In a hybrid system, if both paper and electronic data are going to be maintained and used, this should be specified in the policy. In the hybrid electronic record in which a paper chart is generated and then scanned into the electronic record, policies must specify what will happen to the paper record. The policy must address whether the paper record will be destroyed or maintained in offsite storage. Retention issues must be addressed in the policy. How long will the paper record be maintained in storage before it is destroyed? Will computer-based data be available online or archivally over time?

TRANSCRIPTION

Whether the transcription function is performed inhouse or outsourced, the way in which the transcribed report moves to the EHR is an important issue to consider. The hybrid and electronic

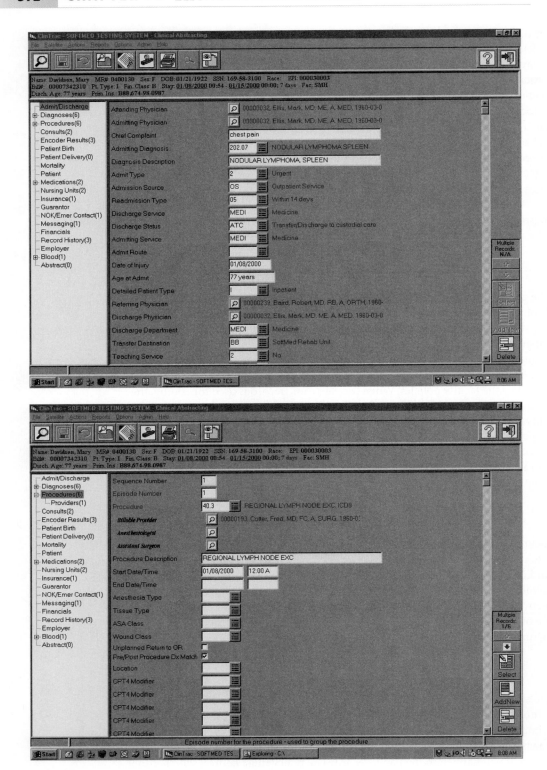

◆ **Figure 12-6**
SoftMed clinical abstract screen. (Courtesy SoftMed Systems, Inc., Bethesda, MD.)

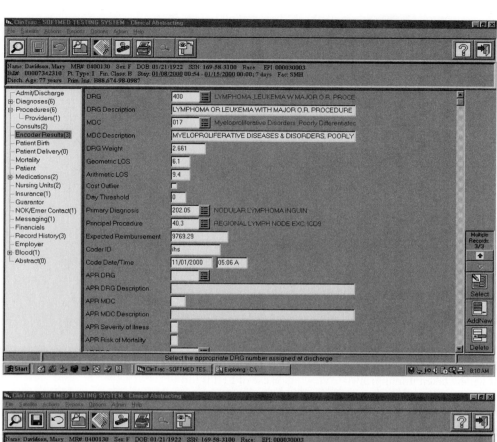

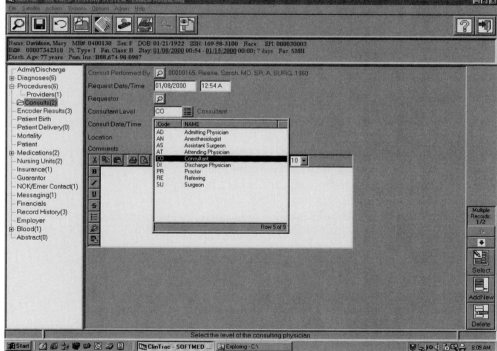

◆ **Figure 12-6 (*cont'd*)**

record will have the transcribed reports available for viewing on the health record as soon as the report is released by the transcriptionist. In some cases, signature deficiencies can be assigned automatically when the document moves from the transcription system to the electronic record system. Another issue to consider is whether the physicians can correct the transcribed reports electronically. If electronic corrections are allowed, how will the different versions of the report be stored? If such corrections are not allowed, how will corrections be made? What about transcribed reports generated from different systems, such as radiology or cardiology? How will these be interfaced?

RELEASE OF INFORMATION

The Health Insurance Portability and Accountability Act (HIPAA) Privacy and Security Rules require health care facilities to have administrative, technical, and physical safeguards in place to ensure privacy and safeguard information whether it is on paper or in an electronic format.

Administrative safeguards include policies and procedures regarding confidentiality and security agreements signed by each staff member, as well as any nonstaff members using the medical record. The Security Rule requires that facilities identify all systems that contain electronic personal health information and perform a risk assessment to identify areas that may pose a security risk. Staff training is an integral part of the Privacy and Security Rule. The following topics are important and should be included in training:

- How to guard against threats of computer viruses or hackers and where to report suspicious activity
- Routine performance of audits to ensure that employees are using PHI on a need-to-know basis and actions that will be taken if inappropriate viewing or use of PHI is found
- Education on how to dispose of PHI information on paper or electronic media such as CD-ROMs or floppy discs
- Management of passwords: how often they will change and sanctions for sharing passwords

Technical safeguards are addressed in detail in the Security Rule. An example of a technical safeguard is a procedure to deny system access immediately upon employee termination. Another example is automatic logoffs: If a computer idles for more than a specific number of minutes, it will automatically log off. Some facilities may also use **encryption** of data as a technical safeguard. Encryption is the most effective way to achieve data security. To read an encrypted file, you must have access to a secret key or password that enables you to read it.

Physical safeguards must be established to protect unauthorized access to areas or systems containing PHI. If a paper-generated record is used, locked doors are used as barriers to protect the information. The following are examples of physical safeguards in an electronic context:

- Placing sensors on portable devices such as laptops or handheld devices that will sound an alarm if they are taken off the premises
- Placing computer monitors in areas that minimize the chance of a stranger viewing confidential information

WORKFLOW ISSUES

In the paper context, *workflow* referred to the way in which the paper record was processed from one HIM function to another or moved from one desk to another. In the electronic context, **workflow** describes how the electronic record moves from one electronic component to another. In the electronic context, once a function is completed, the electronic record may automatically be sent to the appropriate electronic work areas. These electronic work areas are called **queues**. An example of an HIM queue would be the coding queue or the analysis queue. These queues can be further defined (e.g., a coding queue may be called an outpatient coding queue).

When an action is completed in a queue, the workflow program will send the electronic record to the next work area or queue. For example, when a physician dictates an operative report and hits the complete button, the record will then go to the awaiting operative report queue. The reanalysis clerk will manage the work in the awaiting operative report queue and ensure that the transcribed operative report reaches the electronic record.

Workflow issues are complex and must be carefully planned. It must be decided what queues will be included and, more important, which staff members will be responsible for working the numerous queues. In one facility, a queue was identified several months after the electronic health record was implemented. A transcribed report goes to the queue when the HIM interface cannot identify the physician's name. No one was assigned to complete this queue, and HIM personnel believed that another clerical area was taking care of these documents.

A simple example of workflow in an electronic record is listed in Figure 12-7.

Exercise 12-5

Electronic Health Records Management

1. Explain why bar codes are important in an EHR.
2. Define the three different types of authentications in an EHR.
3. List the three types of privacy and security safeguards and give an example of each.
4. What is workflow?
5. List three career opportunities for registered health information technicians with the electronic health record.

CAREER OPPORTUNITIES

As health care organizations begin the transition to the EHR, there will be a greater need for employees with HIM expertise. The health information technologist may find a variety of new careers concentrating on information management, including the following:

- Project management: act as a leader to teams in the process of developing or implementing EHR systems
- Design and development: test new systems, provide training on new systems
- Marketing and sales: sell products and services related to the EHR, provide support to new clients

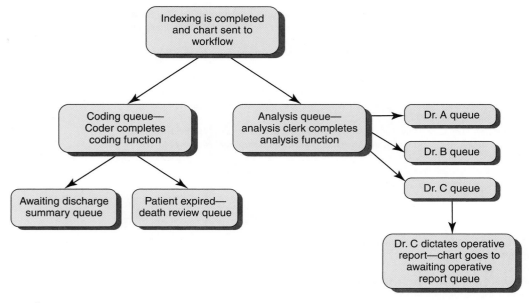

◆ **Figure 12-7**
A simple example of workflow in an electronic record.

Hit-Bit

VeriChip

Another type of PHR is the VeriChip. VeriChip is a subdermal, radio-frequency identification (RFID) device that can be used in a variety of security, financial, emergency identification and other applications. About the size of a grain of rice, each VeriChip product contains a unique verification number that is captured by briefly passing a proprietary scanner over the VeriChip. The standard location of the microchip is in the triceps area between the elbow and the shoulder of the right arm. The brief outpatient "chipping" procedure lasts just a few minutes and involves only local anesthetic followed by the quick, painless insertion of the VeriChip. Once inserted just under the skin, the VeriChip is inconspicuous to the naked eye. A small amount of radio frequency energy passes from the scanner energizing the dormant VeriChip, which then emits a radio frequency signal transmitting the verification number. This number can be used to identify the implanted individual by consulting a registry maintained by the corporation.

- Implementation specialist: help facilities with the implementation of the EHR
- Technical support: provide support to the customers during and after system implementation, including access to facility records and development of a PHR
- Knowledge management: assist with database design and develop reports using databases
- Consumer affairs: educate members of the public about their rights and the appropriate uses of their health information

■ WORKS CITED

AHIMA e-HIM Personal Health Record Work Group. "The Role of the Personal Health Record in the HER." *Journal of AHIMA* 76.7 (2005): 64A-64D.

AHIMA Workgroup on Electronic Health Records Management. "The Strategic Importance of Electronic Health Records Management. Appendix A: Issues in Electronic Health Records Management. *Journal of AHIMA* 75.9 (2004): 80A-80H.

Clinical Research Information System. "The Project: A Clinical Research Information System for NIH." 2006. National Institute of Health 25 July 2006 <http://cris.cc.nih.gov/public/project.html>.

Committee on Data Standards for Patient Safety. "Institute of Medicine Report Identifies Core Capabilities That Should Be a Part of an Electronic Health Record System." 31 July 2003. *National Academies NEWS* 6 June 2005 <http://www4.nas.edu/news.nsf>.

Gater, L. "The RHIO World." 31 July 2003. *For the Record* 25 July 2006 <http://www.fortherecordmag.com/archives/ftr_071805p16.shtml>.

"HL7, SNOMED Sign Associate Charter Agreement Formalization of Relationship Will Advance Healthcare Interoperability Worldwide." 24 June 2005. SNOMED <http://www.h17.org/documentcenter/public/pressreleases/20050623.pdf>.

Medical Transcription Networking Center. "Sample Forms Discharge Summary." 2006. *MT Daily* 25 July 2006 <http://www.mtdaily.com/mt1/miscsample.html>.

Miller, R. G. et al. "Practice Parameter: The Care of the Patient with Amyotrophic Lateral Sclerosis (an Evidence-Based Review). Report of the Quality Standards Committee of the American Academy of Neurology." *Neurology* 52 (1999): 1311.

Stein, Lincoln. "The Electronic Medical Record: Promises and Threats. Web Security: A Matter of Trust." *Web Journal* 2.3 (2006) <http://www.oreilly.com/catalog/wjsum97/excerpt>.

■ SUGGESTED READING

Amatayakul, Margaret K. *Electronic Health Records: A Practical Guide for Professionals and Organizations.* 2nd ed. Chicago: Clinical Research Information Management Association, 2004.

Definitions <http://www.webopedia.com>.

Ferris, Nancy. "Regional Health Information Network Gains Traction." 9 June 2005 *Government Health IT* <http://www.govhealthit.com/article_89134-06-09-05>.

Tegan, Anne, et al. "The EHR's Impact on HIM Functions." *Journal of AHIMA* 76.5 (2005): 56C-H.

WEB SITES

The Institute of Medicine: http://www.iom.org
The Markle Foundation: http://www.markle.org
Health Information Management Systems Society: http://www.himss.org
Health Level Seven: http://www.hl7.org
The Office of the National Coordinator for Health Information Technology: http://www.os.dhhs.gov/healthit/
American Health Information Management Association: http://www.ahima.org

CHAPTER ACTIVITIES

CHAPTER SUMMARY

President George W. Bush would like all health care organizations to use the EHR within the next 10 years. There are many private and federal groups working to make the EHR a reality. Many health care organizations are already using hybrid electronic health records. HIM employees who are already using a hybrid record are already familiar with terms such as *interfacing* and *document imaging.* Health care organizations will be sharing data both interoperably and longitudinally, making health information more accessible to the users and thereby improving the quality of health care. The government is reviewing incentives to decrease the cost of EHR conversion. HIM departments making the transition to an EHR will have to review and revise every function performed in the department. HIM professionals will have to learn the information technology functions to manage the future HIM departments. As the EHR is developed, there will be an increasing need for professionals with HIM knowledge. Job opportunities will be available for project managers, vendor marketing and sales representatives, and database designers.

Review Questions

1. Explain the difference between the paper, hybrid, and electronic health record.
2. Explain the difference between interoperable and longitudinal.
3. List two advantages and two barriers to implementing the EHR. Discuss why what you have listed is advantageous or creates barriers to the use of the EHR.
4. List three HIM functions that will change with the implementation of the EHR and explain the changes.
5. List three careers that the development of the EHR will create.

Assistant Director, HIM

My name is Ann, and I am a HIM implementation specialist in a 250-bed facility, Jameson Hospital. This facility provides acute care, emergency services, ambulatory services, a cancer center, and two offsite rehabilitation centers. Our hospital is one of four hospitals in the city owned by the same corporation. We have approximately 500 physicians on the medical staff.

All four hospitals share a medical record database and use a hybrid medical record. All four hospitals are currently in the process of implementing an EHR. Each hospital has hired an HIM implementation specialist who will work on different HIM applications in the electronic record. I was promoted from clerical supervisor to implementation specialist. This is a very exciting position. It has provided me with an opportunity to learn about the information systems throughout the facility, as well as allowing me to work with many employees from other departments and from the other hospitals.

I am a member of the implementation team at our facility and provide input on HIM functions, forms, and communication. I am working with a joint forms committee with representatives from all four hospitals to revise the record forms to an electronic format. I am also working closely with the vendor and IT department to develop the workflow for the electronic record. I am spending many hours testing the HIM functions for my assigned applications as they are developed. I provide feedback on the results of the application testing to the vendor and implementation committee, who listen carefully to my suggestions for changes. Currently, we are working on the scanning and indexing application. I am developing training materials for the HIM employees at all four hospitals. Several of the file clerks will be performing the scanning and indexing functions. My next application will be working on the bar codes for the revised forms.

This position is allowing me the opportunity to use my computer skills, work with a team, and use my knowledge of HIM workflow and processes. Being part of the team developing the foundation for the EHR is very rewarding.

APPLICATION

Current EHR Activities

Go to the ONCHIT and HL7 Web sites and prepare a brief report on the current actions of each organization as related to the EHR. You should prepare this report as if you were giving it at the next monthly information management meeting at your hospital.

Chapter 13

HIM Department Management

CHAPTER OUTLINE

By the end of this chapter, the student should be able to

- Identify and prioritize health information management department functions and services.

- Organize the appropriate workflow of health information management functions and services.

- Perform job analysis.

- Write job descriptions using the Americans with Disabilities Act requirements.

- Develop plans, goals, and objectives for health information management employees.

- Assess and design an ergonomically sound work environment for health information management personnel.

- For a new health information management department, identify file space, ergonomics, dictation/transcription area, and equipment and supply needs for department functions and services.

- Develop health information management department policies for employee operations and conduct.

- Compare work performance of health information management employees to establish new standards.

- Collect data and report on productivity of a health information management employee and on department productivity and analyze department data for implementation of new productivity standards.

- Evaluate the effectiveness of operations and services in a health information management department.

- Monitor the use of department resources, including inventory, budget, and planning.

- Establish standards for performance of employees in health information management functions and services.

- Develop department policy and procedures for health information management functions and services.

VOCABULARY

delegate	mission	policy
ergonomic	objectives	procedure
full-time equivalent (FTE)	organization chart	productivity
goals	performance improvement plan (PIP)	span of control
job analysis		unity of command
job description	performance standards	vision

his chapter covers the management of health information management (HIM) employees and their roles and responsibilities. It specifically focuses on issues, tools, and techniques unique to HIM. You will learn about human resources, organization, planning, policy and procedures, equipment, supplies, education, and training and development in the context of the HIM department.

Previous chapters focused on the performance of common functions in the HIM department and the many issues, uses, and requirements surrounding health information. As you read this chapter, you are expected to understand the functions of the HIM department and to achieve a level of competence sufficient to perform many of the functions efficiently.

HUMAN RESOURCES

The term *human resources* is most often associated with a department within an organization. The human resource department maintains personnel records; handles employee benefit issues; and advertises for, interviews, hires, disciplines, and terminates facility employees. The human resource department works with the managers in the health care facility, as necessary, when developing job descriptions and performance standards, conducting employee performance evaluations, and handling employee conduct problems, and manages other technical aspects of employment.

As a supervisor, manager, or director of the HIM department, you will be significantly involved in human resource management. Although the human resource department is your consultant on these matters, you will need to know the appropriate methods and tools for managing employees within the HIM department.

The phrase *human resources within the HIM department* refers to the human beings (employees) who are the source of support needed to accomplish health information functions. Employees are resources that can be defined as *assets*. We need humans to perform HIM functions to ensure timely, complete, and accurate health information. Furthermore, the appropriate management of this asset, the employee, has an impact on the entire organization. Management is a skill because different situations call for different measures to accomplish a task. In other words, what works in one facility or with one employee may not always work with another.

In the workplace, people are called *employees, personnel, or associates*. Employees may be classified according to hours worked (full-time or part-time) or by position—that is, management or staff. As shown in Table 13-1, employee classifications by hours worked are full-time, part-time, and temporary (also known as *PRN [as needed], per diem, pool*, etc.). A **full-time equivalent (FTE)** is one who by definition works 32 to 40 hours each week excluding overtime (or in some cases, 64 to 80 hours every 2 weeks), thereby earning full benefits as offered by the health care facility. Full-time status affects employees' benefits in terms of hours earned in paid time off (PTO), vacation, holiday benefits, and retirement options. For example, an employee who works 40 hours each week is considered a full-time employee, and he or she may earn 4 hours of vacation each week. Additionally, the organization might match retirement benefits for the full-time employee at a rate higher than for other classes of employees.

TABLE 13-1	Employee Classifications	
CLASSIFICATION	**COMMON TERMS**	**DESCRIPTION**
Full-time	FTE	Employee who works 32-40 hours each week, or 64-80 hours every 2 weeks, earning full benefits
Part-time	PT	Employee who typically works 16-20 hours each week, occasionally earning benefits at half of the full-time rate
Temporary	Pool, PRN, per diem	Employees scheduled to work as necessary because of an increased workload

A part-time (PT) employee is one who typically works 16 to 20 hours each week, thereby earning benefits at half the weekly rate of a full-time employee, if benefits are earned at all. For example, a PT employee may earn 2 hours of vacation, sick leave, or paid time off for every 20 hours of work. Temporary or per diem employees, on the other hand, rarely earn any type of employee benefit. Per diem employees are scheduled to work as needed in the facility when the amount of work exceeds what the regular employees can accomplish. These employees are valuable to the organization when there is an unexpected excess of work. These categories are discussed in more detail later in the chapter, with regard to the HIM department structure.

The additional employee classification of management or staff can indicate an employee's position and responsibility within the department or organization. Those in management or supervisory positions have responsibility for other employees. Staff employees are responsible for daily tasks and functions, and they report to a supervisor or manager.

Hit-Bit

FTEs

A full-time equivalent (FTE) works 40 hours per week. Often, a department is allowed a number of FTEs that is not even. This fraction typically accounts for the part-time employees. For example: The HIM department is allowed 100 hours each work week for coding. How many FTEs equal 100 hours? The answer is 100 divided by 40 (1 FTE) equals 2.5 FTEs. There are 2.5 FTEs allowed in the coding department each week. We discuss FTEs in more detail later in the chapter.

Exercise 13-1

Human Resources

1. A(n) _____ works 32 to 40 hours each week excluding overtime, earning full benefits as offered by the health care facility.
2. An employee who works 16 to 20 hours each week, occasionally earning partial benefits, is
   a. FTE
   b. PRN
   c. part time
   d. LPN
3. A pool of employees used as needed when work load increases is
   a. FTE
   b. part-time
   c. PRN
   d. coder
4. The department within the health care organization responsible for employee management is the
   a. HIM department
   b. human resources
   c. materials management
   d. operations management
5. The HIM department is allowed 450 hours per week. This equals how many FTEs?
   a. 4.5
   b. 22.5
   c. 11.25
   d. 45

ORGANIZATION CHARTS

One method used by health care facilities to describe the arrangement of departments and positions is the **organization chart.** The organization chart illustrates the relationships among departments, positions, and functions within the organization. To understand an organization chart, you must understand the symbols used in it. The traditional structure of an organization chart resembles a pyramid, in which there are more departments and personnel at the bottom than at the top. An organization chart uses boxes and lines to represent departments and positions within the facility (Figure 13-1). Boxes indicate a department or position. The higher the box is located within the chart, the higher the authority and responsibility of the position or department that it represents. Boxes on the same level indicate similar levels of authority or responsibility. Lines connecting the boxes indicate a relationship. Solid lines indicate a direct relationship. Broken lines indicate an indirect (or shared) relationship. The lines in the organization chart illustrate the subordination of positions in the chain of command. *Chain of command* refers to the order in which decisions are made within the facility. For decisions that require approval, the organization chart describes who must give that approval.

FACILITY ORGANIZATION

The traditional health care facility is composed of departments with specialized personnel or services; these are related to the health care professions discussed in Chapter 1. Figure 13-1 is a useful reference when you are considering the organization chart of a medium-sized acute care facility. The box at the top of the chart represents the ultimate authority and responsibility within the organization. This authority is called the *governing body, board of directors,* or *board of trustees.* Every facility has this type of authority at the top of the organization.

There are typically 8 to 25 members on the board, depending on the size of the facility. Members of the board include the chief executive officer (CEO), members of the medical staff, and members of the community (Abdelhak et al. 1996, p. 23). The board meets regularly to

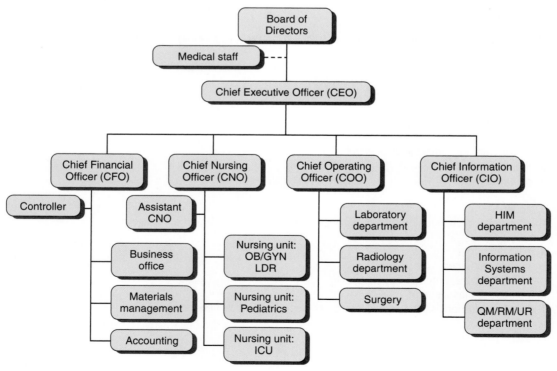

◆ **Figure 13-1**
Health care facility organization chart.

Hit-Bit

For-Profit or Not-For-Profit

All health care facilities have a governing board. A for-profit facility is owned by shareholders. A not-for-profit facility is held "in trust" by the community it serves.

review the business of the health care facility, set direction, and monitor progress. The board has two distinct relationships, as shown in Figure 13-1. One is the board delegates authority to the CEO (also called *administrator* or sometimes *president*) for the daily operations of the facility. The other is the relationship with the facility's medical staff.

The medical staff is the organization of the physicians who practice and participate in the operations of the health care facility. The medical staff has a structure governed by the members of the staff and described in the facility's medical staff bylaws, rules, and regulations. An example of medical staff structure is shown in Figure 13-2.

The CEO, under the governing board, is given the authority to oversee the daily management of the health care facility. The CEO must guide, motivate, and lead the organization under the direction of the governing board.

Below the CEO are several administrative positions. These positions have similar authority and responsibility over specific departments (services) within the organization. These administrators report to the CEO. This level of the administration is also known as the *chiefs, assistant administrators,* or *vice presidents of finance, nursing, information, and quality.*

The personnel responsible for managing specific departments report to the aforementioned administrators. The managers of the departments are known as *directors, department heads,* or *managers.* Below department directors are supervisors and then staff employees. The managers of each department have authority over the supervisors within their departments, and finally the staff employees within each department report to their respective supervisors. Notice how this organization chart indicates the lines of authority and responsibility. The organization chart is a good indicator of the appropriate span of control and unity of command.

Span of Control

In an organization chart, the number of positions or employees shown below the box for an administrator, manager, or supervisor indicate the **span of control** for that position. The phrase *span of control* refers to the number of employees that report to one supervisor, manager, or administrator. The span of control for one supervisor must be appropriate so that management is efficient and effective. Too many varied responsibilities or employees under one supervisor (especially in a large facility) can lead to ineffective management. The appropriate span of control is often determined by the number of employees and their responsibility. A large facility may require

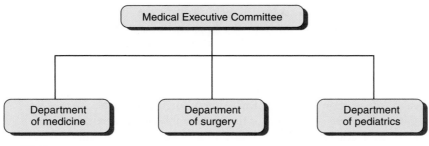

◆ **Figure 13-2**
Medical staff organization chart.

Hit-Bit

Management Styles

The previously discussed topics are affected by the HIM department director's management style. The three major categories of management are autocratic, democratic, and laissez-faire.

The autocratic manager controls everything. Employees function under strict control of this manager. All operations and decisions are overseen by this type of manager. Autocratic managers are sometimes called *micromanagers*, overseeing even the smallest details of the department.

The democratic manager allows all employees to provide input in decision making or operations of the department. The democratic manager seeks input and then typically makes decisions on the basis of this feedback.

The laissez-faire manager allows the employees to run the department and gets involved only when absolutely necessary. This is a true hands-off manager. Chances are, the laissez-faire manager will not pitch in when the work piles up.

more managers than a small facility because of the number of employees needed to accomplish a task or function.

Unity of Command

It is also important that one position (employee) report to one manager. This concept is called **unity of command.** If one employee has two supervisors, the employee might be confused as to which manager's authority is higher or which manager's rules and requests take precedence. If both managers have deadlines, which one must be met first? Who decides? If the employee has only one manager, the employee knows that he or she is accountable to that manager according to the role and responsibility of the position.

Delegation

Delegation describes what a manager does when he or she assigns responsibility to an employee to complete a project or task. When you **delegate**, you give the employee responsibility and the necessary authority to accomplish the project or task. If you delegate a task to an employee, he or she may need some authority to get the job done (e.g., signing forms, making changes in a process, and disciplining employees). Delegation is an important tool that managers use to accomplish multiple tasks. This tool also shows the employee that the manager trusts him or her to do a good job.

HEALTH INFORMATION MANAGEMENT DEPARTMENT ORGANIZATION

Figure 13-3 illustrates the organization of positions within the HIM department. This is an organization chart for a medium-sized HIM department with 30 employees. The box at the top of the chart represents the department director. Ultimately, each HIM department has a top manager responsible for the overall direction of the department. This position may be called *director, manager,* or *department head.* The person in this position has the delegated authority from the administration of the facility to act as the custodian of health information. The director also has the responsibility and authority to manage the daily operations of the HIM department. Figure 13-3 shows a department with one director, one assistant director, three supervisors, and 25 staff employees. Keep in mind that job titles for positions within the HIM department vary among facilities.

In addition, the organization chart in Figure 13-3 shows a department that is organized into three supervised sections of health information functions. Each supervisor is responsible for specific functions within the department. There is a supervisor for the assembly, analysis, release of information (ROI), and filing functions, also known as the clerical, or ROI, supervisor. Another supervisor, called the *coding supervisor,* oversees the coding and abstracting functions. The third supervisor, the *transcription supervisor,* is responsible for the transcription function.

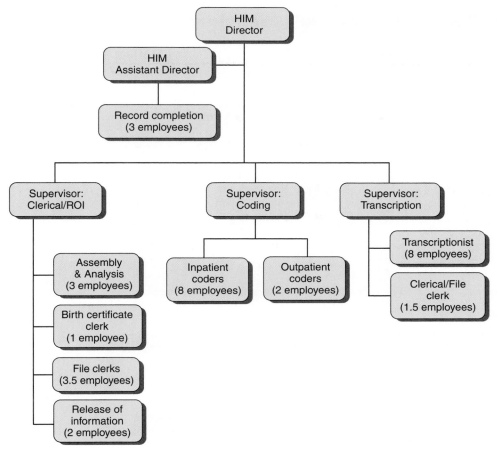

◆ **Figure 13-3**
HIM department organization chart.

Within the HIM department, employees are further identified by the positions that they hold or job functions that they perform. HIM departments have clerical and technical staff positions (Table 13-2). The director of the HIM department or the human resource department determines the title for employee positions. Some titles are generic (e.g., HIM Tech I), whereas other titles describe the employee's responsibilities (e.g., assembly and analysis).

Clerical employees are responsible for the functions known as *assembly, analysis,* and *filing.* Technical employees perform functions such as coding, transcription, record completion, and ROI. (Table 13-2 describes possible job titles.) Such positions are sometimes referred to as *HIM Tech II.* These staff employees typically report to the first or lowest level of management, either the HIM supervisor or a team leader. Responsibilities of the supervisor's positions differ in each department, but they may include scheduling, hiring, training, disciplining, and terminating. The supervisor

Hit-Bit

Exempt or Nonexempt

Exempt employees are salaried; they are not required to punch a time clock. There are some exceptions depending on record-keeping practices. Nonexempt employees are paid according to the number of hours worked.

TABLE 13-2	Staff Positions in the HIM Department		
POSITION	**RESPONSIBILITY/FUNCTION**	**HOURS**	**STATUS**
HIM Director	Daily management of the HIM department including	M-F 8 a.m.–4:30 p.m.	Full-time
Supervisor	Clerical/ROI/filing	M-F 7 a.m.-3:30 p.m.	Full-time
HIM Tech I	Assembly and analysis of all patient records	S-Thur, 6:30 a.m.–3 p.m.	Full-time
HIM Tech I	Birth certificates Saturday assembly/analysis	Tue-Sat, 8 a.m.- 4:30 p.m.	Full-time
HIM Tech I	Filing, loose work	M-F, 12:30 p.m.-9 p.m.	Full-time
HIM Tech II	Inpatient coding	M-F, 8:30 a.m.–5 p.m.	Full-time
HIM Tech II	Outpatient coding	M-Thur, 4 p.m.–9 p.m.	Full-time
HIM Tech II	Release of information	M-F, 8:30 a.m.–5 p.m.	Full-time
HIM Tech II	Record completion	M-F, 7:30 a.m.–4 p.m.	Full-time
Transcriptionist	Pathology transcription and coordination of outside transcription	M-F, 8 a.m.–4:30 p.m.	Full-time

Hit-Bit

Chain of Command

The chain of command refers to the line of authority through which decisions are formerly authorized or processed. An employee should follow the chain of command for approval or decisions related to his or her job in the department, including discussion of disagreements with supervisors.

Exercise 13-2

Organization Charts

1. The _____ is an illustration used to describe the relationship between departments, positions, and functions within an organization.
2. As the new supervisor over the file area, release of information, and assembly and analysis, Sandra feels overwhelmed by the number of projects requiring her attention. One way that Sandra may relieve the pressure from these projects is to _____ some of the projects to her employees.
3. Judy, the physician record clerk in the HIM department, is responsible to Jovan, the supervisor, and Michelle, the director. This situation violates the _____ principle.
4. Janet is a supervisor responsible for eight coding employees; this statement represents Janet's _____.
5. The governing body
   a. has the authority to grant privileges to members of the medical staff
   b. is responsible for quality services provided by the facility
   c. Both A and B are correct
   d. None of the above is correct
6. The amount of work in the HIM department is determined by
   a. the CEO
   b. the department director
   c. admissions
   d. the number of discharges, patient type, and length of stay

is responsible for ensuring that staff employees are performing their functions in a timely manner that is consistent with the policies of the department.

The titles, roles, and responsibilities of positions within the HIM department vary. They are determined by the size, type, and purpose of the health care organization. Smaller facilities with few patient admissions have fewer positions as well as fewer levels of management. However, larger health care facilities have several employees performing one function, and they require more supervisors and levels of management to oversee daily functions.

HEALTH INFORMATION MANAGEMENT DEPARTMENT WORKFLOW

The collection, organization, coding, abstracting, analysis, storage, and retrieval of patient health information are organized into a *workflow* within each health care organization to best suit that facility. Workflow is the order in which the tasks are organized to progress from one function to the next. Efficient workflow allows department employees to accomplish their functions in a timely, accurate, and complete manner.

Because it is not possible to discuss every HIM department scenario, this section covers general workflow concepts such as the management and organization of HIM functions with only a few variations. Variations in the workflow among different facilities are necessary to accommodate the type, size, and structure of each health care facility.

Now it is time to review HIM functions and responsibilities as they are commonly conceived in health care facilities that use paper-based records. *Collection* refers to the retrieval of a health record from the patient care unit for every patient treated by the facility. *Organization* refers to the assembly of the record into a format usable by others; this might mean attaching the record to a file folder labeled appropriately for identification and storage. *Analysis* refers to the review of quantitative or qualitative health information to ensure timely, accurate, and complete records. *Coding* refers to the assignment of alphanumerical or numerical codes to patient diagnoses and procedures for reimbursement and data retrieval. *Abstracting* refers to the method by which the information in the health record is summarized for future reference. *Record completion* refers to the processing of an incomplete record as more health data are entered from appropriate health care personnel. *Storage* refers to the filing methods used to maintain records for future use. *Retrieval* describes the function that locates a record for future use following patient care. *Transcription* refers to the method by which the physician's dictation is turned into a medical report for placement in the patient's record.

These HIM functions occur sequentially and are typically grouped into sections under a supervisor for efficient management (see Figure 13-2). The need for supervisors within a department, as discussed previously, is determined by the number of employees in the HIM department and their varied functions. The fewer the number of employees, the less important the need for supervisors. Typically, supervisors oversee six to twelve employees depending on the functions performed by the group and the employees' need for direct supervision. In other words, if there are twelve transcriptionists, only one supervisor may be necessary. However, if you have twelve employees, six of whom are clerical workers, three of whom are coders, and three of whom are transcriptionists, the department may require three supervisors, one each for the clerical, coding, and transcription sections.

Hit-Bit

HIM Department Identity

The HIM department is also sometimes called the *medical record department* or *health information services*. Names of HIM departments remain diverse across the country.

Now that you have an understanding of the organization of the HIM department, you are ready to consider the workflow.

WORKLOAD AND PRODUCTIVITY

Each department must have a method for determining its workload. The amount of work in the HIM department is determined by the number of discharges and by the type and length of stay. The number of patients discharged each day will be equal to the number of records that must be assembled and organized. The type of record determines the detail required in analysis (e.g., same-day surgery records require less time to review than inpatient stays). The length of stay (LOS) for patients who have been discharged affects the length of time that it will take to assemble the patients' charts. If a patient has an LOS in the facility of 2 days, the record is relatively thin (e.g., approximately 1 inch). However, if the patient remains in the facility for 21 days, the record is relatively thick (approximately 2 to 3 inches) and may require two folders to contain the papers for that one stay. If your facility has many discharges with long LOSs, then the assembly process will take longer than in a facility that has few discharges with short LOSs.

Supervisors may use time studies to determine the appropriate number of personnel for the workload. A time study can be accomplished by monitoring the employee performing the function and the time that it takes to complete the task. If the supervisor is actually present while the employee performs the job, the employee may become nervous or irritated. Likewise, a supervisor does not want to waste valuable time watching employees work. Other methods exist to capture this information without physically watching employees. Employees can fill out forms to indicate their performance, productivity, and time (Figure 13-4).

The standards set for the department must comply with organizational, professional, licensing, and regulatory requirements. These guides determine when many of the functions must be performed (e.g., assembly and analysis within 24 hours of discharge and coding within 48 hours of discharge; Table 13-3). Some internal standards may lead the way for new processes, such as concurrent analysis or coding, to successfully accomplish department functions within the set time frame.

Workload is also affected by the amount of computerization in the HIM department. Sometimes, computerization reduces the complexity of a function, and at other times it increases the steps to complete a function.

Coding Productivity Report
02/20/2006

Coder	IP Total	IP Mcare	IP Non-Mcare	OP Total	ER	OP Refer	OBS	SDS
JBG	22	20	2	40	0	40	0	0
CRB	15	15	0	55	48	0	7	0
TLM	30	25	5	12	0	0	0	12
SNK	32	20	12	5	0	0	0	5

◆ **Figure 13-4**
Productivity report of coders in a HIM department.

TABLE 13-3	**Typical HIM Department Standards***

DEPARTMENT FUNCTION	STANDARD
Assembly and analysis	Completed within 24 hours of patient discharge
Coding and abstracting	Completed within 48–72 hours of patient discharge
Record completion	Completed within 30 days of discharge
Filing	Completed daily
Release of information	Completed within 48–72 hours of receipt of an appropriate authorization or request for information
Transcription	
History and physical	Transcribed within 12 hours of dictation
Consults	Transcribed within 12 hours of dictation
Operative reports	Transcribed within 6 hours of dictation
Discharge summary	Transcribed within 24 hours of dictation

*Note: These standards are for example only; standards in HIM departments may vary.

RETROSPECTIVE PROCESSING

Workflow in the HIM department that performs retrospective processing begins when the patient is discharged from the facility. How does the HIM director decide which functions are performed first? Traditionally, health records were collected, organized, assembled, analyzed, coded, abstracted, completed, and filed (Figure 13-5). Workflow depends on the priorities set within the department. Specifically, the productivity standards for a function may require that one function be performed before another. For instance, if the department is motivated to code the health record within 24 hours of the patient's discharge, the coding function may need to take place before the analysis, and coding may be separated from the abstract function to promote coders' productivity.

CONCURRENT PROCESSING

In concurrent health information processing, the assembly, analysis, coding, and abstracting of the health record occurs while the patient is in the facility. For example, analysis (e.g., review for signatures, forms, content) of the documentation in the health record is performed on the patient care unit. Concurrent analysis of health information is designed to have an impact on the quality of patient care by promoting timely, accurate, and complete documentation of patient health information.

Which functions occur first during concurrent analysis: coding, abstracting, assembly, or analysis? Priority is ultimately determined by the goals and objectives of the HIM department (discussed later in the chapter). The performance of concurrent analysis can include several scenarios. One situation may involve employees' being physically relocated to the patient care units. Another scenario may involve sending HIM employees to the patient care unit to perform the analysis and then report back to the department for follow-up or further processing. One example of this approach is when the HIM clerk goes to the patient care unit to check the chart of each patient who was admitted the previous day. Using the admission report from the previous day, the clerk is able to identify the location of each patient and go to the location to review the chart for the history and physical, physician order signatures, and so on.

Regardless of the method, productivity standards must also be designed to ensure timely processing. Table 13-4 provides an example of the productivity standards for concurrent processing in an HIM department.

ELECTRONIC RECORD PROCESSING

Processing of health information in the computer-based patient record (CPR) environment changes the HIM workflow previously mentioned. The CPR system consists of intelligent computer soft-

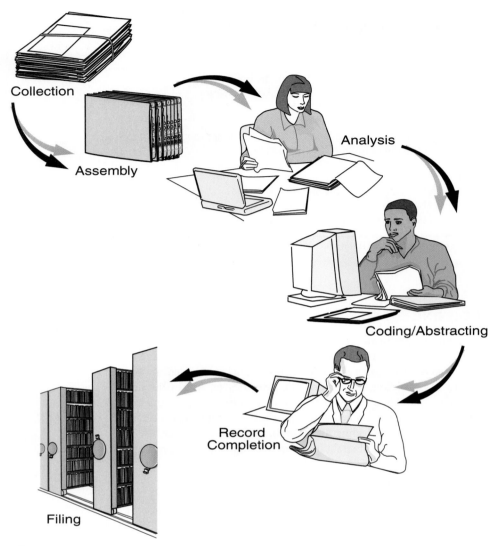

Collection

Assembly

Analysis

Coding/Abstracting

Record
Completion

Filing

◆ **Figure 13-5**
Retrospective processing of health information.

TABLE 13-4	Typical Concurrent Processing Standards*
FUNCTION	**EXAMPLE OF CONCURRENT PROCESSING STANDARD**
Analysis	Initial analysis for patient signatures, forms, history and physical, and physical signatures completed within the first 24 hours of the patient's stay; routine (daily) analysis performed until the patient's discharge
Coding and abstracting	Initial coding performed during the first 24-48 hours of the patient's stay; updated periodically during the patient's stay, as the patient's condition warrants; final coding completed after discharge
Transcription	
History and physical	Transcribed within 12 hours of dictation
Consults	Transcribed within 12 hours of dictation
Operative reports	Transcribed within 6 hours of dictation
Discharge summary	Transcribed within 24 hours of dictation

*Note: These standards are for example only; standards may vary depending upon process.

ware capable of recognizing patient record information and identifying any problems. A system that recognizes the requirements of a timely, accurate, and complete health record removes the need for an employee to review the clinical documentation. The system prompts the users when information is contradictory, incomplete, or required. The CPR system negates or limits the need for quantitative analysis, assuming that the computer recognizes pertinent information. However, analysis of the CPR requires the technical skills of the registered health information technician (RHIT). System maintenance, design, and analysis are part of a process that requires the knowledge of accreditation requirements, coding guidelines, and the clinical aspects of patient care. In fact, the function is likely to resemble that of an auditor or database manager.

Who decides which processing system is best suited for the HIM department? What if a facility would like to change from one processing system to another? These questions are best answered in a discussion on department planning.

Exercise 13-3

Health Information Management Department Workflow

1. List the HIM functions in retrospective processing.
2. _____ is the amount of work produced by an employee in a given time frame.
3. Processing of the health care record after patient discharge is called
   a. retrospective processing
   b. concurrent processing
   c. HIM processing
   d. analysis
4. Processing of the health care record during patient care is called
   a. retrospective processing
   b. concurrent processing
   c. HIM processing
   d. analysis
5. One method of monitoring the amount of work an employee performs is
   a. reviewing the organization chart
   b. reviewing the productivity report
   c. monitoring payroll
   d. limiting employee breaks

DEPARTMENT PLANNING

Planning is a tool used by the HIM department to prepare for the future. Everyone plans for the future; the difference, however, is that some people plan more than others, and some plans are more formal and elaborate than others. Some department plans are formal, written documents; others may be informal, depending on the size, type, or philosophy of the facility. For example, the workflow in a department is a plan (discussed, in the section on the prioritization of department functions). Before employees begin performing the functions of assembly, analysis, and coding, HIM managers must plan to ensure that the work flows smoothly and the department achieves optimal productivity.

The HIM department may also plan for changes or improvements. Managers can plan to implement a new procedure—for example, concurrent coding, purging records, or converting the filing method from straight numerical to terminal digit—or they can plan for optimal use of space. Planning involves analyzing the current situation, determining the goal (i.e, what is to be achieved or accomplished), and designing a strategy to accomplish the goal.

A plan is a guide that describes the manner in which events are expected to take place in the department. For a more thorough explanation of planning, the following example describes a plan to implement the concurrent analysis process.

First consider the following questions: What type of analysis will be performed concurrently? Will it be quantitative, qualitative, or both? Let's begin with quantitative analysis. What do you hope to accomplish by doing this concurrent analysis? You must first analyze how quantitative analysis is presently performed and the effect that it has. Ideally, health records are analyzed within 24 hours of discharge. This means that the first day after a patient's discharge, someone from the HIM department retrieves all discharge records, checks them into the department, assembles them according to the facility policy, and attaches them to a folder marked with the appropriate medical record number for the patient. In concurrent analysis, analysis of patient records begins on the first day of the patient's stay, and then the records are analyzed daily until the patient is discharged.

In health care facilities, formal planning is done annually. This planning is sometimes called *strategic planning* because this is the time when the organization develops a plan of action or strategy for the coming year. Plans are normally guided by the mission or vision of the entire organization.

MISSION

A **mission** statement is a declaration of the organization's purpose. Traditionally, the organization's mission statement shows care and concern for those whom it serves. A mission statement is very important to an organization because it provides a common purpose, which helps the organization unify to serve its community as a team with a specific direction. An example is the mission statement for Diamonte Hospital (our hypothetical acute care facility): "Diamonte Hospital provides high-quality health care through dedication and commitment to excellence."

HIM departments may also have a mission. For example, the HIM department of Diamonte Hospital exists to provide efficient, high-quality health information to all customers to promote high-quality health care in the organization. The mission of the department should be in line with the mission for the entire facility. The following is the mission statement for the HIM department of Diamonte Hospital: "The Health Information Management Department of Diamonte Hospital exists to provide timely, complete, confidential, and secure health information to all users."

VISION

Another common element to be considered when planning in an organization or department is a **vision.** A vision is a statement of what the organization is expected to become, a statement that is above and beyond the mission. For example, the vision may state that while the purpose (mission) is to provide high-quality patient care and to exceed customers' expectations, the vision is to become the leading health care provider in the community. By definition, a vision means unusual foresight or a vivid imaginative conception (*Random House Webster's School and Office Dictionary* 1995). A vision for the HIM department might be to implement a CPR; this would be in line with the vision of the organization, if part of the success of quality patient care and becoming the leading health care provider in the community requires a CPR system.

GOALS AND OBJECTIVES

The goals and objectives of the HIM department are typically more recognizable than its mission and vision statements. The department's goals and objectives should complement the organization's mission and vision. In other words, if the organization is committed to quality, then the HIM goals and objectives should address and support quality. The purpose of the goals and objectives is to keep the department focused and provide a guide for improvement.

Managing the daily operations in an HIM department can be an all-consuming task. Therefore HIM departments annually set **goals** to accomplish new or improved functions. Goals are statements that provide the department with direction or focus. Goals state that the

TABLE 13-5	HIM Department Goals and Objectives*

GOALS	OBJECTIVES
1. Maintain continuous compliance with JCAHO accreditation standards for timely record completion.	1a. The monthly number of delinquent health records will be less than 50% of the average monthly discharges (AMD). 1b. The number of delinquent history and physical records will not exceed 1%. 1c. The number of delinquent operative reports will not exceed 1%.
2. Transcription services will facilitate compliance with JCAHO requirement for timeliness of documentation regarding history and physical records, discharge summary records, consults, and operative reports.	2a. History and physical records will be transcribed within 6 hours of dictation. 2b. Consultation reports will be transcribed within 12 hours of dictation. 2c. Operative reports will be transcribed within 12 hours of dictation. 2d. Discharge summaries will be transcribed within 24 hours of dictation.

*These goals are for example only; they are not all-inclusive.

department will strive to achieve something new. Goals can be annual, short-term, or long-term. Examples of goals for HIM department are listed in Table 13-5.

To reach a goal, the department sets **objectives** to direct how the goal will be achieved. Objectives determine what must be accomplished to achieve the goal. Typically, when the objectives are accomplished, the goal is attained. In this text, each chapter has learning objectives. By reading the chapter, you should be able to complete the objectives. Table 13-5 provides some examples of HIM department objectives.

BUDGET

In addition to managing an efficient and effective HIM department, the HIM director (and supervisors) is responsible for the HIM budget. There are several different types of budget, but for the purposes of this discussion, only capital and operational budgets are pertinent. The capital budget is money set aside to purchase items that are over a certain dollar limit. For example, any purchase over $1500 may be considered a capital purchase item and would need to be part of the capital budget. The specific dollar amount varies depending on the organization. New software for implementation of the electronic health record is an example of an item that may be considered a capital budget item.

The operational budget includes those items necessary to run the department. It includes expenses such as, supply costs, maintenance contract expenses, and utilities. The budget is calculated for a 12-month period, or 1 year. This year, also known as the *fiscal year,* is not always identical to a January-through-December calendar year. For example, a fiscal year may run July 1 through June 30, or October 1 through September 30.

Typically, each department in the organization is responsible for developing and presenting its budget or budgets to the financial administrators for approval. The capital budget is approved separately from the operational budget. Fortunately, when planning for the next year, the department managers are able to use the budget from the previous and current year. This information allows the manager to make sound decisions regarding the proposed budget, which is important because the manager will be held accountable for staying within the budget that is approved for his or her department. The budget contains an estimate for revenue each month and allows the department a set amount of money for each expense (e.g., supplies, employee salaries, contracts). The HIM department is not typically a revenue-generating department.

HIM Department Budget – July (month 7 of Fiscal Year)					
	Budget	YTD-Budget	Actual	YTD-Actual	Difference
Revenue:					
Expenses:					
Salaries	$12000	$84000	$11458	$82880	($1120) or 1.3%
Supplies	$250	$1750	$308	$1800	$50 or −2.9%
Maintenance contract					
Copy machine	$500	$3500	$500	$3500	0%

◆ **Figure 13-6**
HIM Department Budget for July (Month 7 of fiscal year).

However, exceptions exist (e.g., a department that collects charges for copying and ROI or one that offers its transcription or coding services to area physicians for a fee).

Each month, the director (and supervisors) must compare the actual expenses and revenue (if any) with the budgeted expenses and revenue. Figure 13-6 displays limited budget items for the HIM department during the month of July. An actual budget report would include many more line items or expenses. The budget column displays the amount allocated for the particular corresponding expense. The column labeled *actual* displays the actual amount of money spent during the month of July for the corresponding expense. Notice that this information, budget and actual, is also displayed for year to date (YTD) expenses. The YTD information allows the manager to determine whether the budget is being met for the year. This is helpful because sometimes 1 month's expenses will be more or less than the actual budget, and knowing the YTD expenses helps the manager determine whether they will meet the budget for the entire year. The last column displays the difference, or the actual amount that the department is over or under budget.

PRIORITIZATION OF DEPARTMENT FUNCTIONS

Now that you understand the importance of planning for both the facility and the HIM department, you are ready to consider the prioritization of department functions. Prioritization of health information functions can occur once the department has established its goals and objectives. Earlier in the chapter, Table 13-3 provided a list of potential HIM department standards. Standards for department functions are necessary to keep the information flowing. For example, in this textbook HIM functions were discussed in the following order: assembly, analysis, or postdischarge processing (Chapter 5), filing (Chapter 8), and coding (Chapter 6). However, depending on your planning, coding may actually be a function that you want to occur very early in the workflow. Typically, assembly and analysis are the first tasks that you want to accomplish because they organize the record for future processing, especially coding and record completion. An organized record helps coders find the information that they need to assign appropriate codes. The HIM director also wants to make sure that the records are analyzed for deficiencies (i.e., quantitative analysis) as quickly as possible because a record is considered delinquent 30 days after discharge, according to JCAHO requirements. The longer it takes for HIM staff to analyze a record, the less time is available to get the record completed by a physician. The department also sets standards for functions such as ROI and transcription. Timely completion of requests for

Exercise 13-4

Department Planning

1. For the 2005 to 2006 fiscal year, the manager has set a _____ to implement a document imaging system.
2. To reach a desired goal, the department must establish _____, directions for achieving a goal.
3. The purpose of the organization documented in a formal statement is known as the _____.
4. Above and beyond the mission statement, _____ sets a direction for the organization for the future.
5. The HIM director established the following: "The HIM department delinquency percentage will not exceed 50% of average monthly discharges by July 1." This is an example of a(n)
   a. plan
   b. goal
   c. objective
   d. mission
6. In addition, the director stated that the suspension procedure will be performed weekly (as approved in the bylaws). This is an example of a(n)
   a. plan
   b. goal
   c. objective
   d. mission
7. The HIM department is allowed $300 per month for supplies. At the end of the third quarter, the department has spent $3000 on supplies. This means that the HIM department is
   a. under budget YTD by $300
   b. over budget YTD by $300
   c. exactly as it should be on budget for supplies
   d. over budget $250
8. Diamonte Hospital's fiscal year runs July 1 through June 30. Which of the following months are in the third quarter?
   a. January, February, March
   b. April, May, June
   c. July, August, September
   d. October, November, December

ROI can affect continuity of patient care and possibly reimbursement (if the request is related to payment). The transcription section processes the dictated patient health information into a report that is used in communication and decision making during patient care. Timely completion of this function affects patient care.

Department standards set the framework for efficient and effective management of health information. The standards direct the employees within the department workflow to accomplish their tasks in a timely manner. Sometimes, the task directly affects patient care; at other times, the task is part of department workflow. Standards can then be used to evaluate the function of the HIM department.

EVALUATION OF DEPARTMENT OPERATIONS AND SERVICES

It is important that supervisors and managers continually evaluate their departments according to department goals, objectives, and standards. In other words, because goals, objectives, and standards create an environment that promotes the efficient flow of health information, HIM managers use these organizational tools to monitor department progress. If the standard is to assemble and analyze records within 24 hours, then the HIM manager wants to make sure that his or her employees are doing that. Evaluation of goals and objectives takes place annually, but employee-specific productivity should be evaluated at least monthly to ensure quality in the HIM department. (See the discussion on monitoring the quality of health information in Chapter 10.)

HIM managers and supervisors continually monitor the effectiveness and efficiency of the department through employee productivity reports and through quality assurance monitoring. These measures alert the supervisors to any problems. Significant problems can then be addressed as necessary through employee training, performance improvement, or quality improvement efforts.

DEPARTMENT POLICIES AND PROCEDURES

The policies and procedures of a health care facility are documented in paper or computer format so that the employees, customers, accreditation agencies, licensing bodies, regulatory agencies, and legal authorities can recognize the philosophy and methods under which the facility operates. A **policy** is a statement, in broad terms, of what the facility does on a routine basis. For example, a policy might require that a health record be maintained for every patient treated in this facility. The **procedure** is the process of how the policy is carried out. For example, a procedure might require that an assembly clerk retrieve all discharge records from the nursing units immediately following the patients' discharge. Policies and procedures provide details about the following:

- How, when, and why things are done
- Who performs which tasks, jobs, and functions
- Who is responsible for an activity, an authorization, and so forth
- Quality controls and audits
- Historical, routine, and emergency situations

Policies and procedures go together, and indeed they are often documented on the same form. Figure 13-7 shows an example of the previously mentioned policy—that is, a health record is maintained for every patient treated in this facility.

The entire health care organization has policies and procedures that affect everyone in the facility. Each department in the health care facility should have specific policies and procedures that outline their processes, responsibilities, and services. All employees of the facility must have access to the policy and procedures manual. The HIM department manual contains policies and procedures that relate specifically to health information. Figure 13-8 contains a list of contents for an HIM department Policy and Procedures manual.

For example, a policy in the HIM department for coding and abstracting of medical records might read as follows: "The HIM department will maintain accurate diagnosis and procedure indices. The HIM department will maintain appropriate indices by accurately coding all diagnoses and procedures found in the patient's medical records." The procedure then details how coders should go through these records and pull out the primary diagnoses and primary procedures and how they should assign the codes. It should also stipulate or explain how the information is entered into a computer system (e.g., how data are collected for compilation of a patient abstract).

The policy manual is a very important tool. The policies and procedures must be accessible to all members of the organization as necessary for the performance of their jobs. Therefore it is possible to place all policies and procedures on a computerized system, accessible to all employees,

---

Hit-Bit

Computerized Policies and Procedures

Special consideration for a facility's policies in the computerized environment includes securing access to prevent unauthorized people from making changes to policies. It is also important to have a paper copy of the policy statements in case the computer is inaccessible.

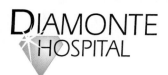

DIAMONTE HOSPITAL

Diamonte, Arizona 89104 ▪ TEL. 602-484-9991

Health Information Management Department
Policy No. 3.01
Health Record Creation and Definition, Unit Medical Record
 Number Assignment

Effective: 01/15/2004   **Reviewed:** 01/2005, 01/2006

Approved:

Policy:

The Health Information Management Department will maintain a health record for all patients receiving treatment at Diamonte Hospital. The record will be kept in accordance with state, federal, accreditation, and professional guidelines. Each patient record will be identified using a unit numbering system.

Procedure:

1. Upon registration at Diamonte Hospital for any service, the patient will be assigned a medical record number and a health record will be initiated.

2. During the patient visit, health information shall be documented in a timely manner on approved facility forms.

3. Following discharge, all patient records will be collected by the Health Information Management Department.

4. The Health Information Management clerk will use the daily ADT (Admission-Discharge-Transfer) reports to verify collection of **all** health records.

5. Records not retrieved the day following discharge will be reported to the Health Information Supervisor immediately, for appropriate action.

Example Policy Only

◆ **Figure 13-7**
Policy and procedure for maintenance of health records for all patients receiving care in a facility.

allowing them to consult the policies on an as-needed basis. This format is attractive to many employees because policy binders on a shelf are often overlooked or even disregarded. The computer is a new avenue for bringing information to the employee. Increasingly, a facility's policies and procedures are being placed on the facility's Web site. This function allows employees and others to view the policies of the facility from the convenience of their homes or offices.

The HIM department director is responsible for ensuring that the departmental policies and procedures are current. This is accomplished by making sure that policies exist for all necessary functions, responsibilities, and services under his or her control. All policies and procedures should be reviewed annually and as significant changes occur in procedures, regulations, or legislation. Review is as simple as reading through each policy and procedure to verify that the contents are accurate, then initialing and dating the review to authenticate the review.

Exercise 13-5

Department Policies and Procedures

1. The following is _____of Diamonte Hospital, an equal opportunity employer: All new hires will be drug tested.
2. A process that describes how to comply with a policy is a _____ .
3. To maintain a high-quality HIM department, the supervisors and managers should
    a. monitor employee dress code
    b. continually evaluate the functions of the HIM department on the basis of the goals and standards set
    c. convert to concurrent processing
    d. never promote from within
4. Policy and Procedures should be
    a. reviewed annually
    b. updated as necessary in accordance with changes in policy or procedure
    c. maintained in an area or manner accessible to all employees
    d. all of the above
5. The HIM department is the only department in the organization that has a policy and procedures manual.
    a. True
    b. False
6. Policy and Procedures should be updated
    a. annually and as needed due to change
    b. only as needed due to change
    c. by the CEO
    d. by the nursing administrator

HEALTH INFORMATION PERSONNEL

Now that you understand how the workflow is organized in the HIM department, it is time to consider the way in which job functions are organized. In the following sections, the organization of the health information functions is discussed in terms of job descriptions with performance standards that communicate the manager's expectation of the employee. Hiring practices and priorities are also discussed.

JOB ANALYSIS

Job analysis is the review of a particular function (e.g., assembly) to determine all of the tasks or components that make up an employee's job. A job analysis is an effective way to assist in the review or creation of an employee job description. When a job analysis is performed, the job tasks are reviewed to ensure that the process works effectively so that employees are not omitting important steps. A job analysis can also ensure that the employee's job fits into the department workflow appropriately. It is important to have the right employee performing the appropriate function at the right time in order to move the work through the HIM department.

Job analysis can be performed by a supervisor or manager working with the employee; together, they review and perform the employee's job function. As the supervisor works with the employee, he or she is able to determine the procedures performed by the employee. The supervisor must document the procedures as performed by the employee so that they can be reviewed in total. Following the supervisor's review of the employee's job (which can take a few hours or even an entire day), the supervisor has actual information with which to develop a job description and performance standards.

Hit-Bit

From Job Analysis to Job Description

If you have involved the employee in a job analysis, the employee should review the job's functions and responsibilities when the job description is complete.

Another effective way to perform a job analysis is to involve the employee by asking the employee to explain how he or she performs the job by using a data collection device. Figure 13-9 is an example of a tool that can be used by the employee to analyze his or her job. The employee uses this form to communicate to the manager in detail what the job involves on a daily basis, using his or her own words. This is similar to having the employee list the job functions on a sheet of paper.

JOB DESCRIPTION

Once the job analysis is complete, it is possible to organize the employee's tasks into a **job description.** The job description is a list of the employee's responsibilities. Each position and employee in the department should have a job description. The job description communicates the expectations of the manager. If an old job description needs to be updated, it is appropriate to give the employee a copy of the current job description for review and updating. Allow the employee to review the job description. This involvement gives the employee an opportunity to see how the job has changed. Job descriptions should be reviewed annually by managers and employees. Employees sign the job description to acknowledge their awareness of their responsibilities and the job functions.

Writing a Job Description

A job description contains several key elements that describe the job specifically. The job description has a heading that briefly describes the position. The heading should include the facility in which the position is located, the title of the position, the supervisor for the position, and the effective date of the job description (Figure 13-10). The remainder of the job description includes information regarding hours worked, the purpose of the job, job responsibilities, description of the environment in which the work is performed, and the abilities or skills that the employee must have to perform job duties or the Americans with Disabilities Act (ADA) requirements.

The job description also contains any numbers, grades, and classification (exempt or nonexempt) used by the human resources department or the organization to describe that position. The job description begins with a statement of the position's duties and responsibilities, explaining who the employee reports to or what type of supervision occurs. Following this statement is a list of the job tasks or functions. A complete job description makes it easier to complete performance standards.

Performance Standards

The job description should include **performance standards.** Performance standards tell the employee how much work should be accomplished within a specific time frame. Additionally, performance standards let the employee know that quality is evaluated in the performance of the job: It is not only important for the employee to complete the job, but the work must be done correctly. Performance standards include requirements for accuracy and quality. Performance standards are used to evaluate the employee after the probationary period, annually, or for merit increases or promotion.

Performance standards must be related to the job description and the productivity required within the department. Table 13-6 provides a list of performance standards relating to the job

Diamonte Health Information Management Department Policy and Procedure Manual	
Table of Contents	
Section 1	**Introduction**
1.01	Purpose
1.02	Responsibility for policy development, update, and approval
1.03	Distribution and access of policies
1.04	Diamonte mission statement
1.05	Diamonte organization chart
1.06	Health information management department mission statement and organization chart
Section 2	**General Department Policies**
2.01	Centralized health information management department
2.02	Scope of service
2.03	Hours of operation
2.04	Confidentiality, privacy, and data security considerations
2.05	Confidentiality statement
2.06	Department orientation
2.07	Training and education of department employees
2.08	Employee competency
2.09	General policies of the health information management department
2.10	Health information management department organization chart
Section 3	**The Health Record**
3.01	Creation and definition, unit medical record number assignment
3.02	Ownership of the health record
3.03	Guidelines for entries into the health record
3.04	Abbreviations list
3.05	Fax copies in the health record
3.06	Completion of discharge summaries
Section 4	**Assembly and Analysis**
4.01	Health record assembly and chart order
4.02	Retrospective record analysis
Section 5	**Storage, Access, and Security**
5.01	Health record storage system
5.02	Security of health information
5.03	Confidentiality and security of computerized information
5.04	Retention schedule for health records and related documents

◆ **Figure 13-8**

Contents of the HIM Department Policy and Procedures Manual.

description shown in Figure 13-10. The employee's performance standard includes a scale that explains how each score is achieved.

Performance standards establish a time frame in which the employee's work is to be completed. For example, the birth certificate clerk is responsible for completing a birth certificate for all newborn admissions according to the facility's policy and state law. Performance standards for this requirement might be stated as follows: "A birth certificate is completed on all newborn admissions according to facility policy and state law prior to the newborn's discharge. If at any time a birth certificate is not completed before the newborn is discharged, the employee has not met the standard, thereby affecting the employee's performance rating."

Employee performance affects the productivity of the entire department. Therefore the standards are developed specifically for each position to ensure that each employee's performance promotes effective and efficient progress in the HIM department.

5.05	Procedure to access health records
5.06	Health record locations
5.07	Removal of health records from the health information management department
5.08	Destruction of records
Section 6	**Record Completion**
6.01	Incomplete chart/record completion process
6.02	Notification of incomplete health records for physicians
6.03	Suspension process
Section 7	**Release of Information**
7.01	General policies for release of information
7.02	Consent for release of information
7.03	Notice of recipient of information, disclosure laws
7.04	Patient's right to health information, copies of health records
7.05	Copy and retrieval fees
Section 8	**Quality of Health Information**
8.01	Monitoring and evaluation of quality in the health information management department
8.02	Record review process/clinical pertinence
8.03	Compliance with regulations and standards
Use of Contract Services or Agencies–Business Associate Agreements	
Job Descriptions	
Safety in the Health Information Management Department	
Materials Safety Data Sheets (MSDS)	

◆ **Figure 13-8 (*cont'd*)**

EMPLOYEE PRODUCTIVITY

Now that you understand a typical HIM employee's job responsibility and how the job is evaluated, you can develop a form or tool to collect information that appropriately supports the employee's evaluation. This method involves collecting information about the employee's performance and **productivity.** There are several ways that this information can be collected: manually, by observation, or by using computerized reports from computer applications. The goal is to have an objective tool that reflects the amount of work performed by the employee. Later, the accuracy and quality of the employee's work can be assessed by sample review of his or her work.

MANUAL PRODUCTIVITY REPORTS

Manual productivity reports can be designed to obtain information about the employee's performance. Figure 13-11 gives a sample form for collection of data on the productivity of a coding employee.

This form contains information to identify the employee, the time frame in which the information is collected, and specifics about the employee's job. Because the employee in our example is responsible for inpatient coding, the form shown in Figure 13-11 collects information about the number of records coded each day. In addition, the form collects information about activities related to the employee's job, including conversations with physicians, problems with chart documentation, and other activities as they occur.

Employee: _____Tim Tall_____
Position: _____file clerk_____
Hours worked: __8:00AM–4:30PM__

Use this form to communicate your job duties or daily routine. Use the comments section to document any unusual occurrences.

	Monday	Tuesday	Wednesday	Thursday	Friday
7:30AM					
8:00AM	Locate charts for coders				
8:30AM					
9:00AM					
9:30AM					
10:00AM					
10:30AM	Organize files				
11:00AM	File				
11:30AM					
12:00noon					
12:30PM					
1:00PM					
1:30PM					
2:00PM					
2:30PM					
3:00PM					
3:30PM					
4:00PM					
4:30PM					
5:00PM					

Comments: _Periodically answer phone calls and bring charts to the floor._

◆ **Figure 13-9**
Job analysis tool.

This form can be developed by reviewing the job description and creating categories for each responsibility. The employee uses the form to collect statistics regarding his or her job performance. The completed form is turned in to the supervisor. The supervisor is then able to review the employee's productivity against the job's performance standards. This information, collected on a regular basis, provides a picture of the employee's job performance for the entire review period. Routine collection of this information over time provides a larger picture of the employee's performance so that the evaluation is not skewed in one direction toward his or her performance over a limited time period.

TABLE 13-6	Performance Standards*	
EMPLOYEE/POSITION	**STANDARD**	**PERFORMANCE RATING SCALE**
Coder	All health records will be coded within 48-72 hours of patient discharge.	Exceeds expectations: 36 or more records coded daily Meets expectations: 28-35 records coded daily Does not meet expectations: Fewer than 28 records coded daily *Supervisor uses daily productivity reports to average the coder's performance*
Coder	Health records will be assigned appropriate and accurate codes according to applicable coding guidelines.	Exceeds expectations: 96%-100% of records reviewed coded appropriately and accurately Meets expectations: 90%-95% of records reviewed coded appropriately and accurately Does not meet expectations: Less than 90% of records reviewed coded appropriately and accurately *Supervisor will review a representative sample of the coder's work to ensure appropriateness and accuracy of coding.*
Assembly/analysis clerk	All patient health records will be assembled and analyzed within 24 hours of patient discharge.	Exceeds expectations: 95%-100% of all records assembled and analyzed within 24 hours of patient discharge Meets expectations: 85%-95% or all records assembled and analyzed within 24 hours of patient discharge Does not meet expectations: Less than 85% of all records assembled and analyzed within 24 hours of patient discharge *Supervisor will routinely assess and document the clerks' productivity to determine score.*
File clerk	Accurate filing of all patient health records will be completed daily.	Exceeds expectations: 100% of all health records filed accurately on a daily basis Meets expectations: 96%-99% of all health records filed accurately on a daily basis Does not meet expectations: Less than 96% of all health records filed accurately on a daily basis *Supervisor will perform routine checks of filing area to determine accuracy; results will be documented to determine file clerk's score.*

* Note: These standards vary in each facility.

COMPUTERIZED PRODUCTIVITY REPORTS

Some of the functions in the HIM department are performed in a computer system that produces a productivity report. The report is maintained by the computer system as the employee logs on to the system and completes job tasks. Some computerized reports not only tell the supervisor how much work is performed but also indicate the time frame in which the work was done. With regard to our coding example, coders are often expected to code a specific number of records within an hourly time frame (i.e., six to eight charts per hour). The software system used by the coders keeps track of productivity without additional effort from the coder.

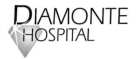

JOB DESCRIPTION

Health Information Management Department
Position Title: Birth Certificate Clerk

Position #: 070530	**Grade:** G2
Reports to: Clerical Supervisor	**Effective:** 01/15/2007

Position Description: Under the general supervision of the Clerical Supervisor, the Birth Certificate Clerk completes a birth certificate, and supporting forms as necessary, for each baby born at Diamonte Hospital. The birth certificates are electronically submitted to the Office of Vital Records, and original certificates with signatures are mailed to the Office of Vital Records in a timely manner. The clerk must maintain a current knowledge of the rules regarding birth certificates. The Birth Certificate Clerk is a member of the Health Information Management department team and maintains knowledge of various other functions in the department to assist as necessary.

Position Qualifications:

Education:	High school diploma
Licensure/Certification/Registration:	None necessary
Experience:	Excellent communication skills. Ability to type 30 WPM. Previous clerical experience preferred. Ability to function in busy office environment with multiple shifting and evolving priorities.

Responsibilities:

1. Monitors Labor and Delivery log and Admission reports to identify all patients requiring a birth certificate.

2. Collects birth certificate information from parent(s) and completes birth certificate accurately. Parent(s) review birth certificate to verify accuracy and sign in appropriate areas.

3. Maintains current knowledge of all birth certificate rules, regulations, and issues. Reviews and implements state laws governing completion of birth certificates.

4. Ensures completion of other forms relating to the birth as necessary, e.g., paternity, social security verification.

5. Maintains current and accurate birth certificate log.

6. Contacts any parents who have left the hospital prior to completion of the birth certificate. Processes new, delayed, or corrected birth certificates.

7. Obtains physician signature on the birth certificate within 1 week of completion.

8. Submits electronic birth certificates immediately following completion, mailing completed original certificate within 15 days of completion.

9. Maintains electronic birth certificate software in working condition; performs backups regularly.

10. Follows established policies and procedures regarding confidentiality and security of health information, infection control, safety and security management, and emergency preparedness.

◆ **Figure 13-10**
Job description.

 E**MPLOYEE** E**VALUATIONS**

Employee evaluations allow management to provide feedback to the employee on the basis of the employee's job performance. Feedback is an important aspect of a manager's communication with employees. The evaluation entails one-on-one communication from the manager about an employee's job performance. Evaluations should be performed at the end of the probationary period and annually thereafter for each employee. Sometimes, the employee's annual evaluation

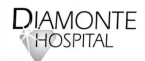

JOB DESCRIPTION, continued

Health Information Management Department
Position Title: Birth Certificate Clerk

Position #: 070530	**Grade:** G2
Reports to: Clerical Supervisor	**Effective:** 01/15/2007

11. Displays a positive and courteous manner toward patients, visitors, customers, and coworkers.

12. Follows all policies and procedures of the facility and HIM department.

13. Completes annual employee in-service and required department training.

Physical Requirements:

Mental and emotional requirements: Employee must be able to manage stress appropriately, work independently, handle multiple priorities.

Working conditions: Employee spends approximately 90% of time inside the health care facility. The work area has adequate lighting, good ventilation, comfortable temperature. Employee work station provided with appropriate access to rest rooms and lunch and break areas.

Physical demands: Employee is responsible for light work—lifting maximum of 20 lb, with frequent lifting or carrying of objects weighing up to 10 lb. Work positions include sitting 50%, standing 20%, walking 20%, lifting/carrying 10%.

Example only

◆ **Figure 13-10 (*cont'd*)**

is tied to a merit pay increase. The result of an evaluation can determine whether an employee receives a 1%, 2%, or 5% increase in pay, and occasionally it affects an employee's promotion.

Routine feedback to employees about their job performance improves effectiveness if there is a problem and makes the employee performance evaluation go more smoothly because the necessary information has been gathered over the entire evaluation period (i.e., over the course of an entire year). If the manager does not gather information over the course of the entire evaluation

	M	Tu	W	Th	F	M	Tu	W	Th	F	M	Tu	W	Th	F	M	Tu	W	Th	F
Coder: _____ **Month/year:** _____																				
Date																				
Inpatient																				
Medicare																				
Non-Medicare																				
Outpatient																				
Observation/surgeries																				
Diagnostics																				
Emergency room																				
Hours worked																				
Physician contacts																				
Other (please comment below)																				
Comments:																				

◆ **Figure 13-11**
Coding productivity sheet.

Hit-Bit

Employee Evaluation

The employee evaluation is not the first communication that the employee receives regarding his or her job performance. Employees are given performance expectations and performance standards when they receive a copy of their job description. Routine communication between the employee and the supervisor should indicate whether the employee's performance is acceptable. The employee evaluation should not be the first occasion on which an employee learns that he or she is not meeting expectations. The manager or supervisor should regularly communicate with the employees, especially when their performance is unacceptable. Poor communication by the management can negatively affect functions in the HIM department.

period and waits instead until the evaluation is due to complete it, the manager may be able to recall only the most recent incidents. If these are not favorable, the manager may not consider the employee's positive performance during the entire evaluation period. In other words, employees should be receiving regular feedback (positive or negative) from the supervisor. Because they have a job description and understand the productivity expectations, evaluations should not be a surprise to employees.

The employee evaluation should be performed in person by the employee's direct supervisor. If at all possible, the employee should sit down with his or her manager to discuss the evaluation; this is an excellent opportunity for feedback and communication. The employee evaluation is the formal summary of the employee's performance (as required in the performance standards) for the evaluation period. It is documented and maintained in the human resource department, and a copy is kept in the employees file maintained by the HIM manager.

Hit-Bit

PIP

The acronym *PIP* stands for various things. For example, CMS has a program called PIP, which stands for periodic interim payments. *PIP* might also stand for preferred Internet provider or performance improvement program. When using an abbreviation or acronym, be sure that you understand the meaning in the context in which it is being used.

What occurs if the evaluation is not favorable? Is the employee immediately terminated for poor performance? Typically, an employee who has successfully completed a probationary period and later performs poorly is put on a **performance improvement plan (PIP).** The PIP informs the employee of the poor performance and describes the consequences of not performing according to the acceptable standards (i.e., termination of employment).

Exercise 13-6

Employee Evaluations

1. A formal list of the employee's responsibilities associated with their job is called a _____.
2. _____ are set guidelines explaining how much work an employee must complete.
3. A _____ involves the review of a function to determine all of the tasks or components that make up an employee's job.
4. Performance standards measure
   a. quantity
   b. quality
   c. A and B
   d. number of employees
5. The job description must contain information about the work environment and the necessary skills and abilities that the employee must have to complete the job. These statements are known as the
   a. salary information
   b. OSHA requirements
   c. ADA information
   d. performance standards
6. The _____ is an opportunity for management to provide feedback to the employee on the basis of the employee's performance.
7. Explain the best method of delivering an employee evaluation.

HIRING HEALTH INFORMATION MANAGEMENT PERSONNEL

Hiring the right employee is a very important task performed by the managers and supervisors in a department. When a person is hired to perform a job, an agreement is made between the organization and the employee. The agreement is that the employee will perform the job required for compensation. Sometimes, finding the right person for the job is quite challenging.

Hit-Bit

Advertising and HIM Associations

Many HIM positions are advertised by word of mouth. Participation in local HIM associations can put you in touch with large numbers of professionals who are potential candidates for open positions in the department.

ADVERTISEMENT

When a position is vacant, whether because the position is new or because someone has resigned, the process of finding a new employee begins. To locate potential candidates for a job, the organization must let others know that the position is open. An open position can be publicized in a number of ways, such as by placing an advertisement in local newspapers, professional journals, or community and association newsletters.

The right advertisement should include all of the qualifications that a candidate should possess. The advertisement must specify how much education is required (e.g., college, high school degree or equivalent) and what type of education (e.g., training in anatomy and physiology, medical terminology, or transcription). The advertisement should also specify (1) the amount of prior experience that a candidate should have, (2) whether the experience needed is specific to a job function or generally related to the HIM field, and (3) the means by which candidates should apply for the position (e.g., by sending a résumé by fax or e-mail or applying in person to the human resources department) (Fig. 13-12). Other information about the position that may be included in the advertisement pertains to employment status: full-time or part-time, the hours worked per week, responsibilities, benefits, and pay scale. Interested candidates should follow the instructions in the advertisement to apply for the position.

APPLICATION

Typically, candidates must complete an application for employment to be considered for a position. All applicants must provide accurate and complete information on this form (Figure 13-13).

Each question on the application must be answered in full. The candidate should not leave any spaces blank, even if he or she believes that the information is covered on the attached résumé. The application should be filled out in ink, and the written portions should be legible and correctly spelled and punctuated. The candidate should always read the question or section carefully before completing the information and carefully consider the best answer before writing it on the application, particularly if it is lengthy or involved. All information must be accurate. References should be current and appropriate; most employers check them before making a final decision. Table 13-7 includes a few suggestions for completing employment applications.

TABLE 13-7	Do's and Don'ts for Filling Out an Employment Application

DO	DON'T
Read the application and question carefully.	Leave sections of the application blank.
Complete the entire application.	Use pencil.
Use ink.	Provide false information.
Write legibly.	
Spell correctly.	

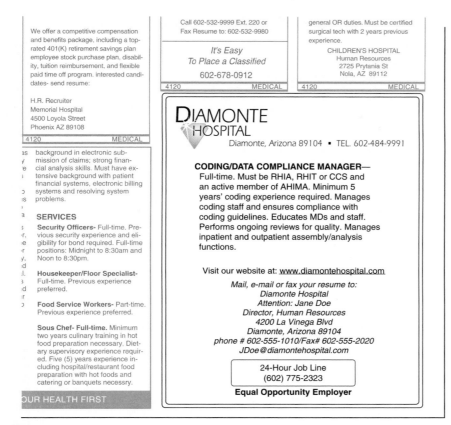

◆ **Figure 13-12**
Newspaper advertisement for HIM personnel.

Hit-Bit

Correspondence to Applicants

For those applicants who are screened but not interviewed, at a minimum, some correspondence should be mailed to the applicants to let them know how their application will be handled. The correspondence may thank candidates for the application before explaining that their qualifications did not match those of the position; in addition, it can inform them that their applications will be kept on file for a specific period in case any future openings occur.

The manager uses the applications to determine who will be interviewed. The applications are carefully reviewed to identify qualified candidates. A legible and complete application is likely to receive a thorough review. Applications that are messy, incomplete, and illegible often receive little attention. Managers review the applications to examine the type of education, training, and experience of each applicant. Those applicants determined to be qualified for the position are contacted for an interview. An applicant should expect that inconsistent, vague, or incomplete information on any part of the application may require further explanation during the interview.

INTERVIEWING

The interview is typically a face-to-face meeting between the applicant and the organization's representative. Each organization has a specific process for performing an interview. Sometimes,

DIAMONTE
HOSPITAL

APPLICATION FOR EMPLOYMENT

This application is not a contract. It is intended to provide information for evaluating your suitability for employment. Please read each question carefully and give an honest and complete answer. Qualified applicants receive consideration for employment without unlawful discrimination because of sex, religion, race, color, national origin, age, disability, or other classification protected by law. Applications will remain active for three months.

PLEASE TYPE OR PRINT ALL INFORMATION

Date: _____

Position(s) applying for: _____

How did you learn about us? ☐ Walk-in ☐ Friend ☐ Relative ☐ Job hotline ☐ Employee ☐ Other
☐ Advertisement (Please state name of publication) _____ Referred by: _____

Name: _____
                   Last   *First*   *Middle initial*

Mailing address: _____
                      City   *State*   *Zip code*

Phone: (____) _____ (____) _____ Social Security #: _____
        Home   *Message*

If related to anyone in our employ, state name and department: _____

If you have been employed under another name, please list here: _____

Are you under 18 years of age?.. ☐ Yes ☐ No

Are you currently employed? .... ☐ Yes ☐ No

May we contact your present employer?.. ☐ Yes ☐ No

Do you have legal rights to work in this country?
  (Proof of legal rights to work in this country will be required upon employment).... ☐ Yes ☐ No

Have you ever been employed with us before? .... ☐ Yes ☐ No *If "yes," give date(s):* _____

Are you available to work: .... ☐ Full-time ☐ Part-time ☐ Shift work ☐ Temporary

Are you available to work overtime if required?...................................... ☐ Yes ☐ No

How flexible are you in accepting varying scheduled hours?.................... ☐ Very flexible ☐ Somewhat flexible
                                                  ☐ Need set schedule

Minimum salary desired: _____

Have you ever been discharged from a job or forced to resign? .... ☐ Yes ☐ No
  Explain: _____

Have you ever been convicted of a felony?
  If "yes," please explain: .... ☐ Yes ☐ No
  Criminal convictions are not an absolute bar to _____
  employment but will be considered with respect
  to the specific requirements of the job for which _____
  you are applying.

◆ **Figure 13-13**
Application for employment.

the applicant is interviewed over the phone or with the human resources department before meeting with the HIM department manager. Other organizations perform a group interview, in which the applicant meets with several different members of the organization at the same time. For the applicant, the interview is an opportunity to learn about the organization and the responsibilities of the position. For the organization, the interview is a way to assess the candidate's qualifications for the position. Interviews may be very formal and structured, informal, or somewhere in between. The interviewer should plan ahead, determine an appropriate location, decide on the style, and write down the questions he or she wants to ask.

All interviews begin with some form of a greeting between the candidate and the interviewer. Experienced interviewers say that they can tell a lot about a candidate within these first few moments. Therefore regardless of your position in the interview process (interviewer or interviewee), be prepared and pay close attention. Greet the other person with a firm handshake, a

EDUCATION

High school: _____ High school graduate/GED: ☐Yes ☐No
_____ Date:_____

College: _____ Graduated: ☐Yes ☐No

Major/field(s) of study: _____ Degree: _____

Date:_____

College: _____ Graduated: ☐Yes ☐No

Major/field(s) of study: _____ Degree: _____

Date:_____

Technical, business, or
correspondence school: _____ Graduated: ☐Yes ☐No

Major/field(s) of study: _____ Degree: _____

Date:_____

Describe any specialized training, apprenticeship, and skills such as computer,
office equipment, etc. _____
_____
_____
_____
_____

LICENSES AND CERTIFICATIONS

Type of license(s)/certification(s): _____ Expiration date: _____

Type of license(s)/certification(s): _____ Expiration date: _____

Type of license(s)/certification(s): _____ Expiration date: _____

Verified by: _____

Date:_____

REFERENCES

(Give name, address, and telephone number of three references that you have known for at least one year who are not
related to you.)

Name: _____ Phone: _____ Years acquainted: _____

Address: _____ Business: _____

Name: _____ Phone: _____ Years acquainted: _____

Address: _____ Business: _____

Name: _____ Phone: _____ Years acquainted: _____

Address: _____ Business: _____

◆ **Figure 13-13** (*cont'd*)

Hit-Bit

The Handshake

The handshake is often part of an introduction. The manner in which you participate in the handshake will make an impression on the other party. A good handshake is assertive and has a firm grip. Try out your handshake on a classmate.

EMPLOYMENT EXPERIENCE

(Please list all employment experience, with most recent employment first. If more space is needed, please use the Additional Employment form.)

Employer: _____   Duties and skills performed:_____

Address: _____   _____

Phone number(s): _____   _____

Job title: _____   _____

Supervisor's name/title: _____   _____

Reason for leaving: _____   _____

Salary received: _____ *hourly / weekly / monthly* _____

Employed from: _____ to _____   _____
         month / year   *month / year*

Employer: _____   Duties and skills performed:_____

Address: _____   _____

Phone number(s): _____   _____

Job title: _____   _____

Supervisor's name/title: _____   _____

Reason for leaving: _____   _____

Salary received: _____ *hourly / weekly / monthly* _____

Employed from: _____ to _____   _____
         month / year   *month / year*

Employer: _____   Duties and skills performed:_____

Address: _____   _____

Phone number(s): _____   _____

Job title: _____   _____

Supervisor's name/title: _____   _____

Reason for leaving: _____   _____

Salary received: _____ *hourly / weekly / monthly* _____

Employed from: _____ to _____   _____
         month / year   *month / year*

Do you expect any of the employers listed above to give you a poor reference? ☐ Yes ☐ No

If yes, explain: _____

_____

◆ **Figure 13-13 (*cont'd*)**

smile, good posture, and pleasantries. Then take your place in the office, either seated at the table or in a chair, and begin the interview.

During the interview in the HIM department, the manager informs the candidate about the position, discussing requirements, environment, and philosophy of the organization or management style. The manager also asks questions to obtain further information about the candidate's qualifications. This exchange gives the candidate and the manager more information with which to develop an opinion about the candidate's suitability for the position. The interview is the opportunity to find out if the candidate is appropriate for the job and a good fit for the department. Figure 13-14 provides a list of the questions often asked during an interview. The same questions are used for each person interviewed for the position.

Although the questions asked in an interview are necessary and inform a manager about a candidate's ability and knowledge, it is often necessary to test the candidate's skills. The inter-

APPLICANT'S STATEMENT

I hereby certify that the statements and information provided are true, and I understand that any false statements or omissions are cause for termination. I agree to submit to a drug test and physical following any conditional offer of employment, and I grant permission to Diamonte Hospital to investigate my criminal history, education, prior employment history, and references, and hereby release all persons or agencies from all liability or any damage for issuing this information.

I understand that this application is current for only **three months**. At the end of that time, if I do not hear from Diamonte Hospital and still wish to be considered for employment, it will be necessary to update my application.

_____   _____
Signature of Applicant   Date

_____
Print Name

DIAMONTE HOSPITAL

◆ **Figure 13-13** (*cont'd*)

viewer must determine whether the candidate can perform the job. For example, if the manager wants to hire a skilled coder, he or she should give real work to the candidate to determine whether the potential coder is capable of handling the work in the organization. Health care workers are also required to pass a criminal background check before being formally offered a position with the organization.

ASSESSMENT

There are at least two different types of applicant assessments—one for skills and the other for aptitude. A skills assessment is designed to identify the applicant's ability to perform the job. The aptitude assessment evaluates the applicant's inclination, intelligence, or appropriateness for a position and the likelihood of his or her fitting into a particular organization or position. The assessment is typically a test given during the interview. Some tests are lengthy. Skills assessments

INTERVIEW QUESTIONS

Tell me a little bit about yourself.

Describe your last job. What did you like or dislike about the job?

What expectations do you have for your supervisor?

Describe your relationship with your former supervisor.

Explain a stressful situation and how you handled it.

What is the one word that best describes you?

Which of your strengths best suit you for this job?

Which of your weaknesses may cause a problem for you in this job?

Do you have any future education goals?

Where do you see yourself in 5 or 10 years?

Are you available to work weekends, evenings, or some holidays?

◆ **Figure 13-14**
Interview questions.

should include exercises that the applicant would encounter on the job; for instance, if the position is for outpatient coding, have the applicant code some of your emergency room or outpatient records. It is not fair practice to assess an applicant with a test that is different from the actual work that he or she will be expected to perform. HIM managers should *always* test the coding skills of an applicant for a coding position and test the typing and terminology skills for a transcription position. Managers and organizations have different screening practices for clerical positions, such as testing filing skills for a file clerk.

OUTSOURCING

It is increasingly common for HIM departments to outsource functions performed within the HIM department. To outsource means to hire a vendor or consultant from outside of the facility to perform the HIM function; another term for this practice may be *to contract out* the function. For example, many facilities use contract coders when they have a backlog or need temporary help during an employee's vacation or sick leave. However some facilities permanently contract out these functions. In other words, they sign a contract for a period of time with a company or consultant who will then perform the function during the contract and bill the facility for the services. The advantage for the facility is the shift of employee management responsibility to the contract company or consultant. The facility holds the company or consultant to the contract, and the company or consultant is responsible for the management of employees performing the function. The facility must be careful to hire a reputable, credible company or consultant and be sure to monitor the outsourced work just as they would that of an on-site employee. Even though a contract exists, the facility remains responsible for the overall quality and integrity of the HIM department.

FAIR EMPLOYMENT PRACTICES

It is extremely important that HIM managers and supervisors comply with appropriate and legal hiring practices. A number of laws pertaining to age, gender, race, religion, and disability affect hiring practices (Table 13-8). Employers must be certain that their hiring practices do not discriminate among candidates. Additionally, employers must be sure that all employees are managed in an appropriate, law-abiding manner.

TABLE 13-8	Employment Laws
LAW	**AREA OF CONCERN**
Age Discrimination in Employment Act (1967)	Protects employees between the ages of 40 and 70 years
Americans with Disabilities Act (ADA) (1990)	Outlaws discrimination against disabled people and ensures reasonable accommodation for them in the workplace
Civil Rights Act (1964)	Prohibits discrimination on the basis of race, color, religion, sex, or national origin and ensures equal employment opportunity
Fair Labor Standards Act (1938)	Sets minimum wage, overtime pay, equal pay, child labor, and record-keeping requirements for employers (Equal Pay Amendment [1963] forbids sex discrimination in pay practices)
Family Medical Leave Act (1993)	Grants unpaid leave and provides job security to employees who must take time off for medical reason for themselves or family members

Modified from Mervat Abdelhak, Sara Grostick, Mary Alice Hanken, and Ellen Jacobs. *Health Information: Management of a Strategic Resource.* Philadelphia: Saunders, 2001, p 572.

Employers are allowed to hold their employees to certain standards; for example, the law allows health care employers to perform a drug screen before making a job offer. An employee working under the influence of certain substances does not have the ability to provide high-quality health care and would expose the employer to liability. Department standards, however, must not contradict the law.

DEPARTMENT EQUIPMENT AND SUPPLIES

The equipment, or tools, needed to perform the functions in the HIM department vary depending on the size of the facility, the type of health care that the facility provides, and the extent to which the information in that facility has been computerized. The equipment most often recognized in an HIM department includes employee work stations (e.g., desks and chairs), filing mechanisms, copiers, fax machines, telephones, computers, and printers. Proper equipment is essential to the functions of the HIM department. Each employee's equipment must be adequate to perform the functions. Old, faulty equipment can have a negative impact on the productivity of an employee, which ultimately affects the entire department. Once an employee has notified the manager of an equipment problem, the manager should be sure to begin the maintenance process in a timely manner.

Hit-Bit

Maintenance Contracts

Equipment such as computer software programs, copiers, and transcription and dictation devices is typically purchased with a maintenance contract option. It is important for managers to update these items and budget for them annually. The maintenance contract provides for repair, assistance, and sometimes replacement of certain equipment. The contract option can usually be purchased at minimal cost for maintenance coverage from Monday through Friday, 9 a.m. to 5 p.m., or for the first 90 days. For a higher fee, the contract may cover the equipment 24 hours per day, 7 days per week, including holidays.

Reference material is another necessary tool for any department providing coding and transcription services. Reference materials should be updated periodically. Table 13-9 provides a list of suggested reference materials for these areas. Additional equipment (e.g., pens, paper, toner, file folders, envelopes, and labels) is commonly referred to as *supplies.* The HIM department should be appropriately equipped and stocked so that employees can effectively perform their jobs. This includes necessary equipment and supplies for contract employees and those employees who work for the facility from their homes.

SUPPLIES

The manager should ensure that the supply of each stocked item is adequate. A lack of supplies can limit the employees' productivity. For example, if you run out of copy paper, you cannot print paper copies of records or reports, thus delaying patient care or insurance requests for timely payment. Orders for additional supplies should be placed in a timely manner to prevent delay, and the manager must stay within the budget for supplies.

Filing

A significant number of supplies are associated with filing, such as folders, color-coded labels, and year-band labels. File folders are typically ordered annually; therefore the manager must consider how many folders will be used every year before purchasing this item. Remember to account for each type of patient that will require a folder—inpatient, outpatient, patients in for observation, and newborns. Of course, the number of folders needed depends on the filing system used, whether serial, unit, or serial-unit. In the unit numbering system, the patient uses the same number for all visits; therefore one folder could conceivably store data for more than one discharge. However,

TABLE 13-9	Suggested Reference Materials for the HIM Department	
REFERENCE	**UPDATES**	**WHO NEEDS THIS REFERENCE MATERIAL?**
Physician's Desk Reference (PDR)	Published annually	One copy each for transcription and coding
Medical dictionary	Updated occasionally	One copy each for transcription and coding
Human disease reference		Coding
Specialized word books (e.g., surgical word book, drug book, abbreviation book)		Transcription
ICD-9-CM coding book	Updated annually October 1	Coding must have current codes as of October 1 each year
Coding Clinic for ICD-9-CM	Quarterly newsletter published by AHA	Coding: provides knowledge and advice on implementation of ICD-9-CM coding guidelines
HCFA Common Procedure Coding System (HCPCS)	Updated annually by HCFA	Coding and the person responsibly for the maintenance of the facility
Current Procedural Terminology (CPT)	Updated annually	Coding: necessary for outpatient and physician's office to have current codes
CPT Assistant	Monthly newsletter published by AHA	Coding: provides examples, explanation, and scenarios for implementation of CPT coding

AHA, American Hospital Association; *HCFA,* Health Care Financing Administration; *HCPCS,* Health Care Financing Administration Common Procedural Coding System.

for serial and serial-unit numbering systems, each patient will need a new folder. To simplify matters, you can assume that each discharge requires a new folder. The number of discharges for the year should almost equal the number of folders used; the manager should order enough extra folders to allow for errors, mistakes, repair of torn folders, and other unforeseen events. Also, be sure to order sufficient quantities of year-band labels and number labels (see Chapter 8).

Copy Machines, Scanners, and Printers

HIM departments rely on copy machines and printers for many different tasks but especially to release information to third parties, transfer patient information to a new facility or health care provider, and provide reports as requested by other departments. Scanners are necessary in departments that use document imaging, as discussed in Chapter 12. Copy machines require an adequate supply of paper and toner. Additionally, the department should have a maintenance agreement for each machine so that it can be serviced routinely. Printers also require paper, as well as ink, which comes in the form of cartridges. Managers must keep a sufficient supply of cartridges on hand so that the department is able to operate efficiently. A good way to stock this supply is always to have one extra ink or toner cartridge for every two printers so that when you run out, you have a replacement. Then you can order a new cartridge before you run out again.

Transcription and Dictation Equipment

Transcription and dictation equipment is important in the communication of patient health information. The dictation equipment is used by the health care professional to record the patient's health information. The transcription equipment is the machine used by the transcriptionist to listen to and type the dictated reports. Transcriptionists use the dictation system to retrieve the recorded voice. They then listen to the voice to type the report. This equipment should have a maintenance agreement, preferably one that ensures 24-hour, 7-day-per-week coverage.

Software

Many of the operations in the HIM department require the use of computer software. Typical software in a HIM department includes the master patient index, chart locator system, ROI form, electronic birth certificate, and encoders and groupers for coding. This software is critical to the operation of the department. Therefore each software system should be maintained in an appropriate environment, on computer equipment sufficient to support the applications, with adequate maintenance contracts for upgrades and support.

Miscellaneous Supplies

Remember to coordinate appropriate ordering practices for even routine supplies, such as pencils, pens, paper, and flags for analysis. An inadequate supply of these critical tools may cause unnecessary delays in the processing of health information.

MONITORING USE OF DEPARTMENT RESOURCES

HIM department managers must carefully monitor the equipment and supplies so that workflow is not affected. Poor equipment management—whether in buying new equipment, maintaining existing equipment, or converting from one system to another—can negatively affect productivity in the department. It is important to maintain adequate supplies for the employee work-

Hit-Bit

Upgrade

An *upgrade*, in computer software terminology, refers to a new version of software that is improved in some way.

force (onsite, contracted, and at home); important supplies include files, labels, printer or copier paper, and toner or ink cartridges. Minor oversights in department equipment and supplies can cause the workflow to backlog. which negatively affects employee performance and sometimes even department budgets. Seemingly minor details play an important role in the management of health information.

ERGONOMICS

Ergonomics is the coordination of the work environment with the worker (*Random House Webster's School and Office Dictionary*, 1995). The work environment should be comfortable, allowing the employee to perform the job as necessary, free from injury or harm. Ergonomics is sometimes thought of as proper body positioning of the employee at his or her desk (Figure 13-15). However, the desk and chair is not the only office equipment that can be adjusted to keep employees free from injury or harm. Other **ergonomic** issues involve lighting, appropriate climate, and the frequency and duration of rest breaks. Because many HIM functions are performed at a computer terminal or desk, appropriate coordination of employees with their work stations is required. Significant time spent in a harmful work environment can compromise employees' health, costing the facility valuable assets when workers' compensation claims are filed.

Areas in the HIM department that require significant ergonomic consideration are the transcription stations and all computer terminals. The height of the chair in relation to the desk or work station must be adjusted correctly to fit each employee, and the general office space should be configured to promote efficient workflow. The lighting, air conditioning, and heating should also be appropriate. The environment must provide safe and appropriate working conditions. For

Exercise 13-7

Ergonomics

1. It is the responsibility of the employer to provide a safe work environment for the employee to perform his or her job function. One way that this can be accomplished is through design of a(n) _____ work space.
2. Which of the following Fair Employment Laws prohibit discrimination based on race, color, religion, or sex?
   a. Fair Labor Standards Act
   b. Civil Rights Act
   c. Americans with Disabilities Act
   d. Age Discrimination in Employment Act
3. Which of the following Fair Employment Laws sets minimum wage, overtime pay, and equal pay?
   a. Fair Labor Standards Act
   b. Civil Rights Act
   c. Americans with Disabilities Act
   d. Age Discrimination in Employment Act
4. Which of the following Fair Employment Laws prohibits discrimination of handicapped people and ensures reasonable accommodation for them in the workplace?
   a. Fair Labor Standards Act
   b. Civil Rights Act
   c. Americans with Disabilities Act
   d. Age Discrimination in Employment Act
5. Identify some HIM functions that may be outsourced.

Anatomy of an Ergonomic Work Station

WORKPLACE ENVIRONMENT

- Most important consideration is working comfortably and efficiently.
- Have sufficient desk area for keyboard, monitor, mouse, document holder, telephone, etc.
- Organize the area so that it reflects the way you use equipment.
- Things you use most often should be within easiest reach.
- Vary your tasks.

- Take frequent breaks.
- If area is shared, be sure all who use it can adjust everything to their needs.
- Document holders should be at the same height and distance from monitor.
- Allow adequate leg room.
- Maintain an unobscured line of sight.

① **Work Surface**
- Proper height and angle
- Neutral postures
- Adjustable
- Standing–prevent slipping, adequate traction
- Sit/stand tools
- Antifatigue floor mats
- Darker, matte finishes are best

② **Storage Areas**
- Good body positions
- Reduce muscular forces
- Avoid excessive reach
- Heavy items between knee and shoulder height
- Frequently used storage closest to worker

③ **Video Display Terminals (VDT) [Monitor]**
- Position to minimize glare and reflections
- Top of screen is slightly below eye level
- Tilted slightly backward (less than 15 degrees)
- Distance from display 18–30 inches
- Perpendicular to windows
- Keep your head upright
- Set contrast and brightness
- Clean the screen (and your glasses)
- Antiglare filters
- Adjustable monitor arm

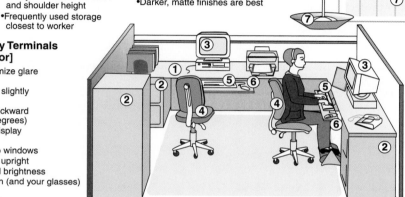

④ **Chairs**
- Comfortable (padded seats that swivel)
- Back and seat are adjustable while seated
- Provide good back support (can add additional cushion if necessary)
- Adjustable arm support
- Back straight
- Knees slightly higher than chair bottom
- Thighs horizontal
- Feet flat on the floor (use a footrest if necessary)
- Change positions occasionally

⑤ **Keyboard**
- Back should be lower than front
- Rounded edges
- Wrist rests (sharp edges, neutral position) same height as front of keyboard
- Type properly: don't force your fingers to stretch to incorrect keystrokes

⑥ **Mouse**
- Keep it on the same level as the keyboard or slightly above
- Keep wrist straight
- Do not stretch your arm; keep mouse within immediate reach
- Use the whole arm to move the mouse ... not just the forearm

⑦ **Lighting**
- Less illumination for computer work
- Indirect lighting is best

Avoid:

Awkward posture

Can include reaching behind, twisting, working overhead, kneeling, bending, and squatting. Deviation from ideal working posture can lead to fatigue, muscle tension, and headaches. **Correct working posture** – arms at sides, elbows bent approximately 90 degrees, forearms parallel to floor, wrists straight.

Repetitiveness

Judgment is based on frequency, speed, number of muscle groups used, and required force. Not all people react to the same conditions, so carefully monitor your personal physical response to repetitiveness.

◆ **Figure 13-15**

Ergonomic environment of an HIM department. (Redrawn from Linda Gaylor. *The Administrative Dental Assistant.* Philadelphia: Saunders, 2003, p 290.)

Hit-Bit

Worker's Compensation

Workers' compensation is the benefit that pays an employee for time away from the work-place because of a work-related injury.

example, if the employee spends a significant amount of time reading, the lighting should be adjusted accordingly. If the employee spends most of the day facing a computer screen, dim or indirect lighting may better protect the employee's eyesight.

WORKS CITED

Abdelhak, Mervat, Sara Grostick, Mary Alice Hanken, and Ellen Jacobs. *Health Information: Management of a Strategic Resource.* Philadelphia: Saunders, 1996.
Random House Webster's School and Office Dictionary. New York: Random House, 1995.

CHAPTER ACTIVITIES

CHAPTER SUMMARY

The management of health information includes the management of the people performing HIM functions. Appropriate organization and management of the department's human resources significantly affect the quality of health information. High-quality health information is necessary in the health care environment to provide good patient care. A good place to begin effective management is in the clear communication of the employee's responsibilities in the job description and performance standards of the position.

HIM supervisors and managers are responsible for the daily operations of the HIM department, as well as future planning in keeping with the facility's mission and vision. To guide the department into the future, HIM managers must plan, set goals and objectives, and continually evaluate the services provided within the department.

Knowledge of health information, combined with management skills, sets the stage for efficient and effective HIM departments.

Review Questions

1. Explain the difference between unity of command and span of control.
2. Explain how to write a job description.
3. What is the purpose of performance standards?
4. List and describe some of the equipment and supplies necessary in the HIM department.
5. Identify some of the issues that must be considered when designing an ergonomic work station.
6. Explain the importance of having maintenance agreements or service contracts on your HIM department equipment.

Health Information Management Director

My name is Mary Catherine, and I am the director of the health information management department at Fullmore Hospital, a 250-bed facility that provides acute care, skilled nursing care, rehabilitation, and a geriatric psychiatric service. The medical staff is divided into five sections: medicine, surgery, OB/GYN, pediatrics, and psychiatric. Our HIM department has 25 employees, 20 FTEs, and 5 part-time employees. I have two supervisors and one assistant director reporting directly to me.

My responsibilities include overseeing the operations of the department and planning and organizing the direction of health information operations. I attend several meetings each month. I am a member of the quality management committee and the risk management committee. I am also the coordinator for the health information management committee. As coordinator, I work closely with the chairman of the committee, a member of the medical staff, to organize the meetings, coordinate record reviews, and compile minutes of the meetings.

I also attend a monthly meeting with all the department directors at which we share important information about our department operations, perform facility-wide strategic planning, and receive communication from administration.

Once a month, I hold a department meeting for all HIM employees. During the meeting, we discuss department business and quality, and employees receive updates about various things that are occurring throughout the facility.

I really enjoy my job. Every day is a new challenge—sometimes from administration, physicians, or employees; at other times, accreditation or federal government requirements present a challenge. Working as a team, we always manage to reach our goals.

Hiring a Coder

You recently lost a coder at your facility. The department director has asked that you, the coding supervisor, create an advertisement for the local newspaper and participate in the interview for this new position. Using your knowledge of hiring practices, create an advertisement for this new position.

Before the interview, document at least three questions that you would like to ask the applicant. Be sure to check the list of appropriate interview questions (see Figure 13-13).

Chapter 14

∾

TRAINING AND DEVELOPMENT

CHAPTER OUTLINE

By the end of this chapter, the students should be able to

- Orient a new employee to the department and his or her job function.
- Orient an employee to a new job procedure.
- Orient medical staff or other facility personnel to the health information management (HIM) department.
- Identify inservice topics for HIM department personnel.
- Develop an inservice topic for presentation.
- Identify continuing education needs for HIM employees.
- Organize an agenda for HIM department meetings.
- Document minutes from an inservice, a continuing education session, or a department meeting.
- Prepare a development plan for HIM staff.
- Assess the training needs for the HIM department.
- Identify key aspects of effective communication.

VOCABULARY

agenda	inservice	probation period
continuing education	memorandum (memo)	training
credentials	minutes	
cross-training	orientation	

well-managed health information management (HIM) department spends considerable time on the training and development of employees. Training involves orientation, education, and practice (practical application) for a particular position or job function. Development is the ongoing improvement of staff personally and professionally. The manager of the HIM department is responsible for the hiring, training, developing, and maintaining of employees who perform the department functions. Occasionally, the responsibility is delegated to supervisors as well. Training is a very important part of any department; well-trained employees provide high-quality service. Training is necessary at many times: at the beginning of employment, as procedures and policies change and processes are improved, and as technology and equipment are improved. Development is equally important because it improves the quality of service. A department that develops its employees is making an investment in the quality of its future service.

In the previous chapter, you learned about hiring the right candidate for a job. In this chapter, you will learn how a manager trains and develops the employee, creating an asset to the organization.

ORIENTATION

When beginning a job at a health care facility, an employee (or a contract employee) needs a few days to learn about the environment and the new job. This is accomplished through **orientation.** The purpose of orientation is to make the employee familiar with the surroundings and convey all the information that is necessary to function on the job and in the organization. One orientation is more general and introduces the employee to the organization; another orientation is specific to the employee's job within the department. Orientation begins with an overall view of the organization and continues with department and job-specific information once the employee reports to the supervisor.

ORGANIZATION ORIENTATION

Typically, before new employees report to their departments, they attend an organization-wide orientation during which they are given information about the organization and have an opportunity to ask questions regarding employment. In most cases, an organization orientation includes the organization chart for the entire facility and the following topics:

- Personnel issues
- Customer service expectations
- Quality
- Building safety and security
- Infection control
- Body mechanics
- Confidentiality
- Tour of the facility

Other topics may include incident reporting, compliance, and the phone and e-mail systems. This orientation should take place before employees begin their job activities; however, because these orientations are sometimes offered only once a month, employees may actually begin work before their organization orientation. It is also important that *all* employees be oriented, including those employees who work from home.

Personnel Issues

Some of the first materials that employees receive during the orientation explain the benefits to which they are entitled as employees of the organization. During this part of the orientation, employees learn about special savings plans and complete necessary forms for income tax and enrollment in special plans or retirement accounts. Because compensation for the job is important, orientation is an opportunity to ask about pay periods, proper completion of payroll forms, and use of the time clock. Employees are also informed of hospital policies and procedures that affect their employment, and they receive a copy of the employee handbook. Information in the employee handbook includes facility dress code, tardy policy, hours earned for vacation and sick leave, grievance procedures, and holidays.

Customer Service

During the initial orientation, the new employee learns about the organization's expectations in relation to all customers. Customer service is an important part of health care, and many facilities use this orientation as an opportunity to instill a positive customer focus in all employees. Employees are encouraged to do the following:

- Identify all of their customers by name
- Greet each customer with a smile
- Provide assistance or find someone who can assist the customer
- Follow up on a customer's request

Employees may have an opportunity to participate in a role-playing exercise in which they learn how to deal with a disgruntled customer.

Quality

As discussed in Chapter 10, quality is critical to all aspects of health care. Because of its importance, employees are informed about the expectations and methods that the organization uses to ensure quality. The orientation should introduce the employee to the quality improvement method of choice. During orientation, new employees learn that everyone in the facility is responsible for quality. Employees are encouraged to identify opportunities to improve quality.

Building Safety and Security

The health care environment should be safe for patients, visitors, and employees. Safety issues are covered in the organization orientation to make the employee aware of the policy and procedures for maintaining a secure environment and for handling situations in the event of an emergency (i.e., the disaster plan). Two commonly discussed topics are fire safety and response to "code" emergencies. A common fire response uses the acronym RACE—rescue, alarm, confine, and extinguish. Employees learn to *rescue* patients, employees, or visitors from the area of the fire. They should go to the closest fire *alarm* and inform the operator of their name and the location

---

Hit-Bit

Customer Satisfaction Survey

Many organizations use a customer satisfaction survey to measure their service to customers. The results are used to improve the quality of customer service, and when the survey results are overwhelmingly favorable, the organization can use them in marketing efforts.

Hit-Bit

Orientation Presentations

Each topic in the organization-wide orientation is typically presented by the employee within the organization who is the authority on that issue. For example, the safety topic is presented by the facility's security officer; body mechanics is presented by a physical therapist; infection control is presented by the infection control nurse; and confidentiality is presented by an HIM professional.

and status of the fire. Then they should *confine* the fire by closing all doors in the area. If possible, they should *extinguish* the fire with a fire extinguisher or other appropriate device.

During a visit to a health care facility, you may have heard the operator announce a "code" over the intercom system. Common codes are code blue for cardiac arrest and code red for fire. These codes alert the employees in the facility to an emergency that is occurring in the facility (Table 14-1). These codes may also be announced as fictitious physician names (e.g., Dr. Red instead of code red, or Dr. Strong for security). All employees must recognize the codes in the facility and know their roles in responding to the emergency.

Infection Control

Health care workers may be exposed to a number of infectious agents. Because of this, several significant topics are covered under the topic of infection control, including hepatitis, acquired immunodeficiency syndrome, and universal (or standard) precautions for blood and body fluids. During this part of the orientation, new employees will learn how to protect themselves and others from infection; the discussion provides information about how these infections are spread and then shares procedures that will help protect employees.

In a discussion about universal precautions for blood and body fluids, employees are informed that one of the best and easiest methods to prevent spread of infection is through washing their hands. Employees are encouraged *always* to wash their hands before and after having contact with a patient, eating, and using the restroom. Universal precautions also include wearing masks and gloves when interacting with potentially infectious material and properly discarding needles and other contaminated objects.

Because some blood-borne organisms can survive for days outside of the body, health care workers are advised to exercise caution while handling items contaminated with body fluids. For example, a paper record contaminated with blood should be filed in a sealed plastic sheath.

Body Mechanics

All employees should maintain proper body mechanics, particularly while sitting at the work station (as mentioned in the section about ergonomics in the previous chapter) and when lifting, pushing, pulling, or transporting patients or equipment. This issue is quite important because employees can be injured if they use poor body mechanics, and injuries are very costly to the entire organization, leading to missed work and reduced productivity.

Confidentiality

Confidentiality has always been an important part of the new employee orientation. HIPAA legislation (see Chapter 11) has increased the need for organizations to ensure that all employees and contractors receive training regarding the confidentiality and security of health information. Typically, this topic is presented by an HIM professional. All employees must recognize the sensitivity of confidential information in a health care facility and the proper manner in which it should be handled. The confidentiality policy is reviewed, and all employees are asked to sign a confidentiality statement, as discussed in Chapter 11 (see Figure 11-1). Additionally, all employees must be made aware any applicable federal and state laws and organization policies regarding patient confidentiality and security.

TABLE 14-1	Emergency Codes
CODE	**EMERGENCY**
Dr. Strong	Security requested in a specific area of the facility
Black	Bomb threat
Red	Fire
Orange	Radiation disaster
Pink	Infant abduction
Blue	Cardiac arrest
Yellow	External disaster

HEALTH INFORMATION MANAGEMENT DEPARTMENT ORIENTATION

After the organization orientation (optimally), employees report to their supervisors in the new work environment for another orientation specific to their jobs and departments. During this orientation, employees become familiar with the work station, the environment, other employees, and the policies and procedures that pertain to their jobs. Each employee is given an opportunity to become acclimated to the work environment, meet the employees that are part of the work group or team, and learn what is expected by management.

During this orientation, the employee is given a copy of the job description, performance standards, rules, and policies and procedures of the HIM department. The employee becomes familiar with the physical layout of the HIM department, including the evacuation route in case of fire, and other related departments within the organization. For example, if the employee is responsible for retrieving information from the emergency room on a daily basis, he or she needs to know where the emergency room is located.

One way to orient employees is to have them sit with employees in each section of the department to familiarize themselves with everyone's tasks. This helps new employees understand the impact of their role in the department.

Employees also need to understand which holidays they may be required to work and how to request time off. Employees should know the hours that they are expected to work. Each employee is given a password with access to appropriate computerized information. Once a password is assigned, employees can begin training on the computer systems associated with their jobs. An excellent way to keep track of everything that must be covered with a new employee is to complete an orientation checklist (Figure 14-1). The employee should initial and date each item as it is completed. This form is kept in the employee's file folder as verification of the orientation for future reference.

CLINICAL STAFF ORIENTATION

Department employees are not the only members of the organization who require an orientation. Clinical staff, physicians, and members of other departments should be familiar with the functions and services of the HIM department. A general orientation explaining HIM department

Hit-Bit

Orientation to New Job Duties

Employees who change positions within an HIM department should be oriented to their new duties and responsibilities.

Hit-Bit

Probation Period

The first 90 days of employment for a new employee are called the **probation period.** During the probation period, employees are allowed ample time to learn their new tasks and responsibilities. At the end of this 90-day period, employees who are performing at an acceptable level are considered permanent.

If at any time during this probation period the employer feels that the employee is not performing as expected, the employee can be released from the job.

DIAMONTE HOSPITAL

Diamonte, Arizona 89104 • TEL. 602-484-9991

EMPLOYEE ORIENTATION CHECKLIST

Employee: _____   Date: _____

Position: _____   Supervisor: _____

The following items have been reviewed with the employee.
(The employee and supervisor should initial and date items as they are reviewed.)

	Employee	Supervisor	Date
Employee identification card policy			
Explanation of payroll procedures, including time clock location			
Absence and tardiness policy			
Employee job description			
Employee performance standards			
Introduction to department employees and physical layout			
Review of department functions			
Review of functions involving related departments			
Departmental Policy and Procedure manual			
Review of specific job-related policies and procedures			
Dress code			
Performance improvement activities			
Security and confidentiality policies			
Review and sign confidentiality statement			
Safety policy, disaster plan, and Safety manual			
Review of break schedule			
Location of restrooms and area to secure belongings			
Password assigned and related policies covered			

Employee signature: _____   Date: _____

Supervisor: _____   Date: _____

Example only. This list is not all-inclusive.

◆ **Figure 14-1**
Employee orientation checklist.

operations will assist these members when they interact with the department. HIM customers need to know the requirements for requesting information or records and the procedures for completing or reviewing records.

Physicians require orientation to the HIM department because they will visit the department to complete their health records and perform research. Physician orientation can be by personal appointment or in the form of a letter (Figure 14-2) introducing or explaining HIM department functions.

Department managers must understand the proper way to request records from the HIM department. Managers often request records for a study or project in which they are involved or to obtain information for a meeting. They need to know how much notice the department needs

> ### Hit-Bit
>
> **Physician Orientation**
>
> Physician orientation is an excellent opportunity to cover information relevant to completion of records, specifically the suspension policy. The suspension policy is typically found in the medical staff bylaws. But even if the orientation is no more than a simple letter of correspondence, it tells the physician how to avoid negative correspondence and unfortunate consequences as a result of delinquent records. Let the physician know whom to contact to gain access to incomplete records and how the HIM department can assist the physician in record completion.

to complete the request. Does the request need to be specific? Does the person requesting the information need to include the patient's name, medical record number, and discharge dates on the request form? When these policies are covered in an orientation, it eliminates a great deal of confusion and stress in the future.

Exercise 14-1

Orientation

1. The term used to describe a training to familiarize a new employee to the job is _____.
2. To become familiar with a new job and surroundings, the employee must attend which of the following?
   a. Training
   b. Orientation
   c. Inservice
   d. Department meeting
3. Which of the following organization orientation topics should be presented by a HIM employee?
   a. Safety
   b. Infection control
   c. Personnel issues
   d. Confidentiality
4. The *R* in the common safety acronym RACE, which is used to describe the employee's expected response to a fire, stands for which of the following words?
   a. Red
   b. Run
   c. Rescue
   d. Reassure

TRAINING

Training is an important part of all jobs. Employees obviously need training when they begin a job, but they need it just as much when processes, procedures, and equipment are changed. Training is the education of employees in new techniques and processes within the organization. It is provided to employees in the health care facility through inservice training sessions and continuing education and helps to ensure the quality of service. You are now ready to learn how a training session is organized.

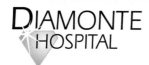

DIAMONTE HOSPITAL   Diamonte, Arizona 89104 • TEL. 602-484-9991

November 30, 2006

Eileen Dombrowski, MD
1101 Medical Center Blvd.
Diamonte, Arizona

Dear Dr. Dombrowski,

On behalf of the Health Information Management department, welcome to Diamonte Hospital. I would like to introduce you to the HIM department staff and the services provided.

Release of information
To obtain copies of health information for a patient under your care, please contact Shelly Pontiac, 565-1411. She will be happy to provide the appropriate forms and process your request.

Coding
Our coding department is supervised by Joanne Davis, CCS. If you have any questions regarding coding, please feel free to contact her.

Request for an old chart for patient care
The unit coordinator will typically request previous records for patients under your care by contacting the Health Information Management department at 565-1400. If you encounter difficulty retrieving a previous patient record, please feel free to contact John Brown, Supervisor.

Medical record completion
In keeping with our policy for timely completion of health records, we will e-mail weekly reminders to your office to notify you of any incomplete records. If you plan to come by our office to complete your records, please call in advance, 565-1455. We will be happy to pull your records and leave them in the physicians' lounge for 48 hours.

I look forward to working with you. If you need any further assistance I can be reached at 565-1416.

Sincerely,

Michelle Parks, RHIA
Director, Health Information Management

◆ **Figure 14-2**
Orientation letter to physicians.

ASSESSMENT OF EDUCATION NEEDS

The first step in planning a training (inservice or continuing education) session involves an assessment. The assessment helps the trainer identify what needs to be taught. Training topics can be identified through the following means:

- A management observation from performance standard reviews
- A survey of employees
- Updated or new equipment
- Process improvement
- Legal or regulatory changes

You learned how to create performance standards in Chapter 13. Performance standards tell employees the amount and the quality of work that they are expected to accomplish. When performing employee evaluations, the manager may determine that additional training is needed in a particular area because of the employees' low performance.

Occasionally, employees may be asked to identify areas in which they would like to acquire more expertise. A survey can identify areas of interest to the employees, and training sessions can be developed accordingly. Surveys may also identify ideal areas for **cross-training**, which teaches employees how to perform job functions that are not part of their job descriptions. Cross-training is a way to prepare a department to handle increased workloads and vacant positions when employees are on a break, are out sick, are on vacation, or leave their position. It can also provide job enrichment for some employees.

With all of the technological advances that occur in today's health care environment, equipment and computer software are continuously being updated and replaced. These changes typically require training so that employees know how to use the new technology in copiers, software, and phone systems.

Another opportunity for training is during the "do" and "act" phases of the PDCA (plan, do, check, act) process improvement method (see Chapter 10). To implement an improved process, all of the employees associated with the process must be trained.

AUDIENCE

An important part of planning a training session is learning about the audience. The presenters do not have to know each person individually, but they should know the participants' backgrounds. Their backgrounds, with regard to education and work-related experience, tell the presenters how to begin the training. When the topic is new to the audience, the presenters begin with an elementary overview of the topic. If participants are knowledgeable about the topic and have practical experience, the training session can be more advanced. Additionally, knowing the backgrounds of participants affects the organization of the presentation—that is, the vocabulary and knowledge pertinent to the audience. In other words, significantly different vocabulary and examples are used to train physicians as opposed to college students.

FORMAT

The format of a training session explains how the information or topic will be presented. For example, will the training take place as a lecture, or will it be hands-on training? Will the presentation include a video or demonstration? Will there be an instructor or a self-guided manual? The format is determined by the topic of the presentation and the audience. If the topic involves procedures and equipment that are completely new to audience members, a demonstration that includes hands-on participation would enhance their understanding. However, an inservice training session in which coding updates are described to coders may require only a few examples or case studies.

The format of the presentation also determines whether the presenter needs to have audiovisual equipment available. If the training session involves a video, then a TV/VCR monitor must be present in the room. Other audiovisual equipment includes overhead projectors, slide projectors, computer equipment with speakers and video capability, and microphones.

ENVIRONMENT

The location of the training session is another element that can be determined by the topic of the presentation and the audience. Training sessions can be held in classrooms, auditoriums, via video conference or the Internet, or in the HIM department. If the training requires demonstration of equipment, the training should happen near the equipment or a demonstration model should be available in the classroom. The location of the training session is also affected by the number of participants. The larger the audience, the more space is required. Sometimes, multiple sessions can be held to accommodate a large number of participants. However, if the number of participants is small, the training session may be held in the HIM department. If audience members are expected to take notes, chairs at tables or desks should be considered. If a computer terminal is used for the training, make sure there is adequate seating for one person per computer.

CALENDAR OF EDUCATION

How often should employees be trained? At a minimum, *all* employees in the facility should receive annual training in customer service, quality, safety, infection control, confidentiality and security, and body mechanics. Additional training sessions can be organized according to the employee's job function or as the need arises.

In the HIM department, there are several positions that require routine training, particularly in the areas of coding and release of information. Coding employees should participate in quarterly training sessions (coding clinics). Inpatient coding changes occur twice a year in April and October; these changes affect all of the employees responsible for inpatient coding. A training session should be organized to inform these employees of any upcoming coding changes that will affect their job. Outpatient coding changes (Current Procedural Terminology [CPT]) occur in January. A training session should be organized accordingly to cover these changes. Additionally, other regulations, such as the implementation of prospective payment systems (PPSs), occur at various times during the year, and require further training sessions. Employees who handle release of information requests should receive annual training, and additional sessions should be organized when there are changes in federal or state laws that affect the release of health information.

It is very important to keep a record of employee attendance at training sessions. The record of the employee's attendance supports the communication of a new policy, procedure, or method required as a part of his or her job.

Use a sign-in sheet to document employee attendance. As a heading at the top of the sign-in sheet, include the topic covered and the objectives that apply. This sign-in sheet can be kept in a binder to record employee education, or the information can be transferred to each employee's file. In addition, the information can be transferred to a computer system to track employee education.

Training is an ongoing process. Often, it is important to involve other departments so that employees learn the necessary information from the appropriate source. Some topics can be coordinated with members of other departments, such as quality management, nursing, infection control, and business. Be sure to include *all* of the employees who are affected by the new information, including employees who work at home.

Exercise 14-2

Training

1. Which of the following is the first step in planning a training, inservice, or continuing education program?
   a. Assessment of education needs
   b. Audience
   c. Area
   d. Inventory of skills
2. Continuing education is critical for coding employees. Which of the following dates is critical in the education of inpatient coders?
   a. January 1
   b. October 1 and April 1
   c. December 1
   d. July 1
3. A general term for education, instruction, or demonstration of how to perform a job is _____.
4. The period of time, also known as a grace period, given to a new employee to learn the job and reach the performance standards associated with that job is known as the _____.

Hit-Bit

Online Training

Because of the increased performance expectations in health care organizations, many employers are looking for efficient and effective methods to train their employees. One method being used is online training. Training that can occur asynchronously, when the employee is available or able to fit it into the work schedule, is one advantage of online methods. Synchronous learning happens when the learner and the instructor are together, whether in person or online. Asynchronous learning can occur as a result of recorded materials or presentations (e.g., Power Point).

 ## INSERVICE EDUCATION

An **inservice** is training for an organization's employees. A training session can be called an inservice when it provides continuing or reinforced education for current employees. An inservice can be part of a monthly department meeting, or it can be held separately to cover a new topic (e.g., use of new equipment). Inservices reinforce and develop new skills and can also be used as a method of cross-training staff. Figure 14-3 provides a list of inservices for HIM employees. All of the elements of a training session apply to the development of an employee inservice.

EDUCATING THE PUBLIC

Health care professionals are often called on to educate the public about changes in laws relating to health care or health information as well as health-related topics, such as cancer awareness, diabetes, and infectious diseases. Therefore each of the topics associated with planning a training session for employees can be modified for use in planning a training session for the public.

 ## CONTINUING EDUCATION

Education does not stop simply because a person has completed a program or obtained employment. Professionals recognize that education will continue over the course of their careers. All

---

EXAMPLES OF INSERVICES

How to use a new copier or printer

How to respond to a fire emergency code, including the use of a fire extinguisher

How to handle a walk-in request for copies of health care records

How to use a clinical pathway

Explanation of a new prospective payment system and how it will affect the organization

◆ **Figure 14-3**
Examples of inservices.

HIM professionals should recognize that their **credentials** are accompanied by a commitment to lifelong learning. In all health care fields, regulations change, technology advances, and processes improve. Because of such changes, you must continue your education as it relates to your job, career, and your special interests (see Table 14-2).

Keeping a record of your continuing education (CE) hours is very important. Because CE periods vary with each association, you may not remember all of the hours that you earned unless

TABLE 14-2	RHIT Core Content Areas	
CORE CONTENT AREA	**DESCRIPTION**	**EXAMPLE**
Technology	Applications of existing and emerging technologies for collection of clinical data, the transformation of clinical data to useful health information, and the communication and protection of information	Attending a presentation explaining the process of converting paper records to a virtual file room
Management Development	Application of organizational management theory and practices as well as human resource management techniques to improve departmental adaptability, innovation service quality, and operational efficiency	Attending an in-service to learn how to use a new employee evaluation system
Clinical Data Management	Application of data analysis techniques to clinical databases to evaluate practice patterns, assess clinical outcomes, and ensure cost-effectiveness of health care services	Attending a meeting of the community health information network to learn how to submit information and interpret results
Performance Improvement	Study of fundamental organizational changes and how they are functionally organized or how they deliver patient care, with special focus on the requisite changes made in health information systems and services	Attending a meeting to learn how to facilitate quality improvement in your organization
External Forces	Knowledge of strategies that organizational and HIM professionals in particular have used to effectively address emerging legislative, regulatory, or other external party action that has the potential to significantly affect the collection and use of health data	Attending a seminar explaining implementation of HIPAA requirements
Clinical Foundations	Understanding of human anatomy and physiology, the nature of disease processes in humans, and the methods of diagnosis and treatment of acute and chronic medical conditions and diseases	Attending a conference on breast cancer
Privacy and Security	Understanding and application of current health care regulations that promote protection and the electronic transmission of health information; to act as the patient's advocate and teach them about their rights with regard to protected health information	Attending a meeting on the implementation of the provider identification number (PIN) for your organization

From American Health Information Management Association: http://www.ahima.org/certification/HIMdomain.asp

you keep a record of your attendance or completion. The easiest method for keeping track of your CE hours is to designate a file folder for material from the meetings you attend, journal article questionnaires submitted, and Web site tutorials completed. If you use a summary form in the file folder, each time you open the folder to file hours, you can also write the hours on the summary sheet (Figure 14-4). This file folder and tracking form are also helpful in the event of an audit of your CE hours. Using this file folder and tracking form makes it easier to fill out the CE form when your continuing education hours are due. Additionally, some organizations, like AHIMA, allow their members to track and maintain a record of their CE hours online. HIM department managers should also maintain a file of all employees' CE activities.

Training and education require communication. Communication must occur between staff employees and management and between management and administration. The following section covers communication in the health care environment.

Continuing education for: _____
No. of hours needed: _____
Cycle ends: _____

Date	Topic/Title	Location	Core Content Area	No. of Hours

◆ **Figure 14-4**
Continuing education tracking form.

Exercise 14-3

Inservice Education

1. _____ indicate a person's specific professional qualifications.
2. To maintain the RHIT credential, the professional must maintain
   a. 20 hours of continuing education each year
   b. 30 hours of continuing education each year
   c. 20 hours of continuing education during a 2-year cycle
   d. 30 hours of continuing education during a 2-year cycle
3. A name for the training provided to employees of an organization is _____.
4. _____ may be required after attaining a position, credential, or degree; this is intended to keep those persons knowledgeable in core content areas.

COMMUNICATION

Communication is an important part of management. Employees in the HIM department communicate daily using written, verbal, physical, and electronic methods. The HIM department also communicates with other departments in the facility—clinicians and physicians, other health care facilities, insurance companies, attorneys, and patients.

Communication should always be clear and appropriate regardless of the parties involved (Figure 14-5).

Communication requires two parties and a message. First, the message must be transmitted to another party. The message can be written, verbal, or electronic or expressed by body language. The first party—called the *sender*—initiates the message. The second party—the *receiver*—is the recipient of the message. This is the basis of all communication. With this understanding, you may consider typical communication within the HIM department. The following sections discuss communication among the following:

- Employees within the HIM department
- Employees within the health care organization
- HIM department personnel and physicians
- HIM department personnel and other departments
- HIM department personnel and outside agencies or parties

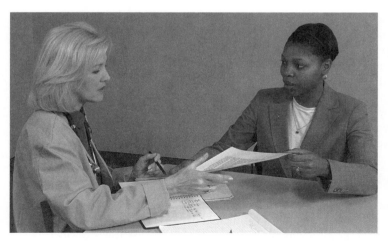

◆ **Figure 14-5**
Communication.

Hit-Bit

Continuing Education

The American Health Information Management Association (AHIMA) includes a **continuing education** requirement as a part of the certification/registration process. To maintain your credential, you must earn continuing education credits pertinent to the HIM profession. The requirement for the Registered Health Information Technician (RHIT) and Registered Health Information Administrator (RHIA) states that the professional must earn 80% of the required hours in a core content area (Table 14-3). AHIMA has designated the following areas as core content for the HIM profession: Technology, Management Development, Clinical Data Management, Performance Improvement, External Forces, Clinical Foundations, and Privacy and Security.

The RHIA must earn 30 continuing education hours every 2 years. The cycle runs January through December of the following year. The RHIT must maintain 20 continuing education hours every 2 years. Therefore the RHIA must have at least 24 (of the 30) hours in any one or multiple core content areas, and the RHIT must have at least 16 of the 20 hours in one or multiple core content areas.

Because certification rules can change, always refer to the AHIMA website for the current requirements.

Continuing education hours can be earned in a variety of ways. Most professionals earn their continuing education hours by attending local, state, or national HIM association meetings. Some may earn the hours by attending meetings within their facility. Yet another method for earning continuing education hours is by reading and responding to the education quizzes found in the *Journal of AHIMA* or visiting the AHIMA Web site.

Additional AHIMA certifications also require a commitment to lifelong learning. The Certified Coding Specialist (CCS) and Certified Coding Specialist—Physician-based (CCS-P) credentials require an annual self-assessment (worth 5 continuing education hours), including health record coding scenarios. Depending on the number and nature of coding changes for that year, the number of multiple-choice questions may be as few as 10 or as many as 30.

Professionals who earn and maintain more than one credential will need to earn 10 additional continuing education hours for each credential but no more than 60 hours per cycle. For example, if Jane has the credentials RHIT and CCS-P, she will need to earn 30 CE credits, 20 for the RHIT and 10 for the CCS-P, in addition to the annual assessment.

EMPLOYEE-TO-EMPLOYEE COMMUNICATION

Communication occurs among employees within the HIM department and throughout the organization. Communication may be verbal, written, or electronic and involve job-related or personal subjects. Positive, appropriate communication among employees enhances productivity.

Most important, communication about or to patients should be kept confidential. Patient health information should be communicated in an appropriate method to employees on a need-to-know basis.

Communication between employees and their immediate supervisors is very important. Employees need to know how their performance is perceived by management. They also need to be informed of changes in their work, processes, and functions that affect their daily operations.

HEALTH INFORMATION MANAGEMENT DEPARTMENT AND PHYSICIANS

The HIM department communicates routinely with physicians regarding record completion, release of information, continuity of patient care, and documentation of health information for utilization or reimbursement. Communication with a physician should be respectful. Consider the physician's time, and make your communication appropriate. Let it be meaningful and brief, if possible, and most important, *clear.*

HEALTH INFORMATION MANAGEMENT DEPARTMENT AND OUTSIDE AGENCIES OR PARTIES

HIM departments often communicate with agents external to the organization. As discussed in Chapter 11, information should be released only according to applicable policy or state or federal law. Communication should be clear, preferably in writing, and should provide information so that the recipient can reply as necessary.

WRITTEN COMMUNICATION

Written communication provides documentation of the message intended for the recipient. Therefore written communication serves two purposes: It conveys a message and records it for later use. A common form of written communication in a health care facility is the memorandum, best known as the *memo*.

Written communication can be on paper or in electronic form. Written paper communication is typically in the form of a memo or letter. Electronic communication is performed via e-mail.

Memos

A **memorandum (memo)** is written or typed communication for informational purposes. A memo is used to provide clear, concise information about a new procedure, process, or policy to all those affected by it (Figure 14-6). The memo is more formal than verbal communication. Memos can be addressed to a group or an individual, but they are not as formal as a letter addressed specifically to an employee.

Memos can also serve as proof of communication to an employee. When a memo is shared with employees in a department, it may be posted in a highly visible and frequented place (e.g., near the time clock or in the break room). At other times, memos are copied for each employee and handed to the employee personally by another staff member. Regardless of the means, the manager wants to be sure that the message is communicated. One easy method for attaining confirmation of the employee's receipt of the memo is to have the employee initial a master copy of the memo. This method allows management to record employees' verification of receipt, and preferably review, of the memo.

Electronic Communication

Today it is extremely common for health care facilities to use a form of electronic communication called *e-mail*. E-mail has changed the way we communicate and is expeditious if all parties are

---

Hit-Bit

E-Mail Etiquette

Do not type an e-mail message using all capital letters. This is considered to be the equivalent of screaming in the e-mail context. Use all-capital words sparingly, only to emphasize a word.

Avoid long messages. Keep the message brief and to the point.

If someone sends you an e-mail message that requires a response, be careful to reply to the sender as appropriate. Include the previous message so that the person knows why you are communicating a specific message.

In a business e-mail, end your message with your name, title, and business address, including phone numbers as appropriate. You want the person to be able to contact you appropriately.

"Snail mail" is the United States Postal Service.

E-mail is not private. Be careful what you send via e-mail. Messages can be read by others or misdirected. Therefore send only what you feel comfortable expressing to the whole world.

Use punctuation appropriately.

E-mail is typically faster than conventional mail. However, the quicker arrival of e-mail does not mean that the intended recipient will actually *read* the message any faster.

connected and responding. E-mail allows a message to be typed and sent via electronic means to another party or parties. The message is then kept in the other party's mailbox until he or she opens the message to receive it. E-mail is convenient because messages can easily be returned, forwarded, or saved. Because e-mail is a form of written communication, it is necessary to use appropriate grammar, punctuation, and etiquette when sending a message via e-mail.

Exercise 14-4

Communication

1. A written/typed communication tool used to communicate or provide information to members of an organization is a _____.
2. A popular form of electronic communication is
   a. memo
   b. e-mail
   c. fax machine
   d. telephone

DEPARTMENT MEETINGS

HIM department meetings are another method of face-to-face communication. Department meetings should be held monthly or more often as the need arises. A good way to schedule the meetings is to set aside one day each month for the meeting (e.g., the last Thursday of each month). When this is done, employees and managers know when to expect the next department meeting. The meeting is an opportunity for department employees to come together to discuss, learn, communicate, and share information. The department meeting is an ideal forum to review policies and procedures (new and old) to ensure that everyone understands the appropriate course of action. The department meeting is also a way to make sure that everyone in the department hears the same message.

If your department is small to medium-sized, a single meeting may suffice to communicate necessary information to all employees. However, if your department is larger, you may need to hold more than one meeting during different shifts so that all employees can attend.

All employees should attend the scheduled monthly HIM department meetings. When employees miss a meeting, they still need to hear the information. Therefore posting or copying minutes from the meeting serves as notification for these employees. Also, employees should initial the attached transmittal memo indicating that they have read the minutes of the meeting.

AGENDA

After the meeting is scheduled, how do you decide what to discuss? Regardless of the style of department meetings (formal or informal), you will need an **agenda** so that you cover all of the necessary topics. Although agendas vary, the agenda in Figure 14-7 is typical for a HIM department. A meeting officially begins with the call to order, whereupon the events of the meeting begin to be recorded. Employees know that it is time to stop the chatter and begin the meeting. Minutes from the previous meeting can be reviewed, depending on the formality of the meeting. Next, any old business from the previous meeting is discussed. Occasionally, topics discussed in a meeting cannot be resolved without further investigation. Such topics will be revisited during the next meeting, when old business is discussed. Topics are typically considered old business until they are resolved, closed, or completed. The next part of the agenda is new business. At this time, new items may be introduced to the meeting, followed by items that are discussed each month, such as reports from sections within the department, quality management activities within the

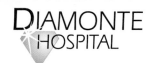

DIAMONTE HOSPITAL

Diamonte, Arizona 89104 • TEL. 602-484-9991

MEMO

TO: Health Information Management Employees

FROM: Michelle Parks, RHIA
        Director, Health Information Management

DATE: May 8, 2006

RE: Monthly Department Meeting

A Health Information Management department meeting will be held Wednesday, May 31, in the hospital auditorium at 2:00 PM.

We will have a brief presentation by the Human Resources department followed by the regular monthly agenda. Please make necessary arrangements to attend this meeting.

Thank you.

◆ **Figure 14-6**
Memo.

department and relating to the department, safety issues, and special announcements from the administration or about the facility.

MEETING

The HIM department meeting should be held in a location commensurate with the size of the department. Be sure to consider the time of the meeting in case it is during the normal hours of operation. This may require that one employee miss the meeting or that you have an alternative method for covering the functions within the department while your employees are at the meeting. Be sure to have a sign-in sheet for all of the employees to record their attendance at the meeting.

HIM DEPARTMENT MEETING AGENDA

I. Call to order
II. Review of minutes
III. Old business
IV. New business
V. In-service
VI. Quality improvement
VII. Announcements
VIII. Adjournment

◆ **Figure 14-7**
HIM department meeting agenda.

Hit-Bit

Robert's Rules of Order

To conduct an orderly meeting, many managers have adopted some form of Robert's Rules of Order. These rules explain how business is conducted during the meeting. Employees become accustomed to a typical order. Meetings are formally called to order, the agenda is followed, and the meeting is concluded with adjournment. The rules explain how debate should proceed and how motions can be made to present new business, make amendments, or vote on issues at hand. Likewise, there is a formal method for keeping track of old business on the agenda until it is resolved to the satisfaction of the meeting members.

Exercise 14-5

Department Meetings

1. _____ are used to record the events, topics, and discussions of a meeting.
2. An _____ is used to organize the topics to be discussed during a meeting.
3. The first item on the monthly HIM department meeting agenda is
   a. call to order
   b. review of old business
   c. new business
   d. adjournment

MINUTES

Appropriate discussion and decisions from each meeting should be recorded for future reference in the **minutes.** When preparing minutes, use the agenda as a guide to be sure that you have recorded the content or discussion surrounding each topic presented at the meeting. Review the minutes shown in Figure 14-8; notice how the content of the topics discussed were recorded just as they were presented at the meeting. Be careful to include only pertinent meeting information

Health Information Management
Department Meeting
October 30, 2006

Employees present:

Employees absent:

Topic/Discussion	Recommendation/Action	Follow-up
I. Call to Order The Health Information Management meeting was called to order by Michelle Parks at 2:00 PM.		
II. Review of Old Minutes The minutes from the September Health Information Management department meeting were reviewed and approved as presented.		
III. Old Business **Uniforms** Employees in the department are interested in adopting a uniform as the dress code. During the previous meeting it was decided that the employees would invite three uniform companies to present at the next meeting. M & R Uniforms, Acorn Uniforms, and B & B Direct presented uniforms, pricing, and payment options to the employees.	After review of the information presented by all uniform companies the employees voted for the uniform and options presented by B & B Direct. The uniform company will return in 2 weeks to take orders and the dress code will take effect in 2 months.	11/2006
IV. New Business **HIPAA** Health Insurance Portability and Accountability Act has taken effect. Policies were presented and reviewed with the employees.		
V. Report Intradepartmental quality Interdepartmental quality		
VI. Safety/In-service		
VII. Announcements		
VIII. Adjournment With no further business to discuss the meeting was adjourned at 2:45 PM.		

_____   _____
Michelle Parks, RHIA   Date

◆ **Figure 14-8**
HIM department meeting minutes.

and participants' comments without mention of the participants' names in the minutes; do not include slander, slang, or irrelevant comments by the participants.

The minutes should clearly recall the events of the meeting as presented, discussed, and decided. The topics presented are documented under the column titled "Topics/Discussion." The decision or action of the meeting members is documented under "Recommendation/Action." The final column, "Follow-up," identifies whether a topic has been closed (i.e., the business for that topic is concluded). Most important, topics that are not finalized should be carried forward to the next meeting until the business is concluded.

MEETING RECORDS

It is important to keep a precise record of each monthly meeting. These records will support any future business, discussion, and accreditation requirements. You can set up a file folder or a binder to organize each month's meeting information. Be sure to keep a copy of the agenda, the sign-in sheet, any attachments or handouts shared with the group, and the final draft of the minutes. The records from these meetings should be kept at least 3 years or as required by legal or regulatory bodies.

WEB SITE

American Health Information Management Association: http://www.ahima.org

CHAPTER ACTIVITIES

CHAPTER SUMMARY

Training and development are critical to the success of the HIM department. These efforts and activities keep HIM employees competent and abreast of all the changing technology, policy, legislative, regulatory, and accreditation requirements. New employees in the organization, whether they are HIM, medical staff, nursing, or other professionals, must be oriented to the organization and trained in HIM-related issues (e.g., confidentiality and security of patient information mandated by HIPAA). Training continues beyond the orientation stage; for example, employees must participate in on-going development efforts to maintain continuing education hours, remain knowledgeable about current requirements (e.g., coding), and become skilled users of new technology that is part of their job responsibilities. Annually, the entire staff must be reminded of the requirements related to their jobs and the entire health care organization. Changes that occur as a result of quality improvement efforts are another reason for continuous training of staff. Development of the employees in the health care organization, through training, continuous education, and communication, creates an environment in which both the employees and the organization are positioned for success.

Review Questions

1. What is the purpose of orientation?
2. List and briefly explain the issues discussed in the organization orientation.
3. Identify two HIM functions that require annual (at a minimum) training of employees.
4. Explain the importance of the meeting agenda and minutes.

HIM Assistant Director

My name is Michelle, and I am the health information management assistant director in a 220-bed facility, Oakcrest Hospital. This facility provides acute care emergency services, skilled nursing, and ambulatory services. Our market share is somewhat unique because we do not provide maternity and pediatric services. Our services are primarily adult and geriatric medicine. We have an HIM department with eight clerical and release of information employees under my responsibility, three coding employees with one coding supervisor, and eight transcription employees with one transcription supervisor.

In our department, things are very organized, to the credit of our department director. New employees participate in the organization orientation before reporting to our department for work. During the first few days of employment, employees are oriented to the department. We begin by explaining the employee's job description and expectations (performance standards). Then the new employee goes through the department, sitting with each employee to learn about other HIM functions and how their jobs are related. Finally, the employee is oriented to his or her new position. During this process, the employee also obtains a password for our computer systems.

I am responsible for organizing our monthly department meetings and choosing the inservice topic. I set up the agenda, copy and distribute any necessary handouts, and record the minutes. In addition, I coordinate any training required by changes in department policy, procedure, equipment, or federal and state mandates. The employees who report to me are cross-trained in several different functions so that we can cover one another for lunch, breaks, vacations, and sick leave.

I really enjoy the training and development aspect of this position. It is rewarding to see a new employee succeed in his or her position or to have an employee move up into a new position because of appropriate training and development.

APPLICATION

Create a Public Education Information Session

Research the current issues associated with health information. Choose a topic that requires education of the local community (the public).

Using the training session information in this chapter, perform an assessment of community education needs. In your preparation, consider the audience, format, and environment in which the education will be provided. Prepare a paper presentation of this information for your instructor.

APPENDIXES

- Physician's Order Form
- Physician's Progress Notes
- Advance Direct Acknowledgment
- Conditions of Admission
- Emergency Room Record
- Face/Registration Sheet
- History and Physical Exam
- Informed Consent
- Intake/Output Record
- Nurses Progress Notes
- Nursing Discharge Summary
- Report of Consultation

○ *PLEASE PUNCH HERE* ○

Diamonte Hospital Phoenix, Arizona 12345-6789 Phone: (999) 123-XXXX Fax: (999) 123-XXXX	Patient Name Label

PHYSICIAN'S ORDER FORM

Date/ Time	Order	Physician's Signature	Date/ Time	Nurse Initials

Physician's Order Form

○ *PLEASE PUNCH HERE* ○

Diamonte Hospital Phoenix, Arizona 12345-6789 Phone: (999) 123-XXXX Fax: (999) 123-XXXX	Patient Name Label

PHYSICIAN'S PROGRESS NOTES

Date	Time	Progress Note	Physician Signature	Discipline

Physician's Progress Notes

DIAMONTE HOSPITAL
Diamonte, Arizona

Advance Directive
Acknowledgment

Instructions: This form should be initiated upon admission to the facility and completed by the admitting RN. All patients receive an Advance Directive Booklet upon admission.

		YES	NO
1.	Is the patient registering him/herself? If NO, please give reason:		
2.	Does the patient have an advance directive? If NO, skip to question 5.		
3.	Does the patient have a living will? Has the patient supplied a copy of the living will ? Placed on chart by _____ Date/Time: _____		
4.	Does the patient have a durable power of attorney for health care? Has the patient supplied a copy of the durable power of attorney for health care? Placed on chart by _____ Date/Time: _____		
5.	Does the patient request additional information or wish to execute an advance directive at this time? If YES, please consult Social Services, x 4435.		

Form completed by _____   Date   Time

Advance Directive Acknowledgment

DIAMONTE HOSPITAL
Diamonte, Arizona

**CONDITIONS of
ADMISSION**

I. **LEGAL RELATIONSHIP BETWEEN DIAMONTE HOSPITAL AND PHYSICIAN**
I understand that many of the physicians on the staff of this hospital, including the attending physician(s), are not employees or agents of Diamonte Hospital but, rather, are independent contractors who have been granted privileges of using its facility for the care and treatment of their patients. I also realize that among those who attend patients at this facility are medical, nursing, and other health care professionals in training who, unless otherwise requested, may be present during patient care as part of their education.

II. **CONSENT TO TREATMENT**
The patient, identified above, hereby consents and authorizes Diamonte Hospital and its staff and the patient's physician(s) to perform or administer the diagnostic and treatment procedures (including, but not limited to, radiology examinations, blood tests and other laboratory examinations and medication) as may be required by the Hospital or as may be ordered by the patient's physician(s). The patient acknowledges that Diamonte Hospital is a teaching institution. The patient agrees that he/she may participate as a teaching subject unless the patient otherwise notes in writing to the contrary.

III. **RELEASE OF RECORDS**
The undersigned authorizes Diamonte Hospital to release any part or all patient medical records to such insurance company (companies), health care plan administrator, workmen's compensation carrier, welfare agency, or their respective authorized auditor or agents, or to any other person or party that is under contract or liable to Diamonte Hospital for all or any part of the hospital charges for this admission. The undersigned further authorizes Diamonte Hospital to release all or part of the patient's medical record or financial record to such physicians involved in the care of the patient, hospital committees, consultants, subsidiaries or physician hospital organizations, including but not limited to any committee, subsidiary, or physician hospital organization in which the patient's physician is a member or their respective agents.

IV. **ASSIGNMENT OF BENEFITS**
In consideration of the care and services to be provided to the patient by Diamonte Hospital, the undersigned assigns and authorizes, whether as agent or patient, direct payment to Diamonte Hospital or hospital-based physicians of all insurance and health plan benefits otherwise payable to or on behalf of the patient for this hospitalization and services. It is understood by the undersigned that he/she is financially responsible for charges not covered by this assignment.

V. **VALUABLES**
The undersigned understands fully that Diamonte Hospital is not responsible for the safety or security of and personal property or valuables.

VI. **PHOTOGRAPHS**
The undersigned hereby authorizes and consents to Diamonte Hospital for the taking of photographs, images, or video tapes of such diagnostic, surgical, or treatment procedures of the patient as may be required by Diamonte Hospital or ordered by the patient's physician(s). With the exception of radiological images, Diamonte is not required to keep videotapes or photographs for any period of time if the medical record contains a record of the surgical, diagnostic, or treatment procedure. The patient hereby consents to the taking of pictures of newborns for possible purchase or for security purposes.

Conditions of Admission

DIAMONTE HOSPITAL
Diamonte, Arizona

EMERGENCY ROOM RECORD

Account No.	FC	Admit Date &Time	Method of Arrival		Religion	Race	Sex
Patient Name			Address			Phone	
DOB	Age	Social Security No.	Employer		Occupation	Phone	
Admitting Physician			Attending Physician				
Guarantor			Address:			Phone	
Nearest Relative		Relation	Address			Phone	
Emergency Contact		Relation	Address			Phone	
Primary Insurance		Address		Group/Plan No.		Phone	
Secondary Insurance		Address		Group/Plan No.		Phone	

CHIEF COMPLAINT

HISTORY	RADIOLOGY
	LABORATORY
PHYSICAL	
DIAGNOSIS	

PHYSICIAN'S SIGNATURE	DATE

Discharge Status	Discharge Disposition

Emergency Room Record

DIAMONTE HOSPITAL
Diamonte, Arizone

FACE/REGISTRATION SHEET

Account No.	FC	Admit Date &Time	PT	Room No.	Discharge Date	Religion	Race	Sex

Patient Name		Address				Phone		

DOB	Age	Social Security No.	Employer		Occupation	Phone		

Admitting Physician	Attending Physician

Guarantor	Address	Phone

Nearest Relative	Relation	Address	Phone

Emergency Contact	Relation	Address	Phone

Primary Insurance	Address	Group/Plan No.	Phone

Secondary Ins	Address	Group/Plan No.	Phone

Principal Diagnosis
_____
_____

Additional Diagnosis
_____
_____
_____
_____
_____

Principal Procedure
_____
_____

Additional Procedures
_____
_____
_____
_____

_____
Attending Physician   Date

Discharge Status	Discharge Disposition

Face/Registration Sheet

DIAMONTE HOSPITAL
Diamonte, Arizona

History

(Page 1 of 2)

Chief Complaint	
History of Present Illness	
History of Past Illness	
Family History	
Social History	
Review of Systems	
General	
Skin	
HEENT	
Neck	
Respiratory	
Cardiovascular	
GI	
GU	
GYN	
Neuropsychiatric	
Musculoskeletal	

History and Physical Exam

DIAMONTE HOSPITAL
Diamonte, Arizona

Physical Exam

(Page 2 of 2)

Blood Pressure	Pulse	Resp.		Temp.	Weight
General					
Skin					
Eyes					
Ears					
Nose					
Mouth					
Throat					
Neck					
Chest					
Heart					
Abdomen					
Genitalia					
Lymphatic					
Blood Vessels					
Musculoskeletal					
Extremities					
Neurological					
Rectal					
Vaginal					
Diagnosis **Plan of Care**					
	Signature			Date	

History and Physical Exam

DIAMONTE HOSPITAL
Diamonte, Arizona

Informed Consent
(example only)

PATIENT CONSENT TO MEDICAL TREATMENT/SURGICAL PROCEDURE
AND ACKNOWLEDGMENT OF RECEIPT OF MEDICAL INFORMATION
READ CAREFULLY BEFORE SIGNING.

TO THE PATIENT: You have been told that you should consider medical treatment/surgery. State law requires this facility to tell you (1) the nature of your condition, (2) the general nature of the procedure/treatment/surgery, (3) the risks of the proposed treatment/surgery, as defined by the State or as determined by your doctor, and (4) reasonable therapeutic alternatives and risks associated with such alternatives.

You have the right, as a patient, to be informed about your condition and the recommended surgical, medical, or diagnostic procedure to be used so that you may make the decision whether or not to undergo the procedure after knowing the risks and hazards involved.

In keeping with the State law of informed consent, you are being asked to sign a confirmation that we have discussed all these matters. We have already discussed with you the common problems and risks. We wish to inform you as completely as possible. Please read this form carefully. Ask about anything you do not understand, and we will be pleased to explain it.

1. Patient name:_____

2. Treatment/procedure:
    (a) Description, nature of the treatment/procedure: _____

    Purpose: _____
    _____

3. Patient condition: Patient's diagnosis, description of the nature of the condition or ailment for which the medical treatment, surgical procedure, or other therapy described in Item 2 is indicated and recommended:
    _____
    _____

4. Material risks of treatment procedure:
    (a) All medical or surgical treatment involves risks. Listed below are those risks associated with this procedure that members of this facility believe a reasonable person in your (patient's) position would likely consider significant when deciding whether to have or forego the proposed therapy. Please ask your physician if you would like additional information regarding the nature or consequences of these risks, their likelihood of occurrence, or other associated risks that you might consider significant but may not be listed below.

        -    See attachment for risks identified by the State
        -    See attachment for risks determined by your doctor

Informed Consent

Page 2 of 3

    (b) Additional risks (if any) particular to the patient because of a complicating medical condition:

_____

_____

    (c) Risks generally associated with any surgical treatment/procedure, including anesthesia are death, brain damage, disfiguring scars, quadriplegia (paralysis from neck down), paraplegia (paralysis from waist down), the loss or loss of function of any organ or limb, infection, bleeding, and pain.

5.   Therapeutic alternatives, risks associated therewith, and risks of no treatment: Reasonable therapeutic alternatives and the risks associated with such alternatives:

_____

_____

ACKNOWLEDGMENT
AUTHORIZATION AND CONSENT

6. (a) No guarantees: All information given me and, in particular, all estimates made as to the likelihood of occurrence of risks of this or alternate procedures or as to the prospects of success are made in the best professional judgment of my physician. The possibility and nature of complications cannot always be accurately anticipated, and therefore there is and can be no guarantee, either express or implied, as to the success or other results of the medical treatment or surgical procedure.

  (b) Additional information: Nothing has been said to me, no information has been given to me, and I have not relied upon any information that is inconsistent with the information set forth in this document.

  (c) Particular concerns: I have had an opportunity to disclose to and discuss with the physician providing such information those risks or other potential consequences of the medical treatment or surgical procedure that are of particular concern to me.

  (d) Questions: I have had an opportunity to ask, and I have asked, any questions I may have about the information in this document and any other questions I have about the proposed treatment or procedure, and all such questions were answered in a satisfactory manner.

  (e) Authorized physician: The physician (or physician group) authorized to administer or perform the medical treatment, surgical procedures or other therapy described in Item 2 is

_____

    (Name of authorized physician or group)

  (f) Physician certification: I hereby certify that I have provided and explained the information set forth herein, including any attachment, and answered all questions of the patient or the patient's representative concerning the medical treatment or surgical procedure, to the best of my knowledge and ability.

_____

    (Signature of physician)   Date   Time

Informed Consent

Page 3 of 3

Consent

I hereby authorize and direct the designated authorized physician/group, together with associates and assistants of his/her choice, to administer or perform the medical treatment or surgical procedure described in Item 2 of this consent form, including any additional procedures or services as they may deem necessary or reasonable, including the administration of any general or regional anesthetic agent, x-ray or other radiological services, laboratory services, and the disposal of any tissue removed during a diagnostic or surgical procedure, and I hereby consent thereto.

I have read and understand all information set forth in this document, and all blanks were filled in prior to my signing. This authorization for and consent to medical treatment or surgical procedure is and shall remain valid until revoked.

I acknowledge that I have had the opportunity to ask any questions about the contemplated medical procedure or surgical procedure described in Item 2 of this consent form, including risks and alternatives, and acknowledge that my questions have been answered to my satisfaction.

_____   _____
Witness   Date/time   Patient or person   Date/time
                                                 authorized to consent

If consent is signed by someone other than patient, indicate relationship: _____

Informed Consent

DIAMONTE HOSPITAL
Diamonte, Arizona

Intake/Output
Record

Date:_____

Time AM/PM	IV Fluid/Rate	Absorbed 7AM-3PM	3PM-11PM	11PM-7AM	Comments:

INTAKE | | | | | | **OUTPUT**

Time	Oral	Tube	IV	Blood	Total	Urine Voided	Catheter	Suction	Drains	Emesis	Total
7AM-3PM											
3PM-11PM											
11PM-7AM											
Total											

IV START/RESTART   Time: IV START/RESTART   Time:

CATHETER SIZE/# USED: /   CATHETER SIZE/# USED: /

TIME	APPEARANCE	SITE
7AM-3PM		
3PM-11PM		
11PM-7AM		

7AM-3PM Shift   3PM-11PM SHIFT

Initials	Signature/Title		Initials	Signature/Title

11PM-7AM Shift

Initials	Signature/Title

Intake/Output Record

DIAMONTE HOSPITAL
Diamonte, Arizona

Date	Time	Problem Number	Nurse's Progress Notes	Nurse Initials

Nurse's Progress Notes

DIAMONTE HOSPITAL
Diamonte, Arizona

**Nursing
Discharge Summary**

Patient Name:

Medical Record No.

(addressograph)

Date of discharge:_____ Time of discharge:_____ Accompanied by:_____
Disposition: ___ Home ___ Death ___ Other (Please specifiy)_____
Discharged: ___ Ambulatory ___ Wheelchair ___ Stretcher ___Ambulance
Vital signs: Blood pressure:_____ Pulse:_____ Resp:_____ Temp:_____
Mental status: ___Alert ___Confused ___Other (specify)_____
Social worker:_____ Phone number:_____

Services Needed
Equipment/Supplies: Company:_____ Phone:_____
Type of service:_____ Date service is to start:_____

Home Health: Company:_____ Phone :_____
Type of service:_____ Date service is to start:_____

Other: Company:_____ Phone:_____
Type of service:_____ Date service is to start:_____

Medication **Dose** **Time of Day** **Special Instruction**
_____
_____
_____
_____

___Medication/diet Counseling for above drugs, signature of dietitian:_____Date:_____
___Prescription given to patient ___Medication from pharmacy returned ___Yes ___No

Diet ___ Regular
___ Other:_____ Diet Instructions:_____
_____ signature of dietitian:_____Date:_____

Treatment/Wound Care ___ No treatments prescribed
Treatment/wound care
Site 1 _____
Site 2 _____
___ Patient instructed ___Significant other Date:_____

Activity
___ Special precautions:_____
___ Gradually resume daily activities
___ Do not lift object heavier than _____
___ Use the following devices to move safely:_____
___ Remain on bed rest except for: ___bathroom ___meals

Follow-up
___ No appointment needed ___ Patient teaching form discussed with patient/family
See doctor_____ on_____Phone_____ Appointment made: Yes/No
See doctor_____ on_____Phone_____ Appointment made: Yes/No
Call doctor if:_____
_____

I have received and understand the above instructions:
Patient signature:_____ Date:_____ Nurse signature:_____Date:_____

Nursing Discharge Summary

DIAMONTE HOSPITAL
Diamonte, Arizona

**Report of
Consultation**

Doctor:_____ has been request to see this patient regarding

___ Second opinion
___ To follow patient for the following condition:_____
___ Surgical treatment
___ Other:_____

Attending Physician Signature:_____Date:_____

Report: ___ Medical record reviewed

_____

_____

_____

_____

_____

_____

_____

_____

_____

_____

_____

_____

_____

_____

_____

_____

_____

_____

_____

Date: **Consulting Physician's Signature:**

Report of Consultation

Appendix B

SAMPLE ELECTRONIC MEDICAL RECORD

The following ten screen shots are samples of an electronic medical record taken from an electronic medical record program by the software company AltaPoint Data Systems. Please go to http://www.altapoint.com/ to see the demo.

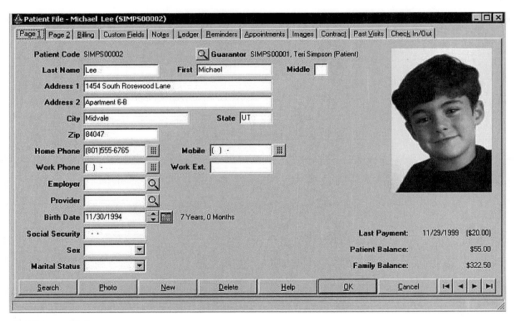

◆ **Figure B-1**
Patient file.

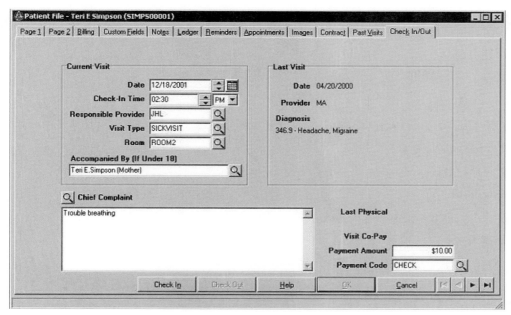

◆ **Figure B-2**
Patient check-in.

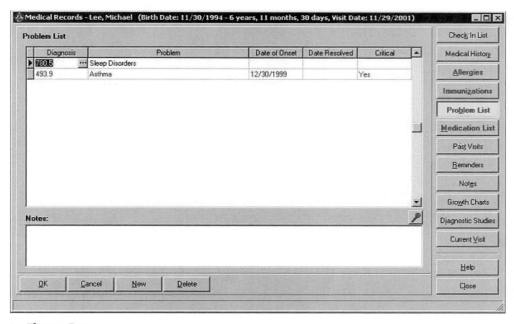

◆ **Figure B-3**
Allergies and problem list.

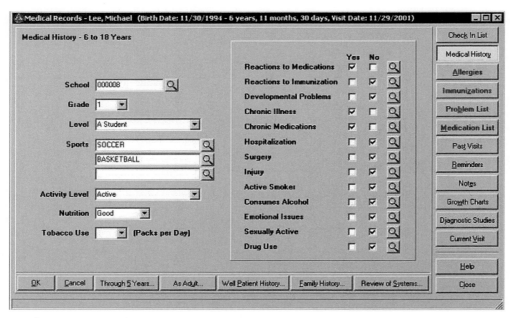

◆ **Figure B-4**
Medical history.

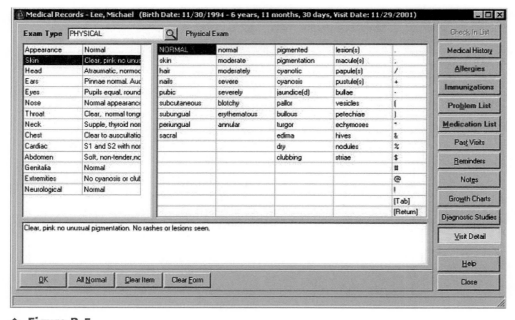

◆ **Figure B-5**
Physical examination.

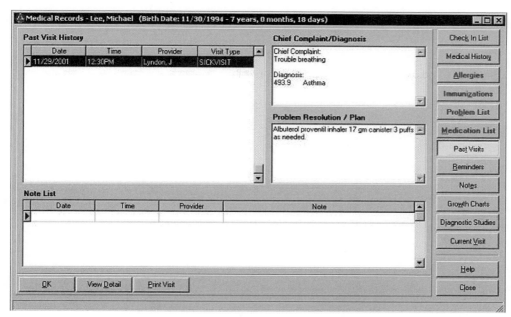

◆ **Figure B-6**
Past visits.

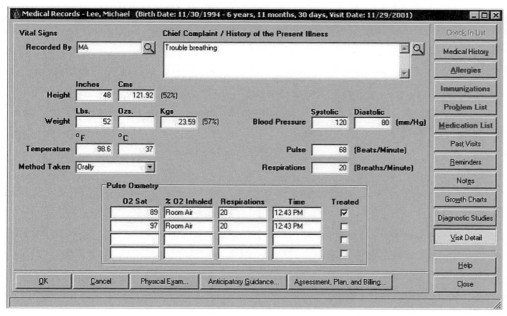

◆ **Figure B-7**
Current visit—vital signs.

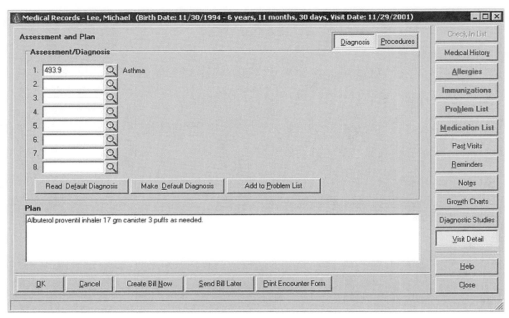

◆ **Figure B-8**
Assessment and plan.

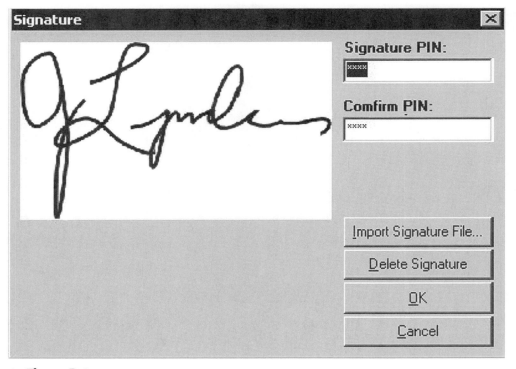

◆ **Figure B-9**
Electronic signatures.

Creekside Clinic
2825 E. Cottonwood Parkway Suite 522
Salt Lake City, UT 84121
(801)555-1122

Patient Visit Record
Page 1
March 1, 2002

Michael Lee
1454 South Rosewood Lane, Apartment 6-B
Midvale, UT 84047

Date/Time In: 03/01/2002 - 10:00AM
Date/Time Out: 03/01/2002 - 10:59AM

Patient ID: SIMPS00002
Birth Date: 11/30/1994
Age: 7 Years, 3 Months

Attending Provider: Lyndon, Jeffery
Vitals Recorded By: Adams, Mitchell
Accompanied By: Teri E.Simpson (Mother)

Chief Complaint:
Trouble breathing

Vitals:

Height:	48in , 121.92cm (54%)	Blood Pressure:	120 / 80
Weight:	52 lbs, 23.59 kgs (57%)	Respirations:	20
Temperature:	98.6F, 37C	Pulse:	68

Pulse Oximetry:	O2 Sat.	O2 Inhaled	Respirations	Time	Treated
	89	Room Air	20	12:43 PM	Yes
	97	Room Air	20	12:43 PM	No

Physical Exam:

Appearance	Normal
Skin	Clear, pink no unusual pigmentation. No rashes or lesions seen.
Head	Atraumatic, normocephalic
Ears	Pinnae normal. Auditory canals clear. Tympanic membranes are normally mobile with landmarks and light reflexes intact.
Eyes	Pupils equal, round react to light and accomodation. Sclerae clear. No discharge or tearing. Extra ocular muscles full ROM.
Nose	Normal appearance. Septum undeviated. No discharge.
Throat	Clear, normal tongue. Tonsils not enlarged. No exudates.
Neck	Supple, thyroid normal size,no adenopathy.
Chest	Clear to auscultation and percussion. Normal appearance.
Cardiac	S1 and S2 with normal physiological split. No murmurs, rubs or heaves.
Abdomen	Soft, non-tender,no masses or organomegaly, bowel sounds normal
Genitalia	Normal
Extremities	No cyanosis or clubbing, peripheral pulses palpable,no orthopedic abnormalities.
Neurological	Normal

Diagnostic Studies:

Far Vision Screen:	(Not Recorded)
Near Vision Screen:	(Not Recorded)
Hearing Screen:	(Not Recorded)

Assessments:
493.9   Asthma

Plan:
Albuterol proventil inhaler 17 gm canister 3 puffs as needed.

Jeffery Lyndon 03/01/2002 10:58AM

◆ **Figure B-10**
Patient visit record.

❧

MINIMUM DATA SET

Numeric Identifier_____

MINIMUM DATA SET (MDS) — *VERSION 2.0*
FOR NURSING HOME RESIDENT ASSESSMENT AND CARE SCREENING

BASIC ASSESSMENT TRACKING FORM

SECTION AA. IDENTIFICATION INFORMATION

1.	RESIDENT NAME⊙				
		a. (First)	b. (Middle Initial)	c. (Last)	d. (Jr/Sr)
2.	GENDER⊙	1. Male		2. Female	
3.	BIRTHDATE⊙	Month — Day — Year			
4.	RACE/⊙ ETHNICITY	1. American Indian/Alaskan Native 4. Hispanic 2. Asian/Pacific Islander 5. White, not of 3. Black, not of Hispanic origin Hispanic origin			
5.	SOCIAL SECURITY⊙ AND MEDICARE NUMBERS⊙ [C in 1st box if non med. no.]	a. Social Security Number b. Medicare number (or comparable railroad insurance number)			
6.	FACILITY PROVIDER NO.⊙	a. State No. b. Federal No.			
7.	MEDICAID NO. ["+" if pending, "N" if not a Medicaid recipient⊙				

8.	REASONS FOR ASSESS-MENT	[Note—Other codes do not apply to this form]
		
		a. Primary reason for assessment
		   1. Admission assessment (required by day 14)
		   2. Annual assessment
		   3. Significant change in status assessment
		   4. Significant correction of prior full assessment
		   5. Quarterly review assessment
		   10. Significant correction of prior quarterly assessment
		   0. *NONE OF ABOVE*
		
		b. *Codes for assessments required for Medicare PPS or the State*
		   1. Medicare 5 day assessment
		   2. Medicare 30 day assessment
		   3. Medicare 60 day assessment
		   4. Medicare 90 day assessment
		   5. Medicare readmission/return assessment
		   6. Other state required assessment
		   7. Medicare 14 day assessment
		   8. Other Medicare required assessment			

9. Signatures of Persons who Completed a Portion of the Accompanying Assessment or Tracking Form

I certify that the accompanying information accurately reflects resident assessment or tracking information for this resident and that I collected or coordinated collection of this information on the dates specified. To the best of my knowledge, this information was collected in accordance with applicable Medicare and Medicaid requirements. I understand that this information is used as a basis for ensuring that residents receive appropriate and quality care, and as a basis for payment from federal funds. I further understand that payment of such federal funds and continued participation in the government-funded health care programs is conditioned on the accuracy and truthfulness of this information, and that I may be personally subject to or may subject my organization to substantial criminal, civil, and/or administrative penalties for submitting false information. I also certify that I am authorized to submit this information by this facility on its behalf.

Signature and Title	Sections	Date
a.		
b.		
c.		
d.		
e.		
f.		
g.		
h.		
i.		
j.		
k.		
l.		

GENERAL INSTRUCTIONS

Complete this information for submission with all full and quarterly assessments (Admission, Annual, Significant Change, State or Medicare required assessments, or Quarterly Reviews, etc.)

⊙ = Key items for computerized resident tracking

☐ = When box blank, must enter number or letter   a. = When letter in box, check if condition applies

Resident_____   Numeric Identifier_____

MINIMUM DATA SET (MDS) — VERSION 2.0
FOR NURSING HOME RESIDENT ASSESSMENT AND CARE SCREENING

BACKGROUND (FACE SHEET) INFORMATION AT ADMISSION

SECTION AB. DEMOGRAPHIC INFORMATION

1.	DATE OF ENTRY	Date the stay began. Note — Does not include readmission if record was closed at time of temporary discharge to hospital, etc. In such cases, use prior admission date

☐☐ — ☐☐ — ☐☐☐☐
Month   Day   Year

2.	ADMITTED FROM (AT ENTRY)	1. Private home/apt. with no home health services 2. Private home/apt. with home health services 3. Board and care/assisted living/group home 4. Nursing home 5. Acute care hospital 6. Psychiatric hospital, MR/DD facility 7. Rehabilitation hospital 8. Other
3.	LIVED ALONE (PRIOR TO ENTRY)	0. No 1. Yes 2. In other facility
4.	ZIP CODE OF PRIOR PRIMARY RESIDENCE	☐☐☐☐☐

5.	RESIDEN-TIAL HISTORY 5 YEARS PRIOR TO ENTRY	(Check all settings resident lived in during 5 years prior to date of entry given in item AB1 above)	
		Prior stay at this nursing home	a.
		Stay in other nursing home	b.
		Other residential facility—board and care home, assisted living, group home	c.
		MH/psychiatric setting	d.
		MR/DD setting	e.
		NONE OF ABOVE	f.

6.	LIFETIME OCCUPA-TION(S) [Put "/" between two occupations]	☐☐☐☐☐☐☐☐☐☐☐☐

7.	EDUCATION (Highest Level Completed)	1. No schooling 5. Technical or trade school 2. 8th grade/less 6. Some college 3. 9-11 grades 7. Bachelor's degree 4. High school 8. Graduate degree
8.	LANGUAGE	(Code for correct response) a. Primary Language 0. English 1. Spanish 2. French 3. Other b. If other, specify ☐☐☐☐☐☐☐☐
9.	MENTAL HEALTH HISTORY	Does resident's RECORD indicate any history of mental retardation, mental illness, or developmental disability problem? 0. No 1. Yes

10.	CONDITIONS RELATED TO MR/DD STATUS	(Check all conditions that are related to MR/DD status that were manifested before age 22, and are likely to continue indefinitely)	
		Not applicable—no MR/DD (Skip to AB11)	a.
		MR/DD with organic condition	
		Down's syndrome	b.
		Autism	c.
		Epilepsy	d.
		Other organic condition related to MR/DD	e.
		MR/DD with no organic condition	f.

11.	DATE BACK-GROUND INFORMA-TION COMPLETED	☐☐ — ☐☐ — ☐☐☐☐ Month Day Year

SECTION AC. CUSTOMARY ROUTINE

1.	CUSTOMARY ROUTINE	(Check all that apply. If all information UNKNOWN, check last box only.)	
	(In year prior to DATE OF ENTRY to this nursing home, or year last in community if now being admitted from another nursing home)	**CYCLE OF DAILY EVENTS**	
		Stays up late at night (e.g., after 9 pm)	a.
		Naps regularly during day (at least 1 hour)	b.
		Goes out 1+ days a week	c.
		Stays busy with hobbies, reading, or fixed daily routine	d.
		Spends most of time alone or watching TV	e.
		Moves independently indoors (with appliances, if used)	f.
		Use of tobacco products at least daily	g.
		NONE OF ABOVE	h.
		EATING PATTERNS	
		Distinct food preferences	i.
		Eats between meals all or most days	j.
		Use of alcoholic beverage(s) at least weekly	k.
		NONE OF ABOVE	l.
		ADL PATTERNS	
		In bedclothes much of day	m.
		Wakens to toilet all or most nights	n.
		Has irregular bowel movement pattern	o.
		Showers for bathing	p.
		Bathing in PM	q.
		NONE OF ABOVE	r.
		INVOLVEMENT PATTERNS	
		Daily contact with relatives/close friends	s.
		Usually attends church, temple, synagogue (etc.)	t.
		Finds strength in faith	u.
		Daily animal companion/presence	v.
		Involved in group activities	w.
		NONE OF ABOVE	x.
		UNKNOWN—Resident/family unable to provide information	y.

SECTION AD. FACE SHEET SIGNATURES

SIGNATURES OF PERSONS COMPLETING FACE SHEET:

a. Signature of RN Assessment Coordinator	Date

I certify that the accompanying information accurately reflects resident assessment or tracking information for this resident and that I collected or coordinated collection of this information on the dates specified. To the best of my knowledge, this information was collected in accordance with applicable Medicare and Medicaid requirements. I understand that this information is used as a basis for ensuring that residents receive appropriate and quality care, and as a basis for payment from federal funds. I further understand that payment of such federal funds and continued participation in the government-funded health care programs is conditioned on the accuracy and truthfulness of this information, and that I may be personally subject to or may subject my organization to substantial criminal, civil, and/or administrative penalties for submitting false information. I also certify that I am authorized to submit this information by this facility on its behalf.

Signature and Title	Sections	Date
b.		
c.		
d.		
e.		
f.		
g.		

☐ = When box blank, must enter number or letter   [a.] = When letter in box, check if condition applies

Resident _____ Numeric Identifier _____

MINIMUM DATA SET (MDS) — *VERSION 2.0*
FOR NURSING HOME RESIDENT ASSESSMENT AND CARE SCREENING
FULL ASSESSMENT FORM
(Status in last 7 days, unless other time frame indicated)

SECTION A. IDENTIFICATION AND BACKGROUND INFORMATION

1.	RESIDENT NAME				
		a. (First)	b. (Middle Initial)	c. (Last)	d. (Jr/Sr)

2.	ROOM NUMBER	

3.	ASSESS- MENT REFERENCE DATE	a. Last day of MDS observation period
		Month — Day — Year
		b. Original (0) or corrected copy of form (enter number of correction)

4a.	DATE OF REENTRY	Date of reentry from most recent temporary discharge to a hospital in last 90 days (or since last assessment or admission if less than 90 days)
		Month — Day — Year

| 5. | MARITAL STATUS | 1. Never married   3. Widowed   5. Divorced
2. Married   4. Separated |
|---|---|---|

6.	MEDICAL RECORD NO.	

7.	CURRENT PAYMENT SOURCES FOR N.H. STAY	(Billing Office to indicate; **check all that apply in last 30 days**)
		Medicaid per diem — a. VA per diem — f.
		Medicare per diem — b. Self or family pays for full per diem — g.
		Medicaid ancillary part A — c. Medicaid resident liability or Medicare co-payment — h.
		Medicare ancillary part B — d. Private insurance per diem (including co-payment) — i.
		CHAMPUS per diem — e. Other per diem — j.

| 8. | REASONS FOR ASSESS- MENT
[Note—**If this is a discharge or reentry assessment, only a limited subset of MDS items need be completed**] | a. Primary reason for assessment
1. Admission assessment (required by day 14)
2. Annual assessment
3. Significant change in status assessment
4. Significant correction of prior full assessment
5. Quarterly review assessment
6. Discharged—return not anticipated
7. Discharged—return anticipated
8. Discharged prior to completing initial assessment
9. Reentry
10. Significant correction of prior quarterly assessment
0. NONE OF ABOVE |
|---|---|---|
| | | b. Codes for assessments required for Medicare PPS or the State
1. Medicare 5 day assessment
2. Medicare 30 day assessment
3. Medicare 60 day assessment
4. Medicare 90 day assessment
5. Medicare readmission/return assessment
6. Other state required assessment
7. Medicare 14 day assessment
8. Other Medicare required assessment |

9.	RESPONSI- BILITY/ LEGAL GUARDIAN	(Check all that apply)
		Legal guardian — a. Durable power attorney/financial — d.
		Other legal oversight — b. Family member responsible — e.
		Durable power of attorney/health care — c. Patient responsible for self — f.
			NONE OF ABOVE — g.

10.	ADVANCED DIRECTIVES	(For those items with supporting **documentation** in the medical record, **check all that apply**)
		Living will — a. Feeding restrictions — f.
		Do not resuscitate — b. Medication restrictions — g.
		Do not hospitalize — c. Other treatment restrictions — h.
		Organ donation — d. NONE OF ABOVE — i.
		Autopsy request — e.	

SECTION B. COGNITIVE PATTERNS

| 1. | COMATOSE | (Persistent vegetative state/no discernible consciousness)
0. No   1. Yes   (If yes, skip to Section G) |
|---|---|---|

2.	MEMORY	(Recall of what was learned or known)
		a. Short-term memory OK—seems/appears to recall after 5 minutes
0. Memory OK   1. Memory problem
		b. Long-term memory OK—seems/appears to recall long past
0. Memory OK   1. Memory problem

3.	MEMORY/ RECALL ABILITY	(Check all that resident was **normally able to recall during last 7 days**)
		Current season — a. That he/she is in a nursing home — d.
		Location of own room — b. NONE OF ABOVE are recalled — e.
		Staff names/faces — c.	

| 4. | COGNITIVE SKILLS FOR DAILY DECISION- MAKING | (Made decisions regarding tasks of daily life)
0. INDEPENDENT—decisions consistent/reasonable
1. MODIFIED INDEPENDENCE—some difficulty in new situations only
2. MODERATELY IMPAIRED—decisions poor; cues/supervision required
3. SEVERELY IMPAIRED—never/rarely made decisions |
|---|---|---|

| 5. | INDICATORS OF DELIRIUM— PERIODIC DISOR- DERED THINKING/ AWARENESS | (Code for behavior in the **last 7 days**.) [Note: Accurate assessment requires conversations with staff and family who have direct knowledge of resident's behavior over this time].
0. Behavior not present
1. Behavior present, not of recent onset
2. Behavior present, over last 7 days appears different from resident's usual functioning (e.g., new onset or worsening) |
|---|---|---|
| | | a. EASILY DISTRACTED—(e.g., difficulty paying attention; gets sidetracked) |
| | | b. PERIODS OF ALTERED PERCEPTION OR AWARENESS OF SURROUNDINGS—(e.g., moves lips or talks to someone not present; believes he/she is somewhere else; confuses night and day) |
| | | c. EPISODES OF DISORGANIZED SPEECH—(e.g., speech is incoherent, nonsensical, irrelevant, or rambling from subject to subject; loses train of thought) |
| | | d. PERIODS OF RESTLESSNESS—(e.g., fidgeting or picking at skin, clothing, napkins, etc; frequent position changes; repetitive physical movements or calling out) |
| | | e. PERIODS OF LETHARGY—(e.g., sluggishness; staring into space; difficult to arouse; little body movement) |
| | | f. MENTAL FUNCTION VARIES OVER THE COURSE OF THE DAY—(e.g., sometimes better, sometimes worse; behaviors sometimes present, sometimes not) |

| 6. | CHANGE IN COGNITIVE STATUS | Resident's cognitive status, skills, or abilities have changed as compared to status of **90 days ago** (or since last assessment if less than 90 days)
0. No change   1. Improved   2. Deteriorated |
|---|---|---|

SECTION C. COMMUNICATION/HEARING PATTERNS

| 1. | HEARING | (With hearing appliance, if used)
0. HEARS ADEQUATELY—normal talk, TV, phone
1. MINIMAL DIFFICULTY when not in quiet setting
2. HEARS IN SPECIAL SITUATIONS ONLY—speaker has to adjust tonal quality and speak distinctly
3. HIGHLY IMPAIRED/absence of useful hearing |
|---|---|---|

2.	COMMUNI- CATION DEVICES/ TECH- NIQUES	(Check all that apply during last 7 days)
		Hearing aid, present and used — a.
		Hearing aid, present and not used regularly — b.
		Other receptive comm. techniques used (e.g., lip reading) — c.
		NONE OF ABOVE — d.

3.	MODES OF EXPRESSION	(Check all used by resident to make needs known)
		Speech — a. Signs/gestures/sounds — d.
		Writing messages to express or clarify needs — b. Communication board — e.
		American sign language or Braille — c. Other — f.
			NONE OF ABOVE — g.

| 4. | MAKING SELF UNDER- STOOD | (Expressing information content—however able)
0. UNDERSTOOD
1. USUALLY UNDERSTOOD—difficulty finding words or finishing thoughts
2. SOMETIMES UNDERSTOOD—ability is limited to making concrete requests
3. RARELY/NEVER UNDERSTOOD |
|---|---|---|

| 5. | SPEECH CLARITY | (Code for speech in the **last 7 days**)
0. CLEAR SPEECH—distinct, intelligible words
1. UNCLEAR SPEECH—slurred, mumbled words
2. NO SPEECH—absence of spoken words |
|---|---|---|

| 6. | ABILITY TO UNDER- STAND OTHERS | (Understanding verbal information content—however able)
0. UNDERSTANDS
1. USUALLY UNDERSTANDS—may miss some part/intent of message
2. SOMETIMES UNDERSTANDS—responds adequately to simple, direct communication
3. RARELY/NEVER UNDERSTANDS |
|---|---|---|

| 7. | CHANGE IN COMMUNI- CATION/ HEARING | Resident's ability to express, understand, or hear information has changed as compared to status of **90 days ago** (or since last assessment if less than 90 days)
0. No change   1. Improved   2. Deteriorated |
|---|---|---|

□ = When box blank, must enter number or letter   [a.] = When letter in box, check if condition applies

Resident _____   Numeric Identifier _____

SECTION D. VISION PATTERNS

1.	VISION	*(Ability to see in adequate light and with glasses if used)* 0. *ADEQUATE*—sees fine detail, including regular print in newspapers/books 1. *IMPAIRED*—sees large print, but not regular print in newspapers/books 2. *MODERATELY IMPAIRED*—limited vision; not able to see newspaper headlines, but can identify objects 3. *HIGHLY IMPAIRED*—object identification in question, but eyes appear to follow objects 4. *SEVERELY IMPAIRED*—no vision or sees only light, colors, or shapes; eyes do not appear to follow objects	
2.	VISUAL LIMITATIONS/ DIFFICULTIES	Side vision problems—decreased peripheral vision (e.g., leaves food on one side of tray, difficulty traveling, bumps into people and objects, misjudges placement of chair when seating self)	a.
		Experiences any of following: sees halos or rings around lights; sees flashes of light; sees "curtains" over eyes	b.
		NONE OF ABOVE	c.
3.	VISUAL APPLIANCES	Glasses; contact lenses; magnifying glass 0. No 1. Yes	

SECTION E. MOOD AND BEHAVIOR PATTERNS

1.	INDICATORS OF DEPRES- SION, ANXIETY, SAD MOOD	*(Code for indicators observed in last 30 days, irrespective of the assumed cause)* 0. Indicator not exhibited in last 30 days 1. Indicator of this type exhibited up to five days a week 2. Indicator of this type exhibited daily or almost daily (6, 7 days a week)	

VERBAL EXPRESSIONS OF DISTRESS

a. Resident made negative statements—e.g., "*Nothing matters; Would rather be dead; What's the use; Regrets having lived so long; Let me die*"

b. Repetitive questions—e.g., "*Where do I go; What do I do?*"

c. Repetitive verbalizations— e.g., calling out for help, ("*God help me*")

d. Persistent anger with self or others—e.g., easily annoyed, anger at placement in nursing home; anger at care received

e. Self deprecation—e.g., "*I am nothing; I am of no use to anyone*"

f. Expressions of what appear to be unrealistic fears—e.g., fear of being abandoned, left alone, being with others

g. Recurrent statements that something terrible is about to happen—e.g., believes he or she is about to die, have a heart attack

h. Repetitive health complaints—e.g., persistently seeks medical attention, obsessive concern with body functions

i. Repetitive anxious complaints/concerns (non-health related) e.g., persistently seeks attention/ reassurance regarding schedules, meals, laundry, clothing, relationship issues

SLEEP-CYCLE ISSUES

j. Unpleasant mood in morning

k. Insomnia/change in usual sleep pattern

SAD, APATHETIC, ANXIOUS APPEARANCE

l. Sad, pained, worried facial expressions—e.g., furrowed brows

m. Crying, tearfulness

n. Repetitive physical movements—e.g., pacing, hand wringing, restlessness, fidgeting, picking

LOSS OF INTEREST

o. Withdrawal from activities of interest—e.g., no interest in long standing activities or being with family/friends

p. Reduced social interaction

2.	MOOD PERSIS- TENCE	One or more indicators of depressed, sad or anxious mood **were not easily altered by attempts to "cheer up", console, or reassure the resident over last 7 days** 0. No mood 1. Indicators present, 2. Indicators present, indicators easily altered not easily altered	
3.	CHANGE IN MOOD	Resident's mood status has changed as compared to status of **90 days ago** (or since last assessment if less than 90 days) 0. No change 1. Improved 2. Deteriorated	
4.	BEHAVIORAL SYMPTOMS	(A) *Behavioral symptom frequency in last 7 days* 0. Behavior not exhibited in last 7 days 1. Behavior of this type occurred 1 to 3 days in last 7 days 2. Behavior of this type occurred 4 to 6 days, but less than daily 3. Behavior of this type occurred daily	

(B) *Behavioral symptom alterability in last 7 days*
0. Behavior not present OR behavior was easily altered
1. Behavior was not easily altered

		(A)	(B)
a.	WANDERING (moved with no rational purpose, seemingly oblivious to needs or safety)		
b.	VERBALLY ABUSIVE BEHAVIORAL SYMPTOMS (others were threatened, screamed at, cursed at)		
c.	PHYSICALLY ABUSIVE BEHAVIORAL SYMPTOMS (others were hit, shoved, scratched, sexually abused)		
d.	SOCIALLY INAPPROPRIATE/DISRUPTIVE BEHAVIORAL SYMPTOMS (made disruptive sounds, noisiness, screaming, self-abusive acts, sexual behavior or disrobing in public, smeared/threw food/feces, hoarding, rummaged through others' belongings)		
e.	RESISTS CARE (resisted taking medications/ injections, ADL assistance, or eating)		

5.	CHANGE IN BEHAVIORAL SYMPTOMS	Resident's behavior status has changed as compared to **status of 90 days ago** (or since last assessment if less than 90 days) 0. No change 1. Improved 2. Deteriorated	

SECTION F. PSYCHOSOCIAL WELL-BEING

1.	SENSE OF INITIATIVE/ INVOLVE- MENT	At ease interacting with others	a.
		At ease doing planned or structured activities	b.
		At ease doing self-initiated activities	c.
		Establishes own goals	d.
		Pursues involvement in life of facility (e.g., makes/keeps friends; involved in group activities; responds positively to new activities; assists at religious services)	e.
		Accepts invitations into most group activities	f.
		NONE OF ABOVE	g.
2.	UNSETTLED RELATION- SHIPS	Covert/open conflict with or repeated criticism of staff	a.
		Unhappy with roommate	b.
		Unhappy with residents other than roommate	c.
		Openly expresses conflict/anger with family/friends	d.
		Absence of personal contact with family/friends	e.
		Recent loss of close family member/friend	f.
		Does not adjust easily to change in routines	g.
		NONE OF ABOVE	h.
3.	PAST ROLES	Strong identification with past roles and life status	a.
		Expresses sadness/anger/empty feeling over lost roles/status	b.
		Resident perceives that daily routine (customary routine, activities) is very different from prior pattern in the community	c.
		NONE OF ABOVE	d.

SECTION G. PHYSICAL FUNCTIONING AND STRUCTURAL PROBLEMS

1.	(A) ADL SELF-PERFORMANCE—*(Code for resident's PERFORMANCE OVER ALL SHIFTS during last 7 days*—Not including setup)*

0. *INDEPENDENT*—No help or oversight —OR— Help/oversight provided only 1 or 2 times during last 7 days

1. *SUPERVISION*—Oversight, encouragement or cueing provided 3 or more times during last 7 days —OR— Supervision (3 or more times) plus physical assistance provided only 1 or 2 times during last 7 days

2. *LIMITED ASSISTANCE*—Resident highly involved in activity; received physical help in guided maneuvering of limbs or other nonweight bearing assistance 3 or more times — OR—More help provided only 1 or 2 times during last 7 days

3. *EXTENSIVE ASSISTANCE*—While resident performed part of activity, over last 7-day period, help of following type(s) provided 3 or more times:
—Weight-bearing support
—Full staff performance during part (but not all) of last 7 days

4. *TOTAL DEPENDENCE*—Full staff performance of activity during entire 7 days

8. *ACTIVITY DID NOT OCCUR* during entire 7 days

(B) ADL SUPPORT PROVIDED—**(Code for MOST SUPPORT PROVIDED OVER ALL SHIFTS during last 7 days; code regardless** of resident's self-performance classification)
0. No setup or physical help from staff
1. Setup help only
2. One person physical assist   8. ADL activity itself did not
3. Two+ persons physical assist   occur during entire 7 days

			(A) SELF-PERF	(B) SUPPORT
a.	BED MOBILITY	How resident moves to and from lying position, turns side to side, and positions body while in bed		
b.	TRANSFER	How resident moves between surfaces—to/from: bed, chair, wheelchair, standing position (EXCLUDE to/from bath/toilet)		
c.	WALK IN ROOM	How resident walks between locations in his/her room		
d.	WALK IN CORRIDOR	How resident walks in corridor on unit		
e.	LOCOMO- TION ON UNIT	How resident moves between locations in his/her room and adjacent corridor on same floor. If in wheelchair, self-sufficiency once in chair		
f.	LOCOMO- TION OFF UNIT	How resident moves to and returns from off unit locations (e.g., areas set aside for dining, activities, or treatments). **If facility has only one floor,** how resident moves to and from distant areas on the floor. If in wheelchair, self-sufficiency once in chair		
g.	DRESSING	How resident puts on, fastens, and takes off all items of **street clothing,** including donning/removing prosthesis		
h.	EATING	How resident eats and drinks (regardless of skill). Includes intake of nourishment by other means (e.g., tube feeding, total parenteral nutrition)		
i.	TOILET USE	How resident uses the toilet room (or commode, bedpan, urinal); transfer on/off toilet, cleanses, changes pad, manages ostomy or catheter, adjusts clothes		
j.	PERSONAL HYGIENE	How resident maintains personal hygiene, including combing hair, brushing teeth, shaving, applying makeup, washing/drying face, hands, and perineum (EXCLUDE baths and showers)		

Resident _____

2.	BATHING	How resident takes full-body bath/shower, sponge bath, and transfers in/out of tub/shower (EXCLUDE washing of back and hair.) *Code for most dependent in self-performance and support.* (A) BATHING SELF-PERFORMANCE codes appear below	(A)	(B)
		0. Independent—No help provided		
		1. Supervision—Oversight help only		
		2. Physical help limited to transfer only		
		3. Physical help in part of bathing activity		
		4. Total dependence		
		8. Activity itself did not occur during entire 7 days *(Bathing support codes are as defined in Item 1, code B above)*		

3.	TEST FOR BALANCE (see training manual)	*(Code for ability during test in the last 7 days)* 0. Maintained position as required in test 1. Unsteady, but able to rebalance self without physical support 2. Partial physical support during test; or stands (sits) but does not follow directions for test 3. Not able to attempt test without physical help	
		a. Balance while standing	
		b. Balance while sitting—position, trunk control	

4.	FUNCTIONAL LIMITATION IN RANGE OF MOTION (see training manual)	*(Code for limitations during last 7 days that interfered with daily functions or placed resident at risk of injury)* (A) RANGE OF MOTION (B) VOLUNTARY MOVEMENT 0. No limitation 0. No loss 1. Limitation on one side 1. Partial loss 2. Limitation on both sides 2. Full loss	(A)	(B)
		a. Neck		
		b. Arm—Including shoulder or elbow		
		c. Hand—Including wrist or fingers		
		d. Leg—Including hip or knee		
		e. Foot—Including ankle or toes		
		f. Other limitation or loss		

5.	MODES OF LOCOMOTION	*(Check all that apply during last 7 days)*	
		Cane/walker/crutch **a.**	Wheelchair primary mode of locomotion **d.**
		Wheeled self **b.**	
		Other person wheeled **c.**	NONE OF ABOVE **e.**

6.	MODES OF TRANSFER	*(Check all that apply during last 7 days)*	
		Bedfast all or most of time **a.**	Lifted mechanically **d.**
		Bed rails used for bed mobility or transfer **b.**	Transfer aid (e.g., slide board, trapeze, cane, walker, brace) **e.**
		Lifted manually **c.**	NONE OF ABOVE **f.**

7.	TASK SEGMENTATION	Some or all of ADL activities were broken into subtasks during **last 7 days** so that resident could perform them 0. No 1. Yes	

8.	ADL FUNCTIONAL REHABILITATION POTENTIAL	Resident believes he/she is capable of increased independence in at least some ADLs **a.**
		Direct care staff believe resident is capable of increased independence in at least some ADLs **b.**
		Resident able to perform tasks/activity but is very slow **c.**
		Difference in ADL Self-Performance or ADL Support, comparing mornings to evenings **d.**
		NONE OF ABOVE **e.**

9.	CHANGE IN ADL FUNCTION	Resident's ADL self-performance status has changed as compared to status of **90 days ago** (or since last assessment if less than 90 days) 0. No change 1. Improved 2. Deteriorated	

SECTION H. CONTINENCE IN LAST 14 DAYS

1.	CONTINENCE SELF-CONTROL CATEGORIES	
	(Code for resident's PERFORMANCE OVER ALL SHIFTS)	
	0. **CONTINENT**—Complete control [includes use of indwelling urinary catheter or ostomy device that does not leak urine or stool]	
	1. **USUALLY CONTINENT**—BLADDER, incontinent episodes once a week or less; BOWEL, less than weekly	
	2. **OCCASIONALLY INCONTINENT**—BLADDER, 2 or more times a week but not daily; BOWEL, once a week	
	3. **FREQUENTLY INCONTINENT**—BLADDER, tended to be incontinent daily, but some control present (e.g., on day shift); BOWEL, 2-3 times a week	
	4. **INCONTINENT**—Had inadequate control BLADDER, multiple daily episodes; BOWEL, all (or almost all) of the time	
a.	BOWEL CONTINENCE	Control of bowel movement, with appliance or bowel continence programs, if employed	
b.	BLADDER CONTINENCE	Control of urinary bladder function (if dribbles, volume insufficient to soak through underpants), with appliances (e.g., foley) or continence programs, if employed	

2.	BOWEL ELIMINATION PATTERN	Bowel elimination pattern regular—at least one movement every three days **a.**	Diarrhea **c.**
			Fecal impaction **d.**
		Constipation **b.**	NONE OF ABOVE **e.**

Numeric Identifier _____

3.	APPLIANCES AND PROGRAMS	Any scheduled toileting plan **a.**	Did not use toilet room/ commode/urinal **f.**
		Bladder retraining program **b.**	Pads/briefs used **g.**
		External (condom) catheter **c.**	Enemas/irrigation **h.**
		Indwelling catheter **d.**	Ostomy present **i.**
		Intermittent catheter **e.**	NONE OF ABOVE **j.**

4.	CHANGE IN URINARY CONTINENCE	Resident's urinary continence has changed as compared to status of **90 days ago** (or since last assessment if less than 90 days) 0. No change 1. Improved 2. Deteriorated	

SECTION I. DISEASE DIAGNOSES

Check only those diseases that **have a relationship** to current ADL status, cognitive status, mood and behavior status, medical treatments, nursing monitoring, or risk of death. (Do not list inactive diagnoses)

1.	DISEASES	*(If none apply, CHECK the NONE OF ABOVE box)*	
		ENDOCRINE/METABOLIC/ NUTRITIONAL	Hemiplegia/Hemiparesis **v.**
			Multiple sclerosis **w.**
		Diabetes mellitus **a.**	Paraplegia **x.**
		Hyperthyroidism **b.**	Parkinson's disease **y.**
		Hypothyroidism **c.**	Quadriplegia **z.**
		HEART/CIRCULATION	Seizure disorder **aa.**
		Arteriosclerotic heart disease (ASHD) **d.**	Transient ischemic attack (TIA) **bb.**
			Traumatic brain injury **cc.**
		Cardiac dysrhythmias **e.**	**PSYCHIATRIC/MOOD**
		Congestive heart failure **f.**	Anxiety disorder **dd.**
		Deep vein thrombosis **g.**	Depression **ee.**
		Hypertension **h.**	Manic depression (bipolar disease) **ff.**
		Hypotension **i.**	
		Peripheral vascular disease **j.**	Schizophrenia **gg.**
		Other cardiovascular disease **k.**	**PULMONARY**
		MUSCULOSKELETAL	Asthma **hh.**
		Arthritis **l.**	Emphysema/COPD **ii.**
		Hip fracture **m.**	**SENSORY**
		Missing limb (e.g., amputation) **n.**	Cataracts **jj.**
		Osteoporosis **o.**	Diabetic retinopathy **kk.**
		Pathological bone fracture **p.**	Glaucoma **ll.**
		NEUROLOGICAL	Macular degeneration **mm.**
		Alzheimer's disease **q.**	**OTHER**
		Aphasia **r.**	Allergies **nn.**
		Cerebral palsy **s.**	Anemia **oo.**
		Cerebrovascular accident (stroke) **t.**	Cancer **pp.**
			Renal failure **qq.**
		Dementia other than Alzheimer's disease **u.**	NONE OF ABOVE **rr.**

2.	INFECTIONS	*(If none apply, CHECK the NONE OF ABOVE box)*	
		Antibiotic resistant infection (e.g., Methicillin resistant staph) **a.**	Septicemia **g.**
			Sexually transmitted diseases **h.**
		Clostridium difficile (c. diff.) **b.**	Tuberculosis **i.**
		Conjunctivitis **c.**	Urinary tract infection in **last 30 days j.**
		HIV infection **d.**	Viral hepatitis **k.**
		Pneumonia **e.**	Wound infection **l.**
		Respiratory infection **f.**	NONE OF ABOVE **m.**

3.	OTHER CURRENT OR MORE DETAILED DIAGNOSES AND ICD-9 CODES	**a.** _____	.		
		b. _____	.		
		c. _____	.		
		d. _____	.		
		e. _____	.		

SECTION J. HEALTH CONDITIONS

1.	PROBLEM CONDITIONS	*(Check all problems present in last 7 days unless other time frame is indicated)*	
		INDICATORS OF FLUID STATUS	Dizziness/Vertigo **f.**
			Edema **g.**
			Fever **h.**
		Weight gain or loss of 3 or more pounds within a 7 day period **a.**	Hallucinations **i.**
			Internal bleeding **j.**
		Inability to lie flat due to shortness of breath **b.**	Recurrent lung aspirations in **last 90 days k.**
		Dehydrated; output exceeds input **c.**	Shortness of breath **l.**
			Syncope (fainting) **m.**
		Insufficient fluid; did **NOT** consume all/almost all liquids provided during **last 3 days d.**	Unsteady gait **n.**
			Vomiting **o.**
		OTHER	NONE OF ABOVE **p.**
		Delusions **e.**	

Resident _____

Numeric Identifier _____

2.	PAIN SYMPTOMS	(Code the *highest level of pain* present in the *last 7 days*)		
		a. FREQUENCY with which resident complains or shows evidence of pain 0. No pain (*skip to J4*) 1. Pain less than daily 2. Pain daily	**b. INTENSITY** of pain 1. Mild pain 2. Moderate pain 3. Times when pain is horrible or excruciating	

3.	PAIN SITE	(If pain present, *check all sites* that apply in *last 7 days*)			
		Back pain	a.	Incisional pain	f.
		Bone pain	b.	Joint pain (other than hip)	g.
		Chest pain while doing usual activities	c.	Soft tissue pain (e.g., lesion, muscle)	h.
		Headache	d.	Stomach pain	i.
		Hip pain	e.	Other	j.

4.	ACCIDENTS	(*Check all that apply*)			
		Fell in **past 30 days**	a.	Hip fracture in **last 180 days**	c.
		Fell in **past 31-180 days**	b.	Other fracture in **last 180 days**	d.
				NONE OF ABOVE	e.

5.	STABILITY OF CONDITIONS	Conditions/diseases make resident's cognitive, ADL, mood or behavior patterns unstable—(fluctuating, precarious, or deteriorating)	a.
		Resident experiencing an acute episode or a flare-up of a recurrent or chronic problem	b.
		End-stage disease, 6 or fewer months to live	c.
		NONE OF ABOVE	d.

SECTION K. ORAL/NUTRITIONAL STATUS

1.	ORAL PROBLEMS	Chewing problem	a.
		Swallowing problem	b.
		Mouth pain	c.
		NONE OF ABOVE	d.

2.	HEIGHT AND WEIGHT	Record (a.) **height in inches** and (b.) **weight in pounds**. Base weight on most recent measure in **last 30 days**; measure weight consistently in accord with standard facility practice—e.g., in a.m. after voiding, before meal, with shoes off, and in nightclothes		
		a. HT (in.)		**b.** WT (lb.)

3.	WEIGHT CHANGE	a. **Weight loss**—5 % or more in **last 30 days**; or 10 % or more in **last 180 days** 0. No 1. Yes	
		b. **Weight gain**—5 % or more in **last 30 days**; or 10 % or more in **last 180 days** 0. No 1. Yes	

4.	NUTRI-TIONAL PROBLEMS	Complains about the taste of many foods	a.	Leaves 25% or more of food uneaten at most meals	c.
		Regular or repetitive complaints of hunger	b.	NONE OF ABOVE	d.

5.	NUTRI-TIONAL APPROACH-ES	(*Check all that apply in last 7 days*)			
		Parenteral/IV	a.	Dietary supplement between meals	f.
		Feeding tube	b.	Plate guard, stabilized built-up utensil, etc.	g.
		Mechanically altered diet	c.		
		Syringe (oral feeding)	d.	On a planned weight change program	h.
		Therapeutic diet	e.	NONE OF ABOVE	i.

6.	PARENTERAL OR ENTERAL INTAKE	(*Skip to Section L if neither 5a nor 5b is checked*)	
		a. Code the proportion of **total calories** the resident received through parenteral or tube feedings in the **last 7 days** 0. None 3. 51% to 75% 1. 1% to 25% 4. 76% to 100% 2. 26% to 50%	
		b. Code the average **fluid intake** per day by IV or tube in **last 7 days** 0. None 3. 1001 to 1500 cc/day 1. 1 to 500 cc/day 4. 1501 to 2000 cc/day 2. 501 to 1000 cc/day 5. 2001 or more cc/day	

SECTION L. ORAL/DENTAL STATUS

1.	ORAL STATUS AND DISEASE PREVENTION	Debris (soft, easily movable substances) present in mouth prior to going to bed at night	a.
		Has dentures or removable bridge	b.
		Some/all natural teeth lost—does not have or does not use dentures (or partial plates)	c.
		Broken, loose, or carious teeth	d.
		Inflamed gums (gingiva); swollen or bleeding gums; oral abscesses; ulcers or rashes	e.
		Daily cleaning of teeth/dentures or daily mouth care—by resident or staff	f.
		NONE OF ABOVE	g.

SECTION M. SKIN CONDITION

			Number at Stage
1.	ULCERS (Due to any cause)	(Record the number of ulcers at each ulcer stage—regardless of cause. If none present at a stage, record "0" (zero). Code all that apply during *last 7 days*. Code 9 = 9 or more.) **[Requires full body exam.]**	
		a. Stage 1. A persistent area of skin redness (without a break in the skin) that does not disappear when pressure is relieved.	
		b. Stage 2. A partial thickness loss of skin layers that presents clinically as an abrasion, blister, or shallow crater.	
		c. Stage 3. A full thickness of skin is lost, exposing the subcutaneous tissues - presents as a deep crater with or without undermining adjacent tissue.	
		d. Stage 4. A full thickness of skin and subcutaneous tissue is lost, exposing muscle or bone.	

2.	TYPE OF ULCER	(For each type of ulcer, *code for the highest stage in the last 7 days* using scale in item M1—i.e., 0=none; stages 1, 2, 3, 4)	
		a. Pressure ulcer—any lesion caused by pressure resulting in damage of underlying tissue	
		b. Stasis ulcer—open lesion caused by poor circulation in the lower extremities	

3.	HISTORY OF RESOLVED ULCERS	Resident had an ulcer that was resolved or cured in LAST 90 DAYS 0. No 1. Yes	

4.	OTHER SKIN PROBLEMS OR LESIONS PRESENT	(*Check all that apply during last 7 days*)	
		Abrasions, bruises	a.
		Burns (second or third degree)	b.
		Open lesions other than ulcers, rashes, cuts (e.g., cancer lesions)	c.
		Rashes—e.g., intertrigo, eczema, drug rash, heat rash, herpes zoster	d.
		Skin desensitized to pain or pressure	e.
		Skin tears or cuts (other than surgery)	f.
		Surgical wounds	g.
		NONE OF ABOVE	h.

5.	SKIN TREAT-MENTS	(*Check all that apply during last 7 days*)	
		Pressure relieving device(s) for chair	a.
		Pressure relieving device(s) for bed	b.
		Turning/repositioning program	c.
		Nutrition or hydration intervention to manage skin problems	d.
		Ulcer care	e.
		Surgical wound care	f.
		Application of dressings (with or without topical medications) other than to feet	g.
		Application of ointments/medications (other than to feet)	h.
		Other preventative or protective skin care (other than to feet)	i.
		NONE OF ABOVE	j.

6.	FOOT PROBLEMS AND CARE	(*Check all that apply during last 7 days*)	
		Resident has one or more foot problems—e.g., corns, callouses, bunions, hammer toes, overlapping toes, pain, structural problems	a.
		Infection of the foot—e.g., cellulitis, purulent drainage	b.
		Open lesions on the foot	c.
		Nails/calluses trimmed during **last 90 days**	d.
		Received preventative or protective foot care (e.g., used special shoes, inserts, pads, toe separators)	e.
		Application of dressings (with or without topical medications)	f.
		NONE OF ABOVE	g.

SECTION N. ACTIVITY PURSUIT PATTERNS

1.	TIME AWAKE	(*Check appropriate time periods over last 7 days*) Resident awake all or most of time (i.e., naps no more than one hour per time period) in the:			
		Morning	a.	Evening	c.
		Afternoon	b.	NONE OF ABOVE	d.

(If resident is comatose, skip to Section O)

2.	AVERAGE TIME INVOLVED IN ACTIVITIES	(When awake and not receiving treatments or ADL care)	
		0. Most—more than 2/3 of time 2. Little—less than 1/3 of time 1. Some—from 1/3 to 2/3 of time 3. None	

3.	PREFERRED ACTIVITY SETTINGS	(*Check all settings* in which activities are preferred)			
		Own room	a.		
		Day/activity room	b.	Outside facility	d.
		Inside NH/off unit	c.	NONE OF ABOVE	e.

4.	GENERAL ACTIVITY PREFER-ENCES (adapted to resident's current abilities)	(*Check all PREFERENCES* whether or not activity is currently available to resident)			
		Cards/other games	a.	Trips/shopping	g.
		Crafts/arts	b.	Walking/wheeling outdoors	h.
		Exercise/sports	c.	Watching TV	i.
		Music	d.	Gardening or plants	j.
		Reading/writing	e.	Talking or conversing	k.
		Spiritual/religious activities	f.	Helping others	l.
				NONE OF ABOVE	m.

Resident _____ Numeric Identifier _____

5.	PREFERS CHANGE IN DAILY ROUTINE	Code for resident preferences in daily routines 0. No change 1. Slight change 2. Major change	
		a. Type of activities in which resident is currently involved	
		b. Extent of resident involvement in activities	

SECTION O. MEDICATIONS

1.	NUMBER OF MEDICA-TIONS	(*Record the number of different medications used in the last 7 days*; enter "0" if none used)	
2.	NEW MEDICA-TIONS	(*Resident currently receiving medications that were initiated during the last 90 days*) 0. No 1. Yes	
3.	INJECTIONS	(*Record the number of DAYS injections of any type received during the last 7 days*; enter "0" if none used)	
4.	DAYS RECEIVED THE FOLLOWING MEDICATION	(*Record the number of DAYS during last 7 days*; enter "0" if not used. Note—enter "1" for long-acting meds used less than weekly)	

a. Antipsychotic	d. Hypnotic	
b. Antianxiety	e. Diuretic	
c. Antidepressant		

SECTION P. SPECIAL TREATMENTS AND PROCEDURES

1.	SPECIAL TREAT-MENTS, PROCE-DURES, AND PROGRAMS	a. SPECIAL CARE—*Check treatments or programs received during the last 14 days*		

TREATMENTS			PROGRAMS	
Chemotherapy	a.		Alcohol/drug treatment program	m.
Dialysis	b.		Alzheimer's/dementia special care unit	n.
IV medication	c.		Hospice care	o.
Intake/output	d.		Pediatric unit	p.
Monitoring acute medical condition	e.		Respite care	q.
Ostomy care	f.		Training in skills required to return to the community (e.g., taking medications, house work, shopping, transportation, ADLs)	r.
Oxygen therapy	g.			
Radiation	h.			
Suctioning	i.			
Tracheostomy care	j.		NONE OF ABOVE	s.
Transfusions	k.			
Ventilator or respirator	l.			

b. THERAPIES - Record the number of days and total minutes each of the following therapies was administered (for at least 15 minutes a day) in the *last 7 calendar days* (Enter 0 if none or less than 15 min. daily)
[Note—count only post admission therapies]
(A) = # of days administered for **15 minutes or more**
(B) = total # of minutes provided in last 7 days

	DAYS (A)	MIN (B)
a. Speech - language pathology and audiology services		
b. Occupational therapy		
c. Physical therapy		
d. Respiratory therapy		
e. Psychological therapy (by any licensed mental health professional)		

2.	INTERVEN-TION PROGRAMS FOR MOOD, BEHAVIOR, COGNITIVE LOSS	(Check all interventions or strategies used in last 7 days—no matter where received)	
		Special behavior symptom evaluation program	a.
		Evaluation by a licensed mental health specialist in **last 90 days**	b.
		Group therapy	c.
		Resident-specific deliberate changes in the environment to address mood/behavior patterns—e.g., providing bureau in which to rummage	d.
		Reorientation—e.g., cueing	e.
		NONE OF ABOVE	f.

3.	NURSING REHABILITA-TION/ RESTOR-ATIVE CARE	Record the NUMBER OF DAYS each of the following rehabilitation or restorative techniques or practices was **provided to the resident for more than or equal to 15 minutes per day in the last 7 days** (Enter 0 if none or less than 15 min. daily.)	

a. Range of motion (passive)		f. Walking	
b. Range of motion (active)		g. Dressing or grooming	
c. Splint or brace assistance		h. Eating or swallowing	
TRAINING AND SKILL PRACTICE IN:		i. Amputation/prosthesis care	
d. Bed mobility		j. Communication	
e. Transfer		k. Other	

4.	DEVICES AND RESTRAINTS	(*Use the following codes for last 7 days*:) 0. Not used 1. Used less than daily 2. Used daily	
		Bed rails	
		a. — Full bed rails on all open sides of bed	
		b. — Other types of side rails used (e.g., half rail, one side)	
		c. Trunk restraint	
		d. Limb restraint	
		e. Chair prevents rising	
5.	HOSPITAL STAY(S)	Record number of times resident was admitted to hospital with an overnight stay **in last 90 days** (or since last assessment if less than 90 days). (*Enter 0 if no hospital admissions*)	
6.	EMERGENCY ROOM (ER) VISIT(S)	Record number of times resident visited ER without an overnight stay **in last 90 days** (or since last assessment if less than 90 days). (*Enter 0 if no ER visits*)	
7.	PHYSICIAN VISITS	In the **LAST 14 DAYS** (or since admission if less than 14 days in facility) how many days has the physician (or authorized assistant or practitioner) examined the resident? (*Enter 0 if none*)	
8.	PHYSICIAN ORDERS	In the **LAST 14 DAYS** (or since admission if less than 14 days in facility) how many days has the physician (or authorized assistant or practitioner) changed the resident's orders? Do not include order renewals without change. (*Enter 0 if none*)	
9.	ABNORMAL LAB VALUES	Has the resident had any abnormal lab values during the **last 90 days** (or since admission)? 0. No 1. Yes	

SECTION Q. DISCHARGE POTENTIAL AND OVERALL STATUS

1.	DISCHARGE POTENTIAL	a. Resident expresses/indicates preference to return to the community 0. No 1. Yes	
		b. Resident has a support person who is positive towards discharge 0. No 1. Yes	
		c. Stay projected to be of a short duration— discharge projected **within 90 days** (do not include expected discharge due to death) 0. No 2. Within 31-90 days 1. Within 30 days 3. Discharge status uncertain	
2.	OVERALL CHANGE IN CARE NEEDS	Resident's overall self sufficiency has changed significantly as compared to status of **90 days ago** (or since last assessment if less than 90 days) 0. No change 1. Improved—receives fewer supports, needs less restrictive level of care 2. Deteriorated—receives more support	

SECTION R. ASSESSMENT INFORMATION

1.	PARTICIPA-TION IN ASSESS-MENT	a. Resident:	0. No 1. Yes	
		b. Family:	0. No 1. Yes 2. No family	
		c. Significant other:	0. No 1. Yes 2. None	
2.	SIGNATURE OF PERSON COORDINATING THE ASSESSMENT:			

a. Signature of RN Assessment Coordinator (sign on above line)

b. Date RN Assessment Coordinator signed as complete

Month	Day	Year

Resident _____   Numeric Identifier _____

SECTION T. THERAPY SUPPLEMENT FOR MEDICARE PPS

1.	SPECIAL TREAT- MENTS AND PROCE- DURES	**a. RECREATION THERAPY**—Enter number of days and total minutes of recreation therapy administered (**for at least 15 minutes a day**) in the **last 7 days** (Enter 0 if none)

(A) = # of days administered for 15 minutes or more
(B) = total # of minutes provided in last 7 days

DAYS (A)   MIN (B)

Skip unless this is a Medicare 5 day or Medicare readmission/ return assessment.

b. ORDERED THERAPIES—*Has physician ordered any of following therapies to begin in FIRST 14 days of stay—physical therapy, occupational therapy, or speech pathology service?*
0. No   1. Yes

If not ordered, skip to item 2

c. Through day 15, provide an estimate of the number of days when at least 1 therapy service can be expected to have been delivered.

d. Through day 15, provide an estimate of the number of therapy minutes (across the therapies) that can be expected to be delivered?

2.	WALKING WHEN MOST SELF SUFFICIENT	*Complete item 2 if ADL self-performance score for TRANSFER (G.1.b.A) is 0,1,2, or 3 AND at least one of the following are present:*

• Resident received physical therapy involving gait training (P.1.b.c)
• Physical therapy was ordered for the resident involving gait training (T.1.b)
• Resident received nursing rehabilitation for walking (P.3.f)
• Physical therapy involving walking has been discontinued within the past 180 days

Skip to item 3 if resident did not walk in last 7 days

(FOR FOLLOWING FIVE ITEMS, BASE CODING ON THE EPISODE WHEN THE RESIDENT WALKED THE FARTHEST WITHOUT SITTING DOWN. INCLUDE WALKING DURING REHABILITATION SESSIONS.)

a. Furthest distance walked without sitting down during this episode.

0. 150+ feet   3. 10-25 feet
1. 51-149 feet   4. Less than 10 feet
2. 26-50 feet

b. Time walked without sitting down during this episode.

0. 1-2 minutes   3. 11-15 minutes
1. 3-4 minutes   4. 16-30 minutes
2. 5-10 minutes   5. 31+ minutes

c. Self-Performance in walking during this episode.

0. *INDEPENDENT*—No help or oversight
1. *SUPERVISION*—Oversight, encouragement or cueing provided
2. *LIMITED ASSISTANCE*—Resident highly involved in walking; received physical help in guided maneuvering of limbs or other nonweight bearing assistance
3. *EXTENSIVE ASSISTANCE*—Resident received weight bearing assistance while walking

d. Walking support provided associated with this episode (code regardless of resident's self-performance classification).

0. No setup or physical help from staff
1. Setup help only
2. One person physical assist
3. Two+ persons physical assist

e. Parallel bars used by resident in association with this episode.

0. No   1. Yes

3.	CASE MIX GROUP	Medicare [ ][ ][ ][ ][ ] State [ ][ ][ ][ ][ ]

Resident _____   Numeric Identifier _____

MINIMUM DATA SET (MDS) - *VERSION 2.0*
FOR NURSING HOME RESIDENT ASSESSMENT AND CARE SCREENING

SECTION W. SUPPLEMENTAL MDS ITEMS

1.	National Provider ID	Enter for all assessments and tracking forms, if available.

If the ARD of this assessment or the discharge date of this discharge tracking form is between July 1 and September 30, skip to W3.

2.	Influenza Vaccine	a. Did the resident receive the Influenza vaccine in this facility for this year's Influenza season (October 1 through March 31)?

0. No (If No, go to item W2b)
1. Yes (If Yes, go to item W3)

b. If Influenza vaccine not received, state reason:
1. Not in facility during this year's flu season
2. Received outside of this facility
3. Not eligible
4. Offered and declined
5. Not offered
6. Inability to obtain vaccine

3.	Pneumo- coccal Vaccine	a. Is the resident's PPV status up to date?

0. No (If No, go to item W3b)
1. Yes (If Yes, skip item W3b)

b. If PPV not received, state reason:
1. Not eligible
2. Offered and declined
3. Not offered

SECTION V. RESIDENT ASSESSMENT PROTOCOL SUMMARY

Numeric Identifier _____

Resident's Name:	Medical Record No.:

1. Check if RAP is triggered.

2. For each triggered RAP, use the RAP guidelines to identify areas needing further assessment. Document relevant assessment information regarding the resident's status.

   - Describe:
     — Nature of the condition (may include presence or lack of objective data and subjective complaints).
     — Complications and risk factors that affect your decision to proceed to care planning.
     — Factors that must be considered in developing individualized care plan interventions.
     — Need for referrals/further evaluation by appropriate health professionals.

   - Documentation should support your decision-making regarding whether to proceed with a care plan for a triggered RAP and the type(s) of care plan interventions that are appropriate for a particular resident.

   - Documentation may appear anywhere in the clinical record (e.g., progress notes, consults, flowsheets, etc.).

3. Indicate under the Location of RAP Assessment Documentation column where information related to the RAP assessment can be found.

4. For each triggered RAP, indicate whether a new care plan, care plan revision, or continuation of current care plan is necessary to address the problem(s) identified in your assessment. The Care Planning Decision column must be completed within 7 days of completing the RAI (MDS and RAPs).

A. RAP PROBLEM AREA	(a) Check if triggered	Location and Date of RAP Assessment Documentation	(b) Care Planning Decision—check if addressed in care plan
1. DELIRIUM			
2. COGNITIVE LOSS			
3. VISUAL FUNCTION			
4. COMMUNICATION			
5. ADL FUNCTIONAL/ REHABILITATION POTENTIAL			
6. URINARY INCONTINENCE AND INDWELLING CATHETER			
7. PSYCHOSOCIAL WELL-BEING			
8. MOOD STATE			
9. BEHAVIORAL SYMPTOMS			
10. ACTIVITIES			
11. FALLS			
12. NUTRITIONAL STATUS			
13. FEEDING TUBES			
14. DEHYDRATION/FLUID MAINTENANCE			
15. DENTAL CARE			
16. PRESSURE ULCERS			
17. PSYCHOTROPIC DRUG USE			
18. PHYSICAL RESTRAINTS			

B.

1. Signature of RN Coordinator for RAP Assessment Process

2. ☐☐ — ☐☐ — ☐☐☐☐
   Month Day Year

3. Signature of Person Completing Care Planning Decision

4. ☐☐ — ☐☐ — ☐☐☐☐
   Month Day Year

RESIDENT ASSESSMENT PROTOCOL TRIGGER LEGEND FOR REVISED RAPS (FOR MDS VERSION 2.0)

Key:
- ● = One item required to trigger
- ❷ = Two items required to trigger
- ✱ = One of these three items, plus at least one other item required to trigger
- @ = When both ADL triggers present, maintenance takes precedence

Proceed to RAP Review once triggered

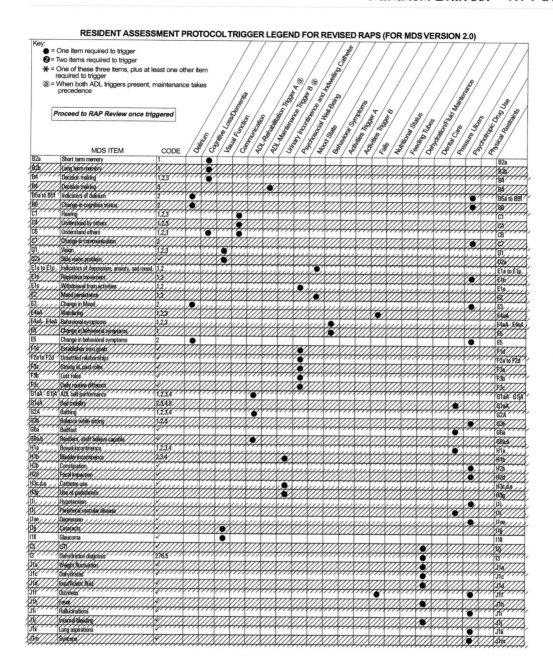

MDS ITEM	Description	CODE
B2a	Short term memory	1
B2b	Long term memory	1
B4	Decision making	1,2,3
B4	Decision making	3
B5a to B5f	Indicators of delirium	2
B6	Change in cognitive status	2
C1	Hearing	1,2,3
C4	Understood by others	1,2,3
C6	Understand others	1,2,3
C7	Change in communication	2
D1	Vision	1,2,3
D2a	Side vision problem	
E1a to E1p	Indicators of depression, anxiety, sad mood.	1,2
E1n	Repetitive movement	1,2
E1o	Withdrawal from activities	1,2
E2	Mood persistence	1,2
E3	Change in Mood	2
E4aA	Wandering	1,2,3
E4aA - E4eA	Behavioral symptoms	1,2,3
E5	Change in behavioral symptoms	2
E5	Change in behavioral symptoms	2
F1d	Establishes own goals	✱
F2a to F2d	Unsettled relationships	✱
F3a	Strong id. past roles	✱
F3b	Lost roles	✱
F3c	Daily routine different	✱
G1aA - G1jA	ADL self-performance	1,2,3,4
G1aA	Bed mobility	2,3,4,8
G2A	Bathing	1,2,3,4
G3b	Balance while sitting	1,2,3
G6a	Bedfast	
G8a,b	Resident, staff believe capable	✱
H1a	Bowel incontinence	1,2,3,4
H1b	Bladder incontinence	2,3,4
H2b	Constipation	
H2d	Fecal impaction	
H3c,d,e	Catheter use	
H3g	Use of pads/briefs	
I1j	Hypertension	
I1l	Peripheral vascular disease	
I1ee	Depression	
I1jj	Cataracts	
I1ll	Glaucoma	
I2j	UTI	
I3	Dehydration diagnosis	276.5
J1a	Weight fluctuation	
J1c	Dehydrated	
J1d	Insufficient fluid	
J1f	Dizziness	
J1h	Fever	
J1i	Hallucinations	
J1j	Internal bleeding	
J1k	Lung aspirations	
J1m	Syncope	

Column headings (RAP categories, left to right): Delirium; Cognitive Loss/Dementia; Visual Function; Communication; ADL-Rehabilitation Trigger A @; ADL-Maintenance Trigger B @; Urinary Incontinence and Indwelling Catheter; Psychosocial Well-Being; Mood State; Behavioral Symptoms; Activities Trigger A; Activities Trigger B; Falls; Nutritional Status; Feeding Tubes; Dehydration/Fluid Maintenance; Dental Care; Pressure Ulcers; Psychotropic Drug Use; Physical Restraints.

RESIDENT ASSESSMENT PROTOCOL TRIGGER LEGEND FOR REVISED RAPS (FOR MDS VERSION 2.0)

Key:
- ● = One item required to trigger
- ❷ = Two items required to trigger
- ✻ = One of these three items, plus at least one other item required to trigger
- @ = When both ADL triggers present, maintenance takes precedence

> Proceed to RAP Review once triggered

MDS ITEM		CODE	Delirium	Cognitive Loss/Dementia	Visual Function	Communication	ADL-Rehabilitation Trigger A @	ADL-Maintenance Trigger B @	Urinary Incontinence and Indwelling Catheter	Psychosocial Well-Being	Mood State	Behavioral Symptoms	Activities Trigger A	Activities Trigger B	Falls	Nutritional Status	Feeding Tubes	Dehydration/Fluid Maintenance	Dental Care	Pressure Ulcers	Psychotropic Drug Use	Physical Restraints	
J1n	Unsteady gait	✓													●						●		J1n
J4a,b	Fell	✓													●						●		J4a,b
J4c	Hip fracture	✓													●						●		J4c
K1b	Swallowing problem																				●		K1b
K1c	Mouth pain	✓																	●				K1c
K3a	Weight loss	1														●							K3a
K4a	Taste alteration	✓														●							K4a
K4c	Leave 25% food	✓														●							K4c
K5a	Parenteral/IV feeding	✓														●	●						K5a
K5b	Feeding tube	✓															●	●					K5b
K5c	Mechanically altered	✓														●							K5c
K5d	Syringe feeding	✓														●							K5d
K6a	Therapeutic diet	✓														●							K6a
L1a,c,d,e	Dental	✓																	●				L1a,c,d,e
L1h	Daily cleaning teeth	No ✓																	●				L1h
M2a	Pressure ulcer	2,3,4													●								M2a
M2a	Pressure ulcer	1,2,3,4																		●			M2a
M3	Previous pressure ulcer	1																		●			M3
M4d	Impaired tactile sense	✓																		●			M4d
N1a	Awake morning												❷	❷									N1a
N2	Involved in activities	0											❷	❷									N2
N2	Involved in activities	2,3										●											N2
N5a,b	Prefers change in daily routine	1,2										●											N5a,b
O4a	Antipsychotics	1-7																			✻		O4a
O4b	Antianxiety	1-7													●						✻		O4b
O4c	Antidepressants	1-7													●						✻		O4c
O4	Diuretic	1-7																●					P4c
P4c	Trunk restraint	1,2													●							●	P4c
P4c	Trunk restraint	2																		●			P4d
P4d	Limb restraint	1,2																				●	P4d
P4e	Chair prevents rising	1,2																				●	P4e

MDS QUARTERLY ASSESSMENT FORM

Numeric Identifier _____

A1.	**RESIDENT NAME**	a. (First) b. (Middle Initial) c. (Last) d. (Jr/Sr)
A2.	**ROOM NUMBER**	
A3.	**ASSESSMENT REFERENCE DATE**	a. Last day of MDS observation period Month — Day — Year b. Original (0) or corrected copy of form (enter number of correction)
A4a	**DATE OF REENTRY**	Date of reentry from most recent temporary discharge to a hospital in last 90 days (or since last assessment or admission if less than 90 days) Month Day Year
A6.	**MEDICAL RECORD NO.**	
B1.	**COMATOSE**	(Persistent vegetative state/no discernible consciousness) 0. No 1. Yes (Skip to Section G)
B2.	**MEMORY**	(Recall of what was learned or known) a. Short-term memory OK—seems/appears to recall after 5 minutes 0. Memory OK 1. Memory problem b. Long-term memory OK—seems/appears to recall long past 0. Memory OK 1. Memory problem
B4.	**COGNITIVE SKILLS FOR DAILY DECISION-MAKING**	(Made decisions regarding tasks of daily life) 0. INDEPENDENT—decisions consistent/reasonable 1. MODIFIED INDEPENDENCE—some difficulty in new situations only 2. MODERATELY IMPAIRED—decisions poor; cues/supervision required 3. SEVERELY IMPAIRED—never/rarely made decisions
B5.	**INDICATORS OF DELIRIUM— PERIODIC DISORDERED THINKING/ AWARENESS**	(Code for behavior in the last 7 days.) [Note: Accurate assessment requires conversations with staff and family who have direct knowledge of resident's behavior over this time]. 0. Behavior not present 1. Behavior present, not of recent onset 2. Behavior present, over last 7 days appears different from resident's usual functioning (e.g., new onset or worsening) a. EASILY DISTRACTED—(e.g., difficulty paying attention; gets sidetracked) b. PERIODS OF ALTERED PERCEPTION OR AWARENESS OF SURROUNDINGS—(e.g., moves lips or talks to someone not present; believes he/she is somewhere else; confuses night and day) c. EPISODES OF DISORGANIZED SPEECH—(e.g., speech is incoherent, nonsensical, irrelevant, or rambling from subject to subject; loses train of thought) d. PERIODS OF RESTLESSNESS—(e.g., fidgeting or picking at skin, clothing, napkins, etc; frequent position changes; repetitive physical movements or calling out) e. PERIODS OF LETHARGY—(e.g., sluggishness; staring into space; difficult to arouse; little body movement) f. MENTAL FUNCTION VARIES OVER THE COURSE OF THE DAY—(e.g., sometimes better, sometimes worse; behaviors sometimes present, sometimes not)
C4.	**MAKING SELF UNDERSTOOD**	(Expressing information content—however able) 0. UNDERSTOOD 1. USUALLY UNDERSTOOD—difficulty finding words or finishing thoughts 2. SOMETIMES UNDERSTOOD—ability is limited to making concrete requests 3. RARELY/NEVER UNDERSTOOD
C6.	**ABILITY TO UNDERSTAND OTHERS**	(Understanding verbal information content—however able) 0. UNDERSTANDS 1. USUALLY UNDERSTANDS—may miss some part/intent of message 2. SOMETIMES UNDERSTANDS—responds adequately to simple, direct communication 3. RARELY/NEVER UNDERSTANDS
E1.	**INDICATORS OF DEPRESSION, ANXIETY, SAD MOOD**	(Code for indicators observed in last 30 days, irrespective of the assumed cause) 0. Indicator not exhibited in last 30 days 1. Indicator of this type exhibited up to five days a week 2. Indicator of this type exhibited daily or almost daily (6, 7 days a week) **VERBAL EXPRESSIONS OF DISTRESS** a. Resident made negative statements—e.g., "Nothing matters; Would rather be dead; What's the use; Regrets having lived so long; Let me die" b. Repetitive questions—e.g., "Where do I go; What do I do?" c. Repetitive verbalizations—e.g., calling out for help, ("God help me") d. Persistent anger with self or others—e.g., easily annoyed, anger at placement in nursing home; anger at care received e. Self deprecation—e.g., "I am nothing; I am of no use to anyone"

E1.	**INDICATORS OF DEPRESSION, ANXIETY, SAD MOOD (cont.)**	**VERBAL EXPRESSIONS OF DISTRESS** f. Expressions of what appear to be unrealistic fears—e.g., fear of being abandoned, left alone, being with others g. Recurrent statements that something terrible is about to happen—e.g., believes he or she is about to die, have a heart attack h. Repetitive health complaints—e.g., persistently seeks medical attention, obsessive concern with body functions i. Repetitive anxious complaints/concerns (non-health related) e.g., persistently seeks attention/ reassurance regarding schedules, meals, laundry, clothing, relationship issues	**SLEEP-CYCLE ISSUES** j. Unpleasant mood in morning k. Insomnia/change in usual sleep pattern **SAD, APATHETIC, ANXIOUS APPEARANCE** l. Sad, pained, worried facial expressions—e.g., furrowed brows m. Crying, tearfulness n. Repetitive physical movements—e.g., pacing, hand wringing, restlessness, fidgeting, picking **LOSS OF INTEREST** o. Withdrawal from activities of interest—e.g., no interest in long standing activities or being with family/friends p. Reduced social interaction
E2.	**MOOD PERSISTENCE**	One or more indicators of depressed, sad or anxious mood were not easily altered by attempts to "cheer up", console, or reassure the resident over last 7 days 0. No mood indicators 1. Indicators present, easily altered 2. Indicators present, not easily altered	
E4.	**BEHAVIORAL SYMPTOMS**	(A) Behavioral symptom frequency in last 7 days 0. Behavior not exhibited in last 7 days 1. Behavior of this type occurred 1 to 3 days in last 7 days 2. Behavior of this type occurred 4 to 6 days, but less than daily 3. Behavior of this type occurred daily (B) Behavioral symptom alterability in last 7 days 0. Behavior not present OR behavior was easily altered 1. Behavior was not easily altered (A) (B) a. WANDERING (moved with no rational purpose, seemingly oblivious to needs or safety) b. VERBALLY ABUSIVE BEHAVIORAL SYMPTOMS (others were threatened, screamed at, cursed at) c. PHYSICALLY ABUSIVE BEHAVIORAL SYMPTOMS (others were hit, shoved, scratched, sexually abused) d. SOCIALLY INAPPROPRIATE/DISRUPTIVE BEHAVIORAL SYMPTOMS (made disruptive sounds, noisiness, screaming, self-abusive acts, sexual behavior or disrobing in public, smeared/threw food/feces, hoarding, rummaged through others' belongings) e. RESISTS CARE (resisted taking medications/ injections, ADL assistance, or eating)	

G1.	**(A) ADL SELF-PERFORMANCE**—(Code for resident's PERFORMANCE OVER ALL SHIFTS during last 7 days—Not including setup)	
	0. INDEPENDENT—No help or oversight —OR— Help/oversight provided only 1 or 2 times during last 7 days 1. SUPERVISION—Oversight, encouragement or cueing provided 3 or more times during last7 days —OR— Supervision (3 or more times) plus physical assistance provided only 1 or 2 times during last 7 days 2. LIMITED ASSISTANCE—Resident highly involved in activity; received physical help in guided maneuvering of limbs or other nonweight bearing assistance 3 or more times —OR—More help provided only 1 or 2 times during last 7 days 3. EXTENSIVE ASSISTANCE—While resident performed part of activity, over last 7-day period, help of following type(s) provided 3 or more times: — Weight-bearing support — Full staff performance during part (but not all) of last 7 days 4. TOTAL DEPENDENCE—Full staff performance of activity during entire 7 days 8. ACTIVITY DID NOT OCCUR during entire 7 days (A)	
a. BED MOBILITY	How resident moves to and from lying position, turns side to side, and positions body while in bed	
b. TRANSFER	How resident moves between surfaces—to/from: bed, chair, wheelchair, standing position (EXCLUDE to/from bath/toilet)	
c. WALK IN ROOM	How resident walks between locations in his/her room.	
d. WALK IN CORRIDOR	How resident walks in corridor on unit.	
e. LOCOMOTION ON UNIT	How resident moves between locations in his/her room and adjacent corridor on same floor. If in wheelchair, self-sufficiency once in chair	
f. LOCOMOTION OFF UNIT	How resident moves to and returns from off unit locations (e.g., areas set aside for dining, activities, or treatments). If facility has only one floor, how resident moves to and from distant areas on the floor. If in wheelchair, self-sufficiency once in chair	
g. DRESSING	How resident puts on, fastens, and takes off all items of street clothing, including donning/removing prosthesis	
h. EATING	How resident eats and drinks (regardless of skill). Includes intake of nourishment by other means (e.g., tube feeding, total parenteral nutrition).	

Resident_____ Numeric Identifier _____

I.	TOILET USE	How resident uses the toilet room (or commode, bedpan, urinal); transfer on/off toilet, cleanses, changes pad, manages ostomy or catheter, adjusts clothes	
J.	PERSONAL HYGIENE	How resident maintains personal hygiene, including combing hair, brushing teeth, shaving, applying makeup, washing/drying face, hands, and perineum (EXCLUDE baths and showers)	

G2. BATHING — How resident takes full-body bath/shower, sponge bath, and transfers in/out of tub/shower (EXCLUDE washing of back and hair.) *Code for most dependent in self-performance.*
(A) BATHING SELF PERFORMANCE codes appear below **(A)**

0. Independent—No help provided
1. Supervision—Oversight help only
2. Physical help limited to transfer only
3. Physical help in part of bathing activity
4. Total dependence
8. Activity itself did not occur during entire 7 days

G4. FUNCTIONAL LIMITATION IN RANGE OF MOTION — *(Code for limitations during last 7 days that interfered with daily functions or placed residents at risk of injury)*

(A) RANGE OF MOTION	(B) VOLUNTARY MOVEMENT
0. No limitation	0. No loss
1. Limitation on one side	1. Partial loss
2. Limitation on both sides	2. Full loss

	(A)	(B)
a. Neck		
b. Arm—Including shoulder or elbow		
c. Hand—Including wrist or fingers		
d. Leg—Including hip or knee		
e. Foot—Including ankle or toes		
f. Other limitation or loss		

G6. MODES OF TRANSFER — *(Check all that apply during last 7 days)*

Bedfast all or most of time	a.	NONE OF ABOVE	f.
Bed rails used for bed mobility or transfer	b.		

H1. CONTINENCE SELF-CONTROL CATEGORIES *(Code for resident's PERFORMANCE OVER ALL SHIFTS)*

0. *CONTINENT*—Complete control [includes use of indwelling urinary catheter or ostomy device that does not leak urine or stool]
1. *USUALLY CONTINENT*—BLADDER, incontinent episodes once a week or less; BOWEL, less than weekly
2. *OCCASIONALLY INCONTINENT*—BLADDER, 2 or more times a week but not daily; BOWEL, once a week
3. *FREQUENTLY INCONTINENT*—BLADDER, tended to be incontinent daily, but some control present (e.g., on day shift); BOWEL, 2-3 times a week
4. *INCONTINENT*—Had inadequate control BLADDER, multiple daily episodes; BOWEL, all (or almost all) of the time

a.	BOWEL CONTINENCE	Control of bowel movement, with appliance or bowel continence programs, if employed	
b.	BLADDER CONTINENCE	Control of urinary bladder function (if dribbles, volume insufficient to soak through underpants), with appliances (e.g., foley) or continence programs, if employed	

H2.	BOWEL ELIMINATION PATTERN	Fecal impaction	d.	NONE OF ABOVE	e.

H3. APPLIANCES AND PROGRAMS

Any scheduled toileting plan	a.	Indwelling catheter	d.
Bladder retraining program	b.	Ostomy present	i.
External (condom) catheter	c.	NONE OF ABOVE	j.
			m.

I2.	INFECTIONS	Urinary tract infection in last 30 days		NONE OF ABOVE	

I3. OTHER CURRENT DIAGNOSES AND ICD-9 CODES — *(Include only those diseases diagnosed in the last 90 days that have a relationship to current ADL status, cognitive status, mood or behavior status, medical treatments, nursing monitoring, or risk of death)*

a. _____ . _____
b. _____ . _____

J1. PROBLEM CONDITIONS — *(Check all problems present in last 7 days)*

Dehydrated; output exceeds input	c.	Hallucinations	i.
		NONE OF ABOVE	p.

J2. PAIN SYMPTOMS — *(Code the highest level of pain present in the last 7 days)*

a. FREQUENCY with which resident complains or shows evidence of pain	b. INTENSITY of pain
0. No pain (*skip to J4*)	1. Mild pain
1. Pain less than daily	2. Moderate pain
2. Pain daily	3. Times when pain is horrible or excrutiating

J4. ACCIDENTS — *(Check all that apply)*

Fell in past 30 days	a.	Hip fracture in last 180 days	c.
Fell in past 31-180 days	b.	Other fracture in last 180 days	d.
		NONE OF ABOVE	e.

J5. STABILITY OF CONDITIONS

Conditions/diseases make resident's cognitive, ADL, mood or behavior status unstable—(fluctuating, precarious, or deteriorating)	a.
Resident experiencing an acute episode or a flare-up of a recurrent or chronic problem	b.
End-stage disease, 6 or fewer months to live	c.
NONE OF ABOVE	d.

K3. WEIGHT CHANGE

a. Weight loss—5 % or more in last 30 days; or 10 % or more in last 180 days
   0. No   1. Yes
b. Weight gain—5 % or more in last 30 days; or 10 % or more in last 180 days
   0. No   1. Yes

K5.	NUTRITIONAL APPROACHES	Feeding tube	b.
		On a planned weight change program	h.
		NONE OF ABOVE	i.

M1. ULCERS (Due to any cause) — *(Record the number of ulcers at each ulcer stage—regardless of cause. If none present at a stage, record "0" (zero). Code all that apply during last 7 days. Code 9 = 9 or more.) [Requires full body exam.]* — **Number at Stage**

a. Stage 1. A persistent area of skin redness (without a break in the skin) that does not disappear when pressure is relieved.
b. Stage 2. A partial thickness loss of skin layers that presents clinically as an abrasion, blister, or shallow crater.
c. Stage 3. A full thickness of skin is lost, exposing the subcutaneous tissues - presents as a deep crater with or without undermining adjacent tissue.
d. Stage 4. A full thickness of skin and subcutaneous tissue is lost, exposing muscle or bone.

M2. TYPE OF ULCER — *(For each type of ulcer, code for the highest stage in the last 7 days using scale in item M1—i.e., 0=none; stages 1, 2, 3, 4)*

a. Pressure ulcer—any lesion caused by pressure resulting in damage of underlying tissue
b. Stasis ulcer—open lesion caused by poor circulation in the lower extremities

N1. TIME AWAKE — *(Check appropriate time periods over last 7 days)* Resident awake all or most of time (i.e., naps no more than one hour per time period) in the:

Morning	a.	Evening	c.
Afternoon	b.	NONE OF ABOVE	d.

(If resident is comatose, skip to Section O)

N2. AVERAGE TIME INVOLVED IN ACTIVITIES — *(When awake and not receiving treatments or ADL care)*
0. Most—more than 2/3 of time   2. Little—less than 1/3 of time
1. Some—from 1/3 to 2/3 of time   3. None

O1. NUMBER OF MEDICATIONS — *(Record the number of different medications used in the last 7 days; enter "0" if none used)*

O4. DAYS RECEIVED THE FOLLOWING MEDICATION — *(Record the number of DAYS during last 7 days; enter "0" if not used. Note—enter "1" for long-acting meds used less than weekly)*

a. Antipsychotic		d. Hypnotic	
b. Antianxiety		e. Diuretic	
c. Antidepressant			

P4. DEVICES AND RESTRAINTS — Use the following codes for last 7 days:
0. Not used
1. Used less than daily
2. Used daily

Bed rails
a. — Full bed rails on all open sides of bed
b. — Other types of side rails used (e.g., half rail, one side)
c. Trunk restraint
d. Limb restraint
e. Chair prevents rising

Q2. OVERALL CHANGE IN CARE NEEDS — Resident's overall level of self sufficiency has changed significantly as compared to status of 90 days ago (or since last assessment if less than 90 days)
0. No change   1. Improved—receives fewer supports, needs less restrictive level of care   2. Deteriorated—receives more support

R2. SIGNATURE OF PERSON COORDINATING THE ASSESSMENT:

a. Signature of RN Assessment Coordinator (sign on above line)

b. Date RN Assessment Coordinator signed as complete

	Month	Day	Year

Resident _____   Numeric Identifier _____

MINIMUM DATA SET (MDS) - *VERSION 2.0*
FOR NURSING HOME RESIDENT ASSESSMENT AND CARE SCREENING

SECTION W. SUPPLEMENTAL MDS ITEMS

1.	National Provider ID	Enter for all assessments and tracking forms, if available.

If the ARD of this assessment or the discharge date of this discharge tracking form is between July 1 and September 30, skip to W3.

2.	Influenza Vaccine	a . Did the resident receive the Influenza vaccine in this facility for this year's Influenza season (October 1 through March 31)?
		0. No (If No, go to item W2b)
		1. Yes (If Yes, go to item W3)
		b. If Influenza vaccine not received, state reason:
		1. Not in facility during this year's flu season
		2. Received outside of this facility
		3. Not eligible
		4. Offered and declined
		5. Not offered
		6. Inability to obtain vaccine
3.	Pneumo- coccal Vaccine	a. Is the resident's PPV status up to date?
		0. No (If No, go to item W3b)
		1. Yes (If Yes, skip item W3b)
		b. If PPV not received, state reason:
		1. Not eligible
		2. Offered and declined
		3. Not offered

USING MICROSOFT EXCEL TO PERFORM CALCULATIONS

When we are working with a small number of items or a simple, two-figure calculation, using a calculator is probably the easiest way to complete the computations. However, when we have a large number of figures or if we are going to be performing the same computation multiple times, it is very useful to know how to use Excel to help with the computations.

In this Appendix, we will explain some common calculations, the purpose of the computations, and how to complete those calculations in Excel.

	A	B	C	D	E	F
1	**Community Hospital**					
2	**First Quarter Discharges**					
3						
4		19,021	*January*			
5		18,945	*Feburary*			
6		21,439	*March*			
7		59,405	*Total First Quarter Discharges*			
8						
9	The formula to obtain the total of 59,405 is: = SUM(B4:B6)					
10	This yields the same result as: = B4+B5+B6					
11						
12	A quarter is 1/4 of a year (3 months)					
13	A fiscal year is the organization's tax year (a business cycle)					
14						
15	In this example, we might want to calculate the					
16	discharges, by quarter, for the entire year:					
17						
18	On the right are the data entry and the formulas. On the left are the results.					
19						
20	As you are preparing your worksheet, you can reveal the formulas by					
21	pressing **Ctrl.** (The Control key and the accent grave, located to the left of					
22	the number 1 on your keyboard.)					
23						
24		**Community Hospital**				
25		**2006 Discharges**				
26						
27	19,021	*January*				19,021
28	18,945	*February*				18,945
29	21,439	*March*				21,439
30	59,405	*Total First Quarter Discharges*				= SUM(A27:A29)
31						
32	18,435	*April*				18,435
33	18,854	*May*				18,854
34	19,146	*June*				19,146
35	56,435	*Total Second Quarter Discharges*				= SUM(A32:A34)
36						
37	20,564	*July*				20,564
38	20,437	*August*				20,437
39	19,111	*September*				19,111
40	60,112	*Total Third Quarter Discharges*				= SUM(A37:A39)
41						
42	19,021	*October*				19,021
43	18,945	*November*				18,945
44	21,439	*December*				21,439
45	59,405	*Total Fourth Quarter Discharges*				= SUM(A42:A44)
46						
47	235,357	*Total Discharges for the Year*				= A30+A35+A40+A45

	A	B	C	D	E	F	G	H
1	Community Hospital							
2	Health Information Department Staffing							
3								
4		75	Total Staff					
5		6	Part-time Staff					
6		69	Full-time Staff					
7	Formula is:	= B4-B5						
8								
9								
10	If you are having problems understanding this calculation, you may not be using the							
11	correct sequence of instructions, because your calculator may require a							
12	different sequence of entries. Some calculators want you to enter the							
13	operation BEFORE the number. Other calculators want you to enter the							
14	operation AFTER the number							
15								

	A	B	C	D	E	F	G	H	I
1		Community Hospital							
2		Full-Time Equivalent Staff							
3									
4									
5		Number	Hours	Total					
6	Part-time	6	20	120	= B6*C6				
7	Full-time	69	40	2760	= B7*C7				
8									
9	Total Hours Worked			2880	= SUM(D6:D7)				
10	Normal Work Hours			40					
11	Full-time Equivalents			72	= D9/D10				
12									
13	FTE = Full-time Equivalents								
14	FTEs = Total number of hours worked per week, divided by number of normal work hours								
15									
16	In this example, we calculated the total hours worked by the part-time employees								
17	and the total hours worked by the full-time employees. We then divided the total								
18	number of hours worked by all employees by the number of hours in the normal work								
19	week. This calculation of Full-time Equivalents provides management with a								
20	number of employees that can be compared to other departments and evaluated								
21	based on other volume measurements, such as number of discharges.								

	A	B	C	D	E	F	G
1		Community Hospital					
2		Patient Census 12/15/06					
3							
4		175	Patients 12/14/05				
5	+	3	Births				
6	−	8	Deaths				
7	+	11	Admitted				
8	−	9	Discharged				
9		172	Patients 12/15/06		= B4 + B5 − B6 + B7 − B8		
10							
11	Be careful with the sequence of instructions in the formula.						
12	In this sequence, the instruction to add or substract goes BEFORE the number to be operated on.						

	A	B	C	D	E	F	G
1	Community Hospital Cafeteria Survey						
2							
3		Total Patients Responding	Liked Food	Percent Who Liked Food			
4							
5	2003	500	394	79%	= C5/B5		
6	2004	2,000	1,645	82%	= C6/B6		
7	Hospital B	20,011	15,492	77%	= C7/B7		
8							
9							
10	Percentages are useful in comparing results between different years or groups.						
11	In this example, Community Hospital is comparing its cafeteria satisfaction						
12	between 2005 and 2006. It is also comparing its cafeteria satisfaction with						
13	a survey taken at another hospital (Hospital B). Because the dissatisfaction						
14	is expressed as a percentage, we can easily see that Community Hospital's						
15	satisfaction results are improving and that they are superior to Hospital B.						
16							
17	Notice that the formula yields a decimal, not a percentage. In order to display the results as a percentage, the cell must be formatted to						
18	recognize the number as a percentage. To format the cell, click on the						
19	following series of options from the main menu at the top of the screen.						
20							
21		Format					
22		Cell					
23		Number					
24		Percentage					
25	Another way to obtain the percentage (without the % sign) is to multiply the decimal times 100 e.g. = C5/B5*100.						
26							

	A	B	C	D	E	F	G	H	I	J	K	L	M	N	O	P	Q
1				Community Hospital													
2				Length of Stay													
3																	
4	1	2	3	3	3	4	4	5	5	6							
5	1	2	3	3	3	4	4	5	5	6							
6	1	2	3	3	4	4	4	5	5	6							
7	1	2	3	3	4	4	4	5	5	6		Computing the answers to					
8	1	2	3	3	4	4	4	5	5	6		various statistical questions:					
9	1	2	3	3	4	4	4	5	5	6							
10	1	2	3	3	4	4	4	5	5	6		How many patients?		250			
11	1	2	3	3	4	4	4	5	5	6			= COUNT(A4:J28)				
12	1	2	3	3	4	4	4	5	5	6							
13	1	2	3	3	4	4	4	5	5	7		What is the average length of stay?				3.864	days
14	1	2	3	3	4	4	4	5	5	7			= AVERAGE(A4:J28)				
15	1	2	3	3	4	4	4	5	5	7			(This is the Mean, which				
16	1	2	3	3	4	4	4	5	5	7			could also be calculated as				
17	1	2	3	3	4	4	4	5	5	7			= SUM(A4:J28)/250				
18	1	2	3	3	4	4	4	5	5	7							
19	1	2	3	3	4	4	4	5	5	7		What is the median length of stay?				4	days
20	1	2	3	3	4	4	4	5	5	7			= MEDIAN(A4:J28)				
21	1	2	3	3	4	4	5	5	5	7							
22	1	2	3	3	4	4	5	5	5	7		What is the mode?				4	days
23	1	2	3	3	4	4	5	5	6	8			= MODE(A4:J28)				
24	1	3	3	3	4	4	5	5	6	8							
25	1	3	3	3	4	4	5	5	6	8							
26	1	3	3	3	4	4	5	5	6	8							
27	1	3	3	3	4	4	5	5	6	9							
28	1	3	3	3	4	4	5	5	6	9							

	A	B	C	D	E	F	G	H	I	J	K	L	M	N	O	P	Q	R	S
1																			
2		Community Hospital										Frequency distribution							
3			Length of Stay																
4												EXCEL will calculate the frequency distribution							
5	1	2	3	3	3	4	4	5	5	6		of a data set. It sorts the data into class intervals							
6	1	2	3	3	3	4	4	5	5	6		that we describe. In this example, we will use the							
7	1	2	3	3	4	4	4	5	5	6		individual lengths of stay as our target, which EXCEL calls "BINS."							
8	1	2	3	3	4	4	4	5	5	6									
9	1	2	3	3	4	4	4	5	5	6		BINS							
10	1	2	3	3	4	4	4	5	5	6		1							
11	1	2	3	3	4	4	4	5	5	6		2							
12	1	2	3	3	4	4	4	5	5	6		3			Step 1: List the BINS in order.				
13	1	2	3	3	4	4	4	5	5	6		4			(THIS BINS ARRAY IS LOCATED				
14	1	2	3	3	4	4	4	5	5	7		5			IN CELLS L10 THROUGH L18.)				
15	1	2	3	3	4	4	4	5	5	7		6							
16	1	2	3	3	4	4	4	5	5	7		7							
17	1	2	3	3	4	4	4	5	5	7		8							
18	1	2	3	3	4	4	4	5	5	7		9							
19	1	2	3	3	4	4	4	5	5	7									
20	1	2	3	3	4	4	4	5	5	7									
21	1	2	3	3	4	4	4	5	5	7		BINS							
22	1	2	3	3	4	4	5	5	5	7		1	= FREQUENCY(A5:J29,L10:L18)						
23	1	2	3	3	4	4	5	5	5	7		2							
24	1	2	3	3	4	4	5	5	6	8		3							
25	1	3	3	3	4	4	5	5	6	8		4			Step 2: Enter the formula.				
26	1	3	3	3	4	4	5	5	6	8		5			Specify the range for the data.				
27	1	3	3	3	4	4	5	5	6	8		6			Specify the range for the BINS.				
28	1	3	3	3	4	4	5	5	6	9		7							
29	1	3	3	3	4	4	5	5	6	9		8							
												9							
												BINS							
												1	= FREQUENCY(A5:J29,L10:L18)						
												2							
												3			Step 3: Click and drag to highlight the				
												4			entire area in which you wish to				
												5			display the results, including the				
												6			formula cell.				
												7							
												8							
												9							
												BINS							
												1	25						
												2	20		Step 4: Press F2. Then, press and hold:				
												3	57		Ctrl Shift Enter				
												4	65						
												5	52						
												6	15		The frequencies of each BIN will appear next to the BIN they represent. These frequencies can then be used to prepare informative tables and graphs.				
												7	10						
												8	4						
												9	2						

	A	B	C	D	E	F
1						
2		Community Hospital				
3		Length of Stay				
4						
5		*Frequencies:*		*Percentage:*		
6		1	25	10%	=C6/$C$15	
7		2	20	8%	=C7/$C$15	
8		3	57	23%	=C8/$C$15	
9		4	65	26%	=C9/$C$15	
10		5	52	21%	=C10/$C$15	
11		6	15	6%	=C11/$C$15	
12		7	10	4%	=C12/$C$15	
13		8	4	2%	=C13/$C$15	
14		9	2	1%	=C14/$C$15	
15		**Total**	250			
16			= SUM(C6:C14)			
17						
18		Notice that we anchored the total in the percentage				
19		formula by placing a dollar sign in front of each				
20		element of the cell.				
21						
22		The graph below is a "Scatter" graph with a line				
23		connecting the dots. It represents the data fields				
24		**B6:B14, D6:D14**				

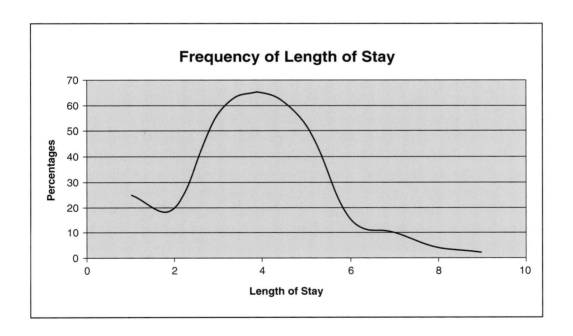

GLOSSARY

ABC	Alternative billing concepts codes used for alternative medicine, such as acupuncture.
Abstract	A summary of the patient record.
Abstracting	The recap of selected fields from a health record to create an informative summary. Also refers to the activity of identifying such fields and entering them into a computer system.
Access	The ability to learn the contents of a record by obtaining it or having the contents revealed.
Accounting of disclosures	The listing of the identity of those to which certain protected health information has been disclosed.
Accreditation	Voluntary compliance with a set of standards developed by an independent agent, who periodically performs audits to ensure compliance.
Accreditation Association for Ambulatory Health Care (AAAHC)	An organization that accredits ambulatory care facilities.
Activities of daily living	Refers to self-care, such as bathing, as well as cooking, shopping, and other routines requiring thought, planning, and physical motion.
Acute care facility	A hospital with an average length of stay less than 30 days, an emergency department, operating suite, and clinical departments to handle a broad range of diagnoses and treatments.
Admission	The act of accepting a patient into care in a hospital. Also refers to the status of a patient. Admission requires a physician's order.
Admission denial	Occurs when the payer or its designee (such as utilization review staff) will not reimburse the facility for treatment of the patient because the admission was deemed unnecessary.
Admission record	The demographic, financial, socioeconomic, and clinical data collected about a patient at registration. Also refers to the document in a paper record that contains these data.
Admitting diagnosis	The reason given by the physician for initiating the order for the patient to be placed into care in a hospital.
Agenda	A tool used to organize the topics to be discussed during a meeting.
Aggregate data	A group of like data elements compiled to provide information about the group.
Algorithm	A procedure (set of instructions) for accomplishing a task.
Allied health professionals	Health care professionals who care for patients or support patient care in a variety of disciplines, including occupational therapy and physical therapy.
Ambulatory patient classifications (APCs)	A prospective payment system for ambulatory care based on medically necessary services.

Ambulatory surgery	Operation performed on an outpatient basis. Also refers to facilities for performing operation on an outpatient basis.
American College of Surgeons (ACS)	National professional organization of surgeons.
Amendment	A change to the original document.
Analysis	The review of a record to evaluate its completeness, accuracy, or compliance with predetermined standards or other criteria.
Assembly	The reorganization of a paper record into a standard order.
Assessment	An evaluation. In medical decision making, the physician's evaluation of the subjective and objective evidence. Also refers to the evaluation of a patient by any clinical discipline.
Assisted living	A type of long-term care in which the resident is significantly independent in activities of daily living and does not need high levels of skilled nursing.
Attending physician	The physician who is primarily responsible for coordinating the care of the patient in the hospital; it is usually the physician who ordered the patient's admission to the hospital.
Audit trail	A computer log of computer processing and access activities.
Authenticate	To take responsibility for data collection or the activities described by the data collection by signature, mark, code, password, or other means of identification.
Average length of stay (ALOS)	The arithmetic mean of the lengths of stay of a group of inpatients.
Bar graph	A chart that represents the frequency of items in the specified categories of a variable.
Baseline	A beginning value; the value at which an activity is originally measured, such as the first blood pressure reading at an initial physician's office visit.
Batch control form	A listing of charts in process, postdischarge, that identified which steps have been completed.
Bed count	The actual number of beds that a hospital has staffed, equipped, and otherwise made available for occupancy by patients.
Behavioral health facility	Medical facility that focuses on the treatment of psychiatric conditions.
Benchmarking	An improvement technique that compares one facility's process with that of another facility with noted superior performance.
Billing	The process of submitting claims or rendering invoices.
Brainstorming	A data-gathering quality improvement tool used to generate information related to a topic.
Business record rule	An exception to the hearsay rule. Allows health records to be admitted as evidence in legal proceedings because they are kept in the normal course of business, recorded concurrently with the events that they describe, and are recorded by individuals who are in a position to know the facts of the events that are described.
Capitation	The systematic reimbursement to a health care provider based on the number of patients contractually in the physician's care, regardless of diagnoses or services rendered.

Case management	The coordination of the patient's care and services, including reimbursement considerations.
Case mix	Statistical distribution of patients according to their utilization of resources. Also refers to the grouping of patients by clinical department or other meaningful distribution.
Case mix index	The arithmetic average (mean) of the relative weights of all cases in a given period.
Census	The actual number of inpatients in a facility at a point in time,. For comparative purposes, usually midnight.
Certification	Approval by an outside agency, such as the federal or state government, indicating that the health care facility has met a set of predetermined standards.
Character	A single letter, number, or symbol.
Charge capture	The systematic collection of specific charges for services rendered to an inpatient.
Chargemaster	The database that contains the detailed description of charges related to all potential services rendered to an inpatient.
Charges	Fees or costs.
Chart locator system	A system for locating records within a facility.
Children's hospital	A specialty facility that focuses on the treatment of children.
Claim	The application to an insurance company for reimbursement.
Classification	Systematic organization of elements into categories. For example, ICD-9-CM is a classification system that organizes diagnoses and procedures into categories, primarily by body system.
Clinic	A facility-based ambulatory care department that provides general or specialized services, such as those provided in a physician's office.
Clinical data	All of the medical data that have been recorded about the patient's stay or visit, including diagnoses and procedures.
Clinical pathway	A predetermined standard of treatment for a particular disease, diagnosis, or procedure designed to facilitate the patient's progress through the facility.
Clinical pertinence	Review of a patient's health record to determine whether the documentation reflects that the care provided to the patient was appropriately related to the diagnosis.
Coding	The assignment of alphanumerical values to a word, phrase, or other non-numerical expression. In health care, coding is the assignment of numerical values to diagnosis and procedure descriptions.
Coding compliance plan	The development, implementation, and enforcement of policies and procedures to ensure that coding standards are met.
Commission on Accreditation of Rehabilitation Facilities (CARF)	An organization that accredits behavioral health and rehabilitation facilities.
Community Health Accreditation Program (CHAP)	An organization that accredits home health agencies.
Comorbidity	A condition that affects the patient's care and/or length of stay and exists at the same time as the principal diagnosis.
Competency	The ability to successfully complete a task or skill.
Completeness	The data quality of existence. If a required data element is missing, the record is not complete.

Compliance	Meeting standards. Also the development, implementation, and enforcement of policies and procedures that ensure that standards are met.
Complication	A condition that arises during hospitalization.
Computer output to laser (COLD)	Forms or reports generated from computer output transferred for storage on laser disk.
Computer-based patient record	Compilation of patient health information in a relational or other computer database.
Computerized patient record	A digital form of the patient's paper health record.
Computerized physician order entry (CPOE)	The term used to describe the computerization or electronic processing of physician's orders.
Concurrent analysis	Any type of analysis (*see* analysis) performed during the patient's stay (after admission but before discharge).
Concurrent coding	Any type of coding (*see* coding) performed during the patient's stay (after admission but before discharge). Concurrent coding must be performed in order to obtain the working diagnosis-related group (DRG).
Concurrent review	Review occurring during the act or event (i.e., during the patient's stay in the facility).
Conditions of Admission	The legal agreement between a hospital and a patient (or the patient's legal agent) to perform routine services. May also include the statement of the patient's financial responsibility and prospective consent for release of information and examination and disposal of tissue.
Conditions of Participation	The terms under which a facility is eligible to receive reimbursement from Medicare.
Confidential communications	The sharing of patient health information.
Confidentiality	Discretion regarding disclosure of information.
Consent	An agreement or permission.
Consultant	A medical professional who provides clinical expertise in a specialty at the request of the attending physician.
Consultation	The formal request by a physician for the professional opinion or services of another health care professional, usually another physician, in caring for a patient. Also refers to the opinion or services themselves as well as the activity of rendering the opinion or services.
Continued stay denial	Similar to admission denial; however, it is the additional payment for the length of stay that is not approved rather than the entire admission.
Continuing education	Education required after attaining a position, credential, or degree intended to keep those persons knowledgeable in their profession.
Continuum of care	The broad range of health care services required by a patient during an illness or for an entire lifetime. May also refer to the continuity of care provided by a health care organization.
Cooperating Parties	The four organizations responsible for maintaining the ICD-9-CM: HCFA, NCHS, AHA, and AHIMA.
Corrective controls	Procedures, processes, or structures that are designed to fix errors when they are detected. Because errors cannot always be fixed, corrective controls also include the initiation of investigation into future error prevention or detection.
Correspondence	Mailing or letters exchanged between parties.
Countersignature	*See* countersigned.

Countersigned	Evidence of supervision of subordinate personnel, such as physician residents.
Court order	The direction of a judge who has made a decision that an order to produce information (on the record) is necessary.
Current Procedural Terminology (CPT)	A nomenclature and coding system developed and maintained by the American Medical Association in order to facilitate billing for physician services.
Credentials	An individual's specific professional qualifications. Also refers to the letters that a professionally qualified person is entitled to list after his or her name.
Cross-training	Training of employees for additional jobs or functions within the department so that they can help with those jobs when necessary.
Custodian	The person entrusted to care for something, i.e., health care records.
Data	The smallest elements or units of facts or observations. Also refers to a collection of such elements.
Data accuracy	The quality that data are correct.
Data collection devices	Paper forms or computer screens designed to capture data elements in a standardized format. Also refers to the physical computer hardware or other tool that facilitates the data collection process.
Data dictionary	A list of details that describe each field in a database.
Data Elements for Emergency Department Systems (DEEDS)	Minimum data set for emergency services.
Data entry	The process of recording elements into a collection device. Generally refers to the recording of elements into a computer system.
Data repository	Where data is stored from different, unrelated software programs.
Data set	A group of data elements collected for a specific purpose.
Data validity	The quality that data reflect the known or acceptable range of values for the specific data.
Data warehouse	Where information from different databases is collected and organized to be used for ad hoc reports and analytical research.
Database	An organized collection of data.
Date-oriented record	*See* integrated record.
Decision matrix	A quality improvement tool used to narrow focus or choose between two or more related issues.
Deductible	A specified dollar amount for which the patient is personally responsible before the payer reimburses for any claims.
Deemed status	The Medicare provision that an approved accreditation is sufficient to satisfy the compliance audit element of the Conditions of Participation.
Defendant	The party or parties against whom the plaintiff has initiated litigation.
Deficiencies	Required elements that are missing from a record.
Deficiency system	The policies and procedures that form the corrective control of collecting the missing data identified in quantitative analysis. Includes the recording and reporting of deficiencies.
Delegate	To transfer a responsibility, task, or project from a manager to a lower level employee.

Delinquent	Status accorded to a record that has not been completed within a specified time frame, such as within 30 days of discharge.
Demographic data	Identification: those elements that distinguish one patient from another, such as name, address, and birth date. Also known as *indicative data.*
Designated record set	A specific portion of the patient's health information, which the patient has the right to access and to request amendment to and restriction of.
Detective controls	Procedures, processes, or structures that are designed to find errors after they have been made.
Diagnosis	Literally, "complete knowledge"; refers to the name of the patient's condition or illness.
Diagnosis-related groups (DRGs)	A collection of health care descriptions organized into statistically similar categories.
Dialysis	The extracorporeal elimination of waste products from bodily fluids (e.g., blood).
Dialysis center	An ambulatory care facility that specializes in blood-cleansing procedures to treat, for example, chronic kidney (renal) failure.
Digital signature	A means to identify the authenticity and integrity of the user's identification.
Digitized signature	An original signature on a report that is then scanned into an electronic document.
Discharge	Discharge occurs when the patient leaves the care of the facility. Also refers to the status of a patient. Discharge may be by physician order, against medical advice, or by death.
Discharge planning	The multidisciplinary, coordinated effort to ensure that a patient is discharged to the appropriate level of care and with the appropriate support.
Discharge register (discharge list)	A list of all patients discharged on a specific date or during a specific time period.
Discharge summary	The recap of an inpatient stay, usually dictated by the attending physician and transcribed into a formal report.
Disclosure	When patient health information is given to someone.
Discounted fee for service	The exchange of cash for professional services rendered, at a rate less than the normal fee for the service.
Discovery	The process of investigating the circumstances surrounding a lawsuit.
Doctor's orders	*See* physician's orders.
Document imaging	Scanning or faxing printed papers into a computer system or optical disk system.
DSM-IV	*Diagnostic and Statistical Manual of Mental Disorders,* 4th edition.
Electronic health record (EHS)	A secure real-time, point-of-care, patientcentric information resource for clinicians "allowing access of patient information when and where needed and incorporating evidence-based decision support.
Electronic health record management	Process by which electronic (e.g., digital) health records are created and preserved for evidentiary (e.g., legal or business) purposes.
Electronic signature	When the authenticator uses a password or PIN to electronically sign a document.

Emancipation	Consideration of a patient as an adult even though the patient is younger than the statutory age.
Encounter	Unit of measure for the volume of ambulatory care services provided.
Encounter form	A data collection device that facilitates the accurate capture of ambulatory care diagnoses and services.
Encryption	Process of making computer information difficult to read to ensure security.
Epidemiology	The study of morbidity (disease) trends and occurrences.
Ergonomic	Alignment of the work environment to accommodate the employee's job function.
Error report	A list of deficient or erroneous data. Usually a computer-generated document.
Ethics	A system of beliefs about acceptable behavior.
Etiology	The cause or source of the patient's condition or disease.
Evidence-based decisions support	Clinical best-knowledge practices used to make decisions for treatments
Exception report	*See* error report.
Exceptions	In HIPAA, uses and disclosures of protected health information for certain public priorities without patient authorization.
Face sheet	The first page in a paper record. Usually contains at least the demographic data and contains space for the physician to record and authenticate the discharge diagnoses and procedures. In many facilities, the admission record is also used as the face sheet.
Family unit numbering	A numerical identification system to identify an entire family's health record using one number and modifiers.
Federal Drug and Alcohol Abuse Regulations	Regulations at the national level addressing requirements for disclosure of chemical and alcohol abuse patient information.
Federal Register	The publication of the proceedings of the United States Congress.
Fee for service	The exchange of cash, goods, or services for professional services rendered at a specific rate, typically determined by the provider and associated with specific activities (such as a physical examination).
Fee schedule	The list of charges that a physician expects to be paid for services rendered. Also, a list of the amounts a payer will remit for certain services.
Field	A collection or series of related characters. A field may contain a word, a group of words, a number, or a code, for example.
File	Numerous records of different types of related data. Files can be large or small, depending on the number of records they contain.
File folder	The physical container used to store the health record in a paper-based system.
Financial data	Elements that describe the payer. For example, the name, address, telephone number, group number, and member number of the patient's insurance company.
Fiscal intermediaries	Organizations that administer the claims and reimbursements for the funding agency. Medicare uses fiscal intermediaries to process its claims and reimbursements.

Flexible benefit account	A savings account in which health care and certain child-care costs can be set aside and paid using pretax funds.
Frequency distribution	The grouping of observations into a small number of categories.
Full-time equivalent (FTE)	An employee who works 32 to 40 hours each week excluding overtime, earning full benefits as offered by the health care facility.
Goals	Desired achievements.
Graph	An illustration of data.
Grouper	The flowchart used to derive the DRG from the ICD-9-CM diagnoses and procedures. Also refers to the computer program that performs this task.
Group practice	Multiple physicians who share facilities and resources and may also cooperate in rendering patient care.
Group practice model HMO	HMO contracts with a group or network of physicians and facilities to provide health care services.
Guarantor	The individual or organization that promises to pay for the rendered health care services after all other sources (such as insurance) are exhausted.
Healthcare Common Procedure Coding System(HCPCS)	The Centers for Medicare and Medicaid Services coding system, of which CPT-4 is level one.
Health data	Elements related to a patient's diagnosis and procedures as well as factors that may affect the patient's condition.
Health information	Organized data that have been collected about a patient or a group of patients. Sometimes used synonymously with the term *health data*.
Health information management (HIM)	The profession that manages the sources and uses of health information, including the collection, storage, retrieval, and reporting of health information.
Health information technology (HIT)	The specialty in the field of health information management that focuses on the day-to-day activities of health information management that support the collection, storage, retrieval, and reporting of health information.
Health Insurance Portability and Accountability Act (HIPAA)	Public law 104-191 addressing the privacy and security of patient information.
Health Level 7	Standards-developing organizations producing standards for particular health care domains such as pharmacy and radiology.
Health maintenance organization (HMO)	Managed care organization characterized by the ownership or employer control over the health care providers.
Health record	Also called *record* or *medical record*. It contains all of the data collected for an individual patient.
Hearsay rule	The court rule that prohibits most testimony regarding events by parties who were not directly involved in the event.
Histogram	A modified bar graph representing continuous data. Each bar represents a class interval; the height of the bar represents the frequency of observations.
History	The physician's record of the patient's chief complaint, history of present illness, pertinent family and social history, and review of systems.
Home health care	Health care services rendered in the patient's home. Also refers to organizations that provide such services.

Hospice	Palliative health care services rendered to the terminally ill, their families, and their friends. Also refers to organizations that provide such services.
Hospital	An organization having permanent facilities that delivers inpatient health care services through 24-hour nursing care, an organized medical staff, and appropriate ancillary departments.
Hybrid record	A record in which both electronic and paper media are used.
ICD-9-CM	*International Classification of Diseases, 9th Revision—Clinical Modification.* The U.S. version of the ICD-9, maintained and updated by the Cooperating Parties.
ICD-10-CM	*International Classification of Diseases, 10th Revision—Clinical Modification.*
ICD-10-PCS	*International Classification of Diseases, 10th Revision, Procedural Coding System;* the U.S. modification to the procedures codes in ICD-10.
ICD-O	*International Classification of Diseases—Oncology.* The coding system used to record and track the occurrence of neoplasms (i.e., malignant tumors, cancer).
Incidence	Number of occurrences of a particular event, disease, or diagnosis or the number of new cases of a disease.
Incomplete system	*See* deficiency system.
Indemnity insurance	Assumption of the payment for all or part of certain, specified services. Characterized by out-of-pocket deductibles and caps on total covered payments.
Independent practice association (IPA) model HMO	The HMO contracts with individual physicians, a portion of whose practices is devoted to the HMO.
Index	A system to identify or name a file or other item so that it can be located.
Indexing	Sorting a record by the different report types, making the viewing of the record uniform.
Indicative data	*See* demographic data.
Indices	Collections of patient data (or a database) specific to a diagnosis, procedure, or physician.
Information	Processed data (i.e., data that are presented in an appropriate frame of reference).
Informed consent	A permission given by a competent individual, of legal age, with full knowledge or understanding of the risks, potential benefits, and potential consequences of the permission.
Infrastructure	Framework that enables interoperability by using standard operating nomenclature, specifications, or protocols.
Inpatient	An individual who is admitted to a hospital with the intention of staying overnight.
Inservice	Training provided to employees of an organization.
Insurer	The party that assumes the risk of paying some or all of the cost of providing health care services in return for the payment of a premium by or on behalf of the insured.
Integrated delivery system	A health care organization that provides services through most or all of the continuum of care.
Integrated record	A paper record in which the pages are organized sequentially, in the chronological order in which they were generated; also known as *date-oriented record* or *sequential record.*

Integrity	The data quality characteristic displayed when alteration of a finalized document is not permitted. Applies to both paper and electronic documents.
Interdepartmental	Relationship between two or more departments (e.g., HIM and the business office).
Interface	Computer setup allowing information to pass from one computer to another.
Interoperable	The ability of the software and hardware on different machines from different vendors to share data.
Intradepartmental	Occurrence or relationship within a department (e.g., assembly and analysis within HIM).
Job analysis	Review of a function to determine all of the tasks or components that make up an employee's job.
Job description	A list of the employee's responsibilities.
Joint Commission on Accreditation of Healthcare Organizations (JCAHO)	The largest and most comprehensive health care accrediting agency.
Jurisdiction	The authority of a court to decide certain cases. May be based on geography, money, or type of case.
Laboratory	The physical location of the specialists who analyze body fluids.
Laboratory tests	Procedures for analysis of body fluids.
Length of stay (LOS)	The duration of an inpatient visit, measured in whole days: the number of whole days between the inpatient's admission and discharge.
Licensed beds	The maximum number of beds that a facility is legally permitted to have, as approved by state licensure.
Licensure	The mandatory government approval required for performing specified activities. In health care, the state approval required for providing health care services.
Line graph	A chart that represents observations over time or between variables by locating the intersection of the horizontal and vertical values and connecting those dots.
Litigation	The term used to indicate that a matter must be settled by the court and the process of engaging in legal proceedings.
Local medical review policy (LMRP)	The outpatient standards for medical necessity defined by the fiscal intermediaries.
Long-term care facility	A hospital that provides services to patients over an extended period of time; an average length of stay is in excess of 30 days. Facilities are characterized by the extent to which nursing care is provided.
Longitudinal	The flow of information electronically from one type of provider to another.
Loose sheets	In a paper health record, documents that are not present when the patient is discharged. These documents must be accumulated and filed with the record at a later date.
Major Diagnostic Categories (MDCs)	Segments of the DRG assignment flowchart (grouper).
Managed care	The blending of the insurance and provider roles.
Marketing	Promoting products or services in the hope that the consumer chooses those products or services over the products or services of a competitor.
Master patient index	A system containing patient and encounter information, often used to correlate the patient to the file identification.

Maximization	The process of determining the highest possible DRG payment.
Mean	The measure of central tendency that represents the arithmetic average of the observations.
Median	The measure of central tendency that represents the observation that is exactly halfway between the highest and lowest observation.
Medicaid	Joint federal/state program for providing access to health care for the poor and the medically indigent.
Medical record	*See* health record; record.
Medical specialty	The focus of a physician's practice, such as pediatrics or oncology. Specialties are represented by Boards, which certify physicians in the specialty.
Medicare	Federally funded health care insurance plan for the elderly and for certain categories of chronically ill patients.
Medications	Chemical substances used to treat disease.
Memorandum (memo)	A communication tool used to inform members of an organization.
Mental health facility	*See* behavioral health facility.
Microfiche	An alternative storage method for paper records on plastic sheets.
Microfilm	An alternative storage method for paper records on plastic film.
Middle-digit filing	A modification of terminal-digit filing in which the patient's medical record number is separated into sets for filing and the first set of numbers is called *secondary*, the second set of numbers is called *primary*, and the third set is called *tertiary*.
Minimum Data Set (MDS)	The detailed data collected about long-term care patients. It is collected several times, and it forms the basis for the RUG.
Minimum necessary	A rule requiring health providers to disclose only the minimum amount of information necessary to accomplish a task.
Minutes	A tool used to record the events, topics, and discussions of a meeting.
Mission	The purpose of the organization documented in a formal statement.
Mode	The measure of central tendency that represents the most frequently occurring observation.
Modifier	A two-digit addition to a CPT code that provides additional information about the service or procedure performed.
Morbidity	Refers to disease.
Mortality	Refers to death.
National Center for Health Statistics (NCHS)	One of the ICD-9-CM Cooperating Parties.
National Center for Injury Prevention and Control (NCIPC)	A component of the CDC that focuses on reducing injuries and the diseases associated with, death from, and sequelae of injuries.
Nomenclature	A formal system of names that pertain to a profession or discipline.
Nonrepudiation	A process that provides a positive identification of the user.

Notice of Privacy Practices	A notice, written in clear and simple language, summarizing a facility's privacy policies and the conditions for use or disclosure of patient health information.
Nurse	A medical professional who has satisfied the academic, professional, and legal requirements to care for patients at state-specified levels. Although usually delivering patient care at the direction of physicians, nurse practitioners may also deliver care independently.
Nursing assessment	The nurse's evaluation of the patient.
Nursing progress notes	Routine documentation of the nurse's interaction with a patient.
Objective	In the SOAP format for medical decision-making, the physician's observations and review of diagnostic tests.
Objectives	Directions for achieving a goal.
Open access	The physician's office scheduling method that allows for patient visits without an appointment. Some versions of open access focus on group visits for certain types of routine care.
Operation	Surgery: An operation consists of one or more surgical procedures.
Operative report	The surgeon's formal report of surgical procedure(s) performed. Often dictated and transcribed into a formal report.
Optical disk	Electronic storage medium; a disk used to store digital data.
Optimization	The process of determining the most accurate DRG payment.
Organization chart	An illustration used to describe the relationship among departments, positions, and functions within an organization.
Orientation	Training to familiarize a new employee with the job.
Outcome and Assessment Information Set (OASIS)	The data set captured for monitoring of home health care.
Outguide	A physical file guide used to identify another location of a file in the paper-based health record system.
Outlier	A patient whose length of stay or cost is far lower or higher than the average expected by the prospective payment system, notably the DRG.
Outpatient	A patient whose health care services are intended to be delivered within 1 calendar day or, in some cases, a 24-hour period.
Outsourced	Refers to services that are provided by external organizations or individuals who are not employees of the facility for which the services are being provided.
Palliative care	Health care services that are intended to soothe, comfort, or reduce symptoms but are not intended to cure.
Patient accounts	The department in a health care facility that is responsible for submitting bills or claims for reimbursement.
Patient care plan	The formal directions for treatment of the patient, which involves many different individuals, including the patient. It may be as simple as instructions to "take two aspirins and drink plenty of fluids," or it may be a multiple-page document with delegation of responsibilities. Care plans may also be developed by discipline, such as nursing.

Payer	The individual or organization that is primarily responsible for the reimbursement for a particular health care service. Usually refers to the insurance company or third party.
Per diem	Each day, daily. Usually refers to all-inclusive payments for inpatient services.
Percentage	Standardization of data so that unlike groups can be compared. Can be calculated by dividing the observations in the category by the total observations and multiplying by 100.
Performance improvement	Also known as quality improvement (QI) or continuous quality improvement (CQI). Refers to the process by which a facility reviews its services or products to ensure quality.
Performance Improvement Plan (PIP)	A plan to explain the required responsibilities and competencies expected of an employee's job performance.
Performance standards	Set guidelines explaining how much work an employee must complete.
Permitted disclosure	Disclosure authorized by the patient, or allowed for treatment, payment, or health care operations.
Personal health record	A patient's own copy of health information documenting the patient's health care history and providing information on continuing patient care.
Personal identification number (PIN)	A unique set of characters that a computer recognizes as belonging to a previous registered individual.
Physiatrist	A physician who specializes in physical medicine and rehabilitation.
Physical examination	The physician's record of examination of the patient.
Physician	A medical professional who has satisfied the academic, professional, and legal requirements to diagnose and treat patients at state-specified levels and within a declared specialty.
Physician's office	A setting for providing ambulatory care in which the primary provider is the physician.
Physician's orders	The physician's directions regarding the patient's care. Also refers to the data collection device on which these elements are captured.
Physician-patient privilege	The legal foundation that private communication between a physician and a patient is confidential. Only the patient has the right to give up this privilege.
Pie chart	A circular chart in which the frequency of observations is represented as a wedge of the circle.
Placebo	A nontherapeutic substance used in clinical drug trials. The patient (and sometimes the physician) does not know whether he or she is receiving the trial drug or the placebo.
Plaintiff	The party who initiates litigation.
Plan of treatment	In the SOAP format for medical decision making, the diagnostic, therapeutic, or palliative measures that are taken to investigate or treat the patient's condition or disease.
Policy	A statement of something that is done or expected in an organization.
Population	An entire group.
Postdischarge processing	The procedures designed to prepare a health record for retention.
Potentially compensable event (PCE)	An event that could cause the facility a financial loss or lead to litigation.

Power of attorney	The legal document that identifies someone as the legal representative to make decisions for the patient when the patient is unable to do so.
Preferred provider organization (PPO)	A managed care organization that contracts with a network of health care providers to render services to the PPO's members.
Premiums	Periodic payments to an insurance company for coverage (an insurance policy).
Prevalence	Rate of incidence of an occurrence, disease, or diagnosis or the number of existing cases.
Preventive controls	Procedures, processes, or structures that are designed to minimize errors at the point of data collection.
Primary caregiver	The individual who is principally responsible for the daily care of a patient at home; usually a friend or family member.
Primary care physician	In insurance, the physician who has been designated by the insured to deliver routine care to the insured and to evaluate the need for referral to a specialist, if applicable. Colloquial use is synonymous with "family doctor."
Primary data	Data taken directly from the patient or the original source. The patient's health record contains primary data.
Principal diagnosis	According to the UHDDS, the condition which, after study, was chiefly responsible for occasioning the admission of the patient to the hospital for care.
Principal procedure	According to the UHDDS, the procedure that was performed for definitive treatment, rather than one performed for diagnostic or exploratory purposes, or was necessary to take care of a complication. If two procedures appear to meet this definition, then the one most related to the principal diagnosis should be selected as the principal procedure.
Privacy	The right of an individual to control access to medical information.
Privacy officer	The designated official in the health care organization who oversees privacy compliance and handles complaints.
Probation period	The period of time (grace period) given to a new employee to learn the job and reach the performance standards associated with that job. During this period, the employee is not considered permanent.
Problem-oriented record	A paper record with pages organized by diagnosis.
Procedure	A process that describes how to comply with a policy. Also, a medical or surgical treatment. Also refers to the processing steps in an administrative function.
Productivity	The amount of work produced by an employee in a given time frame.
Progress notes	The physician's record of each interaction with the patient.
Prospective consent	Permission given prior to having knowledge of the event to which the permission applies. For example, a permission to release information before the information is gathered (i.e., before admission).
Prospective payment	Any of several reimbursement methods that pay an amount predetermined by the payer based on the diagnosis, procedures, and other factors (depending on setting) rather than actual, current resources expended by the provider.
Prospective Payment System (PPS)	The Medicare system for reimbursing acute care facilities based on statistical analysis of health care data.

Protected health information (PHI)	Individually identifiable health information that is transmitted or maintained in any form or medium by covered entities or their business associates.
Provider number	The number assigned to a participating facility by Medicare for identification purposes.
Psychiatrist	A physician who specializes in the diagnosis and treatment of patients with conditions that affect the mind.
Public priority exception	Permitted disclosure in which authorization is not required as long as state law allows the exception.
Qualitative analysis	Review of the actual content of the health record to ensure that the information is correct as it pertains to the patient's care.
Quality assurance (QA)	A method for reviewing health care functions to determine their compliance with predetermined standards that requires action to correct noncompliance and then follow-up review to ascertain whether the correction was effective.
Quality Improvement Organization (QIO)	An organization that contracts with payers, specifically Medicare and Medicaid, to review care and reimbursement issues.
Quantitative analysis	A detective control designed to identify incomplete data. Usually refers to review of the patient health record for complete content and authentications.
Query	To question the database for information or a report.
Queue	Electronic work areas.
Radiology	Literally, the study of x-rays. In a health care facility, the department responsible for maintaining x-ray and other types of diagnostic and therapeutic equipment as well as analyzing diagnostic films.
Radiology tests	The examination of internal body structures using x-rays and other related studies.
Reciprocal services	Professional services exchanged instead of paid for in cash.
Record	A collection of related fields. Also refers to all of the data collected about a patient's visit or all of the patient's visits (*see also* health record).
Record retention schedule	The length of time that a record must be retained.
Referral	The act or documentation of one physician's request for an opinion or services to another health care professional, often another physician, for a specific patient regarding specific signs, symptoms, or diagnosis.
Registry	A database of health information specific to disease, diagnosis, or implant used to improve the care provided to patients with that disease, diagnosis, or implant.
Rehabilitation facility	A health care facility that delivers services to patients whose activities of daily living are impaired by their illness or condition. May be inpatient, outpatient, or both.
Reimbursement	The amount of money that the health care facility receives from the party responsible for paying the bill.
Relative weight	A number assigned yearly by CMS that is applied to each DRG and used to calculate reimbursement. This number represents the comparative difference in the use of resources by patients in each DRG.
Release of information	The term used to describe the HIM department function that provides disclosure of patient health information.

Reliability	A quality exhibited when codes are consistently assigned by one or more coders for similar or identical cases.
Report	The result of a query. A list from a database.
Required disclosure	A disclosure to the patient and to the Secretary of the Department of Health and Human Services for compliance auditing purposes.
Research	The systematic investigation into a matter to find fact.
Resident	A person who after attending college and medical school performs professional duties under the supervision of a fully qualified physician.
Resource Utilization Groups (RUGs)	These constitute a prospective payment system for long-term care. Current Medicare application is a per diem rate based on the RUG III grouper.
Respite care	Services rendered to individuals who are not independent in their activities of daily living for the purpose of temporarily relieving the primary caregiver.
Restriction	Prohibiting access to information.
Retention	The procedures governing the storage of records, including duration, location, security, and access.
Retrospective consent	Permission given after the event to which the permission applies. For example, permission to release information after the information is gathered (i.e., after discharge).
Retrospective review	Review occurring after the act or event (i.e., after the patient is discharged).
Revenue code	A chargemaster code required for Medicare billing.
Right to complain	The patient's right to discuss his or her concerns about privacy violations.
Right to revoke	The right to withdraw consent or approval for a previously approved action or request.
Risk	The potential exposure to loss, financial expenditure, or other undesirable events.
Risk management	The coordination of efforts within a facility to prevent and control inadvertent occurrences.
Rule out	The process of systematically eliminating potential diagnoses. Also refers to the list of potential diagnoses.
Sample	A small group within a population.
Scanner	A machine, much like a copier, used to turn paper-based records into digital images for a computerized health record.
Secondary data	Data taken from the primary source document for use elsewhere.
Sequential record	*See* integrated record.
Serial numbering	A numerical patient record identification system in which the patient is given a new number for each visit and each file folder contains separate visit information.
Serial–unit numbering	A numerical patient record identification system in which the patient is given a new number for each visit; however, with each new admission, the previous record is retrieved and filed in the folder with the most recent visit.
SNOMED-CT	*S*ystematized *nom*enclature of human and veterinary *medi*cine *c*linical *t*erms; a reference terminology that, among other things, links common or input medical terminology and codes with the output reporting systems in an electronic health record.

SOAP format	*Subjective, Objective, Assessment,* and *Plan:* the medical decision-making process.
Socioeconomic data	Elements that pertain to the patient's personal life and personal habits, such as marital status, religion, and culture.
Source-oriented record	A paper record in which the pages are organized by discipline, department, and/or type of form.
Span of control	The number of employees that report to one supervisor, manager, or administrator.
Staff model HMO	When an organization owns the facilities, employs the physicians, and provides essentially all health care services.
Standing orders	The predetermined routine orders that have been designated to pertain to specific diagnoses or procedures. For example, the orders to perform specific blood tests, urinalysis, and x-rays prior to admission for certain surgical procedures. Standing orders must be ordered and authenticated by the appropriate physician.
Statistics	Analysis, interpretation, and presentation of information in numerical or pictorial format derived from the numbers.
Straight numerical filing	Filing folders in numerical order.
Subjective	In the SOAP format of medical decision-making, the patient's description of the symptoms or other complaints.
Subpoena	A direction from an officer of the court.
Subpoena ad testificandum	A direction from an officer of the court to provide testimony.
Subpoena duces tecum	A direction from an officer of the court to provide documents.
Superbill	An ambulatory care encounter form on which potential diagnoses and procedures are preprinted for easy check-off at the point of care.
Surgeon	A physician who specializes in diagnosing and treating diseases with invasive procedures.
Survey	A data gathering tool for capturing the responses to queries. May be administered verbally or by written questionnaire. Also refers to the activity of querying, as in "taking a survey."
Symptom	The patient's report of physical or other complaints, such as dizziness, headache, and stomach pain.
Table	A chart organized in rows and columns to organize data.
Tax Equity and Fiscal Responsibility Act of 1982 (TEFRA)	A federal law with wide-reaching provisions, one of which was the establishment of Medicare PPS.
Terminal-digit filing	A system in which the patient's medical record number is separated into sets for filing, and the first set of numbers is called *tertiary,* the second set of numbers is called *secondary,* and the third set of numbers is called *primary.*
Third party payer	*See* payer.
Timeliness	The quality of data's being obtained, recorded, or reported within a predetermined time frame.
Title XVIII	Amendment to the Social Security Act that established Medicare.
Title XIX	Amendment to the Social Security Act that established Medicaid.
Tracer methodology	JCAHO method of onsite review of open records in which the surveyors follow the actual path of documentation from start to finish.

Training	Education, instruction, or demonstration of how to perform a job.
Treatment	A procedure, medication, or other measure designed to cure or alleviate the symptoms of disease.
Triage	In emergency services, the system of prioritizing patients by severity of illness.
Uniform Ambulatory Care Data Set (UACDS)	The mandated data set for ambulatory care patients.
Uniform Hospital Discharge Data Set (UHDDS)	The mandated data set for hospital inpatients.
Unit numbering	A numerical patient record identification system in which the patient record is filed under the same number for all visits.
Unity of command	Sole management of one employee by one manager.
Universal chart order	Pertaining to a paper health record, the maintenance of the same page organization both before and after discharge.
Use	Employing PHI for a purpose.
Usual and customary fees	Referring to health care provider fees, the rate established by an insurance company, based on the regional charges for the particular service.
Utilization management (UM)	The process that ensures appropriate, efficient, and effective health care for patients.
Utilization review	The process of evaluating medical interventions against established criteria, based on the patient's known or tentative diagnosis. Evaluation may take place before, during, or after the episode of care for different purposes.
Validity	The data quality characteristic of a recorded observation falling within a predetermined size or range of values.
Verification	Confirming accuracy.
Vision	The goal of the organization, above and beyond the mission.
Visit	In ambulatory care, a unit of measuring the number of patients who have been served.
Workflow	The movement of the electronic record from one electronic component to another.
Working DRG	The concurrent DRG. The DRG that reflects the patient's current diagnosis and procedures while still an inpatient.
Wraparound policies	Insurance policies that supplement Medicare coverage.

INDEX

Note: Page numbers followed by b indicate boxes; f, figures; t, tables.